3950

# RANDOMIZED TRIALS IN CANCER:
## A CRITICAL REVIEW BY SITES

*Monograph Series of the European*
*Organization for Research on Treatment of Cancer*
*Volume 4*

# MONOGRAPH SERIES OF THE EUROPEAN ORGANIZATION FOR RESEARCH ON TREATMENT OF CANCER

The Monograph Series of the EORTC deals with selected topics related to cancer treatment. Volumes are usually, but not necessarily, based on the proceedings of an EORTC symposium. The responsibility of the Editorial Advisory Board is to approve the subject of each monograph; the Board does not review individual manuscripts.

# Randomized Trials in Cancer: A Critical Review by Sites

## Monograph Series of the European Organization for Research on Treatment of Cancer
### Volume 4

Editor

### Maurice J. Staquet, M.D.
*EORTC Data Center*
*Institut Jules Bordet*
*Brussels, Belgium*

Raven Press ■ New York

**Raven Press, 1140 Avenue of the Americas, New York, New York 10036**

Made in the United States of America

**Library of Congress Cataloging in Publication Data**
Main entry under title:

Randomized trials in cancer.

(Monograph series of the European Organization for Research on Treatment of Cancer; v. 4)
Includes bibliographies and index.
1. Cancer—Chemotherapy. 2. Antineoplastic agents
—Testing—Statistical methods. 3. Stochastic processes.
I. Staquet, Maurice. II. Series: European
Organization for Research on Treatment of Cancer.
Monograph series of the European Organization for
Research on Treatment of Cancer; v. 4.
RC271.C5R36      616.9'94'061      77–17753
ISBN 0–89004–264–0

# Preface

There are two types of controlled clinical trials: one in which the control group is chosen by randomization, and one in which it is chosen retrospectively from previous results. In a randomized clinical trial, the treatment that a patient receives is selected by a random process in which each patient has an equal probability of receiving any one of the treatments studied. A randomized clinical trial implies that each treatment is started at the same period of time, contrary to the retrospective historical control group approach. A trial with historical controls is a study in which those patients currently being treated are compared to ones found in the literature or to results of previous studies carried out by the same investigators.

The goal of therapeutic studies is to generalize the results observed in the trial to the population of patients under study. However, both ethical and methodological problems may arise. Ethically, the realization of such a study involving human beings must be secondary to the actual care and treatment of the patient. If, however, no curative treatment exists, and both toxicological and pharmacological data indicate that a new treatment may actually be superior to the standard one, then one may ethically carry out a randomized trial on consenting patients. Methodologically, the difficulties are numerous. The generalization of results from the clinical trial to the population studied must be made with caution. Only if the patients treated in each arm of the study are a random sample of the patients in the population under study can the generalization be made. However, the patients included in a therapeutic trial are not necessarily a representative sample of the disease which we wish to study since not all patients have the same probability of entering a study. Only those patients living near centers specializing in the treatment of cancer have a chance of being included. Thus the practice of generalizing the results of a clinical trial to the population under study is open to criticism because the randomization is in fact a randomization among patients who may not be a representative sample to begin with.

There are several possible solutions to this problem. One is to increase the number of centers participating in the study in order to treat patients in as wide a range of institutions as possible. Another is to increase the precision of the results by taking into consideration the distribution of prognostic factors in each treatment arm under study. The process of randomization in fact accomplishes three principal objectives:

1. Randomization eliminates any bias of the investigator in determining which treatment a patient is to receive.
2. Randomization will tend to balance on the average the prognostic factors, whether known or unknown, among the treatment groups.

3. Randomization forms the basis for the validity of the statistical tests of significance.

Some investigators do not believe in the use of randomized controls. In fact, much important therapeutic progress has been made without the use of randomized trials. This is the case for example, when a treatment is clearly superior to previous ones irrespective of a patient's prognostic factors. However, many treatments are thought to be active only on the basis of nonrandomized studies and their true value still remains to be tested.

This book written by clinicians is an attempt to improve the strategy of therapeutic research in cancer. An appraisal of randomized clinical trials carried out in each type of cancer will permit investigators to judge what benefits and what detriments this technique has brought forth and perhaps to judge for themselves what is the best methodology to use in carrying out clinical therapeutic research.

M. Staquet

# Acknowledgment

The EORTC Foundation will receive all royalties from sales of this book. The authors freely gave their time and received no remuneration. We are extremely grateful to all of them.

M. J. Staquet
*European Organization for Research
on Treatment of Cancer
Brussels, Belgium*

# Contents

# Contributors

**Richard A. Bender**
*National Cancer Institute*
*Bethesda, Maryland 20014*

**Stanley J. Birnbaum**
*The New York Hospital-Cornell Medical*
*Center*
*New York, New York 10021*

**Yves Cachin**
*Institut Gustave-Roussy*
*94800 Villejuif, France*

**Stephen K. Carter**
*Northern California Cancer Program*
*Palo Alto, California 94304*

**Bruce A. Chabner**
*National Cancer Institute*
*Bethesda, Maryland 20014*

**Martin H. Cohen**
*Veterans Administration Hospital*
*Washington, D.C. 20422*

**Morton Coleman**
*The New York Hospital-Cornell Medical*
*Center*
*New York, New York 10021*

**André Coune**
*Institut Jules Bordet*
*1000 Bruxelles, Belgium*

**Hugh L. Davis, Jr.**
*National Cancer Institute*
*Bethesda, Maryland 20014*

**Louisette Debusscher**
*Institut Jules Bordet*
*1000 Bruxelles, Belgium*

**Robert L. De Jager**
*Institut Jules Bordet*
*1000 Bruxelles, Belgium*

**Vincent T. DeVita, Jr.**
*National Cancer Institute*
*Bethesda, Maryland 20014*

**Gilbert De Wasch**
*Institut Jules Bordet*
*1000 Bruxelles, Belgium*

**Harry Handelsman**
*National Cancer Institute*
*Bethesda, Maryland 20014*

**Jean-Claude Heuson**
*Institut Jules Bordet*
*1000 Bruxelles, Belgium*

**Jerzy Hildebrand**
*Institut Jules Bordet*
*1000 Bruxelles, Belgium*

**Edwin M. Jacobs**
*Division of Cancer Treatment*
*National Cancer Institute*
*Bethesda, Maryland 20014*

**Ferdy J. Lejeune**
*Institut Jules Bordet*
*1000 Bruxelles, Belgium*

**Wolrad H. Mattheiem**
*Institut Jules Bordet*
*1000 Bruxelles, Belgium*

**Renée Maurus**
*Hôpital Universitaire Saint Pierre*
*1000 Bruxelles, Belgium*

**William P. McGuire**
*National Cancer Institute*
*Bethesda, Maryland 20014*

**Franco M. Muggia**
*National Cancer Institute*
*Bethesda, Maryland 20014*

**Maria G. Nieuwenhuis**
*University Hospital*
*Utrecht, The Netherlands*

**Claire Nouwynck**
*Institut Jules Bordet*
*1000 Bruxelles, Belgium*

**Jacques Otten**
*Hôpital Universitaire Saint Pierre*
*1000 Bruxelles, Belgium*

**Mark W. Pasmantier**
*The New York Hospital-Cornell Medical*
*Center*
*New York, New York 10021*

**Herbert M. Pinedo**
*University Hospital*
*Utrecht, The Netherlands*

**Steven A. Rosenberg**
*National Cancer Institute*
*Bethesda, Maryland 20014*

**Marcel Rozencweig**
*National Cancer Institute*
*Bethesda, Maryland 20014*

**Richard T. Silver**
*The New York Hospital-Cornell Medical*
*Center*
*New York, New York 10021*

**William T. Soper**
*National Cancer Institute*
*Bethesda, Maryland 20014*

**Maurice J. Staquet**
*Institut Jules Bordet*
*1000 Bruxelles, Belgium*

**Pierre A. Stryckmans**
*Institut Jules Bordet*
*1000 Bruxelles, Belgium*

**Daniel D. Von Hoff**
*National Cancer Institute*
*Bethesda, Maryland 20014*

**Robert C. Young**
*National Cancer Institute*
*Bethesda, Maryland 20014*

**Robert Zittoun**
*Hotel-Dieu*
*75004 Paris, France*

*Randomized Trials in Cancer: A Critical Review by Sites,* edited by Maurice J. Staquet, Raven Press, New York © 1978.

# Acute Lymphocytic Leukemia

## Stephen K. Carter

*Director, Northern California Cancer Program, Palo Alto, California 94304*

The treatment of childhood leukemia is one of the great success stories in the history of cancer chemotherapy. Within this story can be seen the sequential steps that have been part of all successful approaches with this modality of treatment. These include the elucidation of active drugs; the combining of active drugs; the development of a high complete response rate; the development of maintenance therapy approaches; the development of sophisticated supportive care; and the utilization of prolonged disease-free survival as a therapeutic end point.

The history of the chemotherapy of childhood leukemia has been a mixture of uncontrolled observations and large-scale controlled clinical trials. A review of all the studies would itself require a book. This chapter reviews some of the highlights of the study, with emphasis on where the trials were controlled as opposed to other experimental design approaches.

The modern era of successful therapy of acute lymphoblastic leukemia began in 1948 with the uncontrolled observation by Farber (11) that aminopterin could induce temporary remission of the disease. Subsequently, methotrexate replaced aminopterin, and in the 1950s 6-mercaptopurine and corticosteroids were added. At this time, survival, which had been 2 to 4 months with supportive care and transfusions only, improved to 6 to 12 months. In the early 1960s, vincristine and cyclophosphamide were introduced, followed by cytosine arabinoside, daunorubicin, and L-asparaginase later in that decade. The observation that each of these drugs had activity was first established in what could be described as uncontrolled phase 2 studies.

In the early 1960s, the combining of drugs began, and prednisone was used in combination with vincristine, 6-mercaptopurine, or cyclophosphamide; remission induction rates in the 80 to 90% range were observed.

The immediate goal of remission induction is to reduce the bulk of leukemic cells as rapidly as possible and allow for return of normal cell production with as little therapy-related toxicity as possible. A secondary goal is to reduce the number of residual leukemic cells to the smallest fraction possible so that further therapy can ultimately lead to eradication of the last leukemic cell.

Received April 30, 1977.

Controlled trials helped establish the optimal way to induce complete remission, and even in today's trials this is still part of some of the complex protocols to be described subsequently.

In Table 1 are listed the drugs shown capable of inducing complete remission (CR) in acute lymphocytic leukemia. As can be seen, these represent a wide range of drugs with differing mechanisms of action. Most of these drugs were discovered to be active in uncontrolled phase 2-like studies.

Childrens Cancer Study Group A evaluated the optimal dosage and schedule of prednisone in a controlled study (36). Two hundred twenty-three previously untreated children were randomized to receive either 2 mg/kg in three divided daily doses (85 patients), 4 mg/kg in three divided daily doses (85 patients), 8 mg/kg every other day (28 patients), or 16 mg/kg every fourth day in a single dose (24 patients). Steroid side effects were minimal in intermittent therapy. Remission rates of 72% (at 2 mg/kg) and 60% (at 4 mg/kg) were obtained with the continuous schedule. With the intermittent schedules, the response rate was 21% (at 8 mg/kg) and 12% (at 16 mg/kg).

One of the building blocks in the strategy of designing protocols with curative intent for acute lymphocytic leukemia has been the information obtained about the residual leukemic population by observing the time of relapse after cessation of treatment. This has been used as a gross bioassay system of the (leukemocidal) effect of a given treatment. In order to accomplish this assay certain assumptions have been made, most of which are supported by a good deal of experimental data. These assumptions, as elucidated by Zubrod, are outlined in Table 2 (51). One of the most crucial assumptions made is the simple concept that one viable

TABLE 1. *Agents capable of producing remission in acute lymphocytic leukemia (pooled data from the literature) (37)*

| Agent | Type of agent | No. of points evaluated | No. achieving CR[a] | %CR[a] | Median duration (months) |
|---|---|---|---|---|---|
| Methotrexate | Antimetabolite of the vitamin folic acid | 73 | 18 | 24 | 6 |
| Prednisone | Adrenal cortical hormone | 863 | 391 | 45 | 2 |
| 6-Mercap-topurine | Antimetabolite of hypoxanthine | 544 | 189 | 35 | 6 |
| Vincristine | Plant alkaloid | 349 | 142 | 41 | 1.5 |
| Cyclophos-phamide | Alkylating agent | 347 | 46 | 13 | ≃3 |
| Daunorubicin | Antibiotic | 82 | 12 | 15 | |
| L-Aspar-aginase | Enzyme | 205 | 101 | 50 | 1–2 |
| Arabinosyl cytosine | Antimetabolite inhibitor of DNA polymerase | 122 | 9 | 7 | |

[a] CR = complete remission.

TABLE 2. *Treatment of acute leukemias: Present assumptions*

1. Total kill of leukemic cells required for cure
2. Leukemic cell population of $\cong 1 \times 10^{12}$
3. Doubling time $\cong$ 4–6 days
4. Exponential growth for majority of cells
5. Exponential cell kill—logarithmic order of cell death for a given dosage of drug
6. Combinations give greater cell kill than single agents

leukemic cell in a favorable anatomic site is eventually lethal and that treatment that fails to eradicate, with or without help from host defense mechanisms, every leukemic cell will fail to cure. If host defense mechanisms will eradicate some number of leukemic cells, then therapy must at least reduce the total cell population to that number.

In 1937, Furth and Kahn carried out single-cell inoculations with a micromanipulator and showed that one viable leukemic cell can be lethal to the mouse (21). The group at Southern Research Institute has repeatedly confirmed this observation (46). They have shown that one leukemic L1210 cell, and its progeny, dividing on the average every half-day, will produce one billion ($10^9$) leukemic cells and kill the host in 15 to 18 days.

Another crucial assumption made is that a given dosage of a given drug kills the same percentage of leukemic cells and not the same number in leukemic cell populations of widely varying sizes (46). This concept of constant percent cell kill is called the "logarithmic order of cell death" or "exponential cell kill" and is a concept discovered around the turn of the century by bacteriologists working with "disinfectants."

The data indicating constant percent cell kill have raised interesting questions regarding how we can best use the available drugs to effect total eradication of the leukemic cell population in man. With a single dose of an agent, the ability to produce complete cell eradication depends on the effectiveness of a drug within dosages of acceptable toxicity. With multiple doses of an agent, the situation becomes more complex and factors such as the cell-kill capability of the agent, generation time of the cancer cells, and period of recovery of the host after a given dosage must all be taken into consideration (52).

It has been estimated based on the degree of organ infiltration and organ size that a child (weighing 30 kg or 66 lb) with acute leukemia, before treatment or after relapse, harbors on the average of about $2.5 \times 10^{12}$ leukemic cells (2,500,000,000,000) (52). The total of $10^{12}$ cells represents a kilogram of leukemic cells in the average child; $10^{13}$ cells would represent 10 kg, which is clearly too much, and $10^{11}$ leukemic cells would represent 100 g, which is too few. The generation time of the acute lymphocytic leukemic cells in humans has been estimated by Ellison and Murphy, and their data indicate a doubling time of about 4 to 5 days (10).

Utilizing a complicated formula and assuming a 4-day generation time, it has been possible, utilizing the duration of unmaintained remission, to make a rough calculation of the cell kill achieved with a given regimen. With vincristine alone for induction, there is a 41-day median duration of remission (15) and this extrapolates back to $10^9$ cells remaining when therapy was stopped. Prednisone alone gives a 60-day median duration of remission and extrapolates back to $10^8$ leukemic cells remaining. Those patients who achieved complete remission on vincristine or prednisone have a 100 or 10,000-fold reduction in the number of leukemic cells based on these calculations. With the VAMP program at the National Cancer Institute, the median time to relapse was 156 days which, if the above assumptions are correct, means that treatment reduced the number of leukemic cells by as much as 10 logs (15).

At the National Cancer Institute beginning in 1962, intensive combination chemotherapy for acute lymphocytic leukemia was pioneered by Freireich, Karon, and Frei (20). They utilized a combination of the four agents most active in inducing complete hematological remission: methotrexate, 6-mercaptopurine, vincristine, and prednisone. Each drug was given at the dose and schedule that had been demonstrated at that time to be most effective for remission induction. The four drugs were given simultaneously over a period of 10 days. The study received the abbreviated name VAMP and is fully detailed in Table 3, which outlines the flow of the protocols at the National Cancer Institute. When complete remission was achieved, additional 10-day courses of therapy were administered, separated by 10-day or longer intervals for recovery from any observed toxicity. After a median of five such consolidation treatments given early in remission, therapy was discontinued. Seventeen consecutive newly diagnosed children were treated with this regimen. Eleven children completed the consolidation treatment of five additional courses after induction, and the median duration of unmaintained remission was 5 months, with 9 of the 11 patients relapsing within 35 weeks.

This study was followed by a program in which remission was induced with the combination of vincristine and prednisone, and consolidation therapy consisting of a 5-day course of methotrexate followed after a 9-day or longer interval by a 5-day course of 6-mercaptopurine and another 9-day or longer interval by cyclophosphamide given in a single dose (19).

This cycle of three compounds was repeated a second time, and thus the protocol was named BIKE because of its bicyclic nature. This study utilized the agents individually, in sequence, allowed the use of a full therapeutic dosage of each compound, and utilized all five of the compounds then known to be of established value in remission induction. After six courses of consolidation, treatment was discontinued and the patient observed (15). Fifteen patients entered this study, and 12 completed the consolidation treatment. The pattern of recurrence and the duration of unmaintained remission for this study was similar to that observed for VAMP (17). It was clear that these protocols had not eradicated the disease, but that the consolidation approach (intensive treatment after the induction of remission) had significantly reduced the residual leukemic load.

TABLE 3. *Sequence of first-line protocols for acute lymphocytic leukemia at the National Cancer Institute*

| Induction | Consolidation | Maintenance |
|---|---|---|
| VAMP<br>VCR, 2 mg/m²/wk × 2<br>MTX, 20 mg/m² q. 4 days<br>6-MP, 60 mg/m²/day p.o.<br>Prednisone, 40 mg/m²/day p.o.<br>Course 10–14 days | 5 Additional<br>VAMP<br>courses | None |
| BIKE<br>VCR, 2 mg/m²/wk<br>Prednisone, 40 mg/m²/day | MTX,<br>15 mg/m²/day × 5 i.v.<br>↓ 9-day rest<br>6-MP,<br>1,000 mg/m²/day × 5 i.v.<br>↓ 9-day rest<br>Cytoxan, 1,000 mg/m²<br>i.v. single dose<br>Six such cycles | None |
| POMP<br>VCR, 2 mg/m²/day × 1<br>MTX, 7.5 mg/m²/day × 5 i.v.<br>6-MP, 600 mg/m²/day × 5 i.v.<br>Prednisolone, 1,000 mg/m²/day<br>× 5 i.v.<br>Courses repeated after<br>9-day intervals | 4 Additional<br>POMP<br>courses | POMP<br>course<br>monthly<br>for 12<br>months |
| New POMP<br>POMP as above plus L-asparagi-<br>nase, 6000 I.U./m²/day × 5 i.v. | Continued POMP<br>for 6 months, then<br>BCNU, 100–150 mg/m²<br>single dose | A. None<br>B. Continued<br>POMP |

VCR = vincristine; MTX = methotrexate; 6-MP = 6-mercaptopurine.

The BIKE study was followed by a third study of intensive therapy called POMP, which incorporated the two major components of the preceding studies. It was a combination chemotherapy program, but the treatment was given in higher doses for shorter periods of time. The four active remission inducing agents (prednisone, Oncovin, methotrexate, and Purinethol) were given simultaneously over a 5-day period, followed by 9 days of rest. The protocol called for a median of two remission reduction courses of treatment given at 2-week intervals. Unlike the VAMP and BIKE studies, where treatment was discontinued after consolidation, a 5-day course of POMP was given monthly for the next 12 months in an attempt to eliminate the leukemic cells remaining after the consolidation treatment. This study required over 14 months from the onset of chemotherapy to the discontinuance of treatment. Thirty-two of 35 consecutive admissions with previously untreated acute lymphocytic leukemia achieved complete remissions.

The POMP regimen resulted in longer remissions (unmaintained and maintained) and longer survival than the low-dose VAMP and BIKE regimens. Analysis of the rate of relapse in the POMP study suggested that the period during which no relapses occurred approximated the period of intensive early treatment, and that subsequently, despite monthly "reinductions" with the same drugs, a constant rate of recurrence was evident (29). This recurrence rate had changed little at the point 14 months from the start of the remission period when all therapy was discontinued (28).

The next study was entitled "New POMP" and consisted of courses of POMP with the addition of L-asparaginase to be repeated as often as possible to a point 6 months following the accomplishment of remission in an attempt to reduce the leukemic cell load. At the end of this 6-month period, 1, 3-bischloro-ethyl nitrosourea (BCNU) was given to attach the remaining cells which might be in nonproliferating state. At this point, randomization occurred to no maintenance or continued therapy with POMP. The last analysis of this study indicates that duration of remission is not been significantly improved over the original POMP results (E. J. Henderson, *personal communication*).

These uncontrolled clinical experiments indicated a possible benefit to intensive induction but left a lot of questions unanswered which required controlled clinical studies.

The Southwest Oncology Group, in their protocol 7220 (12), were able to show that four drugs were not necessarily better than two for induction. The study was designed to compare vincristine and prednisone versus the POMP regimen of prednisone, vincristine, methotrexate, and 6-mercaptopurine. Children with acute lymphoblastic, acute undifferentiated, or acute stem cell leukemia, without prior therapy, were stratified on the basis of initial leukocyte count and age and then randomized between the two inductions. The vincristine and prednisone arm gave a 95% complete remission rate (37 of 39 patients) as compared to 56% (19 of 34 patients) with POMP. The POMP regimen had a higher incidence of sepsis and other toxicities frequently causing therapy interruption, but not unequivocally causing the poor response rate.

Earlier, as indicated, Henderson (28,29) at NCI had achieved a 92% complete remission rate with POMP (32 of 35 patients). This study was the first to compare POMP to standard vincristine plus prednisone in a controlled manner. Why the response rate could not be confirmed is unclear. The major differences between the two studies were time (1967 for Henderson versus 1973 for *SWOG*), and the fact that the SWOG study involved input from a variety of institutions.

If chemotherapy is discontinued when the patient achieves a complete remission, the disease will reappear rapidly, the average duration of such unmaintained remissions being only 2 to 3 months. This would indicate that there are persistent leukemic cells at a concentration lower than can be detected by available means. The early workers found that continuous treatment with folic acid antagonists appeared to be a more satisfactory therapeutic technique than deliberately allowing for a relapse between successive remissions and then giving a repeat course. In 1963, Freireich was the first to delineate a maintenance activity for drugs independent of induction (17). Previously untreated children induced into remission with prednisone were randomly allocated to 6-mercaptopurine or placebo for maintenance. The 6-mercaptopurine-treated patients showed a threefold increase in remission duration over the placebo-treated group, which was statistically significant to a high degree.

Another major advance in leukemia therapy was the discovery of the critical importance of dosage schedule for any given drug. Goldin, in a series of classic experiments, demonstrated in the leukemia L1210 system that methotrexate given every fourth day was superior to daily usage of the drug (27). This superiority was demonstrable only in the early stage of the disease (soon after tumor inoculum), which might be considered analogous to leukemia in remission. In the late or advanced L1210, which is analogous to leukemia in relapse, this schedule-dependency difference was not seen. This schedule sensitivity for methotrexate was then confirmed in man in a series of clinical experiments performed by the Cancer and Leukemia Cooperative Group B (CALGB). Methotrexate for induction therapy was randomly allocated to a daily or intermittent twice-weekly schedule, followed by maintenance on daily or intermittent methotrexate after rerandomization (44). No difference was found in remission induction (31% and 28%), although the twice-weekly methotrexate schedule afforded longer remissions. This confirmation of the findings of Goldin was further confirmed in a series of studies by CALGB, in which previously untreated children were induced with the combination of vincristine plus prednisone and then randomly allocated to various schedules of methotrexate for maintenance (2). In the first study (#6307), the comparison was between 3 mg/m² daily orally and 30 mg/m² twice weekly intramuscularly. A highly significant difference in remission duration favoring the twice weekly parenteral methotrexate over the oral daily dose developed. This study was followed by a study (#6311) in which the importance of the route of drug administration was evaluated (1). In this study, the randomization, after vincristine and prednisone induction, was to methotrexate 30 mg/m² either p.o. or i.v. No evidence of effect of route of administration was found, leaving the proposition that the schedule was the crucial factor. The entire series of CALGB experiments with methotrexate maintenance therapy is outlined in Table 4.

The CALGB looked at unmaintained remission after three intensive 5-day courses of methotrexate given after induction with vincristine plus prednisone and calculated that 120 days of therapy would be needed to achieve complete leukemocidal effect (30). They then designed a program (#6601), outlined in Table 5, including consolidation and intensification treatment with repeated courses of methotrexate, which deliberately lasted 240 days. For comparison purposes there were again only three courses of methotrexate, twice weekly methotrexate for 24 months and a regimen of intermittent inducer doses of vincristine and prednisone given during the 240 days of treatment ("regimen D"). The data from this study demonstrated that the duration of unmaintained remission after 8 months of methotrexate therapy was longer than after three courses, indicating a substantially lowered residual leukemic cell burden. In regimen D, the interspersing of vincristine and prednisone reinduction-type ther-

TABLE 4. *The effect of the schedule of methotrexate when used as remission maintenance in childhood acute leukemia after initial induction with vincristine + prednisone as shown by Cancer and Leukemia Group B (2,28,30)*

| Dosage and schedule | Number of children treated | Median duration of complete remission |
|---|---|---|
| 3 mg/m²/day p.o. | 28 | 3.3 |
| 30 mg/m² twice weekly i.m. | 25 | 17.0 |
| 30 mg/m² twice weekly i.m. | 22 | 8.9 |
| 30 mg/m² twice weekly p.o. | 22 | 10.4 |
| 12–18 mg/m²/day × 5 i.v. re-peated as soon as tolerated (3 courses) | 35 | 5.0 |
| 3 courses as above, then 30 mg/m² twice weekly p.o. | 57 | 18.5 |
| 12–18 mg/m²/day × 5 as above for 8 months | 54 | 10.8 |
| 12–18 mg/m²/day × 5 for 8 months, then 30 mg/m² twice weekly p.o. | 8 | >24 |

apy lengthened the duration of remission even more. In a small group of patients, methotrexate twice weekly was begun after 8 months of the 5-day courses of methotrexate. This group has had an extraordinary duration of remission and survival at last report.

The next first-line protocol of CALGB (#6801, Table 5) attempted to answer the following questions (Lucius Sinks, *personal communication*):

1. If the combination of daunorubicin, vincristine, and prednisone would be more efficient than vincristine plus prednisone for induction of therapy
2. If pretreatment with L-asparaginase before induction with either of the above would enhance the effect
3. To assess the relative value of reinduction treatments during maintenance with daunorubicin, vincristine, and prednisone, as compared to vincristine plus prednisone alone
4. To compare maintenance treatment with methotrexate twice weekly alone versus methotrexate twice weekly combined with daily 6-mercaptopurine

This study has been completed, and the analysis shows daunorubicin to be of no discernable value in combination for either induction or for periodic reinduction during maintenance. The optimal regimen appears to be pretreatment with L-asparaginase, followed by inducation with vincristine plus prednisone and maintenance with the combination of methotrexate and 6-mercaptopurine along with staccato reinforcements with vincristine and prednisone (26).

One of the more recent protocols of CALGB (#7111) is also outlined in Table 5. This complicated protocol has the following objectives (James Holland, *personal communication*):

TABLE 5. *First-line protocols of Cancer and Leukemia Group B in childhood acute leukemia, 1963–1974*

| Protocol number | Induction | Consolidation | Maintenance |
|---|---|---|---|
| 6313 | VCR, 2 mg/m²/wk, + prednisone, a. 40/mg/m²/day b. 120 mg/m²/day | None | a. No treatment b. MTX c. 6-MP d. Cytoxan e. Cyclic MTX-6-MP-cytoxan $e_1$ No treatment $e_2$ BCNU |
| 6601 | VCR, 2/mg/m²/wk, + prednisone, a. 40 mg/m²/day b. 120 mg/m²/day | MTX, 12, 15, or 18 mg/m²/day $\times$ 5 i.v. 3 courses | a. No treatment b. MTX, 30 mg/m²/biw p.o.; treat 2 yr from $M_1$ c. MTX, 12, 15, 18 mg/m²/day $\times$ 5; treat 240 days from $M_1$ d. C + VCR + prednisone, "periodic reinduction" |
| 6801 | a. L-asparaginase, 1,000 IU/kg/day $\times$ 5; then VCR, 2 mg/m²/wk + prednisone, 120 mg/m²/day b. L-asparaginase; then VCR + prednisone as in a. + daunorubicin, 50 mg/m²/wk i.v. c. VCR + prednisone alone d. daunorubicin, vincristine + prednisone | None | a. VCR + prednisone, one week each month b. Same + MTX, 30 mg/m²/biw p.o. c. Same with daunorubicin added to VCR d. 6-MP, 90/mg/m²/day, MTX, 15 mg/m²/day, + VCR + prednisone as in a. e. Same as d. with daunorubicin added |
| 7111 | a. VCR + prednisone (VP) b. VCR + dexamethasone, 6 mg/m²/day p.o. (VD) c. L-asparaginase, 1,000 IU/kg/day $\times$ 10; followed by VP or VD d. L-asparaginase as above concomitantly with VP or VD e. L-asparaginase as above after 3 weeks of VP or VD | MTX, 15 mg/m²/day $\times$ 5 i.m.; 9 day rest and repeat ↓ 6-MP, 600 mg/m²/day $\times$ 5; a day rest and repeat ↓ CNS prophylactic therapy; 2400 R cranial X-ray + i.t. MTX vs. i.t. MTX alone | a. MTX and 6-MP courses as in consolidation followed by BCNU, 150 mg/m² immed. after last dose of 6-MP b. Treatment as above to 1 yr; further $R_x$ to be determined |

TABLE 5. *Continued*

| Protocol number | Induction | Consolidation | Maintenance |
|---|---|---|---|
| 7411 | *Standard Risk* VCR, 2 mg/m²/wk, + prednisone, 40 mg/m²/day, + MTX, 12 mg/m² i.t. day 1, 15, 22, 43, 54, 57, + L-asparaginase, 1,000 I.U./kg/day × 10 day 29–38 vs. same + cranial irradiation 2,400 rads over 16 days status day 43 <br><br> *Increased Risk* Same as above plus daunorubicin, 45 mg/m²/day × 3 day 1–3 of induction | None | a. 6-MP, 90 mg/m²/day p.o. + periodic reinduction with vincristine + prednisone ± daunorubicin <br> b. Cycles of 6-MP, 200 mg/m²/day × 5 p.o. + MTX, 7.5 mg/m²/day p.o., interspersed with periodic reinductions as in a. <br> c. Cycles of MTX, 15 mg/m²/day × 5 p.o., interspersed with periodic reinduction as in a. |

VCR = vincristine; MTX = methotrexate; 6-MP = 6-mercaptopurine;

1. To determine if dexamethasone is at least equal to prednisone in its antileukemic activity and if dexamethasone decreases the occurrence of infection and particularly fatal sepsis during the induction phase
2. To determine in untreated children if the frequency of remissions attained with vincristine and corticosteroids can be increased by addition of asparaginase, and if the position of asparaginase in the treatment schedule (before, during, or after the vincristine and steroid) influences the remission duration
3. To determine the remission duration achieved with prolonged methotrexate and 6-mercaptopurine and BCNU in repeated intensive courses interspersed with periodic inducer doses of vincristine and steroid
4. To determine if the occurrence of CNS leukemia can best be forestalled by the use of intensive i.t. methotrexate or the combination of radiotherapy to the cranium and i.t. methotrexate

The latest protocol of CALGB (#7411; see Table 5) tests the value of cranial irradication and i.t. methotrexate given as part of the induction regimen. It separates standard-risk versus increased-risk children for separate studies, with the latter having daunorubicin added to their induction. Three different maintenance regimens are looked at, so that there are six arms for analysis for each risk category and 12 altogether.

The Children's Cancer Study Group A compared cyclic versus sequential use of drugs as maintenance therapy of remission in acute leukemia (32). Sequential use involved continued treatment with one drug until defined deterioration occurred. Treatment was then begun with the next drug. Cyclic therapy consisted of automatic rotation of each drug at 6-week intervals even though remission continued. The drugs in order of their use were methotrexate, vincristine, prednisone, cytoxan, and 6-mercaptopurine. The median length of maintenance for cyclic therapy was 17.8 months and for sequential was 17.5 months. There was no difference in the length of maintenance with the two methods of drug use.

Krivet et al. (33) reported on a controlled study of children in continuous remission for 2¾ to 3½ years. These children were randomized between continued therapy or no further maintenance. At the time of last report there have been more relapses in the patients discontinuing maintenance therapy, although the total number of children in the study is small (15) and so differences are not significant.

The Children's Cancer Study Group A performed a study in which remission induction was initially tried with prednisone alone at dosages of either 2 or 4 mg/kg/day or 8 mg/kg every other day or 16 mg/kg once in 4 days (Table 6). If one of these regimens was not successful in inducing remission, the patient was given a course of vincristine, and if that was not successful, remission induction was obtained by a combination of 6-mercaptopurine and methotrexate in doses of 2.5 mg/kg/day and 0.1 mg/kg/day p.o., respectively. The patients were then randomly divided into two groups. The control group received 56-day alternating courses of oral 6-mercaptopurine at 2.5 mg/kg/day and oral

TABLE 6. *Two selected protocols of Children's Cancer Study Group A*

| Title | Induction | Consolidation | Maintenance |
|-------|-----------|---------------|-------------|
| "Additive maintenance" | Prednisone, 2 or 4 mg/kg/day or 8 mg/kg e.o.d. or 16 mg/kg q. 4 d If not successful, VCR 0.075 mg/kg/wk $\times$ 6 If not successful, 6-MP 2.5 mg/kg/day p.o. + MTX 0.1 mg/kg/day p.o. | None | a. 56-day alternating courses, 6-MP, 2.5 mg/kg/day p.o. and MTX, 0.1 mg/kg/day p.o. b. Same + actinomycin D 25 gamma/kg i.v., day 28 of 6-MP course, and $HN_2$, 0.2 mg/kg i.v., day 28 of MTX course |
| # 903 | VCR, 2 mg/m²/wk i.v., + prednisone, 60 mg/m²/day p.o. | MTX, 15 mg/m²/ day $\times$ 5 q. 14 d, 4 courses | a. No treatment b. BCG 2 $\times$ wk $\times$ 4 wk then weekly c. MTX, 30 mg/m²/biw + VCR and prednisone as in induction a. for 1 wk each mo. $\times$ 8 |

VCR = vincristine; MTX = methotrexate; 6-MP = 6-mercaptopurine.

methotrexate at 0.1 mg/kg/day. The combination group received in addition a dose of actinomycin D 25 gamma/kg i.v. on day 28 of the 6-mercaptopurine course and nitrogen mustard, 0.2 mg/kg i.v. on day 28 of the methotrexate course. The results are outlined in Table 7 (35).

This study leads to the important conclusion that we may be neglecting the potential role of a variety of agents either discarded for acute lymphatic leukemia in the 1950s or never fully evaluated, such as actinomycin D, nitrogen mustard, and the fluorinated pyrimidines.

This study was followed by another study in which after a methotrexate-plus-prednisone induction, randomization was to six maintenance arms including the two above plus one with actinomycin D during both 56-day maintenance regimens, one with nitrogen mustard during both regimens, one reversing the actinomycin D and nitrogen mustard from the first study, and one utilizing 5-fluorouracil, 10 mg/kg, on day 28 of both the 6-MP and methotrexate courses. The results of the study have not yet been reported in the literature, but long-term remissions are being seen (Dennis Hammond, *personal communication*).

Another protocol of Children's Cancer Study Group A is outlined in Table 6 and involves treatment with vincristine, prednisone, and methotrexate followed by nonspecific immunotherapy with the bacillus of Calmette and Guerin (BCG). The purpose of this study was to evaluate the potential usefulness of this nonspecific immunotherapy in prolonging an unmaintained complete remission induced by chemotherapy and to compare the effect of the BCG immunotherapy early and late in complete remission. This study showed no advantage for BCG maintenance but utilized a different BCG on a different route of administration than described by Mathé.

Several investigators (but most prominently Mathé) have demonstrated that immunotherapy can prolong survival in the mouse leukemic model L1210 (39). Studies in man utilized BCG (40) and killed leukemic cell preparations (47) have indicated an apparent prolongation of unmaintained remission in acute human leukemia. Experiments in animals have indicated that immunotherapy of the BCG type is not effective unless the original leukemic cell population

TABLE 7. *Children's cancer study group additive maintenance study*

| | | Median duration of complete remission in days | |
| --- | --- | --- | --- |
| | Number | Control | Combination |
| Entire group | 135 | 390 | 478.5 = 16 months |
| Patients induced with prednisone only | 104 | 406 | 720 = 24 months |
| Patients induced with VCR or 6-MP + MTX after failing prednisone induction | 31 | 271 | 270 |

VCR = vincristine; 6-MP = 6-mercaptopurine; MTX = methotrexate.

can be significantly reduced to approximately $10^5$ cells. It has not been proven that this is true in man, but it would appear likely.

The Southwest Oncology Group studied the value of periodic reinforcement during maintenance in a controlled study which asked a variety of questions (12). The study compared two induction regimens. Vincristine plus prednisone gave an 83% CR rate (72 of 87 patients) versus 93% (77 of 83 patients) for 6-mercaptopurine and prednisone. When hematologic remission was achieved, patients were randomized to one of three maintenance schedules: 6-mercaptopurine alone, 6-mercaptopurine plus prednisone for 4 weeks every 3 months, or 6-mercaptopurine plus prednisone plus vincristine for 4 weeks every 3 months. Maintenance therapy with 6-mercaptopurine alone following either induction schedule proved to be significantly inferior to therapy with 6-mercaptopurine and periodic reinforcement. When long-term survival was analyzed, there is a slight edge for vincristine plus prednisone. It is interesting to note that in an earlier phase of the analysis with all maintenance arms collapsed there appeared to be a distinct advantage, in terms of survival, for 6-mercaptopurine plus prednisone induction. This points up the hazard of analyzing the studies too early and making definitive conclusions. One has to wait for the survival curves to fully mature, which now will take many years.

The Southwest Oncology Group has studied the value of interrupted versus continuous maintenance therapy (13). They entered 313 patients with childhood acute leukemia previously untreated into a study that began with vincristine and prednisone induction. Of 276 evaluable patients 86% achieved complete bone marrow remission in a median of 35 days. After remissions patients were randomized to one of three oral maintenance therapies: 6-mercaptopurine (75 mg/m²/day), methotrexate (25 mg/m² twice weekly) or cyclophosphamide (100 mg/m²/day). Patients receiving maintenance therapy were further randomized at 2 and 6 months after the start of maintenance either to continue or discontinue study. The results of this study were to clearly establish that continued maintenance beyond 2 and 6 months was important. When patients discontinued maintenance at 2 or 6 months after induction of remission they had significantly shorter lengths of remission than patients continuing on maintenance therapy. There was no significant difference in terms of remission duration among the three drugs studied, although survival tended to favor 6-mercaptopurine.

One of the major developments in the successful treatment of childhood leukemia has been the use of prophylactic treatment of the central nervous system to prevent relapse in that area, which is a pharmacologic sanctuary for so many of the drugs that are standardly used. The controlled clinical trial has played a major role in delineating the value of this approach.

There have been several reports on the use of i.t. methotrexate both in the induction phase of treatment as well as in the maintenance phase of treatment for prophylaxis against meningeal leukemia. Melthorn et al. (42) utilized the drug in a controlled randomized study where 47 patients, with newly diagnosed acute leukemia, either received i.t. methotrexate, or did not, immediately after the diagnosis of systemic disease. Four of the 47 patients were found to have CNS involvement at the time of the original spinal tap and were given i.t. methotrexate and removed from subsequent study groups. Of the remaining 43 patients, 24 received a single dose, 0.9 mg/kg, of methotrexate i.t. within 24 hr of the original diagnosis of systemic disease, while 19 patients acted as controls and received no chemoprophylaxis. Follow-up studies of the CSF were done when clinical signs and symptoms suggested meningeal involvement. Thirteen patients in each group developed meningeal leukemia (54.2% of 24 patients in the treated group; 68.4% of 19 patients in the control group). The difference in the percentage involvement was not considered significant. Average time to onset of CNS involvement in the treated patients was 11.9 months, compared to 7.6 months for the untreated group. This difference was statistically significant. Unfortunately, no data were given on the effect of such therapy on the duration of systemic remission or survival.

Frei et al. (14) was one of the first to employ i.t. methotrexate during the maintenance phase in the treatment of acute lymphocytic leukemia. A summary of their experimental design is shown on Table 8.

There was no intensive phase, and craniospinal irradiation is not used early in remission. However, prophylactic CNS therapy was given at 1 week into remission under Section III of the protocol and then carried out at monthly intervals. Eighty-two percent of the patients achieved a complete remission. The median duration of remission was ≅7½ months. The duration of remission was not affected by i.t. methotrexate at monthly intervals. However, the incidence of meningeal leukemia was ≅ 17% in programs I and II but only 3% in treatment program III.

Similar findings have also been seen by other investigators. Spevak (48), in 1964, found that prophylactic i.t. methotrexate at monthly intervals yielded a median survival of 18.5 months and only a 10% incidence of meningeal leukemia.

TABLE 8. *Experimental design (14)*

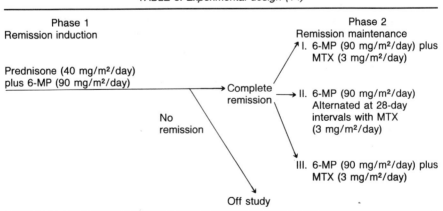

MTX = methotrexate; 6-MP = 6-mercaptopurine.

Unfortunately, this study was not controlled, so whether the i.t. methotrexate directly influenced the remission duration, or decreased the incidence of meningeal leukemia, cannot be determined.

Sullivan and her colleagues (49,50), in the Southwest Chemotherapy Group, reported on a study in which the duration of CNS remissions (following initial intrathecal therapy with methotrexate) were compared among no prophylactic therapy, BCNU therapy every 2 months, and i.t. methotrexate every 2 months. She found that the median duration of CNS remission for the no-therapy group and the BCNU therapy group was $\cong$ 4 months and 3 months, respectively. However, for the i.t. methotrexate-treated group, the median duration of CNS remission was $\cong$ 16 months. However, these findings were in patients in which an original CSF remission had been obtained with i.t. methotrexate. They concluded that "the superiority of the methotrexate regimen is of such degree that it should be considered for all patients with CNS leukemia after remission is achieved." Thus, i.t. methotrexate used every 2 months has a definite advantage over no i.t. prophylactic therapy in maintaining a CNS remission. Since this regimen was not associated with increased morbidity or toxicity, further investigations are currently being carried out.

Over the past 8 years, Pinkel, Mauer, and associates have been using "total therapy" in the treatment of acute lymphocytic leukemia in children. The first pilot study (25) (Total Therapy I) was accomplished with three children in which remission induction with prednisone (Pred) and vincristine (VCR) was followed by daily 6-mercaptopurine (6-MP) orally and weekly VCR and cytoxan (CTX) i.v. During early remission, 500 rads of $^{60}$Co were administered to the entire craniospinal axis. The next 12 children were entered in the second pilot study (22) which utilized VCR and Pred for induction (Total Therapy II). On this regimen 10 of 12 patients went into complete remission. They were subsequently treated with either daily 6-MP or weekly methotrexate combined with VCR and CTX administered every 2 weeks. This group of patients also received craniospinal irradiation with 500 rads of $^{60}$Co. In these two groups of patients, the median duration of complete remission was 8 months and the median survival was 20 months, with 2 patients surviving 5 years or more.

On the basis of these data and the data that was being accrued by other investigators in the field, Pinkel and his associate designed a study (Total Therapy III) that could incorporate an intensive phase and a maintenance phase after remission induction as outlined in Table 9 (23). There were 31 patients in this treatment group. Twenty-seven children (87%) achieved complete remission in a median time of 28 days. The median duration of remission and median survival were about double the previous pilot studies, being 19.5 months and 34 months, respectively. Five patients were still living by 5 years. Central nervous system relapse preceded hematological relapse in 12 patients; whereas in an additional patient, CNS relapse followed a hematological relapse.

The overall incidence of central nervous system leukemia was 46%, which was not smaller than that reported in previous studies from the group. The

TABLE 9. *Total Therapy III for children with acute lymphocytic leukemia (23): design of the study*

| Phase 1<br>Remission induction | Phase 2<br>Intensive therapy | Phase 3<br>Remission Maintenance |
|---|---|---|
| Vincristine,<br>1.5 mg/m²/wk i.v.<br>+<br>prednisone,<br>40 mg/m²/day p.o. → Complete remission → | Methotrexate,<br>10 mg/m²/day i.v. 3 days<br>+<br>6-mercaptopurine,<br>1 g/m²/day i.v. 3 days<br>+<br>cyclophosphamide,<br>600 mg/m²/ i.v. once → | Methotrexate,<br>20 mg/m²/wk i.v.<br>+<br>mercaptopurine,<br>50 mg/m²/day p.o.<br>+<br>cyclophosphamide,<br>200 mg/m²/wk i.v.<br>+<br>vincristine,<br>1.0 mg/m²/wk i.v.<br>+<br>Central nervous system radiation,<br>1,200 rads in 11 days |

No response → Dropped from study

time from diagnosis to the onset of CNS leukemia ranged from 7 to 31 months with a median of ≅ 17 months. Thus, by incorporating an intensive phase, being more vigorous with maintenance therapy, and increasing the dose of CNS radiation, the survival of this group of children was almost doubled. However, central nervous system radiation by the method and dosage used had no influence on the development of CNS leukemia.

To study further the effects of the changes in the Total Therapy III protocol, a fourth study was carried out, Total Therapy IV, where drugs were either administered in full dosages or half dosages during the maintenance phase and craniospinal irradiation was left out altogether (43). The general schema of this protocol is given in Table 10. This protocol was designed to answer the question as to whether or not high doses of the multiple antileukemic drugs were necessary for optimal maintenance of remissions. By eliminating the CNS radiation, this protocol also helped answer another question as to whether or not craniospinal radiation given during early remission prolonged the interval between diagnosis and the development of CNS leukemia. In answer to the first question, the median duration of complete remission was 15 months (as it had been in Total Therapy II) for those receiving the full dosages. However, in those patients receiving half dosages during the maintenance phase, the median duration of complete remission was only 6 months. Also, the survival in the patients receiving the half-dose therapy was 21 months, whereas the survival of those receiving full doses of chemotherapeutic agent was ≅ 34 months. Thus, the absence of CNS radiation did not appreciably alter either remission duration or survival when compared with the results of Total Therapy III.

In answer to the second question, as to the prophylactic effect of CNS radiation

TABLE 10. *Total Therapy IV (43): treatment plan*

| Phase | Purpose | Duration | Drug schedule |
|-------|---------|----------|---------------|
| 1 | Remission induction | 4–6 weeks | VCR, 1.5 mg/m²/week, i.v. Pred, 40 mg/m²/day, p.o. |
| 2 | Intensive chemotherapy | 1 week | MTX, 10 mg/m²/day × 3, i.v. MP, 1 g/m²/day × 3, i.v. Cyclo, 600 mg/m²/day × 1, i.v. |
| 3 | Continuation | 3 years or to hematological relapse | MP, 50 mg/m²/day, p.o. MTX, 20 mg/m²/week, i.v. Cyclo, 200 mg/m²/week, i.v. VCR, 1 mg/m²/week, i.v., or half-dosage of above drugs |

VCR = vincristine;  Pred = prednisone;  MTX = methotrexate;  MP = 6-mercaptopurine; Cyclo = cyclophosphamide.

in the early phase of remission, a clear-cut effect was noted. As will be recalled, the median time from diagnosis to the onset of meningeal leukemia in Total Therapy III was ≅ 17 months, with 46% of the children developing CNS leukemia. In Total Therapy IV, under that section that utilized the same dosages as in Total Therapy III (full dosages), the median time from diagnosis to onset of meningeal leukemia was only ≅ 11 months in 15 of 21 (71%) patients in which CNS leukemia developed. Thus CNS leukemia was delayed and its incidence reduced by the administration of prophylactic radiotherapy in Total Therapy III. That systemic therapy also played a role in delaying the onset of meningeal leukemia was evident by comparing the median time from diagnosis to onset of meningeal leukemia of those at the half dosage and at the full dosage schedule. In those patients who only received half dosage during the maintenance phase, 20 to 21 (95%) developed CNS leukemia in a median time of 5 to 7 months. Thus, development of meningeal leukemia was directly responsible for the decrease in the median time of complete remissions. All subsequent protocols have included CNS prophylaxis either with radiotherapy alone or in combination with IT methotrexate.

Total Therapy V (outlined in Table 11) utilizes the same induction therapy as in the two previous protocols (4). The intensive phase differs only by the addition of prednisone. During early remission and just after the intensive phase, however, a 2½ week phase of CNS prophylaxis is added which includes radiotherapy to the skull (2,500 rads), i.t. methotrexate, 12 mg/m²/wk × 5 doses (with leucovorin protection systemically), and prednisone, 10 mg/m²/day orally × 7 days. The maintenance is similar to the previous full-dosage protocol but is interrupted at 10-week intervals by VCR and Pred reinductions. In the previous study, complete remissions have been most often terminated by nervous system leukemia occurring in the presence of hematological remission. This present therapy schema was designed to explore the possibility that CNS leukemia and thus early termination of complete remission could be prevented by

TABLE 11. *Total Therapy V (4)*

---

*Phase 1—induction (4–6 wk)*
Pred, 40 mg/m²/day orally X 28–42 days
VCR, 1.5 mg/m²/wk i.v. X 4–6 wk

*Phase 2—intensive (1 wk)*
6-MP, 1 g/m²/day i.v. X 3
MTX, 10 mg/m²/day i.v. X 3
Cyclo, 600 mg/m²/day i.v. X 1
Pred, 20 mg/m²/day orally X 7

*Phase 3—CNS (2½ wk)*
Radiotherapy skull, 2,500 rads
MTX i.t., 12 mg/m²/2X/wk X 5 doses
Leucovorin i.m., 12 mg/m²/2X/wk X 5 doses
Pred, 10 mg/m²/day orally X 7

*Phase 4—continuation (2 yr)*
6 MP, 50 mg/m²/d orally
MTX, 20 mg/m²/wk i.v.
Cyclo, 200 mg/m²/wk i.v.

At week 10 and every 10 wk thereafter,
Pred, 40 mg/m²/day orally X 15 days
VCR, 1.5 mg/m²/wk i.v. X 3 doses

---

Pred = prednisone;   VCR = vincristine;   6-
MP = 6-mercaptopurine,    MTX = methotrexate; Cyclo = cyclophosphamide.

administering a moderately high dose of cranial radiotherapy along with i.t. methotrexate early during complete remission.

The results at this time are currently superior to those of any previous treatment program. Complete remissions were successfully attained in 32 of 35 patients (91%) entering this study. Twenty-one of the 32 children who attained remission (64%) are currently in continuous complete remissions for 23 to 30 months (median 25 months). Of 10 children who received all phases of therapy (2 did not due to sepsis in one and varicella in another) and who relapsed from complete remission, only 3 developed nervous system leukemia before hematological relapse and 3 after hematological relapse. Thus only 6 of 32 (19%) children developed CNS leukemia as compared to $\cong 71\%$ in the previous study. The time from diagnosis to onset of meningeal leukemia cannot be determined from the data given. The greater intensity of the CNS therapy in this study may be responsible not only for the reduction of incidence of CNS leukemia, but also for the substantial increase in the duration of complete remission.

Total Therapy VI, from the St. Jude's group, is outlined in Table 12 (3,6). Total Therapy VI is designed to determine the influence of a 1-week course of high-dose intensive chemotherapy on the duration and quality of subsequent chemotherapy-maintained remissions, and evaluate the role of prophylactic craniospinal irradiation in preventing meningeal leukemia and thereby maintaining complete remissions for a longer period of time. A total of 94 patients were randomly allocated between craniospinal irradiation 2,400 rads of $^{60}$Co and

TABLE 12. *Total Therapy VI*

*Remission Induction (4–6 wk) (11,12)*
Pred, 40 mg/m²/day orally × 28–42 day
VCR, 1.5 mg/m²/wk i.v. × 4–6 wk
Dauno, 25 mg/m²/wk i.v. × 4–6 wk

*CR Marrow*
Randomize into two groups:

| Group A | Group B |
|---|---|
| Intensive chemotherapy (7 days) | No intensive chemotherapy |
| 6-MP, 1 g/m²/day i.v. × 3 days | |
| followed by | |
| MTX, 10 mg/m²/day i.v. × 3 days | |
| followed by | No |
| Cyclo, 600 mg/m²/day i.v. × 1 day | delay |
| 2-wk delay | |

*Continuation therapy (3 yr)*
6-MP, 50 mg/m²/day orally
MTX, 20 mg/m²/wk orally
Cyclo, 200 mg/m²/wk orally
At day 70 of this phase add:
VCR, 1.5 mg/m²/wk i.v. × 3 doses (days 1, 8, 15)
Pred, 40 mg/m² orally × 15 days

VCR-Pred course repeated 70 days after final dose of VCR-Pred of each previous course

Four weeks after achieving M-1 marrow patients randomized into Group A (two subgroups) and Group B (two subgroups)

| Group A | | Group B | |
|---|---|---|---|
| A-1 | A-2 | B-1 | B-2 |
| Craniospinal | Craniospinal | Craniospinal | Craniospinal |
| radiotherapy, | radiotherapy, | radiotherapy, | radiotherapy, |
| 2,400 rads | 2,400 rads when CNS | 2,400 rads | 2,400 rads when CNS |
| | leukemia develops | immediately | leukemia develops |

Pred = prednisone; VCR = vincristine; Dauno = daunorubicin; 6-MP = 6-mercaptopurine; MTX = methotrexate; Cyclo = cyclophosphamide.

no prophylactic therapy and intensive chemotherapy or no intensive chemotherapy. All subsequently received identical multiple-drug chemotherapy for at least 1 year. To date there is no difference between the intensive and no intensive chemotherapy. However, the prophylactic CNS radiotherapy section of the protocol already shows a marked difference. CNS leukemia has ended remission in 27 of 49 children (51%) not receiving irradiation prophylactically, compared to only 2 of 45 (6.6%) who received craniospinal irradiation prophylactically. In 7 patients in the irradiated group, the bone marrow was the initial site of relapse, whereas one patient in this group subsequently had a bone marrow relapse following CNS leukemia. In the nonirradiated group, 5 systemic relapses occurred before CNS relapse, whereas 3 occurred after it. Thus, both groups had the same number (8) of bone marrow relapses. Only 4 of 45 patients in the irradiated group had reduction of radiation dosage due to toxicity. Preferentially, chemotherapy was reduced to permit completion of radiotherapy within 4 weeks. The authors concluded that "in children with acute lymphocytic leukemia receiving combination chemotherapy, craniospinal irradiation early in remission delays or prevents CNS leukemia."

Outlined in Table 13 is St. Jude's protocol, Total Therapy VII (5). Total Therapy VII compared the efficacy and toxicity of two therapeutic regimens given early in remission for prophylaxis of nervous system leukemia and thereby for prolongation of continuous complete remissions: cranial radiotherapy plus i.t. methotrexate; and craniospinal radiotherapy. It also determined the efficacy and toxicity of a 15-day course of prednisone and vincristine every 12 weeks during continuation therapy in prolonging continuous complete remissions.

The results of study VII are inferior to those of earlier studies and apparently cannot be explained by the omission of an intensive phase of chemotherapy, the pulses of vincristine and prednisone, the number of agents used during continuation of chemotherapy, or by the type of preventive CNS therapy (41). Furthermore, the induction regimen cannot be implicated as the total reason. The reason is a combination of factors that cannot be determined at this time.

TABLE 13. *Outline of Total Therapy Study VII (6)*

---

*Phase 1—Remission Induction (4–6 wks)*
    Pred, 40 mg/m²/day orally (p.o.)
    VCR, 1.5 mg/m²/wk intravenously (i.v.)

If still either M-2 or M-3 by day 42. Drop from study.

If patient shows progressive leukemia at any time of Phase 1, chemotherapy will be changed in his best interest.

If in remission (M-1 marrow), randomization by Card-Envelope Technique into 4 groups (CM, CMVP, CS, and CSVP) for further therapy with no delay (Phase 2-A and 2-B).

    CM = Cranial radiation + methotrexate (MTX) intrathecally (i.t.)
    CMVP = CM + Pred-VCR pulse
    CS = Craniospinal radiation
    CSVP = CS + Pred VCR pulse

*Phase 2-A—Prophylaxis of Central Nervous System (CNS) Leukemia*
    (2½ or 4 wks)

CM and CMVP—2½ wks:  Cranial radiation, 2,400 rads
                      MTX, 12 mg/m²/twice wk × 5 i.t.
CS and CSVP—4 wks:  Craniospinal radiation, 2,400 rads

*Phase 2-B: Continuation Chemotherapy (2–3 yrs)*

All groups (CM, CMVP, CS, and CSVP):
6-mercaptopurine (6-MP), 50 mg/m²/day p.o.
cyclophosphamide (Cyclo), 200 mg/m²/wk p.o.
methotrexate (MTX), 20 mg/m²/wk p.o.

Groups CM and CMVP receive no p.o. MTX during cranial radiation with i.t. MTX.

*Phase 3: VCR-Pred Pulse*

Groups CMVP and CSVP starting on day 70 after M-1 marrow and every 12 wks from the start of the preceding pulse:

PRED, 40 mg/m²/day × 15 days p.o.
VCR, 1.5 mg/m²/wk × 3 doses i.v.

---

Currently at the St. Jude's Children's Research Hospital, all patients who attain remission after induction therapy are promptly entered on a program of central nervous system prophylaxis. Cranial irradiation is given with a cobolt unit over a period of 2½ weeks. For a child 2 years and older, 2,400 rads are delivered. Between the ages of 1 and 2 years, 2,000 rads are given and if the child is under 1 year of age, 1,500 rads is the dose used. In addition, methotrexate is given intrathecally in a dose of 12 mg/m$^2$ twice weekly for a total of five doses.

The latest protocol of St. Jude's is Total Therapy Study VIII (41). The aims of this protocol are to induce remission with a standard three-drug regimen (prednisone, vincristine, and L-asparaginase), provide for central system prophylaxis (cranial irradiation and intrathecal methotrexate), and then randomize the patients who were disease-free at the end of that time into one of the four groups for continuation therapy. The four groups receive maintenance or continuation therapy with from one to four drugs all given in amounts calculated to be that of maximal biological tolerance. The first group receives methotrexate only. The second also receives 6-mercaptopurine, the third group has added cyclophosphamide as a third drug, and the fourth group a fourth drug, which is cytosine arabinoside. The preliminary results show that the methotrexate alone was dropped early in the study because of the development of subacute leukoencephalopathy in some of the patients. The overall results for the two-, three-, and four-drug regimens to date are similar as far as remission duration and frequency of patients achieving 2½ to 3 years of continuous complete remission, at which time therapy is discontinued.

One of the major problems in the interpretation of clinical trial data in childhood acute leukemia is that we have now reached the successful situation where median survivals of 5 to 7 years are now commonplace, and these must be the end points of new studies. Success has robbed us of the luxury of having end points of complete remission rates and short-term median duration of remission.

The heterogeneity of the material in clinical trials makes comparisons between studies difficult. Karon (34) has shown that a 10 to 20% exclusion at the front end of a study can cause a marked shift in the median duration of remission out at 5 to 10 years. Because small exclusions at the front end make very little difference for periods up to 3 years, the importance of this problem has gone largely unrecognized. This phenomenon is not necessarily restricted to exclusions or induction failures; it can also obtain for any cohort of patients with a certain set of characteristics that result in a survival pattern significantly different from the rest of the population. Among the critical factors that are often ignored in clinical trials and that are rarely analyzable for comparability between different clinical trials are initial white blood count, morphology, age, distribution and degree of leukemia infiltration, and immune status.

The controlled clinical trial has played a major role in delineating the optimal therapeutic approach to childhood leukemia. The initial major advance, which was the ability to induce complete remissions with chemotherapy, did not require a controlled trial, but once this was established the controlled trial became a powerful tool to help establish the optimal approach to induction, the role of maintenance therapy, and the importance of prophylactic treatment of the central nervous system.

## REFERENCES

1. Acute Leukemia Group B (1969): Acute lymphocytic leukemia in children. Maintenance therapy with methotrexate administered intermittently. *JAMA,* 207:923.
2. Acute Leukemia Group B (1965): New treatment schedule with improved survival in childhood leukemia. *JAMA,* 194:75.
3. Aur, R., Hustu, H. O., Ver Zosa, M., and Simone, J. (1971): A comparative study of "prophylactic" craniospinal irradiation in 94 children with acute lymphocytic leukemia (ALL). *Proc. Am. Assoc. Cancer Res.,* 12:19.
4. Aur, R. J. A., et al. (1971): Central nervous system therapy in combination chemotherapy of childhood lymphocytic leukemia. *Blood,* 37(3):272.
5. Aur, R. J. A. (1977): *Personal communication.*
6. Aur, R. J. A., Simone, J. V., Hustu, H. O., and Ver Zosa, M. S. (1977): A comparative study of central nervous system irradiation and intensive chemotherapy early in remission of childhood acute lymphocytic leukemia. *Cancer (in press).*
7. Bernard, J., Boiron, M., Jacquillat, C., and Weil, M. (1968): Rubidomycin in 400 patients with leukemias and other malignancies *(abstract). Twelfth Congr. Int. Soc. Hemat.,* p. 5.
8. Berry, D. H., Pullen, J., George, S., et al. (1975): Comparison of prednisolone vincristine, methotrexate and 6-mercaptopurine vs. vincristine and prednisone induction therapy in childhood acute leukemia. Cancer, 36:98–102.
9. Chevalier, L., and Glidewell, O. (1967): Schedule of 6-MP and effect of inducer drugs on remission maintenance in acute leukemia. *Proc. Am. Assoc. Cancer Res.,* 8:10.
10. Ellison, R. B., and Murphy, M. L. (1964): Apparent doubling time of leukemic cells in marrow *(abstract). Clin. Res.,* 12:284.
11. Farber, S., Diamond, L. K., and Mercer, R. D. (1948): Temporary remissions in acute leukemia in children produced by folic acid antagonist 4-aminopteroyl-glutamic acid (aminopterin). *New Engl. J. Med.,* 238:787.
12. Fernbach, D. J., George, S. L., Sutow, W. W., et al. (1975): Long-term results of reinforcement therapy for children with acute leukemia. *Cancer,* 36:1552–1559.
13. Fernbach, D. J., Griffith, K. M., Haggard, M. E., Holcomb, T. M., Sutow, W. W., Vietti, T. J., and Windmiller, J. (1966): Chemotherapy of acute leukemia in childhood. Comparison of cyclophosphamide and mercaptopurine. *New Engl. J. Med.,* 275:451.
14. Frei, E., III, et al. (1965): The effectiveness of combination of antileukemic agents in inducing and maintaining remission in children with acute leukemia. *Blood,* 26(5):642.
15. Frei, E., III, and Freireich, E. J. (1965): Progress and perspectives in chemotherapy of acute leukemia. In: *Advances in Chemotherapy,* Vol. 2, edited by A. Goldin, F. Hawking, and R. J. Schnitzer, p. 269. Academic Press, New York.
16. Freireich, E. J., Gehan, E., Frei, E., III, Schroeder, L. R., Wolman, I. J., Anbari, R., Bugert, E. O., Mills, S. D., Pinkel, D., Selawry, O. S., Moon, J. H., Gendel, B. R., Spurr, C. L., Storrs, R., Haurani, F., Hoogstraten, B., and Lee, S. (1963): The effect of 6-mercaptopurine on the duration of steroid-induced remissions in acute leukemia: A model for evaluation of other potentially useful therapy. *Blood,* 21:699.
17. Freireich, E. J., Henderson, E. S., and Frei, E., III (1968): *The Proliferation and Spread of Neoplastic Cells. M. D. Anderson Hospital Symposium.* Williams & Wilkins, Baltimore.
18. Freireich, E. J., Henderson, E. S., and Frei, E., III (1968): The treatment of acute leukemia considered with respect to cell population kinetics. In: *The Proliferation and Spread of Neoplastic Cells. M. D. Anderson Hospital Symposium.* Williams & Wilkins, Baltimore.
19. Freireich, E. J., Karon, M., Flatow, F., and Frei, E., III (1965): Effect of intensive cyclic chemotherapy (BIKE) on remission duration in acute lymphocytic leukemia *(abstract). Proc. Am. Assoc. Cancer Res.,* 6:20.

20. Freireich, J., Karon, E. M., and Frei, E., III (1964): Quadruple combination therapy (VAMP) for acute lymphocytic leukemia in childhood *(abstract). Proc. Am. Assoc. Cancer Res.,* 5:20.
21. Furth, J., and Kahn, M. C. (1937): The transmission of leukemia of mice with a single cell. *Am. J. Cancer,* 31:276.
22. George, P., Hernandez, K., Borella, L., and Pinkel, D. (1966): "Total therapy" of acute lymphocytic leukemia in children. *Proc. Am. Assoc. Cancer Res.,* 7:23.
23. George, P., Hernandez, K., Hustu, O., Borella, L., Holton, C., and Pinkel, D. (1968): A study of "total therapy" of acute lymphocytic leukemia in children. *J. Pediatr.,* 72:399.
24. George, P., Hernandez, K., Hustu, O., Borella, L., Holton, C., and Pinkel, D. (1968): A study of "total therapy" of acute lymphocytic leukemia in children. *Pediatr. Pharmacol. Ther.,* 72:399.
25. George, P., and Pinkel, D. (1965): CNS radiation in children with acute lymphocytic leukemia in remission. *Proc. Am. Assoc. Cancer Res.,* 6:22.
26. Glidewell, O. J., and Holland, J. F. (1971): Clinical trials of the Acute Leukemia Group B in acute lymphocytic leukemia. Presented at the 5th International Symposium on Comparative Leukemia Research.
27. Goldin, A., Venditti, J. M., Humphreys, S. R., and Mantel, N. (1956): Modification of treatment schedules in the management of advanced mouse leukemia with amethopterin. *J. Natl. Cancer Inst.,* 17:203
28. Henderson, E. S. (1967): Combination chemotherapy of acute lymphocytic leukemia of childhood. *Cancer Res.,* 27:2570.
29. Henderson, E. S., Freireich, E. J., Karon, M., and Rosse, W. (1966): High dose combination chemotherapy in acute lymphocytic leukemia of childhood *(abstract). Cancer Res.,* 7:30.
30. Holland, J. F., and Glidewell, O. (1970): Complimentary chemotherapy in acute leukemia. In: *Recent Results in Cancer Research,* Vol. 30, p. 95. Springer-Verlag, New York.
31. Howard, J. P., and Tan, C. (1967): Combined daunomycin-prednisone inductions in acute leukemia. *Proc. Am. Assoc. Cancer Res.,* 8:32.
32. Karon, M. (1973): Problems in the evaluation of long-term results. In: *Recent Results in Cancer Research,* Vol. 43, pp. 113–120. Springer-Verlag, New York.
33. Krivit, W., Brubaker, C., Thatcher, L. G., Pierce, M., Perrin, E., and Hartmann, J. R. (1968): Maintenance therapy in acute leukemia of childhood. Comparison of cyclic vs. sequential methods. *Cancer,* 21:352.
34. Krivit, W., Gilchrist, G., and Beatty, E. C., Jr. (1970): The need for chemotherapy after prolonged complete remission in childhood leukemia. *J. Pediatr.,* 76:138–141.
35. Leiken, S. L., Brubaker, C., Hartmann, J. R., et al. (1968): Varying prednisone dosage in remission induction of previously untreated childhood leukemia. *Cancer,* 21:346–351.
36. Leiken, S., Brubaker, C., Hartmann, J., et al. (1969): The use of combination therapy in leukemia remission. *Cancer,* 24:427.
37. Livingston, R. B., and Carter, S. K. (1970): *Single Agents in Cancer Chemotherapy.* IFI/Plenum, New York-Washington-London.
38. Lonsdale, D., Gehan, E. A., Fernbach, D. J., et al. (1975): Interrupted vs. continued maintenance therapy in childhood acute leukemia. *Cancer,* 36:341–352.
39. Mathé, G. (1967): *Rev. Fr. Etud. Clin. Biol.,* 12:912.
40. Mathé, G., et al. (1969): Active immunotherapy for acute lymphoblastic leukemia. *Lancet,* 1:697.
41. Mauer, A. M., and Simone, J. V. (1976): The current status of the treatment of childhood acute lymphoblastic leukemia. *Cancer Treatment Rev.*
42. Melhorn, D. K., Gross, S., Fisher, B. J., and Newman, A. J. (1970): Studies on the use of "prophylactic" intrathecal amethopterin in childhood leukemia. *Blood,* 36:55.
43. Pinkel, D., Hernandez, K., Borella, L., et al. (1971): Drug dosage and remission duration in childhood lymphocytic leukemia. *Cancer,* 27:247.
44. Selawry, O. S., and James, D. (1965): Therapeutic index of methotrexate as related to dose schedule and routes of administration in children with acute lymphocytic leukemia. *Proc. Am. Assoc. Cancer Res.,* 6:54.
45. Simone, J. V., Aur, R. J. A., et al. (1975): Combined modality therapy of acute lymphocytic leukemia. *Cancer,* 35:25.
46. Skipper, H. E., Schabel, F. M., Jr., and Wilcox, W. S. (1964): Experimental evaluation of potential anti-cancer agents. XIII. On the criteria and kinetics associated with "curability" of experimental leukemia. *Cancer Chemother. Rep.,* 35:1.
47. Skrkovich, S. V., Kisljack, N. S., Machonova, L. A., and Begunenko, S. A. (1969): *Nature,* 223:509.

48. Spevak, J. (1964): The prophylaxis of meningeal leukemia with intrathecal methotrexate. *J. Iowa Med. Soc.,* 54(5):238.
49. Sullivan, M. P., Haggard, M. E., Donaldson, M. H., and Krall, J. (1970): Comparison of the prolongation of remission in meningeal leukemia with maintenance intrathecal methotrexate (IT MTX) and intravenous bis-nitrosourea (BCNU). *Proc. Am. Assoc. Cancer Res.,* 11:77.
50. Sullivan, M. P., Vietti, T. J., Fernbach, D. J., Griffith, K. M., Haddy, T. B., and Watkins, W. L. (1970): Clinical investigations in the treatment of meningeal leukemia: Radiation therapy regimens vs. conventional intrathecal amethopterin in childhood leukemia. *Blood,* 36:55.
51. Zubrod, C. G. (1967): Treatment of acute leukemias. *Cancer Res.,* 27:2557.
52. Zubrod, C. G., Schepartz, S., Leiter, J., et al. (1966): The chemotherapy program of the National Cancer Institute: History, plans and analysis. *Cancer Chemother. Rep.,* 50:349.

*Randomized Trials in Cancer: A Critical Review by Sites,* edited by Maurice J. Staquet, Raven Press, New York © 1978.

# Nonlymphocytic Acute Leukemia

Louisette Debusscher and Pierre A. Stryckmans

*Service de Médecine et Laboratoire d'Investigation Clinique Henri Tagnon, Institut Jules Bordet, 1000 Bruxelles, Belgium*

This chapter discusses the contribution of randomized clinical trials to the advancement in treatment of acute nonlymphoblastic leukemia (ANLL). For more than 20 years, it has been realized that the first goal to reach was the achievement of complete remission (CR), since survival appeared to be related directly to this condition. Unlike the acute lymphoblastic leukemia (ALL) situation, this first goal is still hard to attain and further studies to improve the induction treatment must be pursued. The role of randomized trials is shown as remission inducters of the first antimetabolites available, of the corticosteroids (first period), and essentially in the determination of optimal administration schedules for the most efficient drugs introduced later, namely, cytosine arabinoside and daunorubicin, used alone or in different combinations.

The second objective in ANLL treatment is prolongation of the remission status. Even if the percentage of complete remissions obtained has considerably increased, the duration of these remissions does not generally exceed a few months. Some randomized trials have evaluated different modalities of maintenance treatments. Most recently, immunotherapy has been introduced as a new tool to prolong remission duration. Hopefully we shall soon have a correct view of the value of this new weapon thanks to the very numerous randomized clinical trials now in progress.

## INDUCTION TREATMENT IN ANLL

### First Chemotherapeutic Period

The first randomized trials concerning remission induction in ANLL, dating from the late 1950s to the early 1960s, compared different modes of administration of the antimetabolites available, evaluated the value of corticosteroids at different dosages and in combination, and compared different modalities of the first multiple drug combinations.

Received August 30, 1977.

*Evaluation of Different Modes of Administration of Antimetabolites*

The comparison, in 22 ANLL patients, of daily administration of methotrexate (MTX) associated with daily 6-mercaptopurine (6-MP) to daily 6-MP and MTX every third day did not show any difference in frequency of remission, extent of remission, or toxicity. Among the few remitting patients, however, duration of remission and of survival was longer for the continuously treated group (20).

In 1961, the first results on a large number of patients (131 ANLL cases) collected by the Acute Leukemia Group B (ALGB) were published (19). The study compared the effect of 6-MP and methotrexate administered sequentially (after failure of the first drug) or concomittantly. It showed a 15% remission rate (complete and partial) for combination therapy, 21% for 6-MP and 7% for MTX. Responsiveness to the second drug tempted was independent of responsiveness to the first one. However, the survival at 10 weeks was better for patients receiving the combination therapy.

The success in the treatment of adult acute leukemia with divided daily doses of MTX given in 5-day courses and repeated every 10 to 14 days (28) prompted the Southeastern Cancer Chemotherapy Cooperative Study Group to compare randomly on 45 previously untreated leukemic patients this schedule with a generally accepted standard mode of treatment at that time, namely, daily 6-MP and prednisone (60). This trial did not confirm the success of MTX in the previous study. No difference in the number of responses was found between the treatment regimens, and in both groups the number of remissions was very low.

During the years 1963 to 1965, the ALGB conducted a randomized study on the effects of 6-MP versus MTX given intravenously once or twice weekly (14). In ALGB 6308, 74 AML adult patients were randomized among four groups and received: MTX at 40 mg/m² weekly or 20 mg/m² twice weekly, 6-MP at 400 mg/m² weekly or 200 mg/m² twice weekly. Since few toxic side effects were occurring, the doses were increased during the study to 30 mg/m² twice weekly or 80 mg/m² weekly (MTX) and 400 mg/m² twice weekly or 800 mg/m² weekly (6-MP). A second study (ALGB 6411) with higher drug doses was started later: 59 AML patients were allocated to 6-MP, 800 or 1,600 mg/m²; MTX, 40 or 60 mg/m². Both drugs were given intravenously twice weekly. Early in this study, severe marrow depression or severe gastrointestinal toxicity or both were noted in most patients receiving the higher dose of either drug.

The high dose levels had therefore to be discontinued, and randomization continued between the lower doses of the two drugs. Only 4 AML patients remitted completely: 3 with 6-MP twice weekly (2 with 800 mg/m² and 1 with 1,600 mg/m²) and 1 with MTX at 40 mg/m². These studies were published in 1972, at a time when a 50% complete remission (CR) rate could be obtained with more recent drugs. The informative value of these older studies is therefore limited to the toxicity data.

A therapeutic trial conducted by the Veterans Administration Cancer Chemotherapy Study Group comparing the effect of 6-MP and 6-chloropurine (6-CP), published in 1963 (66), confirmed the conclusion of an earlier randomized trial from the late 1950s (15). Both drugs were found to be equally effective when survival and the incidence and duration of hematological and clinical remissions were evaluated. Moreover, toxicity of these two antipurines was similar, except for a suggested increase in the incidence of skin rash in the patients receiving 6-CP.

### Evaluation of the Corticosteroids

In 1962, Shanbrom and Miller (50) compared massive doses of adrenocortical hormones (500 mg prednisolone daily) to conventional doses (50 mg daily) on 57 patients, mostly adults, with various types of acute leukemia. As opposed to the acute lymphoblastic cases, none of the 32 ANLL cases gave evidence of hematologic improvement with steroids, regardless of the dosage. Certain adverse effects of massive steroid therapy were brought out by this study. Eleven patients with ANLL seemed to be made worse by massive steroid therapy, as opposed to only two on conventional dosage. The authors concluded that the corticoids may be harmful in ANLL by accelerating hematologic deterioration and increasing the frequency of complications.

Whether or not this conclusion would hold for corticosteroids combined with an effective chemotherapy can, of course, not be ascertained.

The contribution of corticoids to the therapy of adult acute leukemia was further evaluated by two successive trials conducted by the Working Party of the Medical Research Council. The first study (70), allocating 86 acute myeloblastic leukemia (AML) patients to three treatment regimens—6-MP used either alone or in conjunction with prednisone, low dose (40 mg/day) or high dose (250 mg/day)—confirmed the deleterious effect of high-dose corticoids on survival. In the second study (71), the "high-dose" steroid regimen was omitted, the two other regimens were retained, and a further regimen was instituted in which prednisone alone was administered at a daily dose of 40 mg to allow the comparison of 6-MP and steroids, alone or in combination. In the AML cases, with regard to survival, both steroids alone and mercaptopurine alone were significantly superior to the combination of the two. The unexpected relatively good results with steroids alone can be explained by the subsequent use of antimetabolites after the first 8 weeks of treatment required by the protocol. It should be noted, however, that, unlike the experience of Shanbrom and Miller, of the 39 AML patients, 6 remitted after receiving only steroid therapy.

### Evaluation of Two Dosages of a Four-Drug Regimen

In 1965, the introduction of the four-drug VAMP regimen (29,54) caused the first substantial increase in remission rate and survival in ANLL, but at the price of a relatively high medullotoxicity: Bacterial sepsis was observed in

36% of patients so treated. A comparative trial was designed by Henderson and Serpick (26) in order to establish the value of (a) prophylactic oral antibiotic treatment, and (b) two dose regimens of the chemotherapeutic agents. Eighty patients with AL (66 ANLL and 14 ALL) were randomized separately to high-dose or low-dose 5-day regimens (MTX, 7.5 or 5.0 mg/m²/day; prednisolone, 1,000 or 150 mg/m²/day; vincristine, 2 mg/m² on day 1; and 6-MP, 500 mg/m²/day. Another randomization separated a group treated prophylactically with nonabsorbable oral antibiotics and a control group. The oral antibiotics were neomycin and paromomycin given on alternate weeks at a daily dose of 0.5 g, plus nystatin, 250,000 I.U. throughout. Complete remissions were achieved in 15 of 66 AML patients. Neither prophylactic oral antibiotics (presumably less than optimal by their antimicrobial spectrum and their mode of administration) nor higher doses of prednisolone and methotrexate changed either remission rates or mortality.

In conclusion, all these studies have, evidently, lost most of their interest since the introduction of new drugs and combinations much more effective on the disease than the few antimetabolites and the corticoids available at that time. The few successes obtained then generally do not show any significant differences among the compared treatment schedules. However, they remain extremely valid, not only because their conclusions pointed to some important information (such as the toxicity of massive dosage of corticosteroids) but essentially because they inaugurated a new methodology whereby an effort was made to realize two patient groups as comparable as possible; this was obtained by the use of strict selection and response criteria, and by random allocation of each drug regimen to groups of patients stratified according to the known prognostic factors.

## Cytosine Arabinoside Alone and in Combinations

### Evaluation of Different Modes of Administration of ara-C

In the mid-1960s, a new drug, arabinosyl cytosine (ara-C), a synthetic pyrimidine nucleoside, proved its efficacy on human acute leukemia. As the effectiveness and toxicity of ara-C in leukemic mice varied with the schedule of drug administration (30), the Acute Leukemia Group B initiated two studies (ALB 6503 and ALB 6606) comparing different administration modalities of the drug (12). In ALB 6503, leukemic adult patients in relapse were randomized between two daily doses, 10 mg/m²/day and 30 mg/m²/day, until remission or hypoplastic marrow resulted. It was intended that all patients be treated with continuous infusion for 24 hr a day, but 54% of them received the drug during a 12-hr period because of problems in hospitalizing a large number of patients. As the study proceeded, one of the two initial drug doses, 10 mg/m², was discontinued. Once marrow response occurred and hypocellularity cleared, patients entered the maintenance phase. At first they were randomized into two groups, one receiving no drug and one receiving 30 mg/m$^2$ of ara-C weekly subcutaneously (s.c.). When the use of maintenance drug was shown to be effective (30 weeks median remission duration compared with 5 weeks remission duration in the unmaintained group), the randomization was changed to 30 mg/m$^2$ s.c. once weekly versus twice weekly for maintenance. Table 1 shows the complete remission rates in 98 evaluable AML patients. It must be emphasized that patients were not randomly allocated to the 12- or 24-hr schedule and that the 10-mg/m$^2$/day schedules were discontinued prematurely. Significant, however, is the fact that three times as many days of i.v. infusion were necessary at the lower daily dose to produce an equal drug effect. The twice-weekly maintenance schedule gave poor results (9 weeks median duration of remission), but only 5 patients were entered on this dose.

In the ALB 6606 study, initially patients were randomized between doses of 30 mg/m$^2$/day given over a 1-hr period and the same dose given over a 4-hr period. When it was found that the 1-hr dose was relatively less active in depressing the bone marrow, the randomization was changed to allow for three groups receiving 50 or 100 mg/m$^2$/day in 1 hr or 30 mg/m$^2$/day over 4 hr. Table 1 shows the complete response rate for each subgroup in 82 evaluable AML patients. The maintenance course was randomly assigned to 23 patients (complete and partial responders, different cytological types of acute leukemia); 13 received twice weekly subcutaneous ara-C and 10 received intensive intravenous treatment, 5 days per month. The median duration of remissions was respectively 11½ weeks for the twice-weekly administration group and 14 weeks for the 5-days-per-month group.

TABLE 1. *Arabinosyl cytosine in ANLL: Comparison of different administration schedules*

| Study group | Infusion time (hr/day) | Daily dose (mg/m$^2$) | Evaluable cases (number) | CR number | Reference |
|---|---|---|---|---|---|
| ALB 6503 | 12 | 10 | 12 | 2 | 12 |
|  |  | 30 | 41 | 10 |  |
|  | 24 | 10 | 9 | 2 |  |
|  |  | 30 | 36 | 2 |  |
| ALB 6606 | 1 | 30 | 16 | 3 | 12 |
|  |  | 50 | 20 | 6 |  |
|  |  | 100 | 20 | 5 |  |
|  | 4 | 30 | 26 | 3 |  |

| | Infusion time (hr/course) | Total dose (mg/m$^2$) | Evaluable cases (number) | CR number (%) | Reference |
|---|---|---|---|---|---|
| SWOG | 48 | 800 | 67 | 16 (24) | 52 |
|  | 120 | 1000 | 70 | 27 (38.5) |  |

In conclusion, these two studies, published in 1968, provided interesting information, confirming ara-C as a valuable drug in all types of acute adult leukemia, but it must be deplored that because of some methodological shortcomings, the main goal of these studies, determination of an optimal administration schedule for the drug, was not reached. As a matter of fact, the different treatment groups were probably not comparable because of lack of stratification according to well-known prognostic criteria such as cytological type, and also, some branches of the randomization were given up before they were statistically proved inferior.

More substantial conclusions concerning optimal ara-C administration schedule can be obtained from the study carried out by the adult section of the Southwest Oncology Group (52). One-hundred thirty-seven evaluable adult leukemia patients were randomly assigned to continuous intravenous injection of 800 mg/m$^2$ of ara-C over a period of 48 hr or continuous intravenous infusion of 1,000 mg/m$^2$ over a period of 120 hr. Courses were given at 14-day intervals. Total dose per course was adjusted upward or downward by 25% if so indicated by effects of the previous course. When remission was obtained, the same schedule of ara-C was continued, with total dose per course adjusted to achieve maximum cytopenia compatible with patient safety and welfare. The 120-hr schedule proved substantially more effective in inducing remissions (38% CR) than the shorter 48-hr schedule (24% CR). Although the total dose per course was somewhat larger with the 120-hr schedule, this did not appear to account for the difference in response rates, since dosage increment in the 48-hr schedule carried the dose per course to more than that required in the 120-hr schedule. The median length of remission in both groups was comparable: 62 weeks for patients receiving the 48-hr treatment and 51 weeks for patients on the 120-hr schedule ($p > 0.8$).

Another very important piece of information provided by that study concerns the duration of the remissions: 23% of patients who remitted completely had remissions lasting more than 2 years.

### Comparison Between ara-C Alone and in Combinations

Cytosine arabinoside alone substantially prolongs the life of mice with far-advanced L1210 leukemia, but it is curative only against early disease. However, the drug is synergistic with other antitumor agents and, when used in combination, it proved curative against far-advanced L1210 leukemia. These observations led to investigations of ara-C in combination with other antitumor agents in adults with acute leukemia.

The combination of ara-C and thioguanine (TG) proved highly efficient in a nonrandomized study published in 1969 by Gee, Yu, and Clarkson (23). In order to evaluate the superiority of combination therapy above monotherapy with ara-C, the ALGB (6) allocated randomly 275 unselected patients to receive treatment with ara-C (100 mg/m$^2$/day in a 1-hr drip) alone or combined with thioguanine (2.5 mg/kg oral), mercaptopurine (2.5 mg/kg oral), or daunorubicin (DRB, 45 mg/m$^2$ on days 1 and 2 and repeated on days 10 and 11 if tolerated). Complete remission and partial remission rates for 227 evaluable cases were ara-C, 16.7%; ara-C + TG, 50.0%; ara-C + MP, 32.2%; ara-C + DRB, 36%. In terms of remission induction potency, combination therapy was significantly better than ara-C alone ($p < 0.01$). Ara C + TG was significantly better than ara-C ($p < 0.01$) and ara-C + MP ($p < 0.05$). Ara-C + DRB was significantly better than ara-C ($p < 0.05$), but ara-C + MP was not better than ara-C ($p < 0.20$), nor was ara-C + TG better than ara-C + DRB ($p < 0.20$). In this study, the best induction regimens appeared to be ara-C + TG or ara-C + DRB (Table 2).

The combination of ara-C plus cyclophosphamide produced complete remissions in 40% of patients with a median duration of 5½ months (5). Vincristine sulfate and prednisone were then added to the regimen (COAP). The complete remission rate with the COAP regimen was similar to that obtained with ara-C plus cyclophosphamide, but the median duration of remission was about 11 months (64). Since the apparent superiority of the COAP regimen above ara-C alone might have been due to independent factors such as advances in suppor-

TABLE 2. *Arabinosyl cytosine in ANLL: Alone and in combinations*

| Drug regimens | Patients (number) | Remission (%) | Significance (p) | Reference |
|---|---|---|---|---|
| ara-C | | 16.7[b] | <0.01  <0.01 | |
| ara-C + TG | 275 | 50.0[b] | <0.05 | 6 |
| ara-C + MP | | 32.2[b] | <0.20 | |
| ara-C + DRB | | 36.0[b] | | |
| ara-C | 51 | 31(16)[a] | 0.18 | 4 |
| COAP | 57 | 45(26)[a] | | |
| ara-C | 61 | 11(7)[a] | NS | 53 |
| COAP | 40 | 15(6)[a] | | |
| ara-C | 55 | 16(9)[a] | | |
| ara-C + TG | 53 | 15(8)[a] | NS | 31 |
| ara-C + DRB | 55 | 21(12)[a] | | |
| ara-C | 48 | 25(12)[a] | | |
| ara-C + TG | 70 | 30(21)[a] | NS | 32 |
| ara-C + DRB | 61 | 31(19)[a] | | |

[a] Complete remissions.
[b] Complete + partial remissions.
NS = not significant.

tive care methods, the SWOG initiated a comparative study of the two treatments
(4). One-hundred eight AML patients were randomly allocated to receive ara-
C alone, 200 mg/m$^2$/day for 5 days (rapid i.v. injections every 8 hr), or the
COAP regimen; vincristine, 2 mg i.v. on day 1 of each course, prednisone (25
mg orally 4 times daily for 5 days), ara-C (100 mg/m$^2$ for 5 days), and cyclophosphamide (100 mg/m$^2$/day for 5 days). Both ara-C and cyclophosphamide were
administered by rapid intravenous injection in divided doses every 8 hr. Patients
in complete remission received three additional courses given at 2- to 3-week
intervals as consolidation therapy, followed by a remission maintenance therapy
at approximately 3- to 4-week intervals until recurrence of the disease. Of the
57 AML patients who received the COAP regimen, 26 achieved complete remission (45%), compared to 16 of the 51 patients (31%) on ara-C alone (Table
2). The median duration of complete remission was 62 weeks for the 26 AML
and 6 ALL patients receiving the COAP regimen and 46 weeks for 16 AML
and 2 ALL patients receiving ara-C alone. The median duration of survival
for all patients entered on therapy was 35 weeks for the COAP regimen and
8 weeks for cytarabine alone. This study assessed definitely the value of the
COAP regimen in the treatment of acute leukemia in adults and its superiority
over ara-C alone, at least at the administration schedules used.

This superiority was not confirmed by an ALGB study reported in 1975 by
Stoutenborough and Meyers (53). From 61 previously untreated ANLL treated
by ara-C, 7 achieved CR (11%), compared to 6 treated by COAP (15%). The
remission rate was surprisingly low in this study, but unfortunately we lack
any detailed information to explain the discrepancies with the previous study:
The abstract does not mention the exact drug schedules or the patient selection
criteria, or even if the allocation to treatment regimens was randomized.

The Leukaemia and Hematosarcoma Cooperative Group of the European
Organization for Research on the Treatment of Cancer (E.O.R.T.C.) compared
the CR inductive effect of ara-C (75 to 100 mg/m$^2$ daily, day 1 to 4, one-fifth
of the dose given i.v. and four-fifths by perfusion for 4 hr), ara-C at the same
dose from day 2 to day 5 combined with TG (75 to 100 mg/m$^2$ daily, day 1
to day 5, orally) and ara-C combined with daunorubicin (60 mg/m$^2$ day 1
only, i.v.) on 163 evaluable patients with AML (31). In 29 patients who achieved
CR, a comparison of maintenance treatment using methylglyoxal-bisguanyl-hy-
drazone (MGGH) · 200 mg/m$^2$ weekly i.v. or ara-C 120 mg/m$^2$ weekly s.c.
was made (31). The rates of CR of 16% for ara-C alone, 15% for ara-C and
TG, and 21% for ara-C and DRB are low and not significantly different. Moreover, there was no difference in the duration of remission and survival whatever
the remission induction chemotherapy and whatever the maintenance
chemotherapy.

Since the rate of remissions was very low, a second trial was initiated by
the same group (32) where the modalities of administration of ara-C were those
applied by Clarkson, Dowling, Gee, and Burchenal (7). One-hundred seventy-
nine evaluable AML patients were allocated to ara-C alone (100 mg/m$^2$ iv.

every 12 hr for 7 to 10 days), ara-C plus TG (80 mg/m² every 12 hr for 7 to 10 days, first dose given 6 hr before ara-C), or ara-C plus DRB (60 mg/m² i.v., day 1). The maintenance regimens compared were the same as in the previous trial. Table 2 shows the rates of CR, ranging from 25% with ara-C to 31% with ara-C + DRB and 30% with ara-C + TG. Here again they are not significantly different. If the remission rates seem still rather low, it must be emphasized that, unlike the ALGB trial comparing the same drug combinations (although administered differently), only the CRs are registered here. Moreover, analysis of the results by center revealed much higher CR rates in centers with "intensive hematological care facilities," reaching nearly twice the remission rate of the other centers, that is, 45.5% compared to 25.5%.

As in the previous E.O.R.T.C. trial, the actuarial curves of duration of CR did not show any significant difference between the two maintenance treatments or the induction treatments, the median duration of the first remission being between 8 and 10 months.

In conclusion, the results of these two E.O.R.T.C. trials did not confirm the superiority of ara-C + TG or ara-C + DRB over ara-C alone as remission induction regimens, found in the previous described ALGB study.

## Daunorubicine Alone and in Combinations

In the late 1960s, the value of daunorubicin (DRB) as induction treatment of AML seemed well assessed. Reviewing data on 1,299 patients with acute leukemia treated in the United States and on their own patients with DRB, Bernard et al. concluded that DRB induces a higher complete remission rate than any other drug (3).

The optimal way to administer it was the question of two successive ALGB trials: ALGB protocols 6706 and 6706 A (62). Both studies included all AML patients, regardless of age, prior treatment (except for DRB), and clinical status. In protocol 6706, 124 evaluable patients were allocated at random to receive

TABLE 3. *Daunorubicin in ANLL: Different administration schedules*

| Drug regimens | Number patients | Complete remissions number (%) | Significance (p) | Reference |
|---|---|---|---|---|
| DRB: 60 mg/m²/day × 3 | 44 | 13 | 29 ⎤ | | |
| DRB: 60 mg/m²/day × 5 | 49 | 8 | 16 ⎥ NS | 62 |
| DRB: 60 mg/m²/day × 7 | 31 | 7 | 22 ⎦ | |
| DRB: 60 mg/m²/day × 5 | 61 | 21 | 34 ⎤ 0.14 ⎤ | |
| DRB: 60 mg/m²/week × 2 | 62 | 13 | 20 ⎥ ⎥ 0.02 | 62 |
| DRB: 60 mg/m²/week | 75 | 12 | 16 ⎦ 0.59 ⎦ | |

NS = not significant.

60 mg/m²/day for 3, 5, or 7 consecutive days (Table 3). A difference, although not significant, was noted between the 3-day regimen (29% CR rate) and the 5-day (16% CR) or 7-day (22% CR) regimens.

In protocol 6706 A, 198 evaluable patients received randomly the 5-day regimen or biweekly or weekly DRB injections. Consecutive doses induced more remissions than treatment given on an intermittent schedule, the respective rates of CRs being 34% for 5 daily doses, 20% for semiweekly doses, and 16% for weekly doses. The 5-day courses revealed significantly more activity than weekly administration, but there was no significant difference in survival according to regimen. The maintenance regimens tested did not show any significant difference: In both protocols, median survival from the onset of therapy was 44 weeks for patients in CR and maintained either with ara-C and methyl-guanyl-hydrazone (MGGH) or with 6-MP and MTX.

The results of these two protocols are a patent illustration of the importance of a well-controlled study: In both trials, the investigators were the same, patient characteristics were similar, but in the 5-day consecutive DRB regimen, the percent CR in the first trial was 16% and 34% in the second one. The median survival was 7 weeks in the first study and 16 weeks in the second. This probably reflects increased skill in the use of the drug since, with an equal frequency of leukopenia below $1,000/\mu l$ in both studies, fatal marrow aplasia was less in the second protocol.

The question remained open of whether, in terms of remission induction rates, DRB alone did better than the available combination regimens (Table 4). An answer was furnished to this question by a randomized study conducted by Wiernik and Serpick (69). Forty-three consecutive previously untreated and

TABLE 4. *Daunorubicin in ANLL alone and in combinations*

| Drug regimens | Number patients | Percent remissions[a] | Significance | Reference |
|---|---|---|---|---|
| DRB | 22 | 50 (11) | NS | 69 |
| POMP | 21 | 28 (6) | | |
| DRB | } 523 | 42 | NS | 67 |
| ara-C + TG | | 44 | | |
| DRB + ara-C + TG | | 49 | | |
| DRB | 33 | 49 (16) | NS | 68 |
| DRB + ara-C + TG Pyrimethamine | 33 | 46 (25) | | |
| ara-C + TG | } 206 | 34.4 | NS | 58 |
| DRB + ara-C + TG | | 38.4 | | |
| ara-C + DRB sequentially | 13 | 46 (6) | NS | 39 |
| DRB + ara-C sequentially | 11 | 55 (6) | | |

[a] Complete remissions.
( ) number patients.
NS = not significant.

unselected patients with ANLL were assigned to receive DRB or the so-called POMP combination treatment. DRB was given at a dose of 60 mg/m² i.v. daily for 3 consecutive days. If 5 days after the last dose the marrow was hypocellular without blasts, no further therapy was given. On the contrary, in the presence of residual blasts in the marrow, another 3-day DRB course was given. If the patient did not achieve complete remission after 3 courses of DRB, he was considered an induction failure and crossed over to the POMP regimen. The POMP regimen consisted of vincristine, 2 mg/m² i.v. on day 1; 6-MP, 500 mg/m² i.v. from day 1 to day 5; methotrexate, 5 mg/m² i.v. day 1 to 5; and prednisone, 150 mg/m² p.o. day 1 to 5. The combination of drugs was repeated at 10-day intervals until CR was achieved or a maximum of 5 unsuccessful courses had been administered. No consolidation or intensification therapy was given after either regimen, and remissions were unmaintained. Fifty percent (11 of 22) of the patients treated with DRB alone, and 28% (6 of 21) of the patients treated with POMP achieved complete remission. Although not statistically significant, this strong trend in favor of DRB is still reinforced by the fact that patients who remitted with DRB did so in a median of 19 days, whereas the median time to CR with the POMP regimen was 64 days. The authors do not believe that the minor differences between the two groups (more female patients and a 5-years younger median age in the DRB group) could account for the better results obtained with DRB. The duration of unmaintained remission was not different for the two regimens: 9 weeks in the DRB group and 8 weeks in the POMP group. The survival of remitting patients was also comparable in both groups: 12 months for patients treated with DRB and 11 months for those treated with POMP. This trial illustrates a very important point: Even with a treatment so efficient as to induce CR in 50% of patients, the remissions are very short in the absence of maintenance treatment.

Another important question is whether the results obtained by DRB could be further improved when DRB was associated with other drugs. An ALGB trial (67) compared, on 523 previously untreated AML patients, DRB alone, cytosine arabinoside and thioguanine, and a combination of all three drugs. The complete remission rates were 42% with DRB alone (60 mg/m² daily × 3), 44% with ara-C + TG (100 mg/m² q. 12 hr each until marrow aplasia), and 49% with DRB + ara-C + TG (DRB, 100 mg/m² day 1; ara-C and TG, 100 mg/m² q. 12 hr for 5 days). Remission was maintained with monthly cyclophosphamide and hydroxyurea followed by 7 days of mercaptopurine or thioguanine or half-doses of both. All patients who remitted completely had a median survival of 14+ months. At time of evaluation, the authors concluded that the triple combination treatment might be superior for remission induction in AML. However, this was not definitely proven, since the differences in CR achieved were not statistically significant.

The results of another trial published in 1976 by Wiernik et al. (68), comparing DRB alone with a multiple-drug combination therapy including DRB, confirm the similarity of both regimens for inducing CR. Sixty-six newly diagnosed, unselected, and consecutive ANLL patients were randomly allocated to DRB alone (60 mg/m² daily × 3 i.v.) or DRB (75 mg/m² day 1, i.v.) plus ara-C (75 mg/m² q. 12 hr, days 1 to 5, i.v.), 6-TG (75 mg/m², 12 hr, days 1 to 5, orally), and pyrimethamine (1 mg/kg, days 1 to 5, orally). Patients who achieved CR were treated with two half-dose courses of the successful remission-induction regimen, as consolidation treatment. After the hematologic recovery from that phase, all patients in CR received three monthly courses of cyclophosphamide (1 g/m² in push injection) followed 18 hr later by a 24-hr infusion of 25 g/m² of guanazole. Moreover, the patients in the combination induction-therapy group were given pyrimethamine (2 mg/kg) as a single oral dose given weekly until systemic and/ or central nervous system relapse. Of the patients on single-agent induction therapy, 49% (16 of 33) achieved a CR after a median of 28.5 days. The 46% CRs (15 of 33) with multiple-agent therapy were obtained after a median of 40 days. Median durations of remission for both induction-treatment groups were similar (6.8 and 5.6 months), but the median duration of survival for all treated patients was superior in the single-agent therapy group: 11.6 months versus 5.2 months in the combination therapy group ($p < 0.05$). The incidence of meningeal leukemia was similar in the two groups of patients, a fact that argues against the value of pyrimethamine in the prophylaxis of this complication. Thus, DRB alone proved not inferior to the four-drug combination regimen. On the contrary, the time to CR was less with the single-agent regimen, it was less costly from a platelet transfusion standpoint, and the overall survival time was superior.

Another way to pose the previous question is whether or not the addition of DRB to a drug combination improves the remission rate obtained by the latter. Vogler, Chan, and Kremer (59) reported a trial from the Southeastern Cancer Study group where previously untreated adults with AML were randomized to ara-C (100 mg/m² i.v. push) plus 6-TG (100 mg/m² p.o.) every 12 hr for 10 doses or the same schedule plus DRB (10 mg/m² every 24 hr for 10 doses). Of 51 evaluable patients on the double therapy, 14 achieved a complete remission (27.5%) in a median time of 54 days. Of 55 patients on the triple therapy, 17 achieved a complete remission (31%) in a median time of 37 days. Deaths during the first 6 weeks were 20 with the double combination and 19 with the triple combination. The differences in remission rates are not statistically significant, but the results suggest that the triple therapy produces remissions in a shorter period of time than the double therapy without increased mortality. With increasing numbers of patients entered in this study, the remission rates remained similar (58): From 206 randomized patients, 34. 4% achieved complete remission with ara-C + TG and 38.4% with the triple combination therapy (Table 4).

In an effort to determine the optimal way to combine DRB and ara-C, the two most active agents in AML, Omura (39) tested a clinical application of a mouse model where the leukemic cell kill was greatest when ara-C was given first, less than additive when the two drugs were given simultaneously, and not effective when DRB was given first (11). Patients were sequentially selected without the selected deletion of any patient from the study. Two schedules of DRB and ara-C were compared in the AD sequence, a 5-day continuous infusion of ara-C (100 mg/m$^2$/day) followed 24 or 48 hr later with DRB (100 mg/ m$^2$) i.v. In the DA sequence, DRB (100 mg/m$^2$ i.v.) was followed immediately by a 5-day continuous infusion of ara-C. Six of 13 patients (46%) receiving the AD sequence achieved CR. They required a median dose of 250 mg/m$^2$ DRB and a median time of 45 days to remit completely. Of the 11 patients on DA sequence, there were 6 CRs (55%) obtained with a median dose DRB of 150 mg/m$^2$ in a median time of 33 days. Although this study shows a trend in favor of the DA sequence (in contrast with the results of the mouse model), none of the differences observed were statistically significant.

In conclusion, when considering the CR rates obtained, few differences were observed in the randomized trials comparing DRB alone to the best combination regimens available or in those comparing these combinations to the same where DRB was added. Some of these studies may be criticized for their low numbers of patients, making the demonstration of a significant difference between the regimens compared highly improbable (69,39). From the trials where the number of patients included are high, one may conclude that the regimens evaluated are probably equally active. In these cases, in the absence of a difference in maintenance duration, the best attitude could be to use either DRB in monotherapy, or the combination regimen without DRB, to save the other alternative for further reinduction treatments or eventually remission consolidation therapy courses.

### Remission Induction: Comparison of Different Combination Regimens

Whereas some investigators questioned the value of monotherapy in comparison with multiple-drug induction regimens, others, impressed by the good results of some combinations (23,64), considered that the next objective was to determine which of the combinations could produce the highest remission induction rates.

#### Comparison of Different Dosages of the Same Drugs

ALGB protocol 7021, comparing ara-C and thioguanine at 100 mg/m$^2$/day with the same drugs at 50 mg/m$^2$, showed a higher remission induction rate with the "full" dose scheme. Here again no complete published data are available (15).

Another ALGB study illustrated clearly the influence on the remission induction rate of drug dosages (45). They compared a high-dose therapy schedule of the two most effective drugs available with a somewhat less intensive regimen of the same drugs in a randomized study of AML patients under 60 years. In the "heavy" regimen, ara-C, 100 mg/m$^2$, either by continuous infusion daily or by rapid i.v. injection every 12 hr, was given from day 1 to day 7, with

DRB, 45 mg/m² i.v., daily from day 1 to 3. In the "light" regimen, the drugs were given at the same dosage but ara-C for 5 days and DRB for 2 days only. Forty-three patients were evaluable in each schedule: 77% achieved remission with the 7–3 regimen and 53% with the 5–2 regimen ($p < 0.05$). Unfortunately, the abstract report does not mention the proportion of complete and partial remissions (Table 5).

A study of the Western Cancer Study Group compared two schemas of administration of ara-C and 6-TG. In regimen A, 100 mg/m² of ara-C i.v. and 80 mg/m² of 6-TG p.o. were administered every 12 hr until marrow cellularity was reduced by at least 50%. In regimen B the same drug dosages were administered every 12 hr for 5 days with 5 to 7 day rest intervals between courses. The consolidation regimen consisted of three additional courses of ara-C and 6-TG administered in an identical fashion to the initial induction regimens. Fifteen of 39 (38%) patients on regimen A and 18 of 42 (43%) on regimen B achieved remission (CR + PR). None of both regimens appeared superior: The overall response rate was similar, regimen B proved easier to administer but required greater support.

TABLE 5. *Comparison of different induction regimens in ANLL*

| Drug regimens | Number patients | Percent complete remissions | Significance | Reference |
|---|---|---|---|---|
| ara-C (7) + DRB (3) | 43 | 77 [b] | <0.05 | 45 |
| ara-C (5) + DRB (2) | 43 | 53 [b] | | |
| ara-C + TG (variable duration) | 39 | 38 (15) [b] | NS | 34 |
| ara-C + TG (fixed duration) | 42 | 43 (18) [b] | NS | 34 |
| ara-C + TG | 58 | 30 (17) | NS | 51 |
| Endoxan + ara-C + MTX | 55 | 33 (18) | | |
| TAD | 61 | 49 (30) | <0.05 | 38 |
| AVML | 44 | 27 (12) | | |
| AD + ara-C (seq) <br> AD + ara-C (sim) <br> + prednisone + vincristine | 117 } [a] | 60 (70) } | NS | 35 |
| POMP | 17 | 59 (11) | NS | 36 |
| COAP | 25 [a] | 54 (13) | | |
| ara-C + TG <br> VAMP | 90 } | 46 [b] <br> 29 [b] | NS | 8 |
| ara-C + TG | 69 | 23 (16) | NS | 61 |
| ara-C + CCNU | 60 | 30 (18) | | |
| TAD | 122 | 48 (58) | NS | 54 |
| ara-C (7) + DRB (3) | 52 | 60 (31) | | |

[a] All adult acute leukemia.
[b] Complete and partial remissions.

( ) Number patients.
NS = not significant.

*Comparison of Combinations Empirically Proved Efficient with Combinations
Based on Theoretical Considerations (45)*

The Southern Cooperative Oncology Group (51) analyzed 113 cases of adults
with ANLL treated with ara-C, 100 mg/m$^2$ i.v. q. 12 hr, plus TG, 100 mg/
m$^2$ p.o. q. 12 hr (AT regimen), or with cyclophosphamide, 1.5 g/m$^2$, ara-C,
300 mg/m$^2$, and methotrexate, 80 mg/m$^2$, administered i.v. every 7 days (CAM
regimen). The CAM regimen had the theoretical advantage of combining cell
cycle-nonspecific and cell cycle-specific agents. On the AT regimen, 17 of 58
patients achieved complete remissions and 18 of 55 did so on the CAM regimen.
Median duration of response for CAM and AT were 26 and 25 weeks, respectively. The authors conclude equivalent activity of both regimens, with the advantage of CAM being administered weekly.

Another study was designed by the same group to compare randomly a synchronizing-recruiting therapy (AVML) with a myelotoxic therapy (TAD) in
acute myelogenous adult leukemia (38) The AVML therapy consisted of ara-
C, 100 mg/m$^2$ push i.v. daily (X3), followed by vincristine, 1 mg/m$^2$, and
methotrexate, 50 mg/m$^2$ p.o. q. 6 hr (X4), followed by leucovorin, 5 mg p.o.
q. 6 hr (X9–15). The TAD schedule consisted of ara-C, 100 mg/m$^2$ push i.v.
q. 12 hr (X10), plus thioguanine, 100 mg/m$^2$ p.o. q. 12 hr (X10), plus daunorubicin, 10 mg/m$^2$ i.v. q. 24 hr (X5). With AVML, 12 of 44 (27%) and with
TAD, 30 of 61 (49%) evaluable cases achieved CR. On crossover from AVML
to TAD, 5 of 15 and from TAD to AVML, 0 of 3 patients achieved CR. In
this trial, the AVML schedule based on theoretical ground appeared significantly
less active as an induction regimen than the empirically established TAD
schedule.

In the same sense, the clinical applicability of an animal model has been
tested by the Southwest Oncology Group in a very interestingly elaborated
protocol (35). All adult previously untreated acute leukemia patients were eligible
for the study. Two groups of patients, probably with different prognosis, were
considered separately according to their initial peripheral blood count. If they
had <30,000/cmm circulating blast cells they received initially weekly vincristine, 2 mg/m$^2$ i.v., and daily prednisone, 100 mg p.o. If there was no response
after 10 days, they were randomized to receive adriamycine (AD) and ara-C
either sequentially (SEQ) or simultaneously (SIM): AD at 40 mg/m$^2$ was given
to all patients at day 1, ara-C, 100 mg/m$^2$/day, in continuous infusion from
day 4 to day 9 (SEQ) or from day 1 to 5 (SIM). Patients achieving a CR
with vincristine and prednisone were also randomized to SEQ or SIM for consolidation. In a preliminary analysis of 117 patients, 82 patients received initially
vincristine and prednisone, and 19 of them (23%) achieved a CR. Of the failures,
27 responded to SIM or SEQ. Patients with >30,000/cmm peripheral blood
cells were given randomly SIM or SEQ on diagnosis and vincristine plus prednisone was added. Twenty-two of 35 (63%) achieved a CR. In conclusion, this
program, very effective for the remission induction of AAL with a CR rate of

60% (70 of 117), showed no difference in response rate between SIM or SEQ in any group.

### Comparison of Different Regimens Empirically Proved of Value

McCredie et al. (36) compared two four-drug combinations, both including vincristine and prednisone associated with either methotrexate and 6-mercaptopurine (POMP) or cytosine arabinoside and cyclophosphamide (COAP). Forty-two previously untreated patients with acute adult leukemia, both nonlymphoid and lymphoid types, were randomized to POMP or COAP therapy. With POMP, 11 of 17 (59%) and with COAP 13 of 25 patients (54%) achieved complete remission. Both regimens proved very effective for remission induction in these patients. The surprisingly high remission rate with POMP is probably explanable by the efficacy of this combination on the ALL patients included in this study (47).

The abstract published in 1973 by Crowell et al. (8) comparing ara-C and thioguanine with vincristine, amethopterin, 6-MP, and prednisone (VAMP) could not show any significant difference in the remission induction rate or the survival time of adult acute leukemia. There was, however, a trend in favor of the ara-C plus 6-TG combination (Table 5).

ALGB protocol 7121 was designed to compare the induction and maintenance effectiveness in AML of ara-C plus CCNU with ara-C plus TG which revealed the most effective combination in one of their previous trials (61). One-hundred twenty-nine evaluable patients received by random allocation ara-C, 100 mg/ $m^2$/day by continuous infusion for 5 days, plus either CCNU, 100 mg/$m^2$ orally on day 1 of the first cycle, or TG, 100 mg/$m^2$ orally every 12 hr for 5 days. Patients achieving complete or partial remissions were placed on maintenance by monthly repeating courses of the drugs that produced the remission. CCNU was given every other cycle because of delayed myelosuppression. From 69 patients in the ara-C + 6-TG group, 16 remitted completely (23%) and another 15 partially. From 60 patients on the ara-C + CCNU regimen, 18 achieved a complete remission (30%) and 5 a partial remission. The median duration of remission for the ara-C + 6-TG patients was 18 weeks and for the ara-C plus CCNU patients 40 weeks ($p < 0.05$). This trial confirms the value of CCNU combined with ara-C as remission induction treatment of AML and points to the superiority of this combination above ara-C + 6-TG as maintenance treatment.

ALBG study 7122 compared 5-day courses of continuous infusions of ara-C combined with cyclophosphamide to the same with DRB. Details of this study are not published but some data are mentioned in a review by Ellison et al. in 1973 (16). The remission induction rate with the DRB combination seems higher than with the cyclophosphamide combination.

The Southeastern Cancer Study Group randomized in a ratio of 1:2 the TAD (see above) combination proved efficient in a previous trial (38) with the association of ara-C and DRB at the most efficient dosages of the previously reported ALGB study (45). The CR rates were 58 of 122 (48%) on TAD and 31 of 52 (60%) on ara-C + DRB. This difference was not significant. The randomized evaluation of chemotherapy versus BCG immunotherapy versus no further therapy on these remitting patients will be reported later.

In summary, from these comparisons it seems that the type and the number of drugs that are combined do not necessarily modify greatly the results in terms of percent CRs. On the other hand, the study showing the superiority of the 7–3 days over the 5–2 days ara-C plus DRB indicate that small modifications of the administration schedule and dosage can greatly modify the results. Finally, the comparison ARA-C + CCNU versus ARA-C + TG indicates that similar results in the quantity of CR obtained do not inform us of the quality of these CRs.

### Reinduction Treatment in ANLL in Relapse

Few studies deal with systematic treatment of AML in relapse and most of them are uncontrolled. Levi and Wiernik (33) reported a trial where two poorly evaluated "second-choice" agents were compared randomly for reinduction treatment. Eighteen patients were treated with 5-azacytidine at 200 to 250 mg/$m^2$/day $\times$ 5 intravenously, and 6 achieved a remission (5 complete and 1 partial). Among the 12 patients receiving quanazole at 25 to 30 g/$m^2$/day $\times$ 5 by continuous i.v. infusion, only 1 partial remission was obtained. The authors' conclusions were that 5-aza-acytidine had significant activity in adults with ANLL, even in patients heavily treated before and resistant to previous therapies including ara-C, whereas guanazole lacked significant value in these conditions.

### MAINTENANCE THERAPY IN ANLL

Except for the trials on immunotherapy which will be analyzed separately, very few controlled studies have been conducted in which different modalities of remission maintenance were compared after a uniform standardized induction treatment. Most often, the compared groups vary not only by maintenance but also by induction treatments. The remission durations were mentioned previously in the analysis of the different comparative trials. Generally, in such studies, the maintenance regimens compared do not show any significant difference, except for the 40-weeks median remission duration obtained and maintained by ara-C plus CCNU which is significantly longer than the 18 weeks of remission obtained and maintained by ara-C plus TG ($p < 0.05$) (61).

Three important points must be outlined, however:

1. No randomized trial on a sufficiently large number of patients is available to assess definitely the necessity of maintenance chemotherapy in ANLL. The data from ALGB study 6503 (12) with a median remission of 30 weeks in the ara-C-maintained group compared to 5 weeks in the unmaintained group, al-

though very suggestive, remain unconclusive: The number of patients in each branch are not mentioned, nor are we informed if the remissions considered are all complete. If not, the complete and partial remissions could have been distributed very unequally in each group.

A more suggestive study is a very recent report by Embury et al. (17) on a relatively small number of patients. Twenty-six adult AML patients brought into CR by DRB + ara-C + 6-TG and thereafter consolidated by 2 days ara-C + 6-TG were randomly assigned to receive monthly maintenance chemotherapy or no further treatment. The maintenance courses were identical to the consolidation course, consisting of four 75-mg/m² ara-C infusions (over 4 hr) given every 12 hr and two oral doses of 2.5 mg/kg TG given every 24 hr. The 10.3 months median remission length of the maintained group is significantly longer than the 6.7 months of the unmaintained one ($p < 0.05$).Unfortunately, because of protocol violations, 5 patients in the unmaintained group did not receive any consolidation chemotherapy.

Nevertheless, comparison of the consolidated patients in the maintained (13) and nonmaintained (8) groups indicated that the maintained group still had a significantly longer duration of remission ($p < 0.04$). In spite of the important information given by this trial, the few numbers of patients studied and, mainly, the fact that the efficacy of maintenance therapy was not reflected by increased survival, leave question partly unresolved.

Nevertheless, a general view of the literature argues strongly in favor of maintenance chemotherapy. First, median remission durations of more than a few weeks were observed only when maintenance treatments were applied. Second, even a very effective induction treatment, allowing a 50% CR rate, when not maintained gave only short remissions: 9 weeks median (68).

2. The benefit of consolidation treatment instead of, or in adjunction to, maintenance treatment has not been evaluated by randomized studies. After consolidation treatment (3 courses of ara-C 100 mg/m²/24 hr ×5 plus TG 100 mg/m²/24 hr × 5 + DRB 10 mg/m²/24 hr × 5), the Southeastern Cancer Study Group (40) could not show any difference in the remission durations of 54 patients randomly allocated to either BCNU + ara-C (31 weeks), BCG (32 weeks), or no further treatment (26 weeks). The fair results without any maintenance suggest the efficacy of this consolidation treatment. A similar conclusion can also be drawn from the study of Embury et al. (17).

3. Cytosine arabinoside appears an excellent drug in remission maintenance: A significant proportion of long term remission durations (more than 2 years) were registered in three independent studies where ara-C was used as induction and maintenance regimen—the SWOG study comparing ara-C 120 hr and 48 hr (52), the E.O.R.T.C. study comparing ara-C and methyl-gag maintenance (32), and a nonrandomized trial where 5-day continuous i.v. infusions of ara-C were applied for induction and for maintenance treatment (24). These observations can hypothetically lead to the interesting notion of a selected population of leukemic patients specifically very sensitive to ara-C. It should be worth

examining if these patients do not share some peculiar characteristics. The myelotoxicity of the drugs effective in ANLL limit their long-term use at high dosages. It is therefore not surprising that so many investigators were attracted by the first promising results of immunotherapy in the maintenance therapy of ANLL remissions.

## Immunotherapy in ANLL

Since it has been established that tumor-associated antigens exist in human acute leukemia (21) and that at least some of these antigens are the same for any one type of leukemia, the possibility arose of stimulating the patient's immune system to react against his malignant cells. The first clinical trials evaluating different methods of active specific and nonspecific immunotherapy started in the late 1960s by G. Mathé in LAL. Most of the studies concerned acute leukemia in remission since the animal experiments had suggested that immunotherapy is effective only if the number of malignant cells is small.

### Active Specific and Nonspecific Immunotherapy (Table 6)

A British group (9) published in 1973 the first results of randomized clinical trials on the value of active immunotherapy in the remission maintenance of ANLL.

In a first trial, 40 patients were treated by courses of DRB, 55 mg/m$^2$ on day 1, and ara-C, 70 mg/m$^2$/day from day 1 to day 5 (10 of them received in addition L-asparaginase, 30,000 units/m$^2$ daily for a period up to 28 days, without any influence on the remission rate). Twenty-three who achieved a CR were first submitted to a consolidation treatment: One more course of the induction regimen and 4 to 6 weeks of 6-mercaptopurine (70 mg/m$^2$ orally daily) plus MTX (12 mg/m$^2$ orally twice weekly) and then randomized to

TABLE 6. *Specific and nonspecific active immunotherapy on maintenance in ANLL*

| Maintenance | Number patients | Type of immunotherapy | Median survival (mo.) | Significance | Reference |
|---|---|---|---|---|---|
| C | 22 | Glaxo freeze-dried BCG | 9 | 0.003 | 43 |
| C + I | 28 | Allogeneic, irradiated cells | 17 | | |
| C | 14 | Glaxo BCG | 10 | <0.05 | 46 |
| C + I | 16 | Allogeneic, viable cells | 20 | | |
| C | } 71 | Glaxo BCG | No difference | | 41 |
| C + I | | Allogeneic, irradiated cells | | | |
| C | } 23 | C-parvum | Too early | | 55 |
| C + I | | Allogeneic, irradiated cells | | | |

C = chemotherapy.
I = immunotherapy.

receive the same doses of 6-mercaptopurine and MTX as maintenance therapy or only immunotherapy. Nine patients received immunotherapy given in three ways: intradermal BCG alone, autologous leukemic cells alone, or a combination of allogeneic leukemia cells with BCG. These patients had remission lengths similar to the 13 patients receiving 6-MP and MTX maintenance (115 days with immunotherapy and 120 days with chemotherapy). It would be hazardous to conclude from this study that in AML immunotherapy can be as effective as chemotherapy in maintaining a shortly consolidated remission: The numbers of patients in each group are very small, the groups are not homogeneous (induction regimen with or without asparaginase, different modalities of immunotherapy) and, more important, the maintenance regimen to which the immunotherapy has been compared is certainly far from being optimal. Moreover, the length of remission was calculated from the date the first remission marrow was obtained. Since chemotherapy is then performed as consolidation treatment, the median length of immunotherapeutic treatment alone before relapse is even shorter than the 115 days mentioned.

In a second trial, among 22 patients treated by a slightly modified induction regimen, 7 achieved a CR. In a third trial, 32 patients received the same induction treatment as in trial 1. Sixteen remitted completely. The 23 patients in remission after trials 2 and 3 received an additional 5-day consolidation course of DRB and ara-C and then alternating 5-day courses of ara-C with DRB and ara-C with thioguanine at monthly intervals. These patients were divided into two groups at random, one receiving chemotherapy alone and the other receiving immunotherapy in addition to chemotherapy. The immunotherapy consisted of Glaxo-freeze-dried BCG administered by a 20-needle multiple puncture gun and allogeneic irradiated leukemic cells. The cells were given by weekly subcutaneous and intradermal injections, $10^9$ cells being distributed between three limbs and the BCG given in the fourth limb. All chemotherapy was stopped after 1 year of remission, but immunotherapy was continued in the appropriate group.

The preliminary results on the remission durations reported in 1973 were in favor of the combined therapy group. This trend was confirmed in later reports of the study on larger number of patients (42,43) and became really significant if survival duration was considered: a median of 270 days for 22 patients on chemotherapy alone and 510 days for 28 patients on the combined modality ($p = 0.003$). Interestingly, this increase in survival does not correspond only to the prolongation of the first remission but also to the length of survival after the first relapse: 75 days versus 165 days.

A study from the Leukemia Group of Central Sweden (46) showed a significant prolongation of survival duration by the addition to chemotherapy maintenance of weekly immunotherapy with viable allogeneic leukemic cells and BCG. Thirty patients in remission of ANLL were randomized to either chemotherapy maintenance (14 patients) or chemoimmunotherapy maintenance (16 patients). The median survival time in the chemoimmunotherapy group was 20 months, significantly longer ($p < 0.05$) than in the chemotherapy group (10 months). These results and those from the previously cited British group seem convincing in favor of the usefulness of combined chemoimmunotherapy as maintenance treatment of ANLL. Surprisingly, the British Medical Research Council (41), duplicating the original trial published by Crowther, compared randomly the effectiveness of maintenance by chemotherapy alone and the same chemotherapy with immunotherapy using BCG and irradiated blood cells in 71 ANLL in CR, failed to discover any significant benefit of such immunotherapy. Unfortunately, no detailed published data are available allowing an accurate analysis of this study in comparison with the Royal Marsden's one.

C-parvum and irradiated leukemic cells are evaluated as maintenance treatment adjuvants in a very recent trial of the UCLA Acute Leukemia Study Group (55). The first results on a limited number of patients, favor the chemoimmunotherapy group but are still too preliminary.

### Active Nonspecific Immunotherapy

### BCG (Table 7)

A striking benefit of BCG in prolonging chemotherapy-maintained complete remissions in adult AML was suggested by Gutterman et al. (25). However, this study suffers the criticism of not having been strictly controlled. Some of

TABLE 7. *BCG Immunotherapy on maintenance in ANLL*

| Maintenance | Number patients | Type of BCG | Remission (weeks—median) | Survival (weeks—median) | Reference |
|---|---|---|---|---|---|
| R〈 C | 33 | Tice strain | 24.9[a] ⎱ <0.05 | 78.1 ⎱ NS | 56 |
| C+I | 25 | 1X/week(X4) | 13.3 ⎰ | 93.2 ⎰ | |
| R〈 C | 19 | Glaxo, freeze-dried | No difference | Longer with C+I | 65 |
| C+I | 18 | Intravenous | | | |
| R〈 C | 27 | Pasteur, lyophylized | 55 ⎱ NS | 74 ⎱ NS | 27 |
| C+I | 22 | Scarification | 59 ⎰ | 55+ ⎰ | |
| R〈 C | 24 | Pasteur, immuno-BCG | Too early | | 18 |
| C+I | 20 | Multipunctures gun | | | |
| R〈 C | 17 | Tice strain | 31 ⎤ | 48 ⎱ <0.05 | 40 |
| I | 18 | 2X/week(X4)–1X/mo(XII) Tine technique | 32 ⎬ NS | 101 ⎰ | |
| O | 19 | | 26 ⎦ | ? | |

[a] From onset of maintenance therapy.
C = chemotherapy.
I = immunotherapy.

the following randomized studies are providing data in favor of the effectiveness of BCG alone in the prolongation of remission duration or survival in AML.

The Southeastern Cancer Study Group evaluated the effect of a short course of BCG on remission duration and survival in myeloblastic leukemia (58). Two-hundred six patients were randomly allocated to two induction regimens as described above. The 75 patients achieving CR were rerandomized for a consolidation phase consisting of either continuation of the same induction program (with the exception that ara-C and thioguanine were given 24 hr for 5 days and repeated at intervals of 3 weeks) or a new combination consisting of vincristine (1.4 mg/m²), cyclophosphamide (600 mg/m²), and MTX (2.5 mg p.o.) every 6 hr for 12 doses. These courses were repeated every 14 days. Six cycles of consolidation were given to each group. After the consolidation phase, the 41 patients still in remission were rerandomized to receive BCG followed by MTX or MTX alone (30 mg/m² twice weekly by mouth). Tice-strain BCG containing about $3 \times 10^8$ viable organisms was given by 288 puncture sites (72 sites per limb) weekly for 4 weeks. The composition of the two maintenance groups was similar with regard to induction and consolidation schedules. The median duration of remission from onset of remission was 39.4 weeks for the 18 patients in the BCG + MTX group and 26 weeks for the 23 patients in the MTX group ($p = 0.002$). The median duration of remission after consolidation was 20.4 weeks for the BCG + MTX group and 9.7 weeks for the MTX group ($p = 0.001$). More recent reports of the study, with a larger number of patients in each maintenance group, confirm the same advantage in favor of the BCG-treated patients (56,57). The last evaluation of the study (57) shows still a significant difference in the duration of remission from onset of the maintenance phase: 24.9 weeks for the 25 patients in the BCG + MTX group and 13.3 weeks for the 33 patients in the MTX group ($p < 0.05$). However, the differences in survival are no more really significant: 93.2 weeks in the BCG + MTX group and 78.1 weeks in the MTX group ($p < 0.10$). The 4-year survival curves become similar but when analyzed for the first 20 months of the study, a significantly greater proportion ($p < 0.05$) survives in the BCG + MTX group. This last observation suggests a significant beneficial effect on remission duration and survival of a short course of BCG but a fading of this effect with time.

A significant prolongation of survival correlated with an improved ease to obtain second and third remissions was also noted by Whittaker and Slater using intravenous BCG (65). Thirty-seven of 81 AML adult patients in CR after DRB and ara-C induction treatment were randomized to receive maintenance treatment with DRB plus ara-C (19 patients) or the same chemotherapy plus intravenous Glaxo-BCG (18 patients). Side effects of i.v. BCG were not neglectable: pyrexia, myalgia, headaches, anaphylactic reactions. The most important observation of this study is the improved survival with BCG without any benefit on the duration of first remission, the most striking effect of BCG seeming the facilitation of further remission inductions.

The results of a French group comparing in AML, after consolidation treatment, maintenance therapy by 5-day courses of cyclophosphamide, methylglyoxal, vincristine, and ara-C with the same chemotherapy plus weekly BCG (immuno-BCG Pasteur applied by a 20-multipuncture apparatus), the BCG being stopped 2 weeks before the next chemotherapy course, are too preliminary to be conclusive, and the study is still in progress (18).

The benefit of the addition of BCG to chemotherapy as maintenance treatment in AML could not be demonstrated by a randomized trial from the Southwest Oncology Group (27). Induction regimen (OAP) consisted of courses of oncovin (2 mg i.v. day 1), ara-C (100 mg/m$^2$/day continuous infusion from day 1 through day 10), and prednisone (100 mg p.o. days 1 through 5). After 3 consolidation courses of 5-day OAP, patients were randomized to maintenance 5-day OAP with or without BCG (lyophylized Pasteur BCG applied by scarification). CR rate for AML was 51% (81 of 158). The median length of remission for 27 AML patients on OAP was 55 weeks and for the 22 patients receiving BCG + OAP was 59 weeks ($p = 0.34$). For survival, the median duration from randomization was 74 weeks for OAP and 55 + weeks for OAP + BCG ($p = 0.26$).

As opposed to the previous ones, this study showed no advantage in terms of length of remission or survival for AML patients receiving BCG in addition to chemotherapy. It must be emphasized that numerous differences exist among all these studies. Considering only BCG, major differences can be seen in the strain of the microorganism, its viability, its mode of application (multiple punctures or scarification), its schedule of administration, and so on.

The efficacy of BCG maintenance alone is suggested by a very recent study (40) comparing three groups of patients receiving after a consolidation treatment (which is described above) either no further treatment, BCG, or chemotherapy. Tice-strain BCG is applied on all four limbs by the tine technique biweekly X 4, then monthly X 11. Maintenance chemotherapy consists of monthly 50 mg/m$^2$ BCNU and weekly 100 mg/m$^2$ subcutaneous ara-C. There is no difference in median duration of CR: 31 weeks with chemotherapy, 32 weeks with BCG, and 26 weeks without any treatment. However, on actuarial survival plots, the BCG arm is significantly better than BCNU plus ara-C and no further treatment ($p < 0.05$), with a median survival of 101 weeks with BCG and 48 weeks with chemotherapy.

## Methanol-Extractable Residue (MER)

MER has some theoretical advantages over BCG from which it is derived, as originally pointed out by Weiss (63). In contrast to BCG, MER is nonviable, stable, and subject to precise measurement in dose.

ALGB protocol 7521 (10) is comparing induction chemotherapy with ara-C 100 mg/m$^2$/day in a continuous intravenous infusion for 7 days plus DRB 45 mg/m$^2$/24 hr i.v. for 3 days with the same regimen plus MER in a monthly dose of 1.0 mg, divided into 5 intradermal sites. Of the 255 evaluable AML patients, 25% received MER in induction. The early results of this protocol show that the age-standardized CR rate was 54% for the 22 patients receiving chemotherapy plus MER and 56% for the 85 patients receiving only chemotherapy. An interesting observation is that 50% of patients on chemoimmunotherapy achieved CR after just one course of chemotherapy, whereas only 34% of patients who received chemotherapy alone did so. Patients in CR are randomly allocated to one of four maintenance treatments: 5-day courses of ara-C (100 mg/m²/ 12 hr subcutaneously) plus thioguanine (100 mg/m²/12 hr per o.s.) every 4 weeks, or ara-C plus thioguanine alternating with ara-C, vincristine (2 mg i.v.), and dexamethasone (8 mg/m²/day for 5 days), or the same regimens with monthly MER. In the four regimens, the 3rd, 7th, and 11th courses are substituted by ara-C and DRB. The results of maintenance therapy are still preliminary, but they do show trends of differences between chemoimmunotherapy versus chemotherapy alone, and between the different chemotherapy maintenance arms.

## Other Nonspecific Immunostimulants

Very recent studies, still in progress, are exploring the effectiveness of other nonspecific immunostimulant agents in the treatment of AML.

Gee and Clarkson are conducting a randomized trial where a lipopolysaccharide vaccine derived from *Pseudomonas aeruginosa* is added or not to a sequential multi-drug induction protocol (22). The vaccine is given i.m. at escalating twice-weekly doses ranging from 0.1 to 1.0 ml. With the small number of patients on study, no difference in CR rate was noted: 6 of 13 patients achieving remission with the vaccine, and 7 of 16 patients achieving remission with chemotherapy alone.

The Cancer and Leukemia Group B compared the duration of remission of 67 AML patients on maintenance chemotherapy protocol 7421 (37) and 39 patients randomly allocated to receive the same chemotherapy plus a single injection of Poly I:Poly C (300 mg/m² i.v.). The majority of the patients tested showed significant amounts of serum interferon following Poly I:Poly C treatment, but no difference in response duration between the experimental and control groups has been registered so far.

A Swiss group designed a study to assess the effectiveness of viral oncolysate as adjunct to remission maintenance treatment in AML (48). Forty-four patients achieving CR with ara-C and DRB were randomized to either monthly chemotherapy or the same chemotherapy plus viral oncolysate. The viral oncolysate was prepared by infecting allogeneic leukemic myeloblasts with a leukemia-adapted avian myxovirus (influenza A). After an average follow-up period of 13.5 months there was no difference between the two groups with respect to the probabilities of staying in remission and staying alive.

## Active Specific Immunotherapy

Based on experimental data of successful chemoimmunotherapy with vibrio cholerae neuraminidase (VCN)-treated leukemic cells, an ALGB randomized trial is comparing cyclical maintenance chemotherapy every 4 weeks with the same chemotherapy and VCN-treated allogeneic myeloblasts in ANLL patients in CR after ara-C plus DRB induction (2). The first results are showing an unequivocal trend in favor of the combined maintenance therapy so far as the remission duration is concerned.

## Comparison Between Active Specific Immunotherapy and an Association of Active Specific and Nonspecific Immunotherapy

After the first remission induction with ara-C plus DRB, patients with ANLL are allocated to 3 groups: cyclical chemotherapy alone, cyclical chemotherapy plus intradermal injection of $10^{10}$ neuraminidase-treated myeloblasts in 48 sites every month, or the same chemoimmunotherapy plus 100 $\mu$g of MER given at 10 sites (1). The preliminary results are in favor of the two chemoimmunotherapeutic regimens: Patients on chemotherapy alone show 62% failures at 52 weeks, patients receiving cells in addition show 30% failures at 52 weeks ($p = 0.01$). The remissions maintained by cells + MER are not longer than those treated by cells alone.

In conclusion, two of three studies comparing maintenance treatment by chemotherapy with the same chemotherapy plus BCG and leukemic cells show a significant prolongation of survival in the combined therapy group. Whether both parts of the immunotherapy, or the aspecific or the specific one alone, are accountable for that effect cannot actually be determined. BCG alone, however, seems to show some activity, as suggested by two of three randomized trials where the chemo + BCG-treated group had a prolonged remission or survival duration. Unfortunately, these studies do not give any indication concerning the mechanism by which BCG is acting. It cannot be ruled out that a nonimmunological mechanism was operating, such as the stimulation by BCG of normal hematopoietic precursors (44). One approach to this question should be to seek information about the doses of chemotherapy effectively delivered in each maintenance group to detect a potential protective effect of BCG on the normal marrow, allowing the use of higher doses of drugs in the chemoimmunotherapy group. On the other hand, the very preliminary results of the ALGB trials suggest strongly the activity on remission maintenance of blasts cells alone, at least when their immunogenicity is enhanced (by neuraminidase).

## FINAL COMMENT

Considering the point of view of the clinical investigator, two important concepts remain questionable:

1. Does one of the generally accepted rules of clinical oncology, namely, that polychemotherapy is better than monotherapy for induction of remission, also apply to AML? Some results obtained for induction of AML by daunomycin alone may challenge this concept.

2. Does another rule in clinical oncology, namely, the need for a maintenance therapy, apply to AML with the drugs presently available? This seems to be the case but has never been clearly demonstrated.

Considering the point of view of the clinician, a bold deduction could be to propose the use of daunomycin alone for induction therapy of AML. This could leave many possibilities for induction of relapse. For maintenance there is no solid basis on which to treat or not to treat. However, there is reasonable evidence to propose a combination of chemotherapy and immunotherapy.

## ACKNOWLEDGMENTS

We thank the statisticians of the E.O.R.T.C. Data Center for their help in statistical analysis. This help was made possible by National Institutes of Health grant 2 R10 CA 11488–07.

## REFERENCES

1. Bekesi, J. G., Holland, J. F., Cuttner, J., Glidewell, O., Krull, R., Jarowski, C., Coleman, M., and Silver, R. (1977): Chemoimmunotherapy in acute myelocytic leukemia. *Proc. Am. Assoc. Cancer Res.,* 18:198.
2. Bekesi, J. G., Holland, J. F., Yates, J. W., Henderson, E., and Fleminger, R. (1975): Chemotherapy of acute myelocytic leukemia with neuraminidase treated allogeneic leukemic cells. *Proc. Am. Assoc. Cancer Res.,* 16:121.
3. Bernard, J., Jacquillat, C., Weil, M., Boiron, M., and Tanzer, J. (1970): Present results on daunorubicin. In: *Advances in the Treatment of Acute (Blastic) Leukemias,* edited by G. Mathé, pp. 3–8. Springer-Verlag, New-York. Recent Results in Cancer Research, Vol. 30.
4. Bodey, G. P., Coltman, C. A., Freireich, E. J., Bonnet, J. D., Gehan, E. A., Haut, A. B., Hewlett, J. S., McCredit, K. B., Saiki, J. H. and Wilson, H. E. (1974): Chemotherapy of acute leukemia. Comparison of cytarabine alone and in combination with vincristine, prednisone and cyclophosphamide. *Arch. Intern. Med.,* 133:260–266.
5. Bodey, G. P., Rodriguez, V., Hart, J., and Freireich, E. J. (1970): Therapy of acute leukemia with the combination of cytosine arabinoside (NSC-638 781) and cyclophosphamide (NSC-26271). *Cancer Chemother. Rep.,* 54:255–262.
6. Carey, R. W. (1970): Comparative study of cytosine arabinoside (CA) therapy alone and combined with thioguanine (TG), mercaptopurine (MP) or daunomycin (DN) in acute myelocytic leukemia (AML). *Proc. Am. Assoc. Cancer Res.,* 11:15.
7. Clarkson, B. D., Dowling, M. D., Gee, T. S., and Burchenal, J. H. (1972): In: *Treatment of Acute Myeloblastic Leukaemia,* Vol. 1. Karger, Basel.
8. Crowell, E., Keimowitz, R., Pisciotta, A., and Schloesser, L. (1973): Comparison of cytosine arabinoside and thioguanine (CAT) and vincristine, amethopterin, 6-mercaptopurine, and prednisone (VAMP) therapy in adult acute leukemia (AAL). *Cancer Chemother. Rep.* 57(1):109.
9. Crowther, D., Powles, R. L., Bateman, C. J. T., Beard, M. E. J., Gauci, C. L., Wrigley, P. F. M., Malpas, J. S., Hamilton Fairley, G., and Bodley Scott, Sir Ronald (1973): Management of adult acute myelogenous leukaemia. *Br. Med. J.* 1:131–137.
10. Cuttner, J., Glidewell, O. M. A., and Holland, J. (1976): A comparative study of the value of immunotherapy with MER as adjuvant to induction and two maintenance chemotherapy programs in acute myelocytic leukemia. Immunotherapy of Cancer. Conference held in Bethesda, Oct. 27–29, 1976. Abstract 34, p. 27.

11. Edelstein, M., Vietti, T., and Valeriote, F. (1974): Schedule-dependent synergism for the combination of 1–β-D-arabinofuranosylcytosine and daunorubicin. *Cancer Res.,* 34:293–297.
12. Ellison, R. R., Holland, J. F., Weil, M., Jacquillat, C., Boiron, M., Bernard, J., Sawitsky, A., Rosner, F., Gussoff, B., Silver, R. T., Karanas, A., Cuttner, J., Spurr, C. L., Hayes, D. M. Blom, J., Leone, L. A., Haurani, F., Kyle, R., Hutchison, J. L., Jackson Forcier, R., and Moon, J. H. (1968): Arabinosyl cytosine: A useful agent in the treatment of acute leukemia in adults. *Blood,* 32:507–523.
13. Ellison, R. R., and Hoogstraten, B. (1965): Intravenous 6-mercaptopurine and methotrexate in adults with acute leukemia. *Proc. Am. Assoc. Cancer Res.,* 6:17.
14. Ellison, R. R., Hoogstraten, B., Holland, J. F., Levy, R. N., Lee, S. L., Silver, R. T., Leone, L. A., Cooper, T., Oberfield, R. A., Ten Pas, A., Blom, J., Jacquillat, C., and Haurani, F. (1972): Intermittent therapy with 6-mercaptopurine (NSC-755) and methotrexate (NSC-740) given intravenously to adults with acute leukemia. *Cancer Chemother. Rep.,* 56:535–542.
15. Ellison, R. R., Silver, R. T., and Engle, R. L., Jr. (1959): Comparative study of 6-chloropurine and 6-mercaptopurine in acute leukemia in adults. *Ann. Intern. Med.,* 51:322–338.
16. Ellison, R. R., Wallace, H. J., Hoagland, H. C., Woolford, D. C., and Glidewell, O. J. (1973): Prognostic parameters in acute myelocytic leukemia as seen in the Acute Leukemia Group B. *Adv. Biosci.,* 24:51–69.
17. Embury, S. H., Elias, L., Heller, P. H., Hood, C. E., Greenberg, P. L. and Schrier, S. L. (1977): Remission maintenance therapy in acute myelogenous leukemia. *West. J. Med.,* 126:267–272.
18. Fiere, D., Doillon, M., Martin, C., Vu Van, T., and Revol, L. (1976): Chemo-immunotherapy versus chemotherapy in acute myeloid leukemia. Preliminary results. *Biomedicine,* 25:318.
19. Frei, E., III, Freireich, E. J., Gehan, E., Pinkel, D., Holland, J. F., Selawry, O., Haurani, F., Spurr, C. L., Hayes, D. M., James, G. W., Rothberg, H., Sodee, D. B., Rundles, R. W., Schroeder, L. R., Hoogstraten, B., Wolman, I. J., Traggis, D. G., Cooper, T., Gendel, B. R., Ebaugh, F., and Taylor, R. (1961): Studies of sequential and combination antimetabolite therapy in acute leukemia: 6-Mercaptopurine and methotrexate. *Blood,* 18:431–454.
20. Frei, E., III, Holland, J. F., Schneiderman, M. A., Pinkel, D., Selkirk, G., Freireich, E. J., Silver, R. T., Gold, G. L., and Regelson, W. (1958): A comparative study of two regimens of combination chemotherapy in acute leukemia. *Blood,* 13:1126–1148.
21. Fridman, W. H., and Kourilsky, F. M. (1969): Stimulation of lymphocytes by autologous leukaemic cells in acute leukemia. *Nature,* 224:277–279.
22. Gee, T. S., and Clarkson, B. D. (1976): Pseudomonas aeruginosa vaccine in a treatment protocol for adult patients with acute nonlymphoblastic leukemia. In: Immunotherapy of Cancer. Conference held in Bethesda, 27–29 Oct., 1976, Abstract 35, p. 28.
23. Gee, T. S., Yu, K. P., and Clarkson, B. D. (1969): Treatment of adult acute leukemia with arabinosylcytosine and thioguanine. *Cancer,* 23:1019–1032.
24. Grozea, P. N., Bottomley, R. H., Shaw, M. T., Tu, H., Chanes, R. E., and Condit, P. T. (1975): The role of cytosine arabinoside maintenance in acute nonlymphoblastic leukemia. *Cancer,* 36:855–860.
25. Gutterman, J. U., Hersh, E. M., Rodriguez, V., McCredie, K. B., Mavligit, G., Reed, R., Burgess, M. A., Smith, T., Gehan, E., Bodey, G. P., and Freireich, E. J. (1974): Chemoimmunotherapy of adult acute leukaemia. Prolongation of remission in myeloblastic leukaemia with B.C.G. *Lancet,* 2:1405–1409.
26. Henderson, E. S., and Serpick, A. (1967): The effect of combination drug therapy and prophylactic oral antibiotic treatment in adult acute leukemia. *Clin. Res.* 15:336.
27. Hewlett, J. S., Balcerzak, S., and Gutterman, J. (1976): Remission induction in adult acute leukemia by 10-day continuous intravenous infusion of ARA-C, plus oncovin and prednisone. Maintenance with and without BCG. In: Immunotherapy of Cancer. Conference held in Bethesda, 27–29 Oct., 1976. Abstract 32, p. 26.
28. Huguley, C. M., Jr., Vogler, W. R., Lea, J. W., Corley, C. C., Jr., and Lowrey, M. E. (1965): Acute leukemia treated with divided doses of methotrexate. *Arch. Intern. Med.,* 115:23–28.
29. Karon, M., Freireich, E., and Carbone, P. (1965): Effective combination therapy of adult acute leukemia. *Proc. Am. Assoc. Cancer Res.,* 6:34.
30. Kline, I., Venditti, J. M., Tyrer, D. D., and Goldin, A. (1966): Chemotherapy of leukemia L1210 in mice with 1-β-D-arabinofuranosyl-cytosine hydrochloride. I. Influence of treatment schedules. *Cancer Res.,* 26:853–859.
31. "Leukaemia and Hematosarcoma "Cooperative Group of the E.O.R.T.C. (1973): A comparative trial of remission induction (by cytosine arabinoside, or C.A.R. and thioguanine, or C.A.R.

and Daunorubicin) and maintenance therapy (by C.A.R. or methylgag) in acute myeloid leukae-mia. *Biomedicine,* 18:192–198.

32. "Leukaemia and Hematosarcoma" Cooperative Group of the E.O.R.T.C. (1974): A second comparative trial of remission induction (by cytosine arabinoside given every 12 hours, or C.A.R. and thioguanine, or C.A.R. and daunorubicin) and maintenance therapy (by C.A.R. or methylgag) in acute myeloid leukaemia. *Eur. J. Cancer,* 10:413–418.

33. Levi, J. A., and Wiernik, P. H. (1976): A comparative clinical trial of 5-azacytidine and guanazole in previously treated adults with acute nonlymphocytic leukemia. *Cancer,* 38:36–41.

34. Lewis, J. P., Linman, J. W., Marshall, J., Pajak, T. F., and Bateman, J. R. (1977): Randomized clinical trial of cytosine arabinoside and 6-thioguanine in remission induction and consolidation of adult nonlymphocytic acute leukemia. *Cancer,* 39:1387–1396.

35. McCredie, K. B., Hewlett, J. S., and Kennedy, A. (1976): The chemoimmunotherapy of acute leukemia (CIAL): A cooperative group study. *Proc. Am. Assoc. Cancer Res.,* 17:239.

36. McCredie, K. B., Whitecar, J. P., Burgess, M. A., and Freireich, E. J. (1972): Comparative study of POMP versus COAP in remission induction and maintenance of acute adult leukemia (ALL). *Proc. Am. Assoc. Cancer Res.,* 13:101.

37. McIntyre, O. R., Rai, K., Glidewell, O., and Holland, J. F. (1976): Polyriboinosinic: Polyribocyti-dylic acid (Poly I:Poly C) as an adjunct to remission maintenance therapy in acute myelogenous leukemia. In: Immunotherapy of Cancer. Conference held in Bethesda, 27–29 Oct., 1976. Abstract 36, p. 28.

38. Omura, G. A. (1976): A randomized comparison of synchronizing-recruiting therapy (arabinosyl cytosine, vincristine, methotrexate + leucovorin rescue = AVML) versus myelotoxic therapy (thioguanine + arabinosyl cytosine + daunorubicin = TAD) in acute myelogenous leukemia. *Proc. Am. Assoc. Cancer Res.* 17:29.

39. Omura, G. A. (1976): Sequencing of cytosine arabinoside (NSC–63878) and daunorubicin (NSC–82151) in acute myelogenous leukemia. *Cancer Treatment Rep.,* 60(5):629–631.

40. Omura, G. A., Vogler, W. R., and Lynn, M. J. (1977): A controlled clinical trial of chemotherapy vs. BCG immunotherapy vs. no further therapy in remission maintenance of acute myelogenous leukemia (AML). *Proc. Am. Assoc. Cancer Res.,* 18:272.

41. Peto, R. (1976): Immunotherapy of acute myeloid leukaemia. Immunotherapy of Cancer. Confer-ence held in Bethesda, Oct. 27–29, 1976. Abstract 27, p. 24.

42. Powles, R. L., Crowther, D., Bateman, C. J. T., Beard, M. E. J., McElwain, T. J., Russel, J., Lister, T. A., Whitehouse, J. M. A., Wrigley, P. F. M., Pike, M., Alexander, P., and Hamilton Fairley, G. (1973): Immunotherapy for acute myelogenous leukaemia. *Br. J. Cancer,* 28:365–376.

43. Powles, R. L., Russel, J., Lister, T. A., Oliver, T., Whitehouse, J. M. A., Malpas, J., Chapuis, B., Crowther, D., and Alexander, P. (1976): Immunotherapy for acute myelogenous leukaemia: Analysis of a controlled clinical study 2½ years after entry of the last patient. Immunotherapy of Cancer. Conference held in Bethesda, Oct. 27–29, 1976. Abstract 25, p. 23.

44. Powles, R. L., Russel, J., Oliver, R. T. D., Lister, T. A., Hamilton Fairley, G., and Alexander, P. (1974): Immunotherapy for acute myelogenous leukaemia: A possible mechanism of action. Proc. XI Internat. Cancer Congress, Florence, September 1974.

45. Rai, K. R., Holland, J. F., and Glidewell, O. (1975): Improvement in remission induction therapy of acute myelocytic leukemia. *Proc. Am. Assoc. Cancer Res.,* 16:265.

46. Reizenstein, P., Breuning, G., Engstedt, L., Franzen, S., Gahrton, G., Gullbring, B., Holm, G., Höcker, P., Höglund, S., Hörnsten, P., Jameson, S., Killander, A., Killander, D., Klein, E., Lautz, B., Lindemalm, Ch., Lockner, D., Lönnqvist, B., Mellstedt, H., Palmblad, J., Pauli, C., Skårberg, K. O., Udén, A. M., Vanky, F., and Wadman, B. (1976): Effect of immunotherapy on survival and remission duration in acute, nonlymphatic leukemia. In: Immunotherapy of Cancer. Conference held in Bethesda, 27–29 Oct., 1976, Abstract 26, p. 23.

47. Rodriguez, V., Hart, J. S., Freireich, E. J., Bodey, G. P., McCredie, K. B., Whitecar, J. P., Jr., and Coltman, C. A., Jr. (1973): POMP combination chemotherapy of adult acute leukemia. *Cancer,* 32:69–75.

48. Sauter, Chr., Cavalli, F., Lindenmann, J., Gmür, J., Berchtold, W., Alberto, P., Obrecht, P., and Senn, H. J. (1976): Viral oncolysis: Its application in maintenance treatment of acute myelogenous leukemia. In: Immunotherapy of Cancer. Conference held in Bethesda, 27–29 Oct., 1976. Abstract 29, p. 25.

49. Schabel, F. M., Jr. (1969): The use of tumor growth kinetics in planning "curative" chemotherapy of advanced solid tumors. *Cancer Res.,* 29:2384–2389.

50. Shanbrom, E., and Miller, S. (1962): Critical evaluation of massive steroid therapy of acute leukemia. *N. Engl. J. Med.,* 266:1354–1358.
51. Skeel, R. T., Costello, W., Bertino, J. R., and Bennett, J. M. (1976): Cyclophosphamide, cytosine arabinoside and methotrexate (CAM) vs. cytosine arabinoside and thioguanine (AT) for acute nonlymphocytic leukemia (ANLL) in adults. *Proc. Am. Assoc. Cancer* Res., 17:301.
52. Southwest Oncology Group (1974): Cytarabine for acute leukemia in adults. *Arch. Intern. Med.,* 133:251–259.
53. Stoutenborough, K. A., and Meyers, M. C. (1975): Cytosine arabinoside vs. cyclo-phosphamide, vincristine, cytosine arabinoside and prednisone in the treatment of acute nonlymphocytic leukemia in adults. *Proc. Am. Assoc. Cancer,* 16:258.
54. Thompson, I., Hall, T. C., and Moloney, W. C. (1965): Combination therapy of adult acute myelogenous leukemia. *N. Engl. J. Med.,* 273:1302–1307.
55. UCLA Acute Leukemia Study Group (1977): Chemoimmunotherapy in acute myelogenous leukemia (AML). *Proc. Am. Assoc. Cancer Res.,* 18:139.
56. Vogler, W. R., and Bartolucci, A. A. (1976): The effect of BCG on remission duration and survival in acute myeloblastic leukemia. *Proc. Am. Assoc. Cancer Res.,* 17:109.
57. Vogler, W. R., Bartolucci, A., Omura, G. A., Miller, D., Smalley, R. V., Knospe, W. H. and Goldsmith, A. S. (1976): A randomized clinical trial of BCG in myeloblastic leukemia conducted by the Southeastern Cancer Study Group. In: Immunotherapy of Cancer. Conference held in Bethesda, 27–29 Oct., 1976. Abstract 30, p. 25.
58. Vogler, W. R., and Chan, Y. K. (1974): Prolonging remission in myeloblastic leukaemia by Tice-strain Bacillus Calmette-Guérin. *Lancet,* 2:128–131.
59. Vogler, W. R., Chan, Y. K., and Kremer, W. B. (1973): Comparison of cytosine arabinoside (CA) + 6-thioguanine (TG) to CA + TG + daunorubicin (D) for remission induction in leukemia. *Cancer Chemother. Rep.,* 57(1):100–101.
60. Vogler, W. R., Huguley, C. M., Jr., and Rundles, R. W. (1967): Comparison of methotrexate with 6-mercaptopurine-prednisone in treatment of acute leukemia in adults. *Cancer,* 20:1221–1226.
61. Wallace, H. J., Jr., Hoagland, H. C., Ellison, R. R., Glidewell, O., and Holland, J. F. (1973): CCNU plus cytosine arabinoside (ara-C) treatment of acute myelocytic leukemia compared with thioguanine (TG) plus ara-C. *Proc. Am. Assoc. Cancer Res.,* 14:100.
62. Weil, M., Glidewell, O. J., Jacquillat, C., Levy, R., Serpick, A. A., Wiernik, P. H., Cuttner, J., Hoogstraten, B., Wasserman, L., Ellison, R. R., Gailani, S., Brunner, K., Silver, R. T., Rege, V. B., Cooper, M. R., Lowenstein, L., Nissen, N. I., Haurani, F., Blom, J., Boiron, M., Bernard, J., and Holland, J. F. (1973): Daunorubicin in the therapy of acute granulocytic leukemia. *Cancer Res.,* 33:921–928.
63. Weiss, D. W. (1975): Nonspecific stimulation and modulation of the immune response and of states of resistance by the methanol-extraction residue fraction of tubercle bacilli. *Natl. Cancer Inst. Monogr.,* 35:157–171.
64. Whitecar, J. P., Jr., Bodey, G. P., Freireich, E. J., McCredie, K. B., and Hart, J. S. (1972): Cyclophosphamide (NSC-26271), vincristine (NSC-67574), cytosine arabinoside (NSC-63878) and prednisone (NSC-100231) (COAP) combination chemotherapy for acute leukemia in adults. *Cancer Chemother. Rep.,* 56:543–550.
65. Whittaker, J. A., and Slater, A. J. (1976): The immunotherapy of acute myelogenous leukaemia using intravenous BCG. In: Immunotherapy of Cancer. Conference held in Bethesda, 27–29 Oct., 1976. Abstract 33, p. 27.
66. Whittington, R. M., Rivers, S. L., Doyle, R. T., and Kodlin, D. (1963): Acute leukemia in the adult male. I. Comparative effect of 6-mercaptopurine and 6-chloropurine. *Cancer,* 16:244–248.
67. Wiernik, P. H., Glidewell, O., and Holland, J. F., for Acute Leukemia Group B (1975): Comparison of daunorubicin with cytosine arabinoside and thioguanine, and with a combination of all 3 drugs for induction therapy of previously untreated AML. *Proc. Am. Assoc. Cancer Res.,* 16:82.
68. Wiernik, P. H., Schimpff, S. C., Schiffer, C. A., Lichtenfeld, J. L., Aisner, J., O'Connell, M. J., and Fortner, C. (1976): Randomized clinical comparison of daunorubicin (NSC-82151) alone with a combination of daunorubicin, cytosine arabinoside (NSC-63878), 6-thioguanine (NSC-752) and pyrimethamine (NSC-3061) for the treatment of acute nonlymphocytic leukemia. *Cancer Treatment Rep.,* 60:41–53.

69. Wiernik, P. H., and Serpick, A. A. (1972): A randomized clinical trial of daunorubicin and a combination of prednisone, vincristine, 6-mercaptopurine and methotrexate in adult nonlymphocytic leukemia. *Cancer Res.*, 32:2023–2026.
70. Working Party of the Medical Research Council (1963): Treatment of acute leukaemia in adults: Comparison of steroid therapy at high and low dosage in conjunction with 6-mercaptopurine. *Br. Med. J.*, 1:7–14.
71. Working Party of the Medical Research Council (1966): Treatment of acute leukaemia in adults: Comparison of steroid and mercaptopurine therapy, alone and in conjunction. *Br. Med. J.*, 1:1383–1389.

*Randomized Trials in Cancer: A Critical Review by Sites,* edited by Maurice J. Staquet, Raven Press, New York © 1978.

# Chronic Lymphocytic Leukemia

Robert Zittoun

*Clinique hématologique, Hôtel Dieu, 75004 Paris, France*

Few prospective studies have been performed in chronic lymphocytic leukemia (CLL). The age group of most patients and the long overall survival have combined to retard research on the treatment of this disease. Since the first reports, chlorambucil appeared, among other alkylating agents, as yielding satisfactory antileukemic effect, with relatively slight toxicity (1). It was also noticed that complete remission with disappearance of lymphoid masses and hepatosplenomegaly, and recovery of normal blood picture and bone marrow aspirate was rarely obtained (3). Chlorambucil was reported as potentially inducing bone marrow depression, triggering autoimmune complications such as hemolytic anemia or "idiopathic" thrombocytopenic purpura, and increasing the frequency of cancer in patients submitted to long-term treatment. Consequently, chlorambucil and corticosteroids are generally employed empirically, according to the clinical symptoms and to the physician's own personal experience.

In fact, the problems raised by the management of CLL cannot be solved without considering the great polymorphism of this disease, even if the rare CLL of T-cell origin are excepted, and also the so-called lymphosarcoma cell leukemia. A clinical staging was recently proposed by Rai et al. (8): These authors defined five clinical stages, which have a different prognosis, whether used at diagnosis or during the course of the disease, since these stages can be successive evolutive steps (Table 1). Although some objections could be raised against the confusion in the same stages of cases with enlarged spleen, whether they have lymph nodes enlargement or not, and of cases with hemolytic and aplastic anemia, the prognostic value of this staging makes it a necessary tool for subclassification of CLL before undertaking a randomized trial.

## CHLORAMBUCIL VERSUS OTHER DRUGS

One of the first randomized studies on this topic was performed in CLL by the Southeastern Cooperative Cancer Chemotherapy Group (4): 132 untreated patients, of all clinical stages according to Rai's classification, were enrolled and randomly assigned to one of six regimens. Three drugs, chlorambucil, TEM,

---

Received October 4, 1976.

TABLE 1. *Staging of CLL according to Rai et al. (8)*

| Clinical stage | Criteria | Median survival (months) |
|---|---|---|
| 0 | Blood lymphocytosis $\geq 15,000/mm^3$ Marrow lymphocytosis $\geq 40\%$ | >150 |
| I | ld + lymph nodes enlargement | 101 |
| II | Lymphocytosis + enlargement of spleen and/or liver ± lymph nodes | 71 |
| III | Lymphocytosis + anemia (Hb < 11 g%) ± lymph nodes, spleen, liver enlargement | 19 |
| IV | Lymphocytosis + thrombocytopenia (platelets < 100,000/mm³) ± lymph nodes, spleen, liver enlargement | 19 |

and P32 were used and each was given by two schedules: The continuous regimen, after the first maximum improvement obtained, was continued at regular intervals in the maximum doses tolerated, whereas patients on the intermittent regimen received treatment only at specified signs.

The analysis of the results, in term of the overall response observed after 12 weeks and 6 months, and of the survival rate, have shown that P32 is significantly inferior to chlorambucil and TEM, with only 21% of favorable responses in 12 weeks and 31% at 6 months. There was also a slight difference in favor of chlorambucil over TEM, and, for these agents, of continuous over intermittent treatment, but these differences were not significant. Toxicity, and chiefly thrombocytopenia, was also more pronounced with P32 than with alkylating agents.

Two randomized double-blind trials were later conducted in the same field by Kaung et al. (5,6). Patients selected had more than 15,000 WBC/mm³, enlarged spleen or lymph nodes, and clinical evidence of progressive disease, corresponding to Rai's clinical stages I to IV. Thirty-three and 50% of them had been previously treated. However, the mean clinical and hematological data were similar in the compared groups. Chlorambucil at the starting dose of 0.2 mg/kg/day was compared to cyclophosphamide (2 mg/kg/day) in the first trial, and to streptonigrin (0.04 mg/kg/day) in the second. Few valid conclusions could be drawn, since these studies involved only 39 patients for chlorambucil-cyclophosphamide comparison, and 49 for chlorambucil-streptonigrin. Objective responses appeared more frequent with chlorambucil than with cyclophosphamide (76% versus 44% decrease in organ enlargement), but the differences were not significant, which is not surprising for such a limited number of patients. The rate of response was of similar amplitude (56%) with streptonigrin.

Side effects and chiefly hematologic toxicity were slight, and there was practically no difference between chlorambucil and cyclophosphamide, but the tolerance was far worse for streptonigrin, with significantly higher rate of digestive troubles and thrombocytopenia. The results of crossover studies in the few cases of resistance tested could not lead to definite conclusions.

## CHLORAMBUCIL WITH OR WITHOUT CORTICOSTEROIDS

This was the design of a single, double-blind, randomized trial, by Han et al. (2). But this was also a very short series, with 11 patients under chlorambucil (6 mg/day) and 15 under chlorambucil plus prednisone (30 mg/day). Patients were at various stages of disease, and half of them had been previously treated. However, the two groups were similar for the pretreatment data, and the difference was significant between the 50% tumor-response rate in patients treated by chlorambucil alone and an 87% rate in patients submitted to combined therapy. The lymphocyte response was more frequent, although slower, when prednisone was associated (73% instead of 54%) but not significantly different, as well as improvement in the hematocrit and/or platelet levels (40% versus 22%). Finally, the rate of excellent plus good overall response was significantly higher in the group with combined therapy. An interesting point is that all five patients in the chlorambucil-treated group who exhibited such responses received no previous therapy, whereas 5 of the 13 responding patients in the combination therapy group received previous antileukemic therapy. Prednisone was added in 2 patients who failed to respond to chlorambucil alone, and allowed 1 partial remission. Hematologic toxicity was slight or moderate and temporary in both groups; prednisone allowed a higher total dose of chlorambucil, but induced its own usual side effects.

The duration of maintained remission was the same in both groups (median 9.5 months), and the actuarial survival data did not differ significantly, in spite of a first apparent superiority of the combination treatment.

## TO TREAT OR NOT TO TREAT CLL

Many patients with the milder variants of CLL do not need treatment. The interest of a prolonged therapy by chlorambucil is actually tested in a protocol of the E.O.R.T.C. Leukemia and Hematosarcoma Group. Patients selected for this trial have only slowly progressive disease, no or only slight lymph node and spleen enlargement, anemia or thrombocytopenia, and a WBC count lower than $100,000/mm^3$. The great majority of them correspond to stages 0 and I, according to Rai's classification. After a 6- to 10-month period of observation without treatment, they are randomized between no therapy and a prolonged chlorambucil treatment (3 mg/m²/day/3 months, then continuous maintenance therapy). The results of this trial are not yet published, since the overall survival time for these stages is very long; for 127 randomized patients, the actuarial survival curve gives actually, at 6 years, 60% survival in the untreated patients and 75% in the treated ones, but this difference is not significant. Since chlorambucil doses were adapted in order to avoid bone marrow depression, the mean blood lymphocyte level remained higher than normal in the treated group. At present, the rate of complications such as myeloid decompensation and infection is statistically the same in both groups, as well as the time elapsing between randomization and complications. Mean time elapsing before apparition of a supervening cancer is shorter in the treated group (10 versus 21 months), but this difference is not significant because this event occurred in only 3 treated and 4 untreated patients.

The main difficulty of such a trial was to maintain the same therapeutic attitude throughout the prolonged course of the disease: 21 of 60 patients in the no-therapy group were secondarily treated according to the raised clinical problem, by chemotherapy, radiotherapy, or splenectomy, and 21 of the 67 patients in the treated group received another treatment at some time. Moreover, the general conclusions that could be drawn cannot apply to each individual case, as illustrated by the following observation: Two patients, quite similar for the clinical and hematological data, were randomized nearly at the same time. The first one, untreated, developed a severe myeloid decompensation after 2 years. Chlorambucil had to be started and allowed a complete remission with recovery of bone marrow depression. In the second patient, randomized for treatment, chlorambucil was stopped because of toxic myeloid decompensation, and this patient is actually in a fairly good clinical and hematological status without therapy.

## CONTINUOUS VERSUS INTERMITTENT THERAPY

This is an important problem, as biweekly chlorambucil treatment has given interesting results to Knospe, Loeb, and Huguley (7), with response rate similar to that obtained by the usual daily continuous therapy, but less hematological toxicity. A trial of the Acute Leukemia Group B was recently conducted on this topic by Sawitsky et al. (9) in 96 patients who were in the relatively poor prognosis stages III and IV, that is, anemic and/or thrombopenic. These patients were randomized into one of three treatment schedules: In the first branch, prednisone was given alone, 0.8 mg/kg/day for the first 6 weeks, then 7 consecutive days each month. Chlorambucil was added in the two other branches, continuously in the second (0.08 mg/kg/day), and intermittently in the third (0.4 mg/kg once monthly as starting dose, then up to 1.5 or 2 mg/kg). The results show a superiority of group 3 over 2, and group 2 over 1: The rate of remissions was 47% in the combined therapy with intermittent chlorambucil, 38% in the combined therapy with continuous chlorambucil, and 11% in patients under prednisone alone. Ten percent of patients with the combined therapy showed a complete clinical, hematological, and bone marrow remission. However, although the overall survival rate seems higher than the one previously observed by the same authors in stages III and IV, there was no significant difference of survival duration among the three branches: The median survival rate was 37 months for the best arm, and 21 months for the second one. Toxicity was "minimal," and patients under intermittent chemotherapy tolerated as much as 2 mg/kg single dose of chlorambucil. Age (70 or more), poor performance status, liver enlargement, and thrombocytopenia were initial factors predicting a shorter survival. Finally, and regardless of the chemotherapy employed, increased survival correlated best with some response parameters: improvement in performance status, increase in hemoglobin or platelet levels, and fall in peripheral lymphocytes.

## CONCLUSION

Few conclusions can be drawn if one considers the limited number of randomized trials and the fact that, the more recent ones excepted, they involved relatively few patients. Nevertheless, where therapy appears necessary, the combination chlorambucil-prednisone seems more active than either drug alone. Particularily when there are already manifestations of bone marrow depression, intermittent chlorambucil treatment should be preferred. More experience is needed in order to determine if such treatments can increase the overall survival duration taking into account the clinical stage. Moreover, since the survival of responders to chemotherapy is longer than in the nonresponders, other prospective and randomized studies are needed to test the validity of alternative drugs in chlorambucil-resistant patients, and of other treatments such as localized or titrated total body irradiation, splenectomy, androgenotherapy, and so on. Each therapeutic trial should be limited to a specific clinical stage or a definite clinical problem. The frequency of complications such as spontaneous or toxic bone marrow depression, immune deficiency and infections, or cancer should be tested in large series, according to the treatment schedule. Finally, one has to remember that the overall survival data must be compared to the survival curve of the general population of the same age group, as, even if they reach the best therapeutic procedures, CLL patients can hardly hope for a longer than "normal" survival.

## REFERENCES

1. Galton, D. A. G., Wiltshaw, E., Szur, L., and Dacie, J. V. (1961): The use of chlorambucil and steroids in the treatment of chronic lymphocytic leukaemia. *Br. J. Haematol.,* 7:73–98.
2. Han, T., Ezdinli, E. Z., Shimaoka, K., and Desai, D. V. (1973): Chlorambucil vs combined chlorambucil-corticosteroid therapy in chronic lymphocytic leukemia. *Cancer,* 31:502–508.
3. Han, T., Ezdinli, E. Z., and Sokal, J. E. (1967): Complete remission in chronic lymphocytic leukemia and lymphosarcoma. *Cancer,* 20:243–252.
4. Huguley, C. M. (1962): Long-term study of chronic lymphocytic leukemia: Interim report after 45 months. *Cancer Chemother. Rep.,* 16:241–244.
5. Kaung, D. T., Whittington, R. M., and Patno, M. E. (1964): Chemotherapy of chronic lymphocytic leukemia. *Arch. Intern. Med.,* 114:521–524.
6. Kaung, D. T., Whittington, R. M., Spencer, H. H., and Patno, M. E. (1969): Comparison of chlorambucil and streptonigrin (NSC-45383) in the treatment of chronic lymphocytic leukemia. *Cancer,* 23:597–600.

7. Knospe, W. H., Loeb, V., and Huguley, C. M., Jr. (1974): Bi-weekly chlorambucil treatment of chronic lymphocytic leukemia. *Cancer,* 33:555–562.
8. Rai, K. R., Sawitsky, A., Cronkite, E. P., Chanana, A. D., Levy, R. N., and Pasternack, B. S. (1975): Clinical staging of chronic lymphocytic leukemia. *Blood,* 46:219–234.
9. Sawitsky, A., Rai, K. R., Glidewell, O., Silver, R. T., and participating members of CALGB (Cancer and Leukemia Group B). (1977): A comparison of daily vs. intermittent chlorambucil and prednisone therapy in the treatment of patients with chronic lymphocytic leukemia. *Blood,* 50:1049–1059.

*Randomized Trials in Cancer: A Critical Review by Sites,* edited by Maurice J. Staquet, Raven Press, New York © 1978.

# Chronic Myelocytic Leukemia

## Pierre A. Stryckmans and Louisette Debusscher

*Service de Médecine et Laboratoire d'Investigation Clinique Henri Tagnon, Institut Jules Bordet, 1000 Bruxelles, Belgium*

It has been repeatedly emphasized that only little progress has been made in the treatment of chronic myeloid leukemia (CML). This is obvious when one compares the survival curves obtained recently with the survival data published by Minot, Nuckman, and Isaacs in 1924 (9). One wonders to what extent this is linked to the surprisingly low number of controlled therapeutic studies, only eight of which (2–4, 7, 8, 12–14) have been undertaken on CML patients. These randomized studies constitute the object of the present chapter. It should be noted, however, that a perfect methodology in assigning at random the treatments to compare can only serve to answer the question that has been asked. Evidently, if this question is inadequate or irrelevant to the problem, even the best randomization procedure will be useless to compensate for this insufficiency.

## TREATMENT OF THE CHRONIC PHASE

### Treatments Directed at the Spleen

#### Splenic Irradiation Compared to Busulfan

A controlled trial conducted by the Medical Research Council in Great Britain more than 10 years ago compared radiotherapy over the spleen with busulfan therapy (8). Busulfan was administered orally at a maximum daily dose of 4 mg until the total leukocyte count had fallen between 15 and $20 \times 10^9$/liter (when the treatment was to be discontinued). When the treatment had to be resumed, it was given, if necessarily indefinitely, so as to stabilize the total leukocyte count at approximately $10 \times 10^9$/liter. The precise technique of external radiotherapy was left to the radiotherapists at each center. The radiotherapy was administered in courses, the indications for treatment being left also to the discretion of each radiotherapist.

This study showed a median survival of 28 months for the 54 radiotherapy-treated patients and of 39.5 months for the 48 busulfan-treated patients. This

Received June 7, 1977.

difference was significant ($p < 0.03$). Moreover, (a) whereas 32 of the 54 radio-therapy-treated patients had to receive busulfan because control was unsatisfactory, only 4 of the 48 busulfan patients received radiotherapy, (b) in the busulfan-treated patients the spleen was more often maintained at a small size for long periods, (c) busulfan therapy was much more effective than radiotherapy in sustaining a "normal" hemoglobin concentration during the second year.

Several remarks concerning this study can be made:

(a) This trial has been criticized because it compared busulfan administered on a noncontinuous basis with irradiation administered at long intervals: Thus, the leukocyte counts of the irradiated patients fluctuated more widely than those of the patients treated with busulfan. Although the trial was not a valid comparison of the two therapeutic agents per se, it did compare busulfan with radiotherapy in the manner in which each is usually given. It thus answers a practical question.

(b) While the busulfan treatment was well defined, for radiotherapy the dose, the indication, the frequency, and the modality of each course were apparently left almost completely to the discretion of each radiotherapist. The radiotherapy group could therefore have been treated very inhomogeneously.

(c) Another remark is that, the trial being started in 1959, in more than half of the patients in each group the examination for the $Ph^1$ chromosome was not made. However, all the patients being more than 20 years of age, it is unlikely that a large fraction of the patients were $Ph^1$ negative. Moreover, the randomization procedure is expected to have distributed equally these cases among the two treatment groups.

(d) Since no patients were left untreated as controls, it is difficult to ascertain whether busulfan is better than no treatment in terms of survival or whether radiotherapy is deleterious and shortens the survival.

(e) It should be emphasized that radiotherapy of the spleen inferior to chemotherapy in that particular study might be shown in the future to be very useful if given at small and frequent doses or in combination with chemotherapy.

## Early Splenectomy

The constancy of splenomegaly in CML (17) and the possible role of the spleen in the development of aneuploid clones of leukemic cells (5,10) have led many investigators to propose splenectomy for the treatment of CML. Non-randomized studies by Schwartzenberg et al. (11) and by Spiers et al. (16) respectively on 39 and 26 CML patients in clinical and hematological remission during the chronic phase of their disease showed that this is a relatively safe procedure and suggested a beneficial effect on prognosis of CML. Another large noncontrolled clinical trial on splenectomy in CML was conducted early in the course of disease by the Italian cooperative group on chronic myeloid leukemia (6). This study including 139 patients came to a negative conclusion. The survival in the splenectomized patients was not better than in the other, nonsplenectomized patients. All these data await a final conclusion. At least two groups, the Medical Research Council Leukaemia Unit in Great Britain and the Italian Cooperative Study Group on Chronic Myeloid Leukemia, are presently conducting randomized trials on the effect of early splenectomy in CML. The first group includes already more than 100 patients (A. S. D. Spiers, *personal communication,* 1977) and the second more than 200 patients (S. Tura, *personal communication,* 1977). The follow-up of these patients is still too short to allow any definite conclusion. These studies will hopefully bring an answer to this very important question in the near future.

## Chemotherapy

### Comparison of Busulfan and Chlorambucil

The effects of chlorambucil and busulfan therapy have been studied in parallel in 45 patients with chronic granulocytic leukemia by the Southeastern Cancer Chemotherapy Cooperative Study Group (13). For the 42 evaluable patients, the therapeutic agent, chosen at random, was myleran in 21 cases and chlorambucil in 21 cases. Both agents were administered with the intent to produce either unequivocal evidence of chemotherapeutic effect using the optimal safe dose or depression of bone marrow function as sufficient to indicate that the maximal tolerated amount had been given. Therapy was initiated with a single daily dose of 6 mg of myleran or 12 mg of chlorambucil. After 2 to 4 weeks the respective doses were increased or decreased according to a uniform schedule. Chemotherapy was continued in all instances for 3 months before evaluation of effect of the agent was attempted. The two groups appeared comparable as to age, sex, duration of disease, and the number of previously treated and untreated. The geometric means of the total white cell, platelet, and granulocyte counts were slightly higher in the patients given chlorambucil, suggesting that the basic disease might have been somewhat more severe in this group. An excellent response was defined as the virtual disappearance of all evidence of disease. A good response indicated that leukocytosis, anemia, enlarged lymph nodes, splenomegaly, and the like showed at least 50% improvement induced and maintained by therapy. The results of chemotherapy after an arbitrary period of 3 months were evaluated by the investigators without knowledge of which agent had been given.

The difference in response of the two drugs as evaluated at the end of 3 months was highly significant. All the patients given busulfan had excellent (38%) or good (62%) response. Of the 21 patients given chlorambucil, excellent responses were rare (9.6%), good responses were seen in 48% of the cases, fair responses in 38%, and questionable responses in 4.8%.

### Comparison of Myleran and 6-Mercaptopurine

In 1963 the Southeastern Cancer Chemotherapy Cooperative Study Group studied in a randomized clinical trial the relative effectiveness of 6-mercaptopurine (6-MP) and busulfan for the achievement and maintenance of control of CML (14). Each patient was evaluated after a period of 12 weeks. Eighteen patients received 6-MP and 9 busulfan. The initial dose was a single daily dose of 6 mg of busulfan or 3 mg/kg of 6-MP. After 2 weeks the dose was adapted to achieve complete remission and to avoid severe marrow toxicity.

The two groups, apparently comparable at the beginning of the study, were different at 4 and 12 weeks. This difference was highly significant. The difference was accounted for chiefly by differences in hemoglobin concentration and number of platelets. The excessively high platelet counts exhibited by most patients with CML were usually brought to normal by busulfan. 6-MP often failed to provide adequate control of the high platelet count. There was often a rise in platelet count during the period of study. On the average there was a rise of 1.4 g of hemoglobin/$dl$ during the 12-week study in those patients treated with busulfan but no change in the average hemoglobin in those treated with 6-MP.

When considering the effect of the two drugs on the total leukocyte count and the immature leukocyte count, 6-MP in the dosage used produced a more rapid drop in both of these measurements. After the initial rapid fall, however, there was often considerable fluctuation, making it difficult to maintain full control. The escape of the granulocytes from depression by 6-MP was very rapid. The effect of busulfan was slower but more prolonged. The performance status, bone tenderness, and spleen size improved with both drugs.

In conclusion, considering the overall control of CML, busulfan was superior to 6-MP during a 12-week course of study. Not only were the results obtainable with 6-MP inferior to those with busulfan, but 6-MP was also more difficult to use. This study, however, does not tell us anything about the median survival of the patients treated with those drugs.

### Comparison of Busulfan and Cyclophosphamide

The Veterans Administration Cancer Chemotherapy Group conducted a randomized double-blind study to compare the efficacy of busulfan and cyclophosphamide during the chronic phase of CML (7). On 41 evaluable patients, 20 were allocated to busulfan treatment (0.1 mg/kg/day) and 21 to cyclophosphamide (2 mg/kg/day). The patients of the two groups were remarkably similar in their background and pretreatment data. Both treatments were given for 8 to 12 weeks. Therefore this study can only indicate how many and how easily complete and partial remission can be obtained. Busulfan was found in this respect to be significantly ($p = 0.02$) superior to cyclophosphamide. As a matter of fact, busulfan gave 5 complete remissions and only 1 absence of remission, whereas cyclophosphamide gave no complete remission and absence of remission in 7 patients. The rest were partial or slight remissions. There was also marked difference in the ease of maintenance of remission in the two groups. Seven patients treated with cyclophosphamide relapsed during the period of study, whereas no patient relapsed in the busulfan group ($p = 0.005$).

## Comparison of Busulfan and Dibromomannitol

Canellos et al. (2) have compared dibromomannitol (DBM) to busulfan in the treatment of CML. A total of 40 Philadelphia chromosome-positive cases were treated and 20 patients were randomized to each drug. The two groups were comparable in terms of presenting blood counts and duration from diagnosis to therapy, but as to the age at diagnosis those receiving DBM were younger (median age 34) than those on busulfan (median age 42). The dose of DBM was 250 mg/m$^2$ by mouth daily for the first 3 days followed by reduction of the dose to 150 mg/m$^2$ daily until remission. Busulfan was given as a daily oral dose of 4 mg/m$^2$ and continued until the white blood count was reduced to one-half the initial level, at which point the dose was decreased to 2 mg/m$^2$ daily. Both drugs were discontinued when a remission was obtained. A continuous maintenance treatment was started when there was evidence of reactivation of disease.

Both drugs were effective in inducing remission. The rate of remission was almost the same for both drugs, with 14 remissions with DBM and 15 with busulfan. There was no significant difference in the incidence of blastic transformation, defined as (a) 30% or more blasts in the marrow, (b) refractory anemia and/or thrombocytopenia, (c) splenomegaly, (d) extramedullary myeloblastic infiltrations. The median survival for both groups was about 45 months with 20% of the patients surviving up to 7 years. There was thus no significant difference in the survival between the two agents. The median survival of nonresponders from both groups was 13 months. There was no difference either in the capacity of both drugs to cause, sometimes, severe but nonfatal thrombocytopenia (2 with myleran, 1 with DBM). Certain differences were noted: DBM appeared capable of reducing the white blood count and producing a complete remission more rapidly than busulfan. The median duration from start of treatment to remission was 72 days with DBM and 100 days with busulfan. On the other hand, the overall median duration of the first remission was somewhat longer in the busulfan-treated group. Another difference was that hematologic resistance to busulfan without blastic transformation was not necessarily indicating resistance to DBM.

## Immunotherapy

Immunotherapy of chronic myeloid leukemia was initiated in 1965 by Sokal et al. in Buffalo (12). These authors have immunized patients by intradermal injections of BCG or mixtures of BCG and cultured cells of lines established from blood of patients with advanced myeloid leukemia. Most cases were treated at the same time with intermittent busulfan. A randomized study was undertaken to compare the effectiveness of vaccinations with BCG and cell mixtures with that of BCG alone. At the time of publication, no significant difference was seen between the two groups either in the frequency of serious complications or in survival. It is unfortunate that the BCG in this study was given frequently and at high dose, since this "intensive schedule," as opposed to a less intensive immunotherapy, failed in a nonrandomized study to improve the survival over that of busulfan-treated controls. It is regrettable that the basic question—whether or not immunotherapy is of any value in the treatment of CML—has not yet been answered by a controlled randomized trial.

## TREATMENT OF ADVANCED CML

The first randomized study reviewed in this chapter will remind us that a good methodology in clinical trials is not sufficient. A randomized trial was started by Acute Leukemia Group B for the comparison of four treatment modalities (4). The patients included, in so-called blastic crisis, were randomly assigned to one of the following treatment schedules:

1. 6-Mercaptopurine, "high," 1,200 mg/m$^2$ given i.v. twice weekly
2. 6-Mercaptopurine, "low," 800 mg/m$^2$ given i.v. twice weekly
3. 6-Thioguanine (6-TG) plus azaserine, "high," 80 mg/m$^2$ of 6-TG and 32 mg/m$^2$ of azaserine orally daily
4. 6-Thioguanine plus azaserine, "low," 40 mg/m$^2$ 6-TG and 16 mg/m$^2$ of azaserine

The comparison had to be abandoned rapidly since schedule 1 was rapidly found to be very toxic and schedules 2 and 3 were manifestly ineffective. Of the 17 patients evaluable in group 4, there were no complete remissions and only 2 strikingly brief partial responses. This conclusion emphasizes that there is an urgent need to detect effective drugs and effective drug schedules and that when the efficacy of the treatments is very low there is practically no opportunity to compare them.

Two chemotherapeutic regimens have emerged in recent years. One, comprising the association of 7 drugs, gave 4 complete and 1 partial remission in 9 patients (15). The other was simply associating prednisone (PDN) and vincristine (VCR) as in the classical treatment of acute lymphoblastic leukemia (1). It was unexpected therefore to obtain 8 complete and 8 partial remissions in a group of 50 patients in the blastic transformation of CML. Such results raise immediately the question of the role of each of these two drugs in this combination.

The usefulness of VCR in advanced CML was the object of a clinical trial in which it was randomly administered or not to a group of patients all receiving prednisone and two chemotherapeutic agents (3). Eighty-seven patients with aggressive CML were induced with a combination of hydroxyurea (HU) (30 mg/kg/day), 6-MP (3 mg/kg/day), and PDN (0.75 mg/kg/day). At random, half the patients received in addition one dose of VCR (1.5 mg/m$^2$, i.v.) weekly for 4 weeks. No benefit in response rate could be demonstrated from the use of VCR: Patients receiving VCR achieved a 32% complete plus partial response rate that was not significantly different from 28% for nonreceivers. Responding patients received a maintenance treatment consisting of HU (7 mg/kg/day), 6-MP (0.7 mg/kg), and PDN (0.25 mg/kg/day), with some continuing to receive VCR (1.5 mg/m$^2$ i.v. once a month). The survival of responders and nonresponders considered together was not significantly different for those receiving VCR (11 weeks) and those not receiving VCR (10 weeks). Thus, no additional benefit either in response rate or median survival could be demonstrated from the use of VCR. This conclusion does not necessarily rule out the role of VCR in the combination PDN + VCR. It suggests that other drugs do as well as VCR when associated with PDN. Nevertheless, the association of PDN + VCR being reasonably active, easy to administer, and well tolerated, could be proposed as a reference branch for future randomized studies on the terminal phase of CML.

## SUMMARY

Only six controlled therapeutical trials, all during the last decade, have been conducted on CML patients in the chronic phase of their disease. Such studies showed that in order to obtain a remission in CML, busulfan was significantly better than 6-MP, chlorambucil, and cyclophosphamide. In terms of survival, busulfan was significantly better than splenic irradiation but not really superior to dibromomannitol. Whether or not other chemotherapeutic agents, such as hydroxyurea, cyclophosphamide, 6-thioguanine, 6-mercaptopurine, and so on, could procure a median survival equivalent or better than that obtained by busulfan has never been tested in a controlled manner. The role of adjuvant immunotherapy in CML urgently requires a clear-cut confirmation.

The problems of the usefulness of early splenectomy will probably receive an answer very soon. For the terminal phase of CML the administration of vincristine does not seem to be crucial since in a randomized trial, it was not improving the results obtained by other chemotherapic drugs.

Finally, to encourage the initiation of controlled studies in CML, it should be remembered that in acute lymphoblastic leukemia great progress was made step by step, more than a decade ago, by the systematic use of randomized trials.

## REFERENCES

1. Canellos, G. P., De Vita, V. T., Whang-Peng, J., and Carbone, P. P. (1971): Hematologic and cytogenetic remission of blastic transformation in chronic granulocytic leukemia. *Blood,* 38:671–679.
2. Canellos, G. P., Young, R. C., Nieman, P. E., and De Vita, V. (1975): Dibromomannitol in the treatment of chronic granulocytic leukemia: A prospective randomized comparison with busulfan. *Blood,* 45:197–203.
3. Coleman, M., and Silver, R. T., for the Acute Leukemia Group B (1976): Combination chemotherapy for aggressive chronic granulocytic leukemia. A randomized trial. ASCO, Toronto, 1976, abstract C.265.
4. Hayes, D. M., Ellison, R. R., Glidewell, D., Holland, J. F., and Silver, R. T. (1974): Chemotherapy for the terminal phase of chronic myelocytic leukemia. *Cancer Chemother. Rep.,* 4:233.

5. Hossfeld, D. K., and Schmidt, C. G. (1973): Chromosomal data suggesting a primary role of the spleen in the pathogenesis of chronic myelocytic leukemia (CML) and blastic phase of CML. In: *Chemotherapy of Cancer Dissemination and Metastasis,* edited by S. Garattini and G. Franchi, p. 223. Raven Press, New-York.

6. Italian Cooperative Study Group on Chronic Myeloid Leukemia (1975): A clinical trial of early splenectomy, hydroxyurea and cyclic arabinosyl cytosine, vincristine and prednisone in chronic myeloid leukemia. *Ser. Haemat.* 8(4):121–142.

7. Kaung, D. T., Close, H. P., Whittington, R. M., and Patno, M. E. (1971): Comparison of busulfan and cyclophosphamide in the treatment of chronic myelocytic leukemia. *Cancer,* 27(1):608–612.

8. Medical Research Council's Working Party for Therapeutic Trials in Leukemia (1968): Chronic granulocytic leukaemia: Comparison of radiotherapy and busulfan therapy. *Br. Med. J.,* 1:201.

9. Minot, G. R., Nuckman, J. E., and Isaacs, R. (1924): Chronic myelogenous leukemia: Age incidence; duration and benefit derived. *JAMA,* 82:1486.

10. Mitelman, F., Brandt, L., and Nilsson, P. G. (1974): Cytogenetic evidence for spleen origin of blastic transformation in chronic myeloid leukaemia. *Scand. J. Haematol.,* 13:87–92.

11. Schwarzenberg, L., Mathe, G., Pouillart, P., Weiner, R., Lacour, J., Genin, J., Schneider, M., De Vassal, F., Hayat, M., Amiel, J., Schlumberger, J., Jasmin, C., and Rosenfeld, C. (1973): Hydroxyurea, leucophoresis and splenectomy. *Br. Med. J.,* 1:700.

12. Sokal, J. E., Aungst, C. W., Synderman, M., and Gomez, G. (1977): Immunotherapy of chronic myelocytic leukemia: effects of different vaccination schedules. *Clin. Hematol.,* 6(1):129–139.

13. Southeastern Cancer Chemotherapy Cooperative Study Group (1959): Comparison of chlorambucil and myleran in chronic lymphocytic and granulocytic leukemia. *Am. J. Med.,* 27:424.

14. Southeastern Cancer Chemotherapy Cooperative Study Group, Huguley, Ch. M., Grizzle, J., Rundles, R. W., et al. (1963): Comparison of 6-mercaptopurine and busulfan in chronic granulocytic leukemia. *Blood,* 21:89–100.

15. Spiers, A. D. S., Costello, C., Catousky, D., Galton, D. A. G., and Goldman, J. M. (1974): Chronic granulocytic leukaemia: Multiple-drug chemotherapy for acute transformation. *Br. Med. J.,* II:77–80.

16. Spiers, A. S. D., Baikie, A. G., Galton, D. A. G., Richards, H. G. H., Wiltshaw, E., Goldman, J. M., Catousky, D., Spencer, J., and Peto, R. (1975): Chronic granulocytic leukaemia: Effect of elective splenectomy on the course of the disease. *Br. Med. J.,* 175–179.

17. Wintrobe, M. M. (1974): *Clinical Hematology: Chronic Myelocytic Leukemia,* 7th ed., p. 1501. Lea & Febiger, Philadelphia.

*Randomized Trials in Cancer: A Critical Review by Sites,* edited by Maurice J. Staquet, Raven Press, New York © 1978.

# Multiple Myeloma

Robert L. De Jager

*Service de Médecine et Laboratoire d'Investigation Clinique Henri Tagnon, Institut Jules Bordet, 1000 Bruxelles, Belgium*

Prior to 1968, results of clinical trials were evaluated by improvement of individual clinically relevant parameters. Later response was defined by improvement of a set of parameters, and response was correlated with survival. Prognostic factors were recognized (1,3) and correlated with tumor cell mass. The actual tumor cell mass is measurable, as shown by Durie and Salmon (9), who measured tumor cell burden in 71 patients and established the correlation with clinical factors.

## COMPARISON AMONG SINGLE DRUGS (Table 1)

The Western Cancer Chemotherapy Group reported the first prospective randomized clinical trial in multiple myeloma in 1962 (15). The study compared the effects of prednisone and a placebo, given by the double-blind method, in addition to supportive care and local radiation therapy for palliation of pain when necessary. 33 patients received 40 mg of prednisone daily and 32 a placebo. The two groups were similar for the variables examined: age, sex, time of onset from first symptoms, prior therapy, performance status, hematocrit, BUN, total globulins, calcium, and urinary proteins. Six of 25 patients on prednisone, but none on the placebo, showed an increase in hematocrit greater than 6 vol%. Seven of 25 patients on prednisone, but only 1 of 22 on placebo, showed a fall in globulin $\geq 1.5$ g%. There was, however, no difference in performance status or median survival time from diagnosis (17 months) between the two groups or using a historical control of 600 published cases. This first study suggests that prednisone may affect some parameters of the disease without significant impact on survival.

A double-blind randomized study of ECOG (1958–1961) comparing urethane and placebo failed to demonstrate any significant difference for the selected parameters of activity (11). The shortened survival of urethane-treated patients may in part be explained by unequal distribution of patients with azotemia.

In 1966 the Veterans Administration Cancer Chemotherapy Group reported

---

Received June 30, 1977.

TABLE 1. *Prospective randomized clinical trials in myeloma*

| Treatment | Dose | Criteria[a] | No. treated | Response (%) | Median survival (months) | Cooperative group | References |
|---|---|---|---|---|---|---|---|
| Prednisone | P: 40 mg/day | A | 33 | — | 17 | Western | 15 |
| Placebo | — | | 32 | — | 17 | | |
| Urethane | U: 4.0 g/day | A | 47 | — | (8, 8) 5[b] | ECOG | 11 |
| Placebo | — | | 36 | — | (15, 10.5) 12 | | |
| Melphalan | M: | B | 38 | 37 | — | VA | 17 |
| Cyclo | C: | | 34 | 32 | — | | |
| Melphalan | M: 4 mg/day | Survival only | 38 | — | 18 | Medical Research Council | 16 |
| Cyclo | C: 150 mg/day | | 34 | — | 18 | | |
| Melphalan | M: 0.25 mg/kg/day × 4, q. 6 wk | | 63 | 21 | 18 | | |
| Melphalan + prednisone | M: 0.25 mg/kg/day × 4, q. 6 wk<br>P: 2.0 mg/kg/day × 4, q. 6 wk | B | 75 | 47 | 21 | SWCCG | 2 |
| Melphalan + prednisone | M: 0.25 mg/kg/day × 4, q. 6 wk<br>P: 2.0 mg/kg/day × 4, q. 6 wk | | 79 | 41 | 21 | | |
| Melphalan + prednisone + procarb. | M: 0.20 mg/kg/day × 4, q. 6 wk<br>P: 2.0 mg/kg/day × 4, q. 6 wk<br>PZ: 3.0 mg/kg/day × 9, q. 6 wk | B | 82 | 52 | 23 | SWCCG | 2 |
| | | | Good risk[c] (GR) | | GR + PR | | |
| Melphalan | M: 0.15 mg/kg/day × 7, 0.05 mg/kg/day | | M 35 | 23 | 30 | | |
| Melphalan + prednisone | M: 0.15 mg/kg/day × 7, 0.05 mg/kg/day<br>P: 1.25 mg/kg/day, taper over 8 wk | | MP 42 | 55 | 53 | ALGB | |
| | | | MPT 37 | 65 | 36 | | |
| | | B | Poor risk[c] (PR) | | PR | | |
| Melphalan + prednisone + testosterone | M: 0.15 mg/kg/day × 7, 0.05 mg/kg/day<br>P: 1.25 mg/kg/day, taper over 8 wk<br>T: 10 mg/kg/wk | | M 25 | 28 | 21 | ECOG | 7 |
| | | | M 29 | 31 | 9 | | 27 + |
| | | | MPT 21 | 43 | 4 | | |

| Regimen | Dose | | | | | Group | |
|---|---|---|---|---|---|---|---|
| Anil. mustard | AM: 1 mg/kg/day | | 16 | — | | | |
| Anil. mustard + prednisone | AM: 1 mg/kg/day; P: 1.2 mg/kg/day, taper over 8 wk | A | 17 | — | — | ALGB | 12 |
| Melphalan + prednisone | M: not stated; P: not stated | B | 13 | — | — | | |
| Methotrexate | MTX: 50 mg/m²/day 1 | | | | | Western | 5 |
| → vincristine | VCR: 1.4 mg/m²/day 2 | | 9 | | | | |
| → melphalan | M: 0.05 mg/kg days 3–12 | | | | | | |
| Melphalan | M: 0.05 mg/kg/day | | 38 PR[c] | 16 | 12 | | |
| Melphalan + prednisone | M: 0.05 mg/kg/day; P: 0.6 mg/kg/day, taper over 10 wk | B | 46 PR[c] | 50 | 12 | ALGB | 8 |
| Melphalan + prednisone | M: 0.05 mg/kg/day; P: 0.3 mg/kg/day, taper over 10 wk | | 41 PR[c] | 34 | 12 | | |
| Cyclo + prednisone | C: 600 mg/m² i.v. q. 6 wk; P: 0.8 mg/kg/day, taper over 42 days | B | 20[d] | 5 | — | | |
| Cyclo + prednisone + chloroquine | CPA: 600 mg/m² i.v. q. 6 wk; P: 0.8 mg/kg/day, taper over 42 days; Cq: 250 mg b.i.d. × 10 days | | 18[d] | 5 | — | ALGB | 14 |
| Induction | Remission maintenance: | | | | | | |
| Melph + adriam + pred | | | | 41 | — | | |
| Melph + cyclo + pred | MCBP azathioprine | C | 189 (total) | 50 | — | SWCCG | 18 |
| Melph + cyclo + BCNU + pred | (doses not stated) | | | 33 | — | | |
| BCNU + cyclo + pred | (doses not stated) | B | 104 | 57 | 22 | Southeastern Oncology Group | |
| Melph + pred | | | 9 | 59 | 22 | | |
| BCNU + cyclo + pred | (doses not stated) | B | 48 | 49 | 22 | Eastern Oncology Group | |
| Melph + pred | | | 48 | 32 | 22 | | |

TABLE 1 (Continued)

| Treatment | Dose | Criteria[a] | No. treated | Response (%) | Median survival (months) | Cooperative group | References |
|---|---|---|---|---|---|---|---|
| Melph + pred<br>Mel Cycl BCNU<br>+ → + → + | M: 9 mg/m²/day × 4, q. 4 wk<br>P: 100 mg/day × 4, q. 4 wk | | 79 | 48 | | | |
| Pred Pred Pred | M: 9 mg/m²/day × 4<br>C: 325 mg/m²/day × 4↓ | | 74 | 66 | | National Myeloma Study (Canada) | 4 |
| | B: 150 mg/m², day 1 ↓<br>P: 100 mg/day × 4, q. 4 wk | | | | 24–27 | | |
| Mel + cyclo +<br>BCNU + pred | M: 3 mg/m²/day × 4, q. 4 wk<br>C: 108 mg/m²/day × 4, q. 4 wk<br>B: 50 mg/m², day 1, q. 4 wk<br>P: 100 mg/day × 4, q. 4 wk | | 70 | 66 | | | |
| NaF + NaCl | NaF: 25 mg q.i.d.<br>NaCl: 25 mg q.i.d. | Recalcification of bone | 52 | Useless, possibly detrimental | | | |
| NaF<br>Placebo | NaF: 50 mg q.i.d.<br>— | | 51<br>47 | | — | | 10 |
| All patients: | chemotherapy and radiotherapy as indicated | | | | | | |
| NaF + CaCO₃ | NaF: 50 mg b.i.d.<br>CaCO₃: 1 g q.i.d. | Recalcification of bone | 13 | Useful | — | 13 | |
| Placebo | | | 13 | | | | |
| All patients: | Melphalan: 0.15 mg/kg/day × 7 q. 6 wk<br>Prednisone: 60 mg/day × 7, q. 6 wk | | | | | | |

[a] Response defined by changes in A, individual parameters; B, combination of parameters; C, tumor cell mass.
[b] Previously treated with or without urethane.
[c] Stratification for good-risk (GR) and poor-risk (PR) patients.
[d] Disease resistant to melphalan.

on a double-blind comparison of cyclophosphamide and melphalan (17). The criteria for response recommended by the Chronic Leukemia Task Force were used. The therapeutic activity of the two drugs was similar.

Another comparison of cyclophosphamide and melphalan, both given by a continuous oral schedule, was performed by the Medical Research Council of Great Britain (1964–1968) (16). The conclusion of the trial confirms that no significant difference exists between the effects of these two alkylating agents. The importance of the urea level as a prognostic factor affecting survival was clearly demonstrated in this trial. Median survival times of 33, 20, and 2 months were observed for patients with urea levels less than 40 mg%, between 40 and 79 mg%, and above 80 mg%, respectively.

## COMPARISON AMONG COMBINATIONS OF DRUGS (Table 1)

In 1972, the SWCCG established the usefulness of the melphalan-prednisone combination regimen that has become standard therapy today (2). Although the response rate was increased over melphalan alone, there was little advantage in terms of increase in survival time.

The addition of procarbazin did not result in any additional improvement. At the time, no direct correlation with tumor cell mass was yet possible, and the usual criteria of decline of M-protein peak to 50% of its initial value was decreased to 25%. Only patients achieving this level of response showed an advantage in survival (median survival time of 36 months) over nonresponders (18 months).

Fifteen percent had complete response with disappearance of serum electrophoretic peaks.

The effectiveness of the melphalan-prednisone treatment was confirmed by the report of the ALGB-ECOG study (7). In this trial, patients were classified in two risk categories: good-risk patients met all of the following criteria: BUN less or equal to 30 mg/100 ml, serum calcium less or equal to 12 mg/100 ml, absence of significant infection, WBC greater or equal to 4,000/mm$^3$ and platelets greater or equal to 100,000, expected survival longer than 2 months. Within each risk category, patients were randomly allocated among one of three arms: melphalan alone, melphalan + prednisone, or melphalan + prednisone + testosterone.

Responses are analyzed by parameters: hemoglobin, marrow plasma cell, serum globulin concentration, and urinary protein concentration. Because of difficulty in assessing improvement of bone lesions they were not accepted as criteria for evaluating response, but progression of bone disease was a parameter of relapse. Defining good response as response in over half of those parameters abnormal initially separates a population with significantly better survival than poor response (only one parameter improved) or no response. It is noteworthy that the definition of response is not the same as in the SWCCOG study with regard to decrease in serum globulin concentration: 50% of initial value in the ALBG-ECOG study, 25% of initial value in the SWCCOG study.

The results are that the beneficial effects of adding prednisone to melphalan are statistically significant for good-risk, but not for poor-risk patients. The addition of testosterone produced no additional benefit.

The overall median survival (good- and poor-risk patients) was 27 months. In this trial the value of anemia as a prognostic factor is recognized in the analysis of the data although not used in the initial stratification.

A follow-up study by the ALGB was conducted to evaluate further the melphalan + prednisone combination in poor-risk patients (8). Because of the possibility that prednisone might have increased early mortality, this second study was designed using prednisone doses one-half and one-fourth of those of the initial study. A loading dose of melphalan was also omitted. Although the group receiving melphalan + prednisone at 0.6 mg/kg had a significantly improved response rate, the median survival time was identical for the three regimens (12 months).

Aniline mustard, an alkylating agent effective in plasma cell tumors in BALB/ C mice, was tested by the ALGB (12), but only marginal activity was discovered (4 of 60 parameters improved). The addition of prednisone was beneficial (14 of 55).

Aniline mustard appears inferior to melphalan in its response rate, although the two drugs were not compared directly.

An attempt at combining cell cycle-specific (methotrexate, vincristine) and nonspecific (melphalan) agents in a time-sequential chemotherapeutic regimen was made by the Western Cancer Study Group. The published data (5) of a randomized study comparing this regimen with the combination of intermittent melphalan and prednisone involves too few patients to allow any conclusion.

The study of ALGB (14) comparing cyclophosphamide and prednisone versus cyclophosphamide, prednisone, and chloroquine in melphalan-resistant myeloma confirmed the observation of Bergsagel (4) that some patients resistant to melphalan will respond to cyclophosphamide. No effect of chloroquine could be detected.

Recent trials (6,7) have failed to show combinations of alkylating agents and BCNU to be better than melphalan and prednisone.

The study of the SWCCOG (18), comparing melphalan, adriamycin, prednisone (MAP), melphalan, cyclophosphamide, and prednisone (MCP), and melphalan, cyclophosphamide, BCNU and prednisone (MCBP), is the first one to use the clinical staging based on measurements of tumor cell mass as defined by Durie et al. (9) and to define response quantitatively as a reduction in this tumor cell mass (75%). Response rates appear similar to that of other combination studies, and survival data are as yet not available.

## RECALCIFICATION OF BONE (Table 1)

A randomized study comparing the effect of sodium fluoride on bone recalcification versus placebo was conducted by Harley, Schilling, and Glidewell (10).

No effect was seen. Sodium fluoride given with calcium carbonate was tested against placebo by Kyle et al. (13), all patients being treated with intermittent melphalan and prednisone. Microradiography of bone biopsies and videodensitometry studies revealed significant increases in bone formation and bone mass in the fluoride calcium group, although technetium bone scans and bone densitometry proved insensitive for detection of skeletal changes.

## CONCLUSION

As relevant parameters of disease were recognized, clinical studies were progressively refined and evaluation of treatment made more precise. Although some valuable information could be retrieved from nonrandomized studies if analyzed retrospectively for prognostic factors, the established evidence has been gained by stepwise progression in using prospective randomized trials to establish the relative efficacy of treatment over placebo and combination treatment over single agents. Because of the small number of cases seen annually in individual institutions, it is not surprising that all the clinical trials reviewed are from cooperative groups. For multiple myeloma to date, the situation is similar to that seen in acute myelocytic leukemia. Remissions may be induced by drugs in 40 to 60% of patients but with limited impact on survival: median survival time of 24 months, versus 17 for placebo, responders living longer, that is, median survival time of 36 months. The randomized trials detected the efficacy of melphalan and cyclophosphamide, the improved therapeutic index of melphalan and prednisone over melphalan alone. No further advantage was found in combining alkylating agents and BCNU. Useless agents could be discarded (urethane, chloroquine). The progress in therapeutics was matched by the improved knowledge of the disease provided by definition of prognostic factors, measurement of tumor cell mass, and the design of a clinical staging based on it.

## REFERENCES

1. Alexanian, R. Balcerzak, S., Bonnet, J., Gehan, E., Haut, A., Hewlett, J. S., and Monto, R. W. (1975): Prognostic factors in multiple myeloma. *Cancer,* 36:1192–1201.
2. Alexanian, R., Bonnet, H., Gehan, E., Haut, A., Hewlett, J., Lane, M., Monto, R., and Wilson, H. (1972): Combination chemotherapy for multiple myeloma. *Cancer,* 30:382–389.
3. Bergsagel, D. E. (1975): Plasma cell myeloma: Prognostic factors and criteria of response to therapy. In: *Cancer Therapy: Prognostic Factors and Criteria of Response,* edited by M. Staquet, p. 73. Raven Press, New York.
4. Bergsagel, D. E., Bailey, A. J., Langley, N., MacDonald, N., White, D. E., and Milles, A. B. (1977): Treatment of plasma cell myeloma with prednisone (P.) and sequential, alternating or concurrent schedules of melphalan (M.), cyclophosphamide (CTX) and carmustine (B.C.N.U.). *Proc. Am. Soc. Clin. Oncol.,* 18:329.
5. Brook, J., Prasad, R., and Muthualer, R. (1975): Sequential therapy compared with combination therapy in multiple myeloma. *Arch. Intern. Med.,* 135(1):163–171.
6. Cohen, H. J., Abramson, N., Bartolucci, A., and Bailar, J. (1976): B.C.N.U., cyclophosphamide and prednisone (B.C.P.) vs melphalan and prednisone (M.P.) in myeloma. *Proc. Am. Soc. Clin. Oncol.,* 17:280.
7. Costa, G., Engle, R. L., Schilling, A., Carbone, P., Kochwa, S., Nachman, R. L., and Glidewell, O. (1973): Melphalan and prednisone: An effective combination for the treatment of multiple myeloma. *Am. J. Med.,* 54:589–599.

8. Cuttner, J., Wasserman, L. R., Martz, G., Sonntag, R. W., Kyle R. A., and Silver, R. T. (1975): The use of low-dose prednisone and melphalan in the treatment of poor risk patients with multiple myeloma. *Med. Pediatr. Oncol.,* 1(3):207–216.

9. Durie, B. G. M., and Salmon, S. E. (1975): A clinical staging system for multiple myeloma. *Cancer,* 36:842–854.

10. Harley, J. B., Schilling, A., and Glidewell, O. (1972): Ineffectiveness of fluoride therapy in multiple myeloma. *N. Engl. J. Med.,* 286:1283.

11. Holland, J. F., Hasley, H., Scharban, C., Carbone, P. P., Frei, E., III, Brindley, C. O., Hall, T. I. C., Shnider, B. I., Gold, G. L., Lasagna, L., Owens, A. H., and Miller, S. P. (1966): A controlled trial of methane treatment in multiple myeloma. *Blood,* 27:328–342.

12. Kyle, R. A., Costa, G., Cooper, M. R., Ogawa, M., Silver, R. T., Glidewell, O., and Holland, J. F. (1973): Evaluation of aniline mustard in patients with multiple myeloma. *Cancer Res.,* 33:956–960.

13. Kyle, R. A., Jowsey, J., Kelly, P. J., and Taves, D. R. (1975): Multiple myeloma: Effects of sodium fluoride and calcium carbonate or placebo. *N. Engl. J. Med.,* 293:1334–1338.

14. Kyle, R. A., Seligman, B. R., Wallace, H. J., Silver, R. T., Glidewell, O., and Holland, J. F. (1975): Multiple myeloma resistant to melphalan (NSC-8806) treated with cyclophosphamide (NSC-26271), prednisone (NSC-10023) and chloroquine (NSC-187208). *Cancer Chemother. Rep. Part 1,* 59:557–562.

15. Mass, R. E. (1962): A comparison of the effect of prednisone and a placebo in the treatment of multiple myeloma. *Cancer Chemother. Rep.,* 16:257–259.

16. Report of the Medical Research Council's Working Party for Therapeutic Trials in Leukemia (1971): Myelomatosis: Comparison of melphalan and cyclophosphamide. *Br. Med. J.,* 1:640–641.

17. Rivers, S. (1966): Comparison of cyclophosphamide and melphalan in the treatment of multiple myeloma. *Proc. Am. Assoc. Cancer Res.,* 7:59.

18. Salmon, S. E., Durie, B. G. M., and Alexanian, R., for the Southwest Oncology Group (SWOG) (1975): Combination chemotherapy for multiple myeloma. *Blood,* 46:1039.

19. Salmon, S. E., and Smith, B. A. (1970): Immunoglobulin synthesis and total body tumor cell number in IgG multiple myeloma. *J. Clin. Invest.,* 49:1114–1121.

*Randomized Trials in Cancer: A Critical Review by Sites,* edited by Maurice J. Staquet, Raven Press, New York © 1978.

# Non-Hodgkin's Lymphoma

## Richard A. Bender and Vincent T. DeVita, Jr.

*Division of Cancer Treatment, National Cancer Institute, 9000 Rockville Pike, Building 10, Room 12N226, Bethesda, Maryland 20014*

Malignant lymphomas are now thought to be tumors of the immune system. In 1966, Lukes and Butler (62) separated out Hodgkin's disease in a separate histopathologic classification. This report was followed by others demonstrating the utility of this classification for predicting prognosis. The combination of a satisfactory staging classification developed at Rye, New York, in 1965 and at a conference held at Ann Arbor, Michigan, in 1971 has culminated in rapid and remarkable advances in diagnosis, staging, and therapy of Hodgkin's disease. The remainder of the lymphomas are, unfortunately, referred to by the negative title as the non-Hodgkin's lymphomas. In 1958, Gall and Rappaport (32) described a classification of these diseases, segregating them into those tumors thought to be of lymphocytic origin, those of histiocytic origin, and those containing a mixture of both lymphocytes and histiocytes. In each type they were further subdivided as to whether the histology was predominantly nodular or diffuse. This classification, referred to as the Rappaport scheme, is now in wide use throughout the world (Table 1; 70).

The analysis of the data available from controlled and uncontrolled trials in patients with lymphocytic and histiocytic lymphoma, both nodular and diffuse, as described in the Rappaport classification, is particularly difficult, as the older studies used the early histologic designation of lymphosarcoma, reticulum cell sarcoma, and giant follicular lymphoma. To be useful, a histopathologic language should have three characteristics: It should be clinically relevant, reproducible among a wide variety of pathologists, and scientifically accurate. Currently, there are six histopathologic classifications for the lymphomas other than Hodgkin's disease (5,25,55,63,64,70). Further progress in clinical trials involving these disorders will be hampered unless some common language, one of the six classifications or an amalgamation of the best terms of each of the classifications, is used in future clinical trials. The Rappaport classification is widely used in the United States, and has much to recommend it since it meets two of the three criteria described above. It has been clearly demonstrated by a number of investigators that the classification as described by Rappaport is clinically

---

Received January 4, 1977.

TABLE 1. *Rappaport classification of non-Hodgkin's lymphoma*[a]

| | |
|---|---|
| Malignant lymphoma, undifferentiated, Burkitt's type | Burkitt's tumor |
| Malignant lymphoma, undifferentiated, pleomorphic type | |
| Malignant lymphoma, histiocytic type | Reticulum cell sarcoma |
| Malignant lymphoma, histiocytic-lymphocytic (mixed-cell) type | |
| Malignant lymphoma, lymphocytic type, poorly differentiated | Lymphosarcoma |
| Malignant lymphoma, lymphocytic type, well differentiated | |

[a]Modified from Berard (6).

relevant (2,74). Also, several studies show that with respect to the major subcategorizations within the Rapapport classification, the determination of nodularity or diffuseness of tumor involvement of a lymph node or the recognition of two of the major disease subcategories, nodular poorly differentiated lymphocytic lymphoma (NPDL) and diffuse histiocytic lymphoma (DHL), that the classification is reproducible (15).

The relatively recent recognition that the immune system can be subdivided into a number of population of cells of different derivation with various physiologic functions has highlighted the fact that most of the older classifications based on morphology, including Rappaport's, are scientifically inaccurate (1, 31,42). One classification, that proposed by Lukes and Collins (63), has attempted to circumvent the scientific inaccuracy by subcategorizing lymphomas by their proposed cell of origin. This relatively recent classification, and that described by Lennert et al. (55) based on similar assumptions, have yet to be proven either clinically relevant, with respect to prognosis, or reproducible. Since the information on the immunologic derivation of lymphoma cells is, as yet, incomplete and the techniques are not yet widely available to all clinical investigators, it seems appropriate to depend on the Rappaport classification with an eye toward correcting the scientific inaccuracy at some later date as additional information becomes available. This is particularly true as several large controlled clinical trials are currently under way which are stratified by subcategories in the Rappaport classification.

An accurate appraisal of the extent of the disease is required prior to therapy to assess the results of treatment. Furthermore, restaging following therapy is necessary to evaluate accurately those patients who appear to have complete disappearance of tumor. Agreement as to what studies constitute an adequate staging workup is, therefore, necessary. Considerable work in the staging of Hodgkin's disease (17) has provided the Ann Arbor classification which has been applied to the staging of non-Hodgkin's lymphoma. Unfortunately, the natural history of the group of diseases comprising the non-Hodgkin's lymphomas is quite variable and undermines the usefulness of the Ann Arbor classification. For example, the classification fails to distinguish between the difference in prognosis of the early and late stages of both NPDL and DHL, the two main subcategories in the Rappaport classification. However, like the Rappaport

TABLE 2. *Sequential diagnostic studies used in the staging of malignant lymphomas*[a]

1. Detailed history and physician examination
2. Complete blood count and differential
3. Chest radiography with tomograms, as needed
4. Metastatic bone survey
5. Bipedal lymphangiogram
6. Radioisotopic studies including liver-spleen, bone, and whole-body Gallium scan
7. Bilateral illiac crest bone marrow biopsies
8. Percutaneous liver biopsy
9. Liver biopsies by peritoneoscopy, if negative percutaneously
10. Laparotomy with splenectomy, wedge biopsy of liver, bone marrow biopsy and extensive tissue sampling, as indicated

[a] Modified from Johnson et al. (45).

histopathologic classification, the Ann Arbor staging system provides a widely used and widely acceptable language which can be applied today. The details of a routine staging evaluation are outlined in Table 2. Unfortunately, although it is widely used in clinical trials currently under way, and those under consideration, neither the Ann Arbor classification nor a common method of staging or restaging was used in most of the controlled or uncontrolled trials reported in the literature.

In order to provide background information to allow the reader to interpret the results of controlled clinical trials using the older histopathologic language, a short overview of data available from uncontrolled trials will be provided. Since it was not possible for these reviewers to transfer data from published work into the Rappaport classification or the Ann Arbor staging system, the data are presented as originally described by the authors in the various publications cited. This limits the validity of the conclusions drawn by the authors but, wherever possible, we have tried to distill the essence of the publications that appear applicable across histopathologic classifications. Thus, much of the information is presented in the older designations, lymphosarcoma (LSA), reticulum cell sarcoma (RCS), and giant follicular lymphoma. Further, in many of the studies, patients were staged without the benefit of lymphangiography. Childhood lymphoma, a disease whose natural history is markedly different from the adult variety, will not be discussed (46,84).

## INFORMATION DERIVED FROM PAST APPROACHES TO THERAPY

### Single-Agent Chemotherapy

The chemotherapeutic responsiveness of the lymphocytic and histiocytic lymphomas has been appreciated for some time and has recently been reviewed (13,85). The use of drugs as single agents represented the treatment of choice until the late 1960s, when combination chemotherapy gained prominence. A summary of the experience with single agents for both lymphocytic and histio-

TABLE 3. *Single-agent chemotherapy of histiocytic lymphoma*[a]

| Drug | Average dose | Evaluable patients | Overall response rate (%) | Reference |
|------|--------------|--------------------|---------------------------|-----------|
| Nitrogen mustard | 0.4 mg/kg q. 4 weeks; i.v. | 5 | 20 | 89 |
| | | 6 | 16 | 35 |
| Cyclophosphamide | 3–4 mg/kg q. day X 5; i.v. or p.o. | 11 | 78 | 72 |
| | | 33 | 79 | 80 |
| | | 15 | 66 | 83 |
| | | 66 | 42 | 40 |
| | | 33 | 54 | 18 |
| Vincristine | 0.025–0.075 mg/kg q. week; i.v. | 10 | 100 | 76 |
| | | 58 | 75 | 23 |
| | | 32 | 37 | 18 |
| Vinblastine | 0.10–0.15 mg/kg q. week; i.v. | 5 | 60 | 90 |
| | | 8 | 25 | 8 |
| | | 17 | 35 | 83 |
| Procarbazine | 2–3 mg/kg q. day; p.o. | 4 | 25 | 14 |
| | | 6 | 33 | 37 |
| | | 5 | 20 | 73 |
| Adriamycin | 45–75 mg/m² q. 3 weeks; i.v. | 13 | 54 | 67 |
| | | 50 | 48 | 9 |
| Bleomycin | 10–15 mg/m² 2 X week; i.v. or i.m. | 22 | 36 | 27 |
| | | 20 | 45 | 10 |
| Bis-chlorethyl nitrosourea | 250 mg/m² q. 6–8 weeks; i.v. | 24 | 33 | 19 |
| Imidazole carboxamide | 250 mg/m² q. day X 5; i.v. | 13 | 0 | 30 |
| VM-26 | 30 mg/m² q. day X 5; i.v. | 22 | 36 | 69 |
| VP-16213 | 60 mg/m² q. day X 5; i.v. | 21 | 19 | 69 |

[a] Modified from (13).

cytic lymphomas is found in Tables 3 and 4. Whereas response rates are surprisingly high in some instances, they generally represent only partial regressions of disease lasting 1 to 3 months. However, a common thread of information runs through the response data, and some interesting conclusions have been drawn which are probably valid, in spite of the uncontrolled nature of most of these trials. Complete tumor regressions occurred significantly more frequently in patients with nodular lymphomas, using single drugs, than with diffuse lymphoma and were usually of longer duration. Responses and survival correlated closely with the histopathology of the lymphoma, when the information was available, ranging from a 5% complete response rate in DHL to a 48% complete response rate in NPDL (48). Following the example of Hodgkin's disease and acute lymphocytic leukemia, investigators soon began to combine active single agents into combination chemotherapy protocols for the non-Hodgkin's lymphomas.

TABLE 4. *Single-agent chemotherapy of lymphocytic lymphoma*[a]

| Drug | Average dose | Evaluable patients | Overall response rate (%) | Reference |
|------|-------------|--------------------|---------------------------|-----------|
| Nitrogen mustard | 0.4 mg/kg | 15 | 86 | 7 |
| | q. 4 weeks; i.v. | 17 | 52 | 82 |
| | | 18 | 44 | 41 |
| | | 20 | 60 | 35 |
| Cyclophosphamide | 3–4 mg/kg | 21 | 71 | 88 |
| | q. day × 5; i.v. or p.o. | 56 | 66 | 18 |
| Vincristine | 0.025–0.075 mg/kg | 47 | 38 | 18 |
| | q. week; i.v. | | | |
| Vinblastine | 0.10–0.15 mg/kg | 8 | 12 | 90 |
| | q. week; i.v. | 13 | 23 | 22 |
| Adriamycin | 45–75 mg/m² | 16 | 44 | 67 |
| | q. 3 weeks; i.v. | 44 | 32 | 9 |
| Bleomycin | 10–15 mg/m² | 17 | 41 | 27 |
| | 2 × week; i.v. or i.m. | 17 | 47 | 10 |
| Bis-chlorethyl | 200 mg/m² | 7 | 29 | 71 |
| nitrosourea | q. 6–8 weeks; i.v. | 63 | 19 | 19 |
| Imidazole | 250 mg/m² | 15 | 27 | 30 |
| carboxamide | q. day × 5; i.v. | | | |
| Prednisone | 1–4 mg/kg | 47 | 74 | 58 |
| | q. day; p.o. | | | |
| VM-26 | 30 mg/m² | 12 | 58 | 69 |
| | q. day × 5; i.v. | | | |
| VP-16213 | 60 mg/m² | 7 | 28 | 69 |
| | q. day × 5; i.v. | | | |

[a] Modified from (13).

TABLE 5. *Combination chemotherapy protocols for histiocytic lymphoma*[a]

| Combination | Evaluable patients | CR (%) | Median duration of CR (mo.) | Reference |
|-------------|--------------------|--------|-----------------------------|-----------|
| CVP | 66 | 39 | 5.5 | 61 |
| MOPPr | 8 | 38 | 32+ | 59 |
| COPPr | 17 | 41 | 41+ | 24 |
| VP-araC, MTX (COMA) | 15 | 60 | 10 | 56 |
| CVP-BCNU | 67 | 30 | 21 | 26 |
| BCVP | 17 | 59 | NE | 60 |
| CV-MTX (MEV) | 14 | 93 | 16+ | 52 |
| CHOP | 60 | 68 | NR | 65 |
| HOP | 72 | 67 | NR | 65 |
| BCHOP (BACOP) | 24 | 43 | 8+ | 75 |
| MHBOP (MABOP) | 30 | 55 | 11+ | 13 |

[a] Modified from (13).

Abbreviations: C, cyclophosphamide; V or O, vincristine; P, prednisone; M, nitrogen mustard; PR, procarbazine; ara-C, cytosine arabinoside; MTX, methotrexate; BCNU, bis-chloroethyl nitrosourea; B, bleomycin; H-adriamycin; NE, not evaluable; and NR, not yet reached. Drug doses and schedules are detailed in the cited reference.

TABLE 6. *Combination chemotherapy protocols for lymphocytic lymphoma*[a]

| Combination | Evaluable patients | CR (%) | Median duration of CR (mo.) | Reference |
|---|---|---|---|---|
| CVP | 74 | 50 | 8.6 | 61 |
| CVP | 35 | 57 | 85% at 2 years | 3 |
| CVP | 33 | 39 | 19 | 78 |
| MOPP | 15 | 47 | 11.7+ | 59 |
| COPP | 12 | 25 | 7.5 | 66 |
| BCVP | 31 | 60 | NE | 60 |
| CV-MTX (MEV) | 16 | 56 | 13+ | 52 |
| CHOP | 118 | 72 | NR | 65 |
|  | 7 | 86 | NR | 36 |
| HOP | 114 | 69 | NR | 65 |
| MHBOP (MABOP) | 25 | 64 | 14+ | 13 |

[a]Modified from (13).
See Table 5 for abbreviations. Drug doses and schedules are detailed in the cited reference.

## Combination Chemotherapy

Multiple-drug combinations have been employed for the therapy of lymphocytic and histiocytic lymphoma since the late 1960s, and these are summarized in Tables 5 and 6 for each respective cell type. The influence of histopathologic subtypes is incompletely analyzed in relation to the patient's response to therapy and subsequent survival, further emphasizing the necessity for uniform histopathology, staging, and restaging for evaluation of treatment response.

## Past Radiotherapy Studies

Historical data suggest that approximately 20% of all patients with lymphocytic and histiocytic lymphomas on completion of staging had disease localized to one or two lymphatic areas (47). Survival data reported in the literature consistently show that approximately half of these patients survive 5 years (57). Thus, one can conclude from the early literature that approximately 10% of all patients with the lymphocytic and histiocytic lymphomas were curable by techniques of radiotherapy available in the 1950s and the 1960s. Although it is clear from the available data that radiotherapy is capable of sterilizing tumor in the treatment field in both the histiocytic and lymphocytic lymphomas, the usefulness of radiotherapy alone has been questioned by data now available from a variety of staging studies at major centers throughout the world. These studies, without exception, show that the great majority of patients staged either with laparotomy (33,86) or by a sequence of studies leading up to laparotomy (20) have evidence of widely disseminated disease at presentation not likely to be curable by the application of local radiotherapy. Furthermore, although derived from uncontrolled clinical trials, it can be concluded from the available data, particularly the studies from Stanford (47), that there is little evidence that extending radiation fields to total nodal therapy has influenced relapse-free survival of patients with Stage I and II lymphocytic and histiocytic lymphoma, both nodular and diffuse. Radiotherapy has been used to effect bulk reduction of tumor in patients with more advanced stages of the lymphocytic and histiocytic lymphoma with some success; however, controlled trials have not been conducted in this area. A role for total body irradiation has been suggested by Johnson (43,44), and the results of controlled trials using this modality will be reported later. In general, the true role of radiotherapy *vis-à-vis* chemotherapy of patients with both localized and advanced lymphocytic and histiocytic lymphomas is unclear at the moment and deserves further attention.

## RANDOMIZED CLINICAL TRIALS

### Single-Agent Chemotherapy

There are several randomized clinical trials comparing the effects of single chemotherapeutic agents in lymphocytic and histiocytic lymphomas, and these are summarized in Table 7. With the exception of the study of Solomon et al. (81), all the trials were carried out without stratifying patients according to stage or histopathologic classification, and none employed the Rappaport scheme. Patients were generally classified as LSA or RCS, although one study (18) also stratified according to prior therapy. Further, the definition of a response was unclear. Partial responses ranged from "excellent" or "good" (51) to greater than 20% (82,87) or greater than 33% (83); in some of the studies complete and partial remissions were properly defined, using current criteria, but were not reported separately (35). Only the studies by Carbone and Spurr (18) and Solomon et al. (81) reported partial and complete remissions separately. In addition, careful restaging as a criterion for defining a complete or partial remission was not carried out in any of these studies. Whereas investigators generally employed the drug nitrogen mustard ($HN_2$) in a uniform fashion, there is great variability in the dose and routes of administration for the other commonly used alkylating agent, cyclophosphamide (CTX). However, in spite of these problems with both design and language, a number of conclusions can safely be drawn from these studies (Table 7).

For remission induction, $HN_2$ and CTX emerged as active single agents for both LSA and RCS. The periwinkle alkaloids, vincristine (VCR) and vinblastine (VLB), appear to be less effective than the alkylating agents, although neither 6-diazo-5-oxo-L-norleucine (DON) nor uracil mustard were impressively active. Previously treated patients, particularly those receiving chemotherapy, had lower response rates than patients with no prior therapy. This area was examined in more detail in the study of Carbone and Spurr (18), in which patients previously

TABLE 7. *Randomized single-agent trials in non-Hodgkin's lymphoma*

| Histology | Prior therapy | Agents compared | Maintenance | No. patients | Response rate (%) CR | Response rate (%) PR | Median duration of response (mo.) | Conclusions | Reference |
|---|---|---|---|---|---|---|---|---|---|
| LSA; RCS | RT | DON | No | 19 | 0 | 10 | NE | HN$_2$ superior to DON | 87 |
| | | HN$_2$ | No | | 17 | 30 | | | |
| LSA | NS | CTX | No | 17 | 6 | 66 | NE | CTX not significantly better than HN$_2$ for LSA | 82 |
| | | HN$_2$ | No | 17 | 0 | 54 | | | |
| "Malignant lymphoma" | Chemotherapy; RT | CTX | No | 11 | NE | 45 | NS | In the combined lymphoma group, HN$_2$ appeared to be more effective than CTX and MM | 51 |
| | | HN$_2$ | | 14 | NE | 57 | | | |
| | | MM | | 13 | NE | 54 | | | |
| LSA | Chemotherapy; RT | CTX | No | 12 | 25 | 32 | NE | CTX significantly better than VLB in both histologies | 83 |
| | | VLB | | 6 | 0 | 37 | | | |
| RCS | Chemotherapy; RT | CTX | No | 8 | 0 | 63 | | | |
| | | VLB | | 11 | 8 | 23 | | | |
| LSA | Chemotherapy; RT | HN$_2$ | CLB | 18 | NE | 44 | 7.5 | HN$_2$ and CTX comparable for LSA; CTX "somewhat more efficacious" in RCS | 41 |
| | | CTX | CTX | 19 | NE | 47 | 3 | | |
| RCS | Chemotherapy; RT | HN$_2$ | CLB | 5 | NE | 0 | — | | |
| | | CTX | CTX | 7 | NE | 71 | 3 | | |
| LSA | RT | CTX | No | 17 | NE | 76 | NS | CTX most effective in both LSA and RCS, but median | 34,35 |

| Histology | Prior therapy | Agent | Control | No. | Median (mo.) | % | Ratio | Comments | Ref. |
|---|---|---|---|---|---|---|---|---|---|
| | RT | UM | | 13 | NE | 23 | | survival of all LSA patients treated with CTX (7.3 mo.) was shorter than those treated with HN₂ (14+ mo.) | |
| | | HN₂ | | 20 | NE | 60 | | | |
| RCS | RT | CTX | No | 10 | NE | 40 | | | |
| | | UM | | 6 | NE | 17 | | | |
| | | HN₂ | | 6 | NE | 17 | NS | | 18 |
| LSA | Chemotherapy or none | CTX | CTX | 56 | 10.4 | 58 | 2.8 | CTX more effective than VCR in LSA, but not in RCS. Untreated patients responded better than previously treated patients. Duration of CR not affected by maintenance, but duration of PR is. | |
| | | VCR | Placebo | 47 | 6.3 | 32 | 1.6 | | |
| | | | CTX | | | | 4 | | |
| | | | Placebo | | | | 1 | | |
| RCS | Chemotherapy or none | CTX | CTX | 33 | 12 | 39 | 3.2 | | |
| | | VCR | Placebo | 32 | 12 | 25 | 1.2 | | |
| | | | CTX | | | | 2.5 | | |
| | | | Placebo | | | | 1 | | |
| LSA | Chemotherapy; RT | HN₂ | No | 18 | 5.6 | 44 | 16.5 | VLB and HN₂ are comparable in RCS or LSA as initial inducing agents. Duration of HN₂ responses in LSA significantly longer than with CTX. Nodular PDL was most responsive histology. | 81 |
| | | VLB | | 23 | 4.4 | 30 | 2.3 | | |
| RCS | Chemotherapy; RT | HN₂ | No | 26 | 7.7 | 27 | 3.6 | | |
| | | VLB | | 20 | 10 | 35 | 2.3 | | |

The abbreviations used are identical to those used in Tables 5 and 6 with the following additions: LSA, lymphosarcoma; RCS, reticulum cell sarcoma; RT, radiotherapy; DON, 6-diazo-5-oxo-L-norleucine; CLB, chlorambucil; UM, uracil mustard; MM, mannitol mustard; CR, complete remission; PR, partial remission; NS, not stated; and PDL, poorly differentiated lymphocytic lymphoma.

TABLE 8. *Randomized combination chemotherapy trials in non-Hodgkin's lymphoma*

| Histology | Prior therapy | Agents compared | Maintenance | No. patients | Response rate (%) CR | Response rate (%) PR | Median duration of response (mo.) | Conclusions | Reference |
|---|---|---|---|---|---|---|---|---|---|
| LSA | RT | CTX, CVP-high, CVP-low | MTX or placebo | 14, 16, 21 | 21, 31, 38 | 21, 69, 52 | NE | CVP better than CTX for LSA but only CVP-high better than CTX for RCS. CVP-high vs. CVP-low only better in RCS. MTX no better than placebo for maintenance. | 39 |
| RCS | RT | CTX, CVP-high, CVP-low | MTX or placebo | 11, 13, 13 | 9, 31, 31 | 36, 54, 23 | NE | | |
| LSA | NS | V, SN-CTX, P; V, CTX, P, SN; VP | No, No, CTX | 63, 60, 65 | 38, 45, 54 | 33, 33, 31 | NS | VP with CTX maintenance offers the best control of LSA and RCS. There were no significant differences among response durations. | 38 |
| RCS | NS | V, SN-CTX, P; V, CTX, P, SN; VP | No, No, CTX | 52, 47, 47 | 33, 43, 43 | 25, 19, 31 | NS | | |
| LSA | Chemotherapy; RT | COP | COP, None | 17, 15 | 50 | 38 | 10.7, 4.7 | Only maintenance randomized. For LSA, COP maintenance significantly prolonged length of CR. For RCS, no difference observed. | 61 |
| RCS | | COP | COP, None | 11, 8 | 39 | 39 | 5.3, 5.5 | | |
| NHL-ST. IA and IIA Lymphocytic | NS | NS | BCG, None | 7, 5 | NE, NE | NE, NE | 20, 7.5 | Only maintenance randomized. BCG appeared to prolong remission duration but the difference is not statistically significant. | 79 |
| Histiocytic | NS | NS | BCG, None | 5, 2 | NE, NE | NE, NE | 7, 1.5 | | |
| DHL ST. III and IV | NS | CTX, P; CVP | No, No | NS, NS | 23, 32 | 14, 14 | NS | VCR or BCNU add nothing to CTX, P but increase hematologic | 4, 53 |

| Diagnosis/Stage | Prior therapy | Treatment | Maintenance | No. | | | Survival (mos) | Comments | Ref |
|---|---|---|---|---|---|---|---|---|---|
| NHL ST. III and IV | No | CVP-BCNU | No | NS | 33 | 18 | | toxicity. Median survival same for all treatment groups. CHOP and HOP are essentially comparable. Nodular lymphomas more likely to achieve CR than diffuse. Of CR, histiocytic more likely to relapse. Maintenance arms identical to date. | 21,65,77 |
| | | CHOP | COP OP-ara-C | 142 | 64 | 22 | NR | | |
| | | HOP | COP OP-ara-C | 145 | 57 | 26 | NR | | |
| Lymphocytic- ST. III and IV | NS | CVP | No | 23 | 43 | NE | 13+ | The survival in either arm was not different. The response rate for either therapy was similar for NPDL, but single agent therapy was less effective for DPDL. | 50 |
| | | C-V-P | No | 22 | 46 | NE | 20+ | | |
| NHL-ST. IV Histiocytic | RT | CVP | No | 13 | 38 | NS | 6 | CVP better than HBP for lymphocytic but not histiocytic lymphoma. Nodular lymphoma had higher CR than diffuse with CVP but not HBP. | 12 |
| | | HBP | | 14 | 43 | NS | 2.5 | | |
| Lymphocytic | | CVP | | 11 | 55 | NS | 5 | | |
| | | HBP | | 11 | 36 | NS | 5 | | |
| NHL ST. III and IV | Chemotherapy; RT | CVP | CV None | 54 | 43 | 39 | 8.4 | CVP gave better CR rate, duration of first remission, and survival than CV. Response rate not influenced by histology, but survival is. Maintenance with CV prolonged disease-free interval, but not survival. | 54 |
| | | CV | CV None | 59 | 17 | 53 | 5.4 | | |
| Lymphocytic- ST. III and IV | Chemotherapy; RT | CP | CVP-BCNU CLB | 135 | 19 | 37 | NR | Overall CR and PR comparable with CP and BCNU-P. Nodular lymphomas responded equally well with CP or BCNU-P, but diffuse lymphomas responded significantly better to CP (73% vs. 44%). Prior chemotherapy significantly reduced CR rate. | 28 |
| | | BCNU-P | CVP-BCNU CLB | 138 | 23 | 44 | NR | | |

TABLE 8 (Continued)

| Histology | Prior therapy | Agents compared | Maintenance | No. patients | Response rate (%) | | Median duration of response (mo.) | Conclusions | Reference |
|---|---|---|---|---|---|---|---|---|---|
| | | | | | CR | PR | | | |
| NHL-ST. III and IV Lymphocytic | Chemotherapy | MTX-HBOP (6)<br>MTX-HBOP (2) | Yes | 14<br>11 | 64<br>18 | 22<br>18 | 15<br>14 | For histiocytic lymphoma 2 cycles as effective as 6 cycles. In lymphocytic lymphoma, 6 cycles much more effective. CR in nodular or diffuse histology were equally likely. Median duration of CR same for 6 or 2 cycles, but longer in nodular vs. diffuse histology. | 11 |
| Histiocytic | | MTX-HBOP (6)<br>MTX-HBOP (2) | Yes | 29<br>28 | 55<br>50 | 24<br>25 | 9<br>7 | | |
| Lymphocytic-ST. III and IV | Chemotherapy; RT | CVP-BCNU,<br>HN₂ | CLB<br>CLB, P<br>CTX<br>CTX, P | 33 | 75 | 13 | 22 | No benefit for 5-drug combination over 2-drug combination in design where all patients placed on maintenance. P added nothing to CTX or CLB for maintenance. | 49 |
| | | HN₂, P | CLB<br>CLB, P<br>CTX<br>CTX, P | 30 | 77 | 14 | 22+ | | |
| NHL-DHL | NS | CVP + ara-C<br>MOPP | Same<br>Same | 70<br>38 | 34<br>32 | —<br>— | 28.7<br>13.6 | The overall response rates to CVP with or without ara-C comparable to MOPP in total pt. group. Separate analysis of CVP with or without ara-C data not available. | 21 |
| NPDL | | CVP + ara-C<br>MOPP | Same<br>Same | 14<br>11 | 64<br>36 | —<br>— | 24<br>NR | | |

The abbreviations used are identical to those used in Tables 5–7 with the following additions: SN, streptonigrin; ST, Stage; NHL, non-Hodgkin's lymphoma; DHL, diffuse histiocytic lymphoma; DPDL, diffuse, poorly differentiated lymphocytic lymphoma; NPDL, nodular PDL; and MTX-HBOP (2) or (6), 2 or 6 cycles of induction chemotherapy.

treated with either RCS or LSA failed to achieve a complete remission (CR) with either CTX or VCR induction. Moreover, the partial remission (PR) rate in this group was one-third or less than the PR rate in the no-prior-treatment group. Cross-resistance was examined in the study of Solomon et al. (81) using a crossover design so that $HN_2$ induction failures were reinduced with VLB and vice versa. None of the LSA patients initially treated with $HN_2$ and crossed over to VLB responded to therapy, whereas 50% of the group initially failing VLB induction subsequently responded to $HN_2$. For RCS, 25% of patients who initially failed $HN_2$ induction subsequently responded to VLB, whereas 36% of VLB induction failures subsequently responded to $HN_2$. The author concluded that VLB and $HN_2$ were comparable for initial induction in the therapy of RCS or LSA. They were able to subclassify their patients by histology, thus allowing an analysis of differential response rates. Twenty-five patients with DHL, 11 with diffuse, poorly differentiated lymphocytic lymphoma (DPDL), and 13 with NPDL were evaluated. The authors concluded that the behavior of NPDL was distinct from DHL and DPDL in that a greater proportion of patients could be induced into a CR or PR with either VLB or $HN_2$.

Maintenance chemotherapy following remission induction is built into the studies by both Jacobs et al. (41) and Carbone and Spurr (18); however, only the latter investigators examined its role in a randomized fashion. Following induction chemotherapy with either vinca alkaloids or alkylating agents, patients were randomized to one of three maintenance arms: placebo, daily oral CTX, or intermittent intravenous CTX. They concluded that the duration of CTX-maintained remissions was at least twice as long as those maintained by a placebo. Intermittent CTX appeared superior to daily CTX for maintenance in LSA, with median survivals of 120 weeks versus 59 weeks, respectively, and 64% versus 28% of patients alive at 2 years. Similar differences for the RCS group were not apparent, with median survivals of 47 and 36 weeks, respectively. Statistical analyses, however, were not reported by the authors. The authors concluded that whereas the duration of PR was affected by maintenance, the duration of CR were not. Thus, the single-agent trials establish a role for alkylating agent therapy, emphasize the importance of achieving a complete response on survival, suggest differences in response based on histology, and imply some role for maintenance therapy, particularly in patients achieving only a PR to induction.

### Combination Chemotherapy

Many of the studies employing combination chemotherapy are either still in progress or have been reported only in preliminary or abstract form, precluding a detailed analysis in many cases. Data from all the published studies are presented in Table 8. The earlier studies (38,39) do not stratify patients by stage in the Ann Arbor classification or by histopathology in any classification, making conclusions drawn from the data open to question. Of the studies that do report

initial stage and histology, the work of Lenhard and Pocock (53) and that of
Kaufman et al. (49) do not stratify response by initial stage of disease. Only
the studies by Bonadonna et al. (11,12) and by the Southwestern Group (21,65,77)
allow a separate analysis of response for histiocytic and lymphocytic histology.
However, the significance of the nodularity or diffuseness of the tumor is somewhat obscured by small patient numbers in the Bonadonna study. Similarly,
small patient numbers obscure a detailed analysis of the maintenance arms in
the study of Kaufman et al. (49). An evaluation of the effectiveness of a particular
drug combination requires knowledge of the CR and PR rates, as well as the
median durations of response and survival from the onset of chemotherapy.
Further, rigorous restaging of patients following induction therapy to allow
accurate assessments of CR and PR rates is essential. Only Bonadonna et al.
(12) rigorously restaged their patients. Such a lack of restaging would be likely
to spuriously elevate complete remission rates. This might explain the 75 to
77% CR rate reported by Kaufman et al. (49) with a lower (57%) figure reported
by Bagley et al. (3) in a similar population of patients who had been restaged
following induction chemotherapy.

Induction chemotherapy was examined in a number of these randomized
trials. The only trial comparing a single agent (CTX) with a three-drug combination (CTX, VCR, and prednisone, P) showed superiority for the latter (39).
Moreover, this observation is consistent with the improved activity of combinations over single agents using "historical" controls. The study by Kennedy et
al. (50) compared successive CTX, VCR, and P with the same three-drug combination (CVP) in advanced lymphocytic lymphoma and observed no difference
in overall survival. However, attention to histologic subclassification revealed
that the response rate for either therapy was comparable for NPDL, but that
single agents were less effective for DPDL. The role of VCR in the CVP combination was questioned in a study by Lenhard and Pocock (53). In advanced DHL,
CTX, and P gave a 23% CR rate compared to 32% for CVP with identical
PR rates. The CR rates do not differ significantly from each other or from
that obtained by adding a nitrosourea, BCNU, to the CVP combination. More
recently, CVP was compared with CTX-VCR with clear superiority demonstrated for the three-drug combination (54). In yet another variation, CTX-P
was compared with BCNU-P for remission induction in advanced lymphocytic
lymphoma. Whereas overall CR and PR rates were comparable (19% and 23%,
respectively), diffuse lymphomas responded significantly better (73% versus
44%) to CTX-P (28). These conclusions should be tempered by the fact that
the response rates and survival data reported by these authors appears worse
for both types of treatment than that reported by others. Studies by Bonadonna
et al. (11) and Kaufman et al. (49) were designed to examine the role of the
intensity of remission induction in achieving a CR. Its role in survival could
not be interpreted, as both studies had maintenance arms. Bonadonna et al.
used a five-drug combination randomizing to two or six cycles for induction.
Although the data are preliminary, they concluded that two cycles were as

effective as six in histiocytic lymphoma, but that six were much more effective in lymphocytic lymphoma. However, statistical analyses have not been reported. Kaufman et al. compared another five-drug combination with a two-drug combination in lymphocytic lymphoma and found no advantage for the more intensive induction. However, the effect of maintenance on DPDL, NPDL, and DHL appears to vary with each respective histology, as will be discussed, and compounds a simple interpretation of these data.

Cross-resistance of drug combinations was examined by Bonadonna et al. (12) using two combinations, CVP and HBP (adriamycin, bleomycin, and P) made up of drugs that are different and have different mechanisms of action. They observed that 68% of patients responded to CVP initially, whereas only 43% responded after failing HBP. Similarly, 81% of patients responding to HBP initially, whereas only 75% responded after failing CVP. The authors conclude that this data suggests lack of cross-resistance between the two combinations. As the pattern of DPDL and NPDL is one of CR followed by relapse and eventual refractoriness to the primary combination, the availability of an active secondary induction combination is extremely useful.

The role of maintenance drug treatment after induction of either a CR or PR was examined by several investigators. Hoogstraten et al. (39) were not able to demonstrate a significant effect of drug maintenance in LSA or RCS, but did observe that the median duration of methotrexate-maintained remissions was twice as long as those maintained by a placebo (100 versus 49 days, respectively). Luce et al. (61) induced all their patients with an identical combination, but randomized all CR patients to maintenance chemotherapy or no further therapy. They observed a difference approaching significance ($p = 0.06$) for LSA, but no difference in median duration of CR for the disease they called RCS. Sokal, Aungst, and Snyderman (79) examined the effect of immunotherapy on remission duration. They accrued patients already in remission at varying times following their initial treatment, either radiotherapy or chemotherapy, and randomly allocated them to receive BCG vaccinations or no therapy. They observed that for all malignant lymphomas, including Hodgkin's disease, a significant prolongation of the mean time to relapse occurred in the BCG group; however, when only non-Hodgkin's lymphomas were examined, a significant difference was not observed. These observations are mentioned because of the paucity of immunotherapy data in the literature and must be viewed as inconclusive. The practice of selecting patients at various times after treatment for their illness automatically preselects a population of patients who have remained disease-free beyond the high-risk period of recurrence and is not to be recommended in clinical trials evaluating adjuvant treatment. The role of maintenance chemotherapy is also being examined in an ongoing Southwestern Group Study (21, 65,77). Following either HBP or HBP-CTX induction, patients achieving a CR were randomized to CVP or VCR, arabinosyl cytosine (ara-C), and P maintenance. Of 115 patients maintained on COP, 75% remained in CR at 1 year. For the 108 patients maintained on VCR, ara-C, and P, 60% remained at 1 year. Although these results do not differ, further analysis by histology is required. The study by Lenhard et al. (54) examined the role of CTX-VCR maintenance versus none in advanced-stage non-Hodgkin's lymphoma. Maintenance was found to prolong the duration of either a CR or PR and thus extend mean remission times from 4.8 months to 12.8 months for maintained patients. However, the overall survival was 46.4 months and 47.8 months, respectively, and does not differ significantly. This observation is quite consistent with the previously reported (29,91) observation in Hodgkin's disease that maintenance therapy prolongs the disease-free interval without affecting survival. The study of Ezdinli et al. (28) compares the role of a four-drug "intensive" maintenance with a single alkylating agent, chlorambucil (CLB) in remission duration of lymphocytic lymphoma. Of 115 patients who achieved either a CR or PR, 53 received the four-drug combination and 62 received CLB. For PR patients, 49% relapsed on CLB versus 16% on the four-drug combination ($p < 0.05$). For CR patients, 17% relapsed on CLB versus 7% on the four-drug combination, but these results do not differ significantly. The study by Kaufman et al. (49) examines the role of prednisone plus an alkylating agent in the maintenance of remissions in advanced lymphocytic lymphomas. The authors observed that 63% of those patients receiving an alkylating agent plus prednisone versus 68% of those receiving an alkylating agent alone were in remission at 18 months. These same authors also examined the role of prior treatment, either radiotherapy or chemotherapy, on remission duration and found that 80% of patients receiving no prior treatment versus 47% receiving prior treatment were in remission at 12 months ($p < 0.01$). They extended this analysis to examine the role of histology on remission duration and survival and found that nodular or diffuse histologies did not predict for a better response to treatment.

These studies suggest that several drug combinations are active in the non-Hodgkin's lymphomas and that tumor histology is an important determinant of which combinations are most active. Moreover, CR and PR rates and durations of CR and survival are closely correlated with histology. The role of maintenance seems to be limited to patients achieving only a PR to treatment in that their disease-free interval is favorably influenced. However, convincing evidence that maintenance, as opposed to reinduction at the time of progression, is superior is lacking.

### Chemotherapy—Radiotherapy

Four studies have been reported in this area, but two are too preliminary to allow conclusions to be drawn (Table 9). The remaining studies from Stanford (68) and the National Cancer Institute (16,92) are not yet complete, but a number of conclusions may be drawn from the data. The Stanford study (68) is well stratified and well designed and examines only Stage IV favorable histology lymphocytic lymphoma patients who have been carefully staged before treatment and restaged before assessing the completenes of their response. The authors

TABLE 9. *Randomized chemotherapy-radiotherapy trials in non-Hodgkin's lymphoma*

| Histology | Prior therapy | Regimens compared | Maintenance | No. patients | Response rate (%) | | Median duration of response (mo.) | Conclusions | Reference |
|---|---|---|---|---|---|---|---|---|---|
| | | | | | CR | PR | | | |
| Lymphocytic ST. IV (DWDL, NML, and NPDL) | No | CVP CVP-TLI CTX or CLB(SA) | CVP CVP CTX or CLB | 23 20 20 | 78 65 55 | 22 30 40 | NR NR NR | All three arms are equally effective in achieving responses and prolonged disease-free survivals. CVP-TLI is no better than CVP or SA and is more toxic. | 68 |
| NHL-ST. II, III, and IV | No | CVP or COPP RT | No No | 50 49 | 54 80 | 32 10 | 21-nodular 11-diffuse 26-nodular 17-diffuse | There is no overall difference in remission induction or survival at 4 years of follow-up with CVP or RT. Also, nodular vs. diffuse or subgroups of Stage IV do equally well on either treatment. | 16,92 |
| Lymphocytic & Histiocytic-ST. I, I$_E$, II and II$_E$ | No | IFR IFR-CVP | No No | 26 27 | 69 78 | NE NE | NR NR | No difference in relapse rate between either arm to date. Lymphocytic and histiocytic histologies did equally well. New lesions occurred more frequently in diffuse vs. nodular histology. | 13 |
| NHL-ST. III & IV | No | CVP or COPP TBI + CVP or COPP | No No | 16 18 | 67 64 | NS NS | NR NR | Follow-up is too short for meaningful conclusions (median = 14 mo.), but initial response rates are similar to either modality alone. | 92 |

Abbreviations not previously used in Tables 5–8 are as follows: DWDL, diffuse well-differentiated lymphocytic lymphoma; NML, nodular mixed lymphoma; TLI, total lymphoid irradiation; SA, single alkylating agent; RT, radiotherapy including 21 total body (TBI), 11 total nodal, and 17 hemibody; and IFR, involved field radiotherapy.

randomized patients to chemotherapy with CVP, split-course CVP, and total nodal radiation therapy, or single-agent therapy with CLB. They suggest that all three treatment programs are effective in achieving "excellent" responses and prolonged disease-free survival, but hasten to point out that the addition of radiotherapy to combination chemotherapy does not appear to improve the duration of CR and may be beginning to have ($p = 0.07$) an adverse effect on survival compared to CVP alone or single-agent therapy. Current data show that the CR rate with CVP in this study is 85% compared to 65% with CLB and that remission induction with CVP is more rapid than with CLB. It should be noted that the complete remission rate with CLB is higher than that reported in controlled or uncontrolled studies in the past, which may be a function of patient selection. CVP and CLB appear to be equally effective at this time in influencing survival in these histologies, but these data are too preliminary to draw conclusions about the effects of treatment on survival.

The study from the National Cancer Institute (16,92) again reflects attention to histology and stage in that patients are stratified by the histopathologic scheme of Rappaport. In this study there is a difference in the assessment of the duration of complete response as the radiotherapy patients did not have repeated bone marrow and liver biopsies to determine if they were, in fact, truly disease-free. The authors, therefore, emphasize the complete remission rates in the two arms of the study (total body radiation versus CVP chemotherapy), and the overall survival at 4 years. The study was limited to patients who had DPDL, NPDL, nodular mixed, or nodular histiocytic lymphoma. At the 4-year point, there is comparable survival both in the nodular and diffuse lymphomas with either therapeutic modality, although there was an early difference in disease-free survival in the radiation therapy group that could be explained by the lack of precise restaging. The authors conclude that "there appears to be no advantage of one therapy over the other" in either achieving remission or in survival for those histologies studied.

The study of Bonadonna et al. (13) addresses the problem of early dissemination of "localized" non-Hodgkin's lymphoma following initial involved field radiotherapy. In a study begun in 1972, they randomized patients with limited-stage disease to receive radiation alone or radiation plus chemotherapy. To date, the CR rate and relapse rates do not differ in either arm, but additional follow-up will be required to see if they diverge with time. Of equal importance is the curability of these "limited"-stage disease patients, a point that will be indirectly answered by this study.

## NEW DIRECTIONS IN THERAPY

It is clear from the aforementioned studies that in spite of the fact that many thousands of patients have been placed on clinical trials, many of which were uncontrolled, little precise information is available. This is largely due to the failure of various authors to use the common approach to histopathologic subclassification, staging, restaging, and criteria for response. Recognition and correction of these defects alone in the design of future trials would very likely yield a wealth of new information on which to build additional clinical trials.

Currently, the following points can be stated with some confidence in spite of the weakness of the data. The lymphocytic lymphomas, particularly in the nodular form, are the more indolent of the non-Hodgkin's lymphomas. In most studies they comprise the group designated as "favorable histology." However, the best management for patients with various stages of lymphocytic lymphoma remains unclear. For patients with localized disease, nodular and diffuse, it appears certain that radiation therapy can cure a small fraction of patients, probably not more than 10 to 15% of the entire patient population that presents at any institution. Because of the indolent nature of these disorders, the median survival and 5- and 10-year survivals of patients who are not cured are still quite good. Thus, although it appears appropriate to examine the effect of some of the available drug combinations in conjunction with radiotherapy in the early stages of the lymphocytic lymphomas, particularly in the diffuse variety, these patients should be separated out from histiocytic lymphomas because of the differences in the natural history of the two diseases. Since there is no evidence that extending radiotherapy from an involved field to a total nodal field has any beneficial effect in terms of relapse-free or overall survival, it would appear most appropriate to examine the effect of involved field radiotherapy plus chemotherapy in comparably staged patients. Several such studies are now in progress.

The data previously reviewed suggest that for patients with advanced (Stages III and IV) lymphocytic lymphoma, both of the nodular and diffuse variety, combination chemotherapy produces a higher CR rate and that complete remissions are important in the overall survival of the patients. Recent data from Stanford suggest that single-agent chemotherapy may have greater efficacy than has been previously appreciated and this point remains to be clarified in further detail. There are now several drug combinations (Table 6) that have been shown to produce comparable overall response and CR rates. No single combination emerges as clearly superior in patients with advanced diffuse and nodular lymphocytic lymphoma. Since one of the prerequisites for the design of adjuvant chemotherapy studies should be the use of a known quantity, that is, a combination known to have a predictable effect in patients with advanced disease, it seems appropriate to recommend that such adjuvant studies employ one of the combinations listed in Table 6. Further information on which of the therapies is superior could be obtained by controlled clinical trials evaluating the efficacy of these combinations *used as reported by the authors.* The latter point is emphasized because of the propensity of the clinical investigators to partially adopt another's treatment program but to modify the dose and schedule of drugs, thus diluting the validity of any comparisons between the studies. Clearly, the use of current drug combinations in patients with advanced-stage lymphocytic lymphoma does not provide sufficient evidence to be confident that any of these patients are being cured of their disease, although one study (92) points out that more than 20% of patients with advanced nodular, poorly differentiated lymphocytic lymphoma remain relapse-free at 5 years of follow-up. Furthermore, with regard to radiotherapy, athough existing evidence does not suggest that further benefit can be derived from extending the treatment fields, it should be pointed out that the staging employed in the studies from which this information was derived was often inadequate. Thus, further studies in adequately staged patients should be used to reassess this point.

For the histiocytic lymphomas, several points can be gleaned from the literature. Uncontrolled trials suggest that, as in lymphocytic lymphoma, a small proportion of patients with localized disease can be cured by radiotherapy and that the addition of wide-field radiotherapy does not appear to provide any benefit. Clear separation between Stages I and II has been reported by the Stanford group; the 5-year disease-free survival for Stage I at Stanford and worldwide appears to hover around the 50% point for diffuse histiocytic lymphoma, whereas in patients with Stage II there is a sharp break in the curve with a disease-free survival of approximately 26%. In patients with Stage III and IV disease, there are now a number of drug combinations that have been shown to produce CR rates ranging from 30 to 93% (Table 5). The variability in CR rates may result from differences in sites of tumor involvement among patient populations. A most interesting phenomenon has been noted in these studies; a significant fraction of those patients who achieved a CR have remained free of disease for periods of follow-up extending up to 10 years. Most of these studies have also noted that all adverse events, namely, relapse and death, tend to occur within the first 2 years of study as opposed to the nodular and diffuse lymphocytic lymphomas which demonstrate a prolonged and continuous rate of relapse over 5 to 6 years. Therefore, there is substantial evidence that a significant fraction of patients with advanced (Stages III and IV) diffuse histiocytic lymphoma are curable with currently available drug combinations (24). A similar observation has been made in an uncontrolled trial by Young and co-workers in patients with nodular histiocytic lymphoma (92).

These observations should have a profound effect on the design of controlled clinical trials in patients with localized diffuse and nodular histiocytic lymphoma. It is clear from the data that the reported beneficial results in patients with advanced disease exceed those achievable in patients with Stage II disease in spite of the fact that the volume of tumor in the two categories of patients is strikingly different. In the view of these authors, there is sufficient evidence to hypothesize that currently available combination chemotherapy programs might be more beneficial than radiotherapy even in the management of patients with localized lymphomas, and this hypothesis should be tested in controlled clinical trials. For patients with Stage I diffuse histiocytic and nodular histiocytic lymphoma, randomization between involved field radiotherapy and involved field radiotherapy plus chemotherapy would seem appropriate. The chemotherapy selected for the latter studies should be one of the existing drug combinations already shown to produce durable complete remissions (Tables 5 and 8). For patients with Stage II disease, the role of chemotherapy *alone* should be evaluated. Such a study would involve randomization among three arms: involved field radiotherapy alone, involved field radiotherapy plus combination chemotherapy, and combination chemotherapy alone.

Although at least 10 drug combinations have been studied in patients with advanced diffuse histiocytic disease, there have been insufficient controlled clinical trials to determine the relative efficacy of any of the combinations. As mentioned earlier, this would be important information since it would allow investigators to select, with some confidence, the most efficacious combination for use in the adjuvant situation. It should be stressed again that it would be deemed an incorrect approach to an adjuvant study to select a totally unknown drug combination under the assumption that it would be as efficacious as those already shown to produce durable complete remissions. Therefore, controlled clinical trials testing the relative efficacy of C-MOPP (66), BACOP (75), CHOP (21), HOP (21), COMA (56), and MEV (52) would seem most appropriate. Selection of a standard "best" combination program would also assist in the development of clinical trials to identify combinations of new drugs or new premutations of existing drugs with or without immunotherapy in an attempt to improve the results of treatment in advanced disease. Rapid movement of a drug combination from those patients with advanced disease to studies in those with localized disease would be facilitated by development of such information in controlled clinical trials.

The efficacy of immunotherapy has not been fully studied in patients with lymphoma. As many patients in all subcategories of lymphoma achieve complete remissions with existing treatment and, therefore, have a reduced tumor volume, they provide particularly suitable subjects in whom to assess the role of immunotherapy on the maintenance of remission. Such studies are in progress and more should be developed.

Finally, the question of drug maintenance treatment has been addressed in some trials, but these studies suffer from the defect of not including an unmaintained control arm in patients who achieve a complete remission to determine not only if different forms of maintenance might be more beneficial, but if maintenance therapy itself is likely to be of benefit in each of the subcategories of non-Hodgkin's lymphoma. Studies directed at these problems will help to answer many nagging questions.

## SUMMARY

Interpretation of data from controlled and uncontrolled clinical trials in patients with non-Hodgkin's lymphoma has been severely hampered by the lack of a uniform language used by clinical investigators throughout the world. The recognition of this problem has led, in recent years, to the development of adequately designed controlled clinical trials which should yield valuable information. Many of these trials are either in their early stages or have been reported only in abstract form, which has hampered the interpretation of the data, in our view. Nonetheless, it is safe to conclude the following: (a) radiotherapy is effective in sterilizing tumor in a treatment field; (b) a number of chemotherapeutic agents have been developed that appear to have effects on both lymphocytic and histiocytic lymphoma alone, and (c) these effects appear to be magnified when the drugs are used in combination; (d) for patients with advanced, diffuse histiocytic lymphoma, the results from combination trials suggest that some patients may be cured with drug combinations; (e) the ability to achieve a significant fraction of complete remissions in patients with advanced non-Hodgkin's lymphoma offers a unique opportunity for testing the efficacy of immunotherapy as a form of final irradiation of cells or maintenance of drug-induced remissions; and (f) the availability of effective chemotherapy in patients with advanced disease offers the opportunity to test the effects of these programs in patients with localized disease treated with radiotherapy.

It is hoped that these conclusions will provide fertile ground for the development of future clinical trials that, hopefully, will rapidly advance the therapy of patients with non-Hodgkin's lymphoma.

## REFERENCES

1. Aisenberg, A. C., and Long, J. C. (1975): Lymphocyte surface characteristics in malignant lymphoma. *Am. J. Med.,* 58:300–306.
2. Anderson, T., Bender, R. A., Fisher, R. I., DeVita, V. T., Chabner, B. A., Bernard, C. W., Norton, L., and Young, R. C. (1977): Combination chemotherapy in non-Hodgkin's lymphoma: The results of long-term follow-up. *Cancer Treat. Rev.,* 61:1057–1066.
3. Bagley, C. M., DeVita, V. T., Berard, C. W., and Canellos, G. P. (1972): Advanced lymphosarcoma: Intensive cyclical combination chemotherapy with cyclophosphamide, vincristine, and prednisone. *Ann. Intern. Med.,* 76:227–234.
4. Bennett, J. M., Lenhard, R. E., Ezdinli, E., Johnson, G. J., Carbone, P. P., and Pocock, S. J. (1977): Chemotherapy of non-Hodgkin's lymphomas: The Eastern Cooperative Oncology Group experience. *Cancer Treatment Rev.,* 61:1079–1084, 1977.
5. Bennett, M. H., Farrer-Brown, G., Henry, K., and Jelliffe, A. M. (1974): Classification of non-Hodgkin's lymphomas. *Lancet,* II:405–406.
6. Berard, C. W. (1972): Histopathology of lymphoreticular disorders—conditions with malignant proliferative response—lymphoma. In: *Principles of Hematology,* edited by W. J. Williams, E. Beuther, A. J. Erslev, and R. W. Rundles, pp. 901–912. McGraw-Hill, New York.
7. Bierman, H., Shimkin, M., Mettier, S. R., Weaver, J., Berry, W. C. and Wise, S. P. (1949): Methyl-bis (beta-chlorethyl) amine in large doses in the treatment of neoplastic diseases. *Calif. Med.,* 71:117–125.
8. Bleehen, N. M., and Jelliffe, A. M. (1965): Vinblastine sulphate in the treatment of malignant disease. *Br. J. Cancer,* 19:268–273.
9. Blum, R. H., and Carter, S. K. (1974): Adriamycin. A new anticancer drug with significant clinical activity. *Ann. Intern. Med.,* 80:249–259.
10. Blum, R. H., Carter, S. K., and Agre, K. (1973): A clinical review of bleomycin—A new antineoplastic agent. *Cancer,* 31:903–914.
11. Bonadonna, G., DeLena, M., Lattuada, A., Milani, F., Monfardini, S., and Beretta, G. (1975): Combination chemotherapy and radiotherapy in non-Hodgkin's lymphomata. *Br. J. Cancer,* 31:481–488.
12. Bonadonna, G., DeLena, M., Monfardini, S., Rossi, A., Brambilla, C., Uslenghi, C., and Lucali, R. (1975): Combination usage of adriamycin (NSC-123127) in malignant lymphomas. *Cancer Chemother. Rep.,* 6:381–388.

13. Bonadonna, G., and Monfardini, S. (1974): Chemotherapy of non-Hodgkin's lymphomas. *Cancer Treat. Rev.,* 1:167–181.
14. Brunner, K. W., and Young, C. W. (1965): A methylhydrazine derivative in Hodgkin's disease and other malignant neoplasms. Therapeutic and toxic effects studied in 51 patients. *Ann. Intern. Med.,* 63:69–86.
15. Byrne, G. E., Rappaport, H. (1977): Classification of non-Hodgkin's Lymphoma: Histologic features and clinical significance. *Cancer Treat. Rev.,* 61:935–944.
16. Canellos, G. P., DeVita, V. T., Young, R. C., Chabner, B. A., Schein, P. S., and Johnson, R. E. (1975): Therapy of advanced lymphocytic lymphoma. A preliminary report of a randomized trial between combination chemotherapy (CVP) and intensive radiotherapy. *Br. J. Cancer,* 31:474–480.
17. Carbone, P. P., Kaplan, H. S., Musshoff, K., et al. (1971): Report of the committee on Hodgkin's disease staging classification. *Cancer Res.,* 31:1860–1861.
18. Carbone, P. P., and Spurr, C. (1968): Management of patients with malignant lymphoma. A comparative study with cyclophosphamide and vinca alkaloids. *Cancer Res.,* 28:811–822.
19. Carter, S. K., Schabel, F. M., Broder, L. E., and Johnston, T. P. (1972): 1,3-Bis-(2-chlorethyl)-1-nitrosourea (BCNU) and other nitrosoureas in cancer treatment: A review. *Adv. Cancer Res.,* 16:273–332.
20. Chabner, B. A., Johnson, R. E., Canellos, G. P., Hubbard, S. P., Johnson, S. K., and DeVita, V. T. (1976): Sequential nonsurgical and surgical staging of non-Hodgkin's lymphoma. *Ann. Intern. Med.,* 85:149–154.
21. Jones, S. E., and Moon, T. E. (1977): Chemotherapy of non-Hodgkin's Lymphoma: 10 year's experience in the Southwest Oncology Group. *Cancer Treat. Rev.,* 61:1067–1078.
22. Cooperative study—neoplastic disease. Treatment with vinblastine. *Arch. Intern. Med.,* 116:846–852, 1965.
23. Desai, D. V., Ezdinli, E. Z., and Stutzman, L. (1970): Vincristine therapy of lymphomas and chronic lymphocytic leukemia. *Cancer,* 26:352–359.
24. DeVita, V. T., Canellos, G. P., Chabner, B. A., Schein, P. S., Hubbard, S. P., and Young, R. C. et al. (1975): Advanced diffuse histiocytic lymphoma, a potentially curable disease. Results with combination chemotherapy. *Lancet,* 1:248–250.
25. Dorfman, R. E. (1975): The non-Hodgkin's lymphomas. In: *The Reticuloendothelial System,* edited by J. W. Rebuck, C. W. Berard, and M. R. Abell. Pp. 262–281. Williams & Wilkins, Baltimore.
26. Durant, J. R., Loeb, V., Dorfman, R., and Chan, Y. (1975): 1,3-Bis-(2-chlorethyl)-1-nitrosourea (BCNU), cyclophosphamide, vincristine and prednisone (BCOP). A new therapeutic regimen for diffuse histiocytic lymphoma. *Cancer,* 36:1936–1944.
27. Frei, E., Luce, J. K., Gamble, J. F., Coltman, C. A., Constanzi, J. J., Talley, R. W., Monto, R. W., Wilson, H. E., Hewlett, J. S., Delaney, F. C., and Gehan, E. A. (1972): Bleomycin in reticuloses. *Br. Med. J.,* 1:285–286.
28. Ezdinli, E., Pocock, S., Berard, C. W., Aungst, G. W., Silverstein, M., Horton, J., Bennett, S., Bakemeier, R., Stolbach, L., Perlia, C., Brunk, S. F., Lenhard, R. E., Klaassen, D. J., Richter, J., and Carbone, P. P. (1976): Comparison of intensive versus moderate chemotherapy of lymphocytic lymphomas. A progress report. *Cancer,* 38:1060–1068.
29. Frei, E., Luce, J. K., Sosin, H., Brunning, R. D., and Kersey, J. H. (1973): Combination chemotherapy in advanced Hodgkin's disease: Induction and maintenance of remission. *Ann. Intern. Med.,* 79:376–382.
30. Frei, E., Luce, J. K., Talley, R. W., Vaitkevicius, V. K., and Wilson, H. E. (1972): 5-(3,3-dimethyl-1-triazeno) imidazole-4-carboxamide (NSC-45388) in the treatment of lymphoma. *Cancer Chemother. Rep.,* 56:667–670.
31. Gail-Peczalska, K. J., Bloomfield, C. D., Coccia, P. F., Sosin, H., Brunning, R. D., and Kersey, J. H. (1975): B and T cell lymphomas. Analysis of blood and lymph nodes in 87 patients. *Am. J. Med.,* 59:674–685.
32. Gall, E. A., and Rappaport, H. (1958): Seminar on diseases of lymph nodes and spleen. In: *Proceedings of 23rd Seminar of the American Society of Clinical Pathology,* edited by J. R. McDonald, p. 1–107.
33. Goffinet, D. R., Castellino, R. A., Kim, H., Dorfman, R. F., Fuks, Z., Rosenberg, S. A., Nelson, T., and Kaplan, H. S. (1973): Staging laparotomies in unselected previously untreated patients with non-Hodgkin's lymphomas. *Cancer,* 32:672–681.
34. Gold, G. L., Salvin, L. G., and Shnider, B. I. (1962): A comparative study with three alkylating

agents: mechlorethamine, cyclophosphamide, and uracil mustard. *Cancer Chemother. Rep.,* 16:417–419.

35. Gold, G. L., Schnider, B. I., Salvin, L. G., Schneiderman, M. A., Colsky, J., Owens, A. H., Krant, M. J., Miller, S. P., Frei, E., Hall, T. C., Spurr, C. L., McIntyre, O. R., Hoogstraten, B., and Holland, J. F. (1970): The use of mechlorethamine, cyclophosphamide, and uracil mustard in neoplastic disease: A cooperative study. *J. Clin. Pharmacol.—New Drugs,* 10:110–120.
36. Gottlieb, J. A., Gutterman, J. U., McCredie, K. B., Rodriguez, V., and Frei, E. (1973): Chemotherapy of malignant lymphoma with adriamycin. *Cancer Res.,* 33:3024–3028.
37. Hansen, M. M., Hertz, H., and Videback, A. (1966): Use of a methyl hydrazine derivative (Natulan) especially in Hodgkin's disease. *Acta. Med. Scand.,* 180:211–224.
38. Hayes, D. M., and Glidewell, O. (1971): Intensive combination chemotherapy for lymphosarcoma and reticulum cell sarcoma. *Blood,* 38:803.
39. Hoogstraten, B., Owens, A. H., Lenhard, R. E., Glidewell, O. J., Leone, L. A., Olson, K. B., Harley, J. B., Townsend, S. R., Miller, S. P., and Spurr, C. L. (1969): Combination chemotherapy in lymphosarcoma and reticulum cell sarcoma. *Blood,* 33:370–378.
40. Hyman, G. A., and Cassileth, P. A. (1966): Efficacy of cyclophosphamide in the management of reticulum cell sarcoma. *Cancer,* 19:1386–1392.
41. Jacobs, E. M., Peters, F. C., Luce, J. K., Zippin, C., and Wood, D. A. (1969): Mechlorethamine HCl and cyclophosphamide in the treatment of Hodgkin's disease and the lymphomas. *JAMA,* 203:392–398.
42. Jaffe, E. S., Shevach, E. M., Frank, M. M., Berard, C. W. and Green, I. (1974): Nodular lymphoma—Evidence for origin from follicular B lymphocytes. *N. Engl. J. Med.,* 290:813–819.
43. Johnson, R. E. (1972): Remission induction and remission duration with primary radiotherapy in advanced lymphosarcoma. *Cancer,* 29:1473–1476.
44. Johnson, R. E. (1975): Total body irradiation (TBI) as primary therapy for advanced lymphosarcoma. *Cancer,* 35:242–246.
45. Johnson, R. E., DeVita, V. T., Kun, L. E., Chabner, B. A., Chretien, P. B., Berard, C. W., and Johnson, S. R. (1975): Patterns of involvement with malignant lymphoma and implications for treatment decision making. *Br. J. Cancer,* 31:237–241.
46. Jones, B., and Klingberg, W. G. (1963): Lymphosarcoma in children. *J. Pediatr.,* 63:11–20.
47. Jones, S. E., Fuks, Z., Kaplan, H. S., and Rosenberg, S. A. (1973): Non-Hodgkin's lymphomas V. results of radiotherapy. *Cancer,* 32:682–691.
48. Jones, S. E., Rosenberg, S. A., Kaplan, H. S., Kadin, M. E., and Portman, R. F. (1972): Non-Hodgkin's lymphomas II. Single agent chemotherapy. *Cancer,* 30:31–38.
49. Kaufman, J. H., Ezdinli, E., Aungst, C. W., and Stutzman, L. (1976): Lymphosarcoma. A comparison of extended to conservative chemotherapy. *Cancer,* 37:1283–1292.
50. Kennedy, B. J., Hill, J., Bloomfield, C., Kiang, D. Fortuny, I., and Theologides, A. (1975): Combination (COP) versus successive single agent chemotherapy (C-O-P) in lymphocytic lymphoma. *Proc. Am. Assoc. Cancer Res.,* 16:142.
51. Laszlo, J., Grizzle, J., Jonsson, U., and Rundles, R. W. (1962): Comparative study of mannitol mustard, cyclophosphamide, and nitrogen mustard in malignant lymphomas. *Cancer Chemother. Rep.,* 16:247–250.
52. Lauria, F., Baccarani, M., and Fiacchini, M. (1975): Methotrexate, cyclophosphamide and vincristine (MEV regimen) for non-Hodgkin's lymphoma. *Eur. J. Cancer,* 11:343–349.
53. Lenhard, R. E., and Pocock, S. (1975): Combination chemotherapy in histiocytic lymphomas. A comparison of three multi-drug regimens. *Proc. Am. Assoc. Cancer Res.,* 16:236.
54. Lenhard, R. E., Prentice, R. L., Owens, A. H., Bakemeier, R., Horton, J. H., Shnider, B. I., Stolbach, L., Bernard, C. W., and Carbone, P. P. (1976): Combination chemotherapy of the malignant lymphomas. A controlled clinical trial. *Cancer,* 38:1052–1059.
55. Lennert, K., Stein, H., and Kaiserling, E. (1975): Cytological and functional criteria for the classification of malignant lymphomata. *Br. J. Cancer,* 31:29–43.
56. Levitt, M., Marsh, J. C., DeConti, R. C., Mitchell, M. S., Skeel, R. T., Farber, L. R., and Bertino, J. R. (1972): Combination sequential chemotherapy in advanced reticulum cell sarcoma. *Cancer,* 29:630–636.
57. Lipton, A., and Lee, B. J. (1971): Prognosis of Stage I lymphosarcoma and reticulum-cell sarcoma. *N. Engl. J. Med.,* 284:230–233.
58. Livingston, R. B., and Carter, S. K. (eds.) (1970): *Single Agents in Cancer Chemotherapy.* Plenum Press, New York.

59. Lowenbraun, S., DeVita, V. T., and Serpick, A. A. (1970): Combination chemotherapy with nitrogen mustard, vincristine, procarbazine, and prednisone in lymphosarcoma and reticulum cell sarcoma. *Cancer,* 25:1018–1025.

60. Luce, J. K., DeLaney, F. C., and Gehan, E. A. (1973): Remission induction chemotherapy of disseminated malignant lymphoma with combination bleomycin, cytoxan, vincristine, and prednisone. *Proc. Am. Assoc. Cancer Res.,* 14:66.

61. Luce, J. K., Gamble, J. F., Wilson, H. E., Monzo, R. W., Issacs, B. L., Palmer, R. L., Coltman, C. A., Hewlett, J. S., Gehan, E. A., and Frei, E. (1971): Combined cyclophosphamide, vincristine and prednisone therapy of malignant lymphoma. *Cancer,* 28:206–217.

62. Lukes, R. J., and Butler, J. J. (1966): The pathology and nomenclature of Hodgkin's disease. *Cancer Res.,* 26:1063–1081.

63. Lukes, R. J., and Collins, R. D. (1975): New approaches to the classification of the lymphomata. *Br. J. Cancer,* 31:1–28.

64. Mathe, G., Rappaport, H., O'Connor, G. T., and Torloni, H. (1976): *Histological Diseases of Hematopoietic and Lymphoid Tissues.* WHO International Histological Classification of Tumors, Geneva, No. 14.

65. McKelvey, E. M., Gottlieb, J. A., Wilson, H. E., Haut, A., Talley, R. W., Stephens, R., Lane, M., Gamble, J. F., Jones, S. E., Grozea, P. N., Gutterman, J., Coltman, C., and Moon, T. E. (1976): Hydroxyldaunomycin (Adriamycin) combination chemotherapy in malignant lymphoma. *Cancer,* 38:1484–1493.

66. Mukherji, B., Yagoda, A., Oettgen, H. F., and Krakoff, I. H. (1971): Cyclic chemotherapy in lymphoma. *Cancer,* 28:886–893.

67. O'Bryan, R. M., Luce, J. K., Talley, R. W., Gottlieb, J. A., Baker, L. H., and Bonadonna, G. (1973): Phase II evaluation of adriamycin in human neoplasia. *Cancer,* 32:1–8.

68. Portlock, C. S., Rosenberg, S. A., Glatstein, E., and Kaplan, H. S. (1976): Treatment of advanced non-Hodgkin's lymphomas with favorable histologies: Preliminary results of a prospective trial. *Blood,* 47:747–756.

69. Pouillart, P., Hayat, M., Schwarzenberg, L., Amiel, S. L., Mathe, G., and Tubiana, M. (1975): Non-Hodgkin's malignant lymphomata in adults. Chemo-radiotherapy in Stages III and IV. *Br. J. Cancer,* 31:505–511.

70. Rappaport. H. (1966): Tumors of the hemopoietic system. In: *Atlas of Tumor Pathology, Section III, Fasc. 8.* Armed Forces Institute of Pathology, Washington, D.C.

71. Rege, V. B., and Lehnhard, R. E. (1969): BCNU [1,3-bis (2-chloroethyl)-1-nitrosourea; NSC-409962] Its effectiveness and toxicologic data in the treatment of advanced Hodgkin's disease (HD), lymphosarcoma (LYS) and reticulum cell sarcoma (RCS). *Proc. Am. Assoc. Cancer Res.,* 53:92.

72. Rundles, R. W., Laszlo, J., Garrison, F. E., and Hobson, J. B. (1962): The antitumor spectrum of cyclophosphamide. *Cancer Chemother. Rep.,* 16:407–411.

73. Samuels, M. L., Leary, W. V., Alexanian, R., Howe, C. D., and Frei, E. (1967): Clinical trials with N-isopropyl-(2-methy-hydrazino)-P-Toluamide hydrochloride in malignant lymphoma and other disseminated neoplasia. *Cancer,* 20:1187–1194.

74. Schein, P. S., Chabner, B. A., Canellos, G. P., Young, R. C., Berard, C. W., and DeVita, V. T. (1974): Potential for prolonged disease-free survival following combination chemotherapy of non-Hodgkin's lymphoma. *Blood,* 43:181–189.

75. Schein, P., DeVita, V. T., Hubbard, S. P., Chabner, B. A. Canellos, G. P., Berard, C. W., and Young, R. C. (1976): Bleomycin, adriamycin, cyclophosphamide, vincristine, and prednisone (BACOP) combination chemotherapy in the treatment of advanced diffuse histiocytic lymphoma. *Ann. Intern. Med.,* 85:417–422.

76. Shaw, R. K., and Brunner, J. A. (1964): Clinical evaluation of vincristine (NSC-67574). *Cancer Chemother. Rep.,* 42:45–48.

77. Skarin, A. T., Frei, E., Moloney, W. C., and Gutterman, J. U. (1975): New agents and combination chemotherapy of non-Hodgkin's lymphoma. *Br. J. Cancer,* 31:497–504.

78. Skarin, A. T., Pinkus, G. S., Myerowitz, R. L., Bishop, Y. M., and Moloney, W. C. (1974): Combination chemotherapy of advanced lymphocytic lymphoma. Importance of histologic classification in evaluating response. *Cancer,* 34:1023–1029.

79. Sokal, J. E., Aungst, C. W., and Snyderman, M. (1974): Delay in progression of malignant lymphoma after BCG vaccination. *N. Engl. J. Med.,* 291:1226–1230.

80. Solidoro, A., and Saenz, R. (1966): Effects of cyclophosphamide (NSC-26271) on 127 patients with malignant lymphoma. *Cancer Chemother. Rep.,* 50:265–270.

81. Solomon, J., Jacobs, E. M., Bateman. J. R., Lukes, R. J., Weiner, J. W., and Donohue, D. M.

(1973): Chemotherapy of lymphoma with mechlorethamine and vinblastine. *Arch. Intern. Med.,* 131:407–417.

82. Spear, P. W., and Patno, M. E. (1962): A comparative study of the effectiveness of HN$_2$ and cyclophosphamide in bronchogenic carcinoma, Hodgkin's disease, and lymphosarcoma. *Cancer Chemother. Rep.,* 16:413–415.

83. Stutzman, L., Ezdinli, E. Z., and Stutzman, M. A. (1966): Vinblastine sulfate vs. cyclophosphamide in the therapy of lymphoma. *J. Am. Med. Assoc.,* 195:173–178.

84. Sullivan, M. P. (1962): Leukemic transformation in lymphosarcoma of childhood. *Pediatrics,* 589–599.

85. Ultmann, J. E. (1970): Current status: The management of lymphoma. *Semin. Hemat.* 7:441–460.

86. Veronesi, U., Musumeci, R., Pizzetti, F., Gennari, L. and Bonadonna, G. (1974): The value of staging laparotomy in non-Hodgkin's lymphomas (with emphasis on the histiocytic type). *Cancer,* 33:446–469.

87. Veterans Administration Cancer Chemotherapy Group (1959): A clinical study of the comparative effect of nitrogen mustard and DON in patients with bronchogenic carcinoma, Hodgkin's disease, lymphosarcoma, and melanoma. *J. Natl. Cancer Inst.,* 22:433–439.

88. Wall, R. L., and Conrad, F. G. (1961): Cyclophosphamide therapy. Its use in leukemia, lymphoma and solid tumors. *Arch. Intern. Med.,* 108:456–482.

89. Wintrobe, M. M., and Huguley, C. M. (1948): Nitrogen-mustard therapy for Hodgkin's disease, lymphosarcoma, the leukemias, and other disorders. *Cancer,* 1:357–382.

90. Wright, T. L., Hurley, J., Korst, D. R., Monto, R. W., Rohn, R. J., Will, J. J., and Louis, J. (1963): Vinblastine in neoplastic disease. *Cancer Res.,* 23:169–179.

91. Young, R. C., Chabner, B. A., Canellos, G. P., Schein, P. S., and DeVita, V. T. (1973): Maintenance chemotherapy for advanced Hodgkin's disease in remission. *Lancet,* 1:1339–1343.

92. Young, R. C., Johnson, R. E., Canellos, G. P., Chabner, B. A., Brereton, H. D., Berard, C. W., and DeVita, V. T. (1977): Advanced lymphocytic lymphoma: Randomized comparisons of chemotherapy and radiotherapy alone or in combination. *Cancer Treatment Rev.,* 61:1153–1159.

*Randomized Trials in Cancer: A Critical Review by Sites,* edited by Maurice J. Staquet, Raven Press, New York © 1978.

# Hodgkin's Disease

Marcel Rozencweig, Daniel D. Von Hoff, Hugh L. Davis, Jr., Edwin M. Jacobs, Franco M. Muggia, and Vincent T. DeVita, Jr.

*Division of Cancer Treatment, National Cancer Institute, Bethesda, Maryland 20014*

Hodgkin's disease is one of the malignancies showing the most rapid improvement in therapeutic results over the last 15 years. Summarizing the Toronto experience from 1928 to 1954, Peters (61) reported a 5-year survival rate of 40%, all stages included; this rate dropped to 15% in stage III, which corresponded to the current stages III and IV. Recent results indicate that a 5-year survival above 85% can be achieved in stages I through IIIA (68), whereas this figure reaches 65% in the remaining cases (21). A better understanding of the natural course of Hodgkin's disease, together with the development of new radiotherapy techniques and appropriate combination chemotherapy, are the basis for this dramatic improvement.

Reliable methods of assessing abdominal involvement only became available during the 1960s. Lymphangiography revealed a high incidence of previously unsuspected, and thus untreated, invasion of paraaortic and pelvic lymph nodes, heralding the first four-stage classification, which was proposed at the Rye Conference (65). Lymphangiograms also provided the first convincing evidence of a consistent tendency of Hodgkin's disease to spread by contiguity within the lymphatic system (45). This observation led in turn to a rationalization of the concept of prophylactic radiotherapy (30,43,61). Knowledge of the natural spreading of Hodgkin's disease was further enhanced by the introduction of staging laparotomy plus splenectomy, a procedure yielding more accurate findings than the previous clinical staging, particularly with regard to the status of the spleen.

Prognostic implications ascribed to staging have resulted in its wide use as a guide for therapeutic decisions in Hodgkin's disease. The latest Ann Arbor staging system (11), derived from that adopted at the Rye Conference, takes into consideration the extent and distribution of the disease as well as the presence or absence of constitutional signs and symptoms (Table 1). The current histopathologic classification of the disease was defined by Lukes et al. (53) and considers the following histologic subtypes: lymphocytic predominance (LP),

Received September 16, 1977.

TABLE 1. *Ann Arbor staging system for Hodgkin's disease*

| Stage | Criteria |
|---|---|
| I | Involvement of a single lymph node region (I) or a single extralymphatic organ or site ($I_E$) |
| II | Involvement of two or more lymph node regions on the same side of the diaphragm (II) or localized involvement of extra lymphatic organ or site and of one or more lymph node regions on the same side of the diaphragm ($II_E$) |
| III | Involvement of lymph node regions on both sides of the diaphragm (III), which may also be accompanied by localized involvement of extralymphatic organ or site ($III_E$) or by involvement of the spleen ($III_S$) or both ($III_{SE}$) |
| IV | Diffuse or disseminated involvement of one or more extralymphatic organs or tissues with or without associated lymph node enlargement |

Each stage is subclassified to indicate the absence (A) or presence (B) of (1) unexplained loss of more than 10% of the body weight during the 6 months previous to admission; (2) unexplained fever with temperature above 38°C, and (3) night sweats.

From Carbone et al. (11).
This staging classification, whether based on clinical (CS) or pathologic (PS) findings, applies only to patients at the time of disease presentation and prior to definitive therapy.

nodular sclerosis (NS), mixed cellularity (MC), and lymphocytic depletion (LD). This classification is also closely correlated with the course of the disease, and its impact on treatment selection has been increasing. Additional predictive parameters, primarily age and sex, have been identified. In fact, all of the prognostic factors in Hodgkin's disease are interrelated, and their individual significance remains difficult to ascertain because their apparent influence may vary greatly with the quality of staging and the type of treatment (69).

High dose levels and wide-field irradiation were suggested to substantially prolong survival in Hodgkin's disease when only kilovoltage X-ray equipment was available (30,61). The usefulness of these techniques was firmly established after the introduction of megavoltage beam energies, allowing safe delivery of higher doses on more sharpened fields. A tumoricidal dose in the range of 3,500 to 4,000 rads was identified (44), and various types of fields were investigated. However, definition of these fields has varied somewhat from one study to another. Roughly, involved field (IF) irradiation usually includes involved and immediately surrounding nodal areas. Extended field (EF) encompasses IF and adjacent nodal areas, including at least a "mantle" field for supradiaphragmatic areas and an "inverted Y" field for infradiaphragmatic areas. Limited extended field (LEF) is intermediate between IF and EF, whereas total nodal (TN) irradiation is directed to both the "mantle" and the "inverted Y" field. Classically, the "mantle" field covers in contiguity the cervical, supraclavicular, infraclavicular, axillary, hilar, and mediastinal nodes down to the level of the diaphragm. The "inverted Y" field covers the spleen or splenic pedicle, as well as the celiac, paraaortic, iliac, inguinal, and femoral nodes.

The most appropriate extent of treatment fields according to well-defined prognostic factors remains a matter of conjecture. However, the importance of that question has been somewhat reduced by the introduction of highly effective combination chemotherapy and the potential of the combined modality approach in nodal disease.

A large number of cytotoxic drugs have been active in Hodgkin's disease as single agents (4,14). Their initial integration into various combinations culminated in the development of the MOPP regimen at the National Cancer Institute. Following the initial report of DeVita and Serpick (22), the MOPP combination has rapidly become a standard treatment for patients not potentially curable by radiotherapy. Experience with this treatment at the National Cancer Institute has been recently reviewed (21). From 1964 to 1976, 194 advanced disease patients, most of them previously untreated, received the MOPP combination. The complete response rate was 81% in all patients, 100% in asymptomatic patients and 77% in symptomatic patients. All asymptomatic patients remained in remission, whereas 60% of symptomatic patients who achieved complete remission remain disease-free at 5 years; 65% of all patients were alive at 5 years and 58% at 10 years. These results illustrate the high probability of cure that can at present be obtained in the disseminated stage of the disease.

Randomized trials have been used extensively in Hodgkin's disease. Our analysis will document their contributions in confirming results of uncontrolled studies and, to a lesser extent, in testing unique innovations. This analysis is based on published reports of completed or still ongoing clinical studies.

## RANDOMIZED TRIALS IN STAGE I AND II HODGKIN'S DISEASE

### Trials Comparing Radiotherapy Techniques

Randomized trials have investigated the respective value of IF, EF, and TN irradiation in stage I and II disease (Table 2). None of these trials was restricted to patients who underwent surgical staging, and the only conclusions possible are for clinical stages I and II. Results indicate an overall superiority of the TN technique, at least in the prevention of relapses. Most of these randomized trials failed to detect any significant difference in survival, presumably because of effective secondary treatments.

At Stanford University, Kaplan and Rosenberg first compared IF and EF radiotherapy in clinical stages I and II (46,47). The doses were 4,000 rads in known involved areas and 3,000 to 3,500 rads in adjacent areas. The EF was usually a "mantle" field which, in the presence of mediastinal involvement, was completed by irradiation of the retroperitoneal lymph nodes down to the level of iliac bifurcation in females and including the pelvic nodes in males. In 97 asymptomatic patients, no significant therapeutic difference was detected at 10 years (31). In 21 patients with clinical stages IB and IIB, EF therapy significantly prolonged the relapse-free interval as well as survival. In this latter group, 80% of the patients were free of relapse at one year following EF versus

TABLE 2. *Randomized trials of radiotherapy in stage I–II Hodgkin's disease*

| Investigators and treatment arms | Initial disease stage | Significant difference[a] in | |
|---|---|---|---|
| | | Relapse-free survival | Survival |
| Kaplan and Rosenberg (46) | CS I–II | EF = IF (A patients) | EF = IF (A patients) |
| A. IF | | EF > IF (B patients) | EF > IF (B patients) |
| B. EF | | | |
| Radiotherapy Hodgkin's Disease Group (62) | CS + PS I–II | EF > IF | EF = IF |
| A. IF | | | |
| B. EF | | | |
| Jellife (40) | CS + PS IA and IIA | No results | No results |
| A. IF | | | |
| B. EF | | | |
| Rosenberg and Kaplan (66) | CS + PS IA and IIA | TN > IF | TN = IF |
| A. IF | | | |
| B. TN | | | |
| Jellife (40) | CS + PS IB and IIB | No results | No results |
| A. IF | | | |
| B. TN | | | |
| Johnson et al. (41) | CS I–II | TN > EF | TN = EF |
| A. EF | | | |
| B. TN | | | |

[a]Difference reported with $p > .05$.

less than 30% following IF radiotherapy; the respective 4-year survival rates were 90% versus less than 40%. It is noteworthy that many patients with constitutional symptoms assigned to EF treatment had mediastinal involvement and their treatment was essentially similar to that of the TN technique. Upon relapse, patients initially treated with IF radiotherapy were randomized to either palliative or radical radiotherapeutic dose groups. The influence of this subsequent trial on the overall survival following IF therapy is unknown.

IF and EF radiotherapy were also compared in a large-scale cooperative study of the Radiotherapy Hodgkin's Disease Group (62). Surgical staging was introduced after the onset of the study. Interpretation of the results is difficult because the extent of the fields to be used in the EF group was changed during the trial. In supradiaphragmatic disease, paraaortic and splenic fields were initially irradiated only in the presence of mediastinal involvement and systematically thereafter. A dose of at least 3,500 rads in 3 to 4 weeks was given to all prescribed fields. Four hundred sixty-seven patients entered the trial and were followed for periods ranging from 8 months to 6 years. The treatment groups were similarly distributed with regard to disease stages, presence or absence of symptoms, histology, age, sex, and type of staging. Following IF and EF radiotherapy the 4-year extension-free survival from the time of initial evaluation was 47% and 61%, respectively, which was a statistically significant difference. These results were not subdivided into categories A and B. The 4-year survival rates for IF and EF radiotherapy were 82 and 83%, respectively, in patients at risk by that time; there was no difference between or within stages I and II with or without constitutional signs or symptoms. Survival was also similar in both treatment groups by type of staging.

At Stanford University (66), IF and TN radiotherapy were compared in 62 symptomatic patients after surgical staging in over 80% of them. The results revealed a significant advantage in relapse-free interval with the TN approach but no significant difference as yet in survival. As estimated from actuarial curves, the disease-free survival after IF treatment was less than 40% versus 80% after TN treatment, with 90% of all patients still alive at 8 years (31).

At the National Cancer Institute, Johnson et al. (41,42) evaluated EF versus TN radiotherapy in patients who had clinical stage I or II. EF therapy included the "mantle" or the "inverted Y" field and para-aortic nodes were treated when the mediastinum was involved. Irradiation to the involved fields consisted of 4,000 rads in 4 to 7.5 weeks, whereas 3,000 to 4,000 rads were given to uninvolved areas. At the time of the latest report, most of the cases had been followed for at least 3 years. The trial was rapidly discontinued for patients with NS disease due to a relatively favorable clinical course observed after EF radiotherapy. The actuarial survival curve for the entire group of NS patients was plateauing at 91% from the second through the sixth year. In patients with other histologic subtypes, the nodal relapse rate was significantly reduced following TN irradiation as compared to EF radiotherapy (11 versus 36%). When relapses in all sites were considered, the same trend was still apparent but the difference was no longer significant. The projected 6-year survival rates also favored the TN technique (91 versus 57%), but these survival data were not analyzed statistically.

## Combined Radiotherapy and Chemotherapy

Several randomized trials have attempted to determine if the successful prophylactic radiotherapy directed to minimal nodal involvement could be replaced or complemented by chemotherapy, with an additional benefit in extranodal disease (Table 3). Most of these studies were flawed by inconsistent staging procedures, a small number of patients, and/or reporting of combined results involving additional stages.

In clinical stages I and II, the role of adjuvant chemotherapy with single agents has been tested by Thompson Hancock et al. (82) and the European Organization for Research on Treatment of Cancer (E.O.R.T.C.) (26). Thompson Hancock et al. began their study prior to the era of lymphangiography and megavoltage radiotherapy. No benefit was noted with adjuvant chemotherapy, but it was limited to a single administration of nitrogen mustard ($HN_2$).

TABLE 3. *Randomized trials with combined radiotherapy and chemotherapy in stage I–II Hodgkin's disease[a]*

| Investigator and treatment arms | Initial disease stage | No of pts. | Significant difference [b] in disease-free interval |
|---|---|---|---|
| Thompson Hancock et al. (82) <br> A. LEF <br> B. As in A + HN$_2$ (single dose) | CS I–II <br> A and B | 108 | RT + CT = RT |
| E.O.R.T.C. (26) <br><br> A. EF <br> B. As in A + VLB/2 yr | CS I–II <br> A and B | 296 | RT + CT > RT |
| Thompson et al. (81) <br><br> A. CTX, VCR, PCZ/2 yr <br> B. As in A + TN | CS IIB, <br> IIIB, IV | 24 | CT + RT > CT |
| Grasso et al. (33) <br><br> A. IF <br> B. As in A + CHL, VCR, VLB, <br> PCZ, Pred/6 months | (I) CS <br> IA and IIA | 101 | RT + CT > RT <br> (I) + (II) |
| A. TN <br> B. As in (I) B | (II) CS IB, <br> II–III, A and B | | |
| Wiernik and Lichtenfeld (86) <br><br> A. EF <br> B. IF + MOPP (3 cycles) <br> C. MOPP (3 cycles) + IF | CS I–II, <br> A and B | 22 | RT + CT = CT + RT = RT |
| De Lena et al. (20) <br><br> A. MABOP (2 or 6 cycle) + RT <br> B. As in A + sequential CT | CS + PS IIB, <br> IIIB & III$_s$ | | No results |
| Rosenberg and Kaplan (67) <br><br> A. EF <br> B. IF + MOPP (6 cycles) | (I) PS IA and IIA | 86 | RT + CT > RT <br> (I) + (II) |
| A. EF <br> B. As in A + MOPP (6 cycles) | (II PS IA and IIA | | |
| A. TN <br> B. As in A + MOPP (6 cycles) | (III) PS IB and <br> IIB | 50 | RT + CT = RT |
| A. TN + liver irradiation <br> B. TN + MOPP (6 cycles) | (IV) PS II$_s$ | | |
| O'Connell et al. (57) <br><br> A. EF <br> B. EF + MOPP (6 cycles) | PS I–II, A and B <br> IIIA | 72 | RT + CT > RT |
| Thompson et al. (81) <br> A. TN <br> B. As in A + CTX, VCR, PCZ/ <br> 1 yr | PS IIA and IIIA | 22 | RT + CT > RT |

[a] Additional studies have investigated the role of chemotherapy combined with radiotherapy in various lymphomas at unspecified stages (76,79)

[b] Difference reported with $p > 0.05$.

In the E.O.R.T.C. trial, all patients received EF radiotherapy but the irradiated fields were not extended beyond the diaphragm when regions adjacent to the diaphragm were invaded. Two hundred ninety-six patients, who were clinically in complete remission following radiotherapy, were randomized to either no further treatment or weekly intravenous administration of vinblastine (VLB) for 2 years. The percentage of patients free of disease was significantly greater with the combined treatment modalities. However, this difference in recurrence rate did not remain significant when relapses in the paraaortic lymph nodes and in the spleen were excluded from the analysis, suggesting that VLB would have played no role after more extensive radiotherapy (83). Results by cell type showed that VLB was effective in both NS and MC cases, but the prolongation of disease-free interval was significant only in MC presentations. Whatever the histological findings, actuarial survival curves were similar in both treatment groups up to 10 years (26). This E.O.R.T.C. study demonstrated the tolerance of long-term single-agent chemotherapy following radiotherapy. This adjuvant treatment showed "prophylactic" potential, especially for unfavorable disease, but no clear effect on extranodal disease or overall survival. The role of adjuvant combination chemotherapy, more accurate staging, and larger-field radiotherapy naturally became the next question to be elucidated.

Three comparative trials using combination chemotherapy and radiotherapy in clinical stages I and II failed to provide useful information. Only abstracts are presently available to analyze findings in various disease stages by Thompson et al. (81) at St. Jude Children's Hospital and by Grasso et al. (33) at Roswell Park Memorial Institute. These reveal an overall superiority of the combined modalities but give few details relevant to stages I and II. Wiernik and Lichtenfeld (86) at the Baltimore Cancer Research Center detected no benefit of the combined approach over EF radiotherapy alone. However, the trial included only 22 patients, which precludes a definitive conclusion.

Interim results are available for trials of adjuvant chemotherapy, all using drug combinations, in patients who underwent surgical staging.

At Stanford University (67), the MOPP regimen (six cycles) is being tested in combination with various radiotherapeutic programs designed according to pathologic stages, histology, and site of involvement. Patients with pathologic stages IA and IIA are divided into two groups. The first group includes patients with LP or NS histologic subtypes, without involvement of the low left neck, left infraclavicular region, left axilla, or paraaortic lymph nodes. In this "favorable" group, patients are randomized to either IF radiotherapy followed by chemotherapy or to EF radiotherapy limited to the "mantle" or the "inverted Y" field. Patients with pathologic stages IA and IIA, MC or LD histologic subtypes, or involvement of unfavorable site are treated by EF radiotherapy with or without subsequent MOPP treatment. EF irradiation includes the paraaortic lymph nodes and the splenic pedicle in supradiaphragmatic presentations. In this study, all symptomatic patients receive TN irradiation with or without chemotherapy. Patients having histologic invasion of the spleen who are randomized to radiotherapy alone receive additional liver irradiation at an estimated dose of 2,500 to 3,000 rads. The combination of intensive radiotherapy and chemotherapy, although difficult, appeared feasible, but these investigators subsequently deleted the use of prednisone in the MOPP regimen for patients receiving mediastinal irradiation, because of the apparent potentiation of radiation pneumonitis or pericarditis encountered with abrupt corticosteroids withdrawal. Results were recently provided for the 87 asymptomatic and 50 symptomatic stage I and II patients now involved in the trials (68). In asymptomatic stages I and II patients receiving adjuvant chemotherapy, a significant improvement was noted in freedom from relapse ($p < .02$) but not yet in survival. At 6 years, the actuarial relapse-free rates were 86 versus 70% and the corresponding survival rates 97 versus 87%. However, in symptomatic patients, no difference was detected in freedom from relapse or survival. The 8-year relapse-free and survival rates, with or without adjuvant chemotherapy, were 86 versus 81% and 92 versus 87%, emphasizing the striking effectiveness of TN irradiation in pathologic stages IB and IIB.

The preliminary findings at Stanford University point to several emerging factors. The similarity in end results among asymptomatic and symptomatic patients indicate that the presence of symptoms is unlikely to worsen the prognosis in patients classified in stage I or II after careful pathologic staging. The 6-year relapse-free survival in asymptomatic and symptomatic patients without adjuvant chemotherapy was 70 and 81%, respectively. Although this difference is not significant, it suggests that suboptimal initial radiotherapy might have been used in asymptomatic patients. Adjuvant combination chemotherapy appears to prolong the disease-free interval in pathologic stages I and II. This improvement is statistically significant only within the group of asymptomatic patients, and has not yet been translated into a clear survival benefit. In spite of the practical difficulties encountered with this aggressive therapeutic approach, the relative merits of the MOPP combination as adjuvant versus secondary treatment requires further assessment. Survival rates over 85% at 6 years may be achieved in pathologic stages I and II, A and B, with radiotherapy alone, followed by secondary treatment upon relapse. A trend toward a survival gain is presently apparent with adjuvant MOPP therapy, but a considerable number of patients and at least a 10-year follow-up might be required for this difference eventually to reach statistical significance.

The remaining trials cited in Table 3 have not yielded additional firm information for pathologic stages I and II. At the Baltimore Cancer Research Center (57), 72 evaluable patients with pathologic stages I through IIIA received EF radiotherapy alone or followed by the MOPP regimen. Failure on radiotherapy or noncompletion of at least three courses of chemotherapy excluded patients from final analysis. Actuarial curves indicated a highly significant improvement in complete remission duration with the combined modalities, the estimated disease-free survival being approximately 94 versus 71% 3 years after completion of radiotherapy. Little data are available by disease stages. Within a follow-up period of 2 to 5 years, relapse rates for radiotherapy alone and radiotherapy plus chemotherapy were 28% (8 of 29) versus 16% (3 of 18) in stages I–II and 42% (5 of 12) versus 0% (0 of 13) in stage IIIA disease. This suggests that most of the observed difference in remission duration may have been related to the difference in results obtained in stage III patients. No deaths had occurred among evaluable stage I–II patients at the time of the report.

At St. Jude Children's Research Hospital (81), 22 pathologic stage II and III asymptomatic patients were randomized to TN radiotherapy alone or with a three-drug combination chemotherapy. Only 4 patients relapsed or failed to remit; all were initially treated with radiotherapy alone. Data were not broken down by stages of disease.

## RANDOMIZED TRIALS OF RADIOTHERAPY WITH OR WITHOUT CHEMOTHERAPY IN STAGE III HODGKIN'S DISEASE

Several randomized trials have attempted to establish the relative value of radiotherapy and chemotherapy alone or in combination in stage III Hodgkin's disease. An exploratory trial was first undertaken by the Acute Leukemia Group B (35,36). One hundred four evaluable patients received TN irradiation alone, TN irradiation followed by chemotherapy, chemotherapy alone, or chemotherapy followed by either IF or TN radiotherapy. TN irradiation was selected as initial radiotherapy in view of the promising results yielded by this technique as compared to low-dose IF radiotherapy at Stanford University (46,47). Chemotherapy consisted of a combination of $HN_2$ and VLB. Among the 22 patients treated with this chemotherapy regimen alone, there were 10 complete remissions and 9 partial remissions, with an overall median duration of 3 months. With the other therapeutic options, the complete response rates varied from 75 to 90% and no benefit in remission duration was detected with the combined modality treatment as compared to radiotherapy alone. The small number of patients per treatment arm, use of suboptimal chemotherapy, and lack of detailed analysis of the remission durations make these data of little use in drawing firm conclusions.

A therapeutic superiority of radiotherapy over chemotherapy was found in pathologic stage IIIA in a multiinstitutional study by radiotherapists sponsored by the British National Lymphoma Investigation (8). Eighty-one patients were randomly allocated to TN irradiation or a modified MOPP program. The intended tumor dose was 4,000 rads in 4 weeks to involved node regions and 3,500 rads in 4 weeks to the apparently uninvolved node regions. In the chemotherapy group, patients achieving complete remission received three additional cycles of MOPP, and all patients were treated with at least six cycles of this regimen. Both treatment groups were similar with respect to histology, age, and sex. Radiotherapy and chemotherapy yielded complete remission rates of 95% and 74%, respectively ($p < .05$). It is noteworthy that, in this trial, the remission induction rate for stage IIIA patients treated with MOPP was strikingly lower than that reported by others (21). Up to 4 years no difference could be detected in disease-free survival of the complete responders in either treatment group, and the survival of the entire group of patients entered in the trial did not appear to be affected by the type of initial therapy.

The ability of adjuvant combination chemotherapy to prolong the disease-free interval over that achieved by radiotherapy alone in asymptomatic patients has been documented by three studies already cited (see Table 3). At Stanford University (67,68), treatment options for pathologic stages IIIA and B were similar to those defined earlier for pathologic stages IB and IIB, that is, TN radiotherapy with or without adjuvant MOPP chemotherapy. The estimated tumor dose to "mantle" and "inverted Y" fields was 4,400 rads delivered in 4 weeks; uninvolved regions were treated with 3,500 to 4,000 rads. Additional liver irradiation with 2,500 to 3,000 rads was used in patients who had splenic involvement and were randomized to receive radiotherapy alone. The actuarial curves for freedom from relapse indicated a statistically significant benefit of the combined modalities over radiotherapy alone for up to 8 years in 60 asymptomatic patients and 44 symptomatic patients (Figure 1). The estimated 8-year

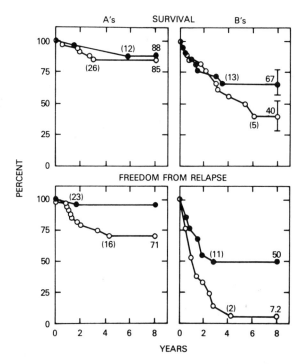

**FIG. 1.** Stanford trial (68). Actuarial survival and freedom from relapse curves following total nodal radiotherapy (○————○) versus total nodal radiotherapy plus adjuvant MOP (P) chemotherapy (●————●) in pathologic stage III Hodgkin's disease with (B) (44 patients) and without (A) systemic symptoms (60 patients). ( ) indicate number of patients at risk at the final calculations, no events occurring thereafter. Standard errors shown for the final calculation at that point.

relapse-free rates were, respectively, 96 versus 71% in stage IIIA patients and 50 versus 7% in stage IIIB patients. Adjuvant chemotherapy also appeared to prolong survival, with 8-year actuarial survival rates of 88% in asymptomatic and 67% in symptomatic patients; however, these latter results were not significantly better than those achieved with radiotherapy as initial treatment.

The Stanford results in asymptomatic patients are supported by similar findings in other studies. Grasso et al. (33) reported in clinical stage IIIA a 3-year relapse-free survival of 37% with TN irradiation and 100% with TN irradiation followed by a combination of chlorambucil (CHL), vincristine (VCR), VLB, procarbazine (PCZ), and prednisone ($p < 0.05$). However, irradiation alone appeared to be unusually ineffective in this trial. O'Connell et al. (57) used subtotal nodal radiotherapy alone, or followed by a MOPP combination, in 25 evaluable patients with pathologic stage IIIA. The respective recurrence rates were 42 versus 0% within an observation period of 8 to 42 months following completion of radiotherapy. Four patients, all of them treated with radiotherapy alone, were dead at the time of the report.

Finally, radiotherapy has also been used for consolidation between induction and maintenance chemotherapy (20,83). Very little data are available for these trials.

Thus, at this point, it appears that the relative value of radiotherapy and chemotherapy in stage IIIA Hodgkin's disease remains controversial. The induction potential of these treatment modalities has been compared in a single trial, suggesting a superiority of radiotherapy in terms of complete remission rate. In this trial, however, complete responses after chemotherapy were seen in only 74% of the patients, which was a relatively low figure for stage IIIA disease treated with the MOPP regimen.

Excellent results have been achieved in stage IIIA by initial TN irradiation with freedom from relapse and survival rates of approximately 70 and 85% at 8 years. Adjuvant chemotherapy may significantly increase the relapse-free rate, but an effect on survival has not yet been detected. However, as discussed earlier for stages I and II, larger numbers of patients and longer periods of observation may be needed in view of the outstanding results obtained without adjuvant treatment. In stage IIIB, TN irradiation fails to control substantially the course of the disease. At this stage, the role of radiotherapy used as an adjuvant to chemotherapy remains to be evaluated.

## RANDOMIZED TRIALS OF CHEMOTHERAPY IN ADVANCED HODGKIN'S DISEASE

### Single-Agent Chemotherapy

The vast majority of randomized trials comparing single agents were initiated before 1970, and their relevance is often narrowed by the inadequacies in study design common to that period.

TABLE 4. Randomized trials of single-agent chemotherapy[a]

| Investigators and treatment arms | Total no. of patients | No. of responders | | Overall response rate (%) | Remission duration (weeks) |
|---|---|---|---|---|---|
| | | Complete | Partial | | |
| Spear and Patno (74) | | | | | |
| A. HN$_2$, 0.4 mg/kg or 0.2 mg/kg/ day $\times$ 2 q. 4 wk i.v. | 33 | 2 | 12 | 42 | — |
| B. CTX, 8 mg/kg/day $\times$ 5 q. 4 wk i.v. | 33 | 0 | 13 | 39 | — |
| Gold et al. (32) | | | | | |
| A. HN$_2$, 0.2 mg/kg/day $\times$ 2 q. 2 wk i.v. | 26 | — | — | 65 | — |
| B. CTX, 15 mg/kg/wk i.v. | 19 | — | — | 53 | — |
| C. Uracil mustard, 0.15 mg/kg/ wk p.o. | 20 | — | — | 30 | — |
| Alison and Whitelaw (1) | | | | | |
| I | | | | | |
| A. HN$_2$, 0.4 mg/kg then 0.2 mg/ kg/q. 4 wk i.v. | 29 | 9 | 5 | 48 | 35 |
| B. VLB, 10 mg/wk i.v. | 32 | 9 | 13 | 69 | 31 |
| II | | | | | |
| A. As IA after progression on IB | 26 | 4 | 5 | 35 | 33 |
| B. As IB after progression on IA | 24 | 5 | 7 | 50 | 35 |
| Solomon et al. (73) | | | | | |
| I | | | | | |
| A. HN$_2$, 0.4 mg/kg i.v. ($\pm$maintenance CHL) | 44 | 2 | 28 | 68 | 36 |
| B. VLB, 0.10–0.25 mg/kg/wk i.v. | 41 | 2 | 24 | 63 | 33 |
| II | | | | | |
| A. As IA after progression on IB | 17 | 1 | 7 | 47 | 50 |
| B. As IB after progression on IA | 21 | 0 | 11 | 52 | 17 |
| Carbone et al. (12) | | | | | |
| A. CTX, 15 mg/kg i.v. | 86 | 12 | 34 | 53 | |
| A1. Maintenance CTX | | | | | 32 |
| A2. No maintenance | | | | | 5 |
| B. VLB, 0.10–0.30 mg/kg/wk i.v. | 88 | 18 | 39 | 65 | |
| A1. Maintenance CTX | | | | | 34 |
| A2. No maintenance | | | | | 5–6 |
| ALGB 6953 (71,85) | | | | | |
| A. BCNU, 200 mg/m$^2$ q. 6 wk i.v. | 28 | — | — | 36[b] | 3 |
| B. CCNU, 100 mg/m$^2$ q. 6 wk p.o. | 26 | — | — | 69[b] | 10 |
| ALGB 7252 (85) | | | | | |
| A. CCNU, 100 mg/m$^2$ q. 6 wk p.o. | 27 | — | — | 52[c] | — |
| B. Methyl CCNU 150 mg/m$^2$ q. 6 wk p.o. | 19 | — | — | 26[c] | — |

[a] Studies including at least 25 patients per treatment arm.
[b,c] Difference statistically significant, but complete data are not available for analysis.

HN$_2$ has been the most widely investigated single agent. It has been compared to a number of drugs, including 6-diazo-5-oxo-L-norleucine or DON (84), thioTEPA (6,89), cytoxan (CTX) (32,39,49,59,74,80), and VLB (1,27,73). Other trials have compared uracil mustard and prednisone (28), CTX and VLB (12,77), CCNU and BCNU or MeCCNU (71,85), and streptonigrin and CHL (48).

Dose scheduling has been studied with VCR (13) and BCNU (64). One trial has investigated the value of CHL as maintenance therapy following induction with $HN_2$ (70).

Few trials have randomized at least 25 evaluable patients with Hodgkin's disease per treatment arm (Table 4), and only one of them (12), performed jointly by the Eastern Cooperative Oncology Group and the Acute Leukemia Group B, has yielded major conclusions.

Carbone et al. (12) reported the results of this cooperative group study, which compared CTX and VLB and also further investigated the value, previously suggested by Scott (70), of maintenance chemotherapy. Patients were stratified according to prior or no prior chemotherapy and were similarly distributed in both treatment groups with respect to performance status, age, and sex. Responders on day 42 of treatment were further randomized to maintenance or reinduction with CTX upon relapse. Progressive disease on day 28, or unchanged disease on day 42, was treated with the alternate single agent. No overall difference was found between the two induction regimens in terms of response rate. However, in patients without prior chemotherapy, the response rates to CTX and VLB were 54 and 75% ($p < .05$). Remission duration was similar with either treatment but was prolonged by maintenance therapy, especially in complete responders. Thus, maintained complete and partial remissions lasted 1 year and 2 months, respectively, whereas unmaintained complete and partial remissions lasted 3 months versus 1 month. No survival advantage was seen for maintenance versus reinduction chemotherapy, but these data were not given separately for complete and partial remissions. Finally, this trial also identified participating institutions as a major prognostic factor in cooperative clinical trials. For example, a statistically significant difference in median response rates was achieved between institutions including more than 10 versus 10 or fewer patients in the trial.

In summary, this trial pointed to the influence of prior therapy on response, the correlation between completeness of response and remission duration, and the influence of institutional variability in cooperative clinical trials. This trial also established the influence of maintenance therapy on length of complete response after brief induction treatment, emphasizing the need for prolonged induction regimens. The lack of effect on overall survival might have reflected a selection of poor-risk patients but also emphasized the role of retreatment and the basic limitations of single agent programs.

### Single-Agent versus Combination Chemotherapy

Two of the most active agents in Hodgkin's disease, VLB and $HN_2$, have been tested against combination regimens incorporating these drugs (Table 5). These trials definitely established the superiority of combination chemotherapy.

The Eastern Cooperative Oncology Group (50) compared VLB with two dose levels of a combination of VLB, CTX, and prednisone. The treatments

TABLE 5. *Single-agent versus combination*

| Investigator and treatment arms | Total no. of patients | No. of responders Complete | No. of responders Partial | Response rate (%) | Median disease-free interval (months) | Survival (months) |
|---|---|---|---|---|---|---|
| Lenhard (50) | | | | | | |
| A. VLB, 0.1–0.3 mg/kg i.v. weekly | 30 | 2 | 22 | 80 | 4.2 | 30[a] |
| B. VLB, 0.2 mg/kg i.v. weekly CTX, 10 mg/kg i.v. weekly Pred, 1 mg/kg/day p.o. | 32 | 12 | 17 | 91 | 6.2 | 30 |
| C. VLB, 0.06 mg/kg i.v. weekly CTX, 3.3 mg/kg i.v. weekly Pred, 0.33 mg/kg/day p.o. | 21 | 3 | 9 | 52 | | 30 |
| Huguley et al. (37) | | | | | | |
| A. HN$_2$, 0.2 mg/kg/day $\times$ 2 i.v., then 0.1–0.2 mg/kg i.v. biweekly | 47 | 6 | 6 | 26 | 12 | 13[b] |
| B. HN$_2$, 0.2 mg/kg i.v. day 1 and 8 every 4 weeks VCR, 1.4 mg/m$^2$ i.v. day 1 and 8 every 4 weeks PCZ, 50 mg day 1, 100 mg day 2, then 100 mg/m$^2$/$\times$ 8 every 4 weeks Pred, 40 mg/m$^2$/day $\times$ 14 every 4 weeks at first and fourth course only | 61 | 29 | 11 | 66 | 15 | 38 |

[a] Mean.
[b] Median.

were given weekly and evaluated after 8 weeks; when a remission was obtained, no further treatment was given despite the conclusions of their previous study indicating the insufficiency of brief induction therapy. During the trial, the low-dose combination was found to be less effective and was discontinued. As compared to VLB, the high-dose combination yielded a significantly greater rate of complete remission (38% versus 7%) with longer median disease-free intervals (6.2 versus 4.2 months), but the average survival was approximately 30 months with both treatments.

The trial carried out by the Southeastern Cancer Study Group (37) was designed specifically to determine if the apparently superior results of combination chemotherapy were due to the use of a combination of drugs or the intensity and long duration of treatment. One hundred seventy-nine patients with clinical stages III or IV, A and B, were entered into the study. After stratification by extent of prior therapy and bone marrow status, patients were randomized to either HN$_2$ for 12 doses or to a MOPP-type combination (6 cycles) slightly different from the one developed by DeVita, Serpick, and Carbone (23). The latter regimen use less HN$_2$ (6 mg/m$^2$ days 1 and 8) and more PCZ (100 mg/m$^2$/day $\times$ 14) (see Table 5). One hundred eight patients (60%) were judged

TABLE 6. *Complete remission rate with MOPP according to pretherapeutic variables*

| Variable | Number of patients | Complete response rate (%) |
|---|---|---|
| Symptoms | | |
| Absent | 98 | 83 |
| Present | 349 | 67 |
| Age | | |
| 50 years or less | 161 | 75 |
| More than 50 | 27 | 48 |
| Prior therapy | | |
| None | 284 | 77 |
| RT a/o CT | 256 | 68 |
| Histology | | |
| LP | 13 | 77 |
| NS | 115 | 70 |
| MC | 95 | 78 |
| LD | 35 | 63 |
| Sex | | |
| Male | 281 | 68 |
| Female | 140 | 73 |

RT = radiotherapy, CT = chemotherapy, LP = lymphocyte predominance, NS = nodular sclerosis, MC = mixed cellularity, LD = lymphocyte depletion.

Cumulative results compiled from Bonadonna et al. (5), Cooper et al. (18), De Vita et al. (23), Frei et al. (29), Greenberg et al. (34), Huguley et al. (37) Lowenbraun et al. (51), Moore et al. (54), Nixon and Aisenberg (56), Olweny et al. (58), and Ziegler et al. (88).

evaluable, 42 being ineligible by protocol stipulation and 29 because of failure to complete a full course of therapy. Both treatment groups were evenly distributed according to the major prognostic factors identified for response to chemotherapy, that is, prior treatment, age, and presence or absence of constitutional signs and symptoms (Table 6). Both the complete and partial remission rates at the end of the treatment were significantly higher for MOPP than for $HN_2$. The minimum posttherapy follow-up was 18 months. In patients achieving complete remission, the curves of unmaintained remission duration, as well as survival curves, were similar for both treatment groups. Patients who failed to respond or relapsed on $HN_2$ were usually treated with an MOPP combination. The survival curves of the entire treatment groups were significantly different, with median values of 38 months for all patients initially treated with MOPP and 13 months for those receiving $HN_2$ alone.

Other investigations have taken place to test the respective value of single-agent versus combination chemotherapy (9,40,63), but the available data are not sufficient to allow comment.

Thus, effective combination chemotherapy as exemplified by the MOPP program was conclusively shown more effective than $HN_2$. This result is not surprising in view of the abundant historical data describing the limitations of single agent therapy. The ECOG trial reached similar conclusions using a less effective three-drug regimen, an observation of historical interest since the duration of treatment was inadequate by current standards.

## Combination Chemotherapy

With the exception of studies dealing with two-drug combinations among small numbers of patients (55,75), all randomized trials investigating the relative value of combination chemotherapy for induction treatment have generally used the MOPP combination versus closely related regimens (Table 7).

The British National Lymphoma Investigation Group (7), the Acute Leukemia

TABLE 7. *The MOPP regimen versus other combination chemotherapy as induction treatment in advanced Hodgkin's disease*

| Investigator and treatment arm | Total no. of patients | Response rate (%) | |
|---|---|---|---|
| | | Complete | Complete and partial |
| British National Lymphoma Investigation (7) | | | |
| A. MOPP | 49 | 80 | 96 |
| B. HN₂, VCR, prednisone | 41 | 44 | 86 |
| Nissen et al. (55) | | | |
| A. MOPP | — | — | 88 |
| B. BCNU, VCR, prednisone | — | — | 71 |
| C. VCR, PCZ, prednisone | — | — | 69 |
| D. BCNU, VCR, PCZ, prednisone | — | — | 91 |
| Hum et al. (38) | | | |
| A. MOPP | 20 | 35 | 85 |
| B. CCNU, VLB, prednisone | 19 | 63 | 84 |
| Stutzman and Glidewell (78) | | | |
| A. MOPP | 81 | 61 | ≥90 |
| B. PCZ, prednisone, VCR, CHL, VLB | 77 | 49 | ≥90 |
| C. CHL, VLB, prednisone/VCR, PCZ | 89 | 61 | ≥90 |
| Coltman et al. (15) | | | |
| A. MOPP | 30 | 57 | — |
| B. MOPP + BLM (low dose) | 27 | 89 | — |
| C. MOPP + BLM (high dose) | 27 | 67 | — |
| Cooper et al. (19) | | | |
| A. MOPP | — | — | — |
| B. HN₂, VLB, PCZ, prednisone | — | — | — |
| C. CCNU, VCR, PCZ, prednisone | — | — | — |
| D. CCNU, VLB, PCZ, prednisone | — | — | — |
| Bennett et al. (3) | | | |
| A. MOPP | 115 | 69 | 80 |
| B. BCNU, CTX, VLB, PCZ prednisone | 115 | 68 | 82 |
| Bonadonna et al. (5) | | | |
| A. MOPP | 29 | 62 | 79 |
| B. ADM, BLM, VLB, DTIC | 27 | 70 | 81 |

Group B (55), and the Western Cancer Study Group (38) have used three-drug combinations that generally showed lower activity than the MOPP combination. Little information is available for these trials, especially with regard to patient selection, stratification criteria, or response by prognostic factors.

The British National Lymphoma Investigation Group (7) has designed a trial to establish the role of prednisone in the MOPP regimen. Patients were randomized to the four-drug combination, including prednisone, or to the same combination without prednisone (MOP). The steroid was given in each cycle and not only in the first and the fourth cycle as reported in the original regimen (23). There was a highly significant difference in the complete remission rates favoring the MOPP combination and emphasizing the role of prednisone in this regimen.

More than 500 patients with stage IIIB and IV have been entered into the study of the Acute Leukemia Group B (55) comparing MOPP to either BCNU, VCR, PCZ, and prednisone (BOPP) or BCNU, VCR, and prednisone (BOP) or VCR, PCZ, and prednisone (OPP). After 6 months of induction chemotherapy, responders received one of three maintenance regimens until relapse: CHL, a combination of CHL, VCR, and prednisone, or VLB alone. Final analysis of the data is not available, but the latest report indicated a significant superiority in overall response rates of the four-drug regimens over the three-drug combinations. The latter combinations were then discontinued and the study of the other combinations was pursued with the modification of randomly decreasing the dosage of VCR to one-half the usual dose in half of the patients entering the protocol. It is unfortunate that this trial with such a large accrual will be of no help in defining if maintenance therapy, still of unproven value after MOPP-related regimens, should be used at all.

In another trial of the Acute Leukemia Group B (78), 247 evaluable patients, after stratification for prior or no prior therapy, were randomized to MOPP or a five-drug regimen given either sequentially or by alternating of a two-drug and a three-drug combination. Treatment groups were reported to be similar in size for stage, prior response, sex, age, and duration of disease, but distribution of patients by prognostic factors was not given. The complete remission rate was 49% for the sequential schedule and 61% for the two other treatments. These responses were not detailed by pretreatment characteristics. The median duration of response to MOPP was 11 months versus 7 months for either of the other regimens. Furthermore, 4 years after the study was closed for entry, relapses occurred in 54% with MOPP versus 75% with the other regimens, a difference that was statistically significant. At the time of the report, no differences in survival rates were apparent among the three treatment groups, the median survival time being approximately 30 months in all instances.

Other combinations of four or more drugs have been developed and compared to the MOPP regimen. These combinations have used other alkylating agents, nitrosoureas, and VLB. As seen in a trial previously described in this section (55), the substitution of BCNU for $HN_2$ apparently did not improve the therapeutic results of the original combination. However, two trials (15,19) have detected apparently enhanced effectiveness with newer combinations. Unfortunately, both trials used maintenance treatments without untreated controls after induction chemotherapy. These data are preliminary and must await further confirmation.

The Southwest Oncology Group (15) undertook a study to determine the comparative effectiveness of MOPP alone and in combination with either low- or high-dose bleomycin (BLM). Complete responses were maintained for 18 months with MOPP (two schedules) or radiotherapy plus MOPP. The distribution of patients in the three induction regimens was comparable with respect to pathologic stage, age, and prior therapy. An interim report indicated a significant difference in the rate of complete remissions between patients who received MOPP (57%) and MOPP plus low dose BLM (89%).

Cooper et al. (19) published in an abstract results of four programs of the Acute Leukemia Group B, that is, MOPP and three related combinations in which either $HN_2$ or VCR, or both, were replaced by CCNU and VLB, respectively. A maintenance program using VLB alone or with periodic four-drug reinduction was also investigated in this trial. Of the 438 patients randomized, only 327 were evaluated at the time of the report. According to these partial results, the frequency of complete responses ranged from 55 to 59%; the toxicity appeared to be reduced and the remission duration significantly prolonged with the combination of CCNU, VLB, PCZ, and prednisone (CVPP) as compared to the MOPP regimen.

Improvement of tolerance to the MOPP regimen has also been found by the Eastern Cooperative Oncology Group (3) with a five-drug combination (BCVPP). This combination was obtained by substituting CTX for $HN_2$, VLB for VCR, and by adding BCNU in the standard MOPP combination. Unlike the MOPP program, intravenous medication including CTX, VLB, and BCNU was administered only once every 4 weeks. Complete responders were to receive six additional courses of BCVPP, BCG, or no further therapy. Results of the maintenance phase are still coded (2). In the induction phase, there was no significant difference in the rate of complete remission. BCVPP produced a very low incidence of neurologic toxicities and far fewer instances of gastrointestinal disturbances, including nausea, vomiting, or diarrhea. However, hematologic side effects were more pronounced with this regimen.

Along the same line, it must be mentioned that combinations of CTX, VLB, PCZ, and prednisone with or without CCNU have been studied in South America (60) but cannot yet be assessed.

Finally, Bonadonna et al. (5) developed a combination with four drugs not used in the standard MOPP program. This combination included adriamycin (ADM), BLM, VLB, and DTIC (ABVD), and was also given in monthly cycles. In a preliminary report of a controlled study randomizing MOPP versus ABVD, 56 previously untreated patients were evaluable for the analysis of remission induction. Treatment groups had been stratified for stage (IIB, IIIB, IIIS, and IV) and histology. Complete remission occurred in 62% of the patients treated with MOPP and in 70% of those given ABVD. Complete and good partial responses were consolidated with low-dose radiotherapy followed by six additional cycles of the induction treatment in patients with extranodal disease. Data concerning crossover therapy after remission induction failure were available for 10 patients. ABVD elicited 2 complete responses in 5 patients for 2 and 5 months, whereas no complete remission was seen with MOPP.

In summary, the toxicity of $HN_2$ and VCR in the MOPP program may be alleviated with the use of other alkylating agents, nitrosoureas, and VLB, apparently with no loss of antitumor activity. Promising results have been achieved in patients with no prior treatment by using the ABVD regimen, and its degree of cross-resistance with the MOPP combination is being explored. The various studies comparing induction regimens of combination chemotherapy are essentially characterized by a lack of firm data presently available. There is some evidence that the MOPP combination is superior to a three-drug combination. It has been suggested that the effectiveness of the MOPP program can still be increased by adding BLM or substituting CCNU for $HN_2$ and VLB for VCR, but confirmation of these findings is needed.

In a previous section of this chapter, it was shown that maintenance treatment can prolong the duration of remissions induced by short-term, single-agent induction, especially in complete responders. Several trials have specifically investigated the value of maintenance therapy in patients achieving complete response with more aggressive induction regimens (Table 8). Thus far, results obtained with maintenance chemotherapy following optimal induction therapy have been disappointing.

A combination of CTX, VCR, and prednisone (COP) was selected by Luce et al. (52) as induction treatment. If complete remission was achieved with six courses given at 2-week intervals, four additional courses were given at the same schedule. Patients still in complete remission after 10 courses of induction treatment were randomized to no further treatment or continued treatment with COP at 4-week intervals until relapse. Patients relapsing during unmaintained remission were treated again with the induction regimen. This study included patients with Hodgkin's disease and other lymphomas, and randomization to maintenance or no maintenance was made without respect to type of disease, resulting in an uneven distribution of patients with Hodgkin's disease between the treatment groups. Complete remission was achieved in 36% of the patients with Hodgkin's disease, and the median duration of complete remission from time of randomization was significantly longer with COP maintenance. At the time of the report, more than 90% of the patients in complete remission after induction treatment were alive at 80 weeks, and the effect of maintenance treatment on survival could not be analyzed.

In 1973, the National Cancer Institute (87) and the Southwest Oncology Group (29) published conflicting interim results on the potential of maintenance therapy in complete responders following induction with the MOPP regimen. At the National Cancer Institute, 57 patients with clinical stages IIIB and IV were selected for the study. Eight of the patients had prior extensive radiotherapy,

TABLE 8. *Maintenance treatment following complete remission on combination chemotherapy*[a]

| Induction therapy | Maintenance treatment | No. of patients | Median disease-free interval (weeks) | Reference |
|---|---|---|---|---|
| COP every 2 weeks | A. COP every 4 weeks | 11 | 42 | 52 |
| (10 cycles) | B. 0 | 20 | 19 | |
| MOPP every 4 weeks | A. MOPP 10 cycles/15 | | | 87 |
| (6 cycles) | months | 20 | >208 | |
| | B. BCNU 200 mg/m² X 5/15 | 16 | >208 | |
| | months | 21 | >208 | |
| | C. 0 | | | |
| MOPP every 4 weeks | A. MOP 9 cycles/18 months | 35 | >150 | 17 |
| (6 cycles) | B. 0 | 40 | 150 | |
| BCVPP every 4 weeks[b] | A. BCVPP 6 cycles/6 months | 21 | >208 | 25 |
| | B. MOPP 6 cycles/6 months | 29 | >208 | |
| | C. 0 | 51 | >208 | |

COP = cytoxan, vincristine, prednisone; MOPP = mechlorethamine, vincristine, procarbazine, prednisone; BCVPP = BCNU, cytoxan, vinblastine, procarbazine, prednisone.
[a] Various other studies were designed to test the value of maintenance therapy, but minimal or no results are available for analysis. The maintenance regimens have included single agents (16,19,55), sequential regimens (20,24), combination chemotherapy (3,15), single-agent or sequential regimens plus reinduction with combination chemotherapy (19,20,55), chemotherapy and radiotherapy (5,15), and immunotherapy (2,72).
[b] Results available only for patients without prior major treatment.

most of them 2 to 6 years before MOPP induction treatment. None of the remaining 49 patients had been treated before entering the trial. The MOPP induction therapy consisted of six cycles, or more if evidence of continued response short of a complete remission occurred after six cycles. Two additional cycles of therapy were given after complete remission. Within 3 months of entering complete remission, as assessed by extensive staging procedures, patients were randomly allocated to either no further therapy or maintenance with MOPP or BCNU. Each group was similar with regard to sex ratio, previous therapy, stage, histology, mean absolute lymphocyte counts before starting therapy, mean time to complete remission, and mean number of cycles of MOPP given. After a median follow-up time of 2.75 years, ranging from 6 years to less than 1 year, the percentage of relapses without maintenance and with MOPP or BCNU maintenance was 24%, 25%, and 13%, respectively. No statistical difference could be found in disease-free survival curves up to 3.5 years, and the median duration of complete remission, calculated from the end of induction therapy, was projected to be greater than 48 months in each group. One death occurred in each group, and it was too early to estimate if survival was influenced by maintenance therapy.

In the study undertaken by the Southwest Oncology Group (29), remission induction also consisted of six courses of MOPP, or more if only partial remission was achieved at that time. Seventy-five clinical stage III or IV patients entered the study, 49 with no prior treatment and 26 with prior radiotherapy and/or chemotherapy. Those allocated to maintenance received two more courses of MOPP at 4-week intervals, followed by treatment every 8 weeks for at least 2 years. Prednisone was not given during remission maintenance therapy. Groups were similar with regard to stages, age, histologic cell types, sex ratio, and prior therapy. After a follow-up ranging from 3 to 5 years, relapses in the maintained and the unmaintained group occurred in 31 and 53%, respectively. The fraction of patients remaining in complete remission was significantly higher in the maintenance group than in the no maintenance group. However, there was evidence that the unmaintained remission curve was leveling off at 3 years. These results were recently updated after follow-up of 7.2 years (17). The median duration of maintained complete remission was not yet reached; the median for unmaintained complete remission was 150 weeks. The difference between the two groups was no longer significant. The respective survival estimates at 7.2 years for maintenance and no maintenance treatment were 48 versus 58%, strongly suggesting that there will be no survival advantage with maintenance therapy.

The Southeastern Cancer Study Group (25) has randomized patients in complete remission on BCVPP induction therapy to either no further treatment or to six more courses of BCVPP or MOPP. Stratification was made according to prior therapy. A benefit of maintenance therapy was seen only in patients with no major therapy prior to the trial. In this category of patients, estimates based on data obtained with a follow-up of 1 to 4 years indicated that the probability of remaining disease-free 3 years after completion of therapy was approximately 87 and 67% for maintained and unmaintained patients. The corresponding probability of 4-year survival was 97% and 67%, respectively. These differences in duration of remission and survival were statistically significant. However, a multivariate analysis of the data showed that these results were related to an imbalance of prognostic variables and not to the maintenance treatment. Age was identified as the major factor influencing the disease-free interval, whereas high lymphocyte counts and favorable histology (LP or NS) were the significant determinants in survival.

Thus, a role for maintenance chemotherapy could not be established in any trial following a MOPP or a MOPP-related induction regimen. These trials proved to be difficult, as reflected by the small number of patients studied (Table 8). In fact, larger accrual will probably be needed to detect a possible therapeutic benefit of maintenance therapy in an unselected population, and, *a fortiori,* in subsets of patients with well-defined prognostic variables.

## RANDOMIZED TRIALS INVOLVING RADIOTHERAPY IN STAGE IV HODGKIN'S DISEASE

Two trials involving radiotherapy for stage IV Hodgkin's disease have been initiated at Stanford University (47). Patients with liver involvement and no other extranodal disease are randomly treated by MOPP (six cycles) or by

TN irradiation plus liver irradiation. In all other stage IV presentations, randomization is to either MOPP (six cycles) or a "split course" of MOPP with TN radiotherapy given between the second and the third cycle of chemotherapy. Little data are available for these trials (31).

## RANDOMIZED TRIALS INVOLVING IMMUNOTHERAPY IN HODGKIN'S DISEASE

Two controlled trials have used immunotherapy as maintenance therapy in Hodgkin's disease. Conclusive data are not available from either trial.

At Roswell Park Memorial Institute (72), stage I-IIIA lymphomas in complete or partial remission following "standard treatment" were randomized to receive BCG or no therapy. The standard treatments had been given at various intervals prior to the BCG administration. This interval was longer than 1 year in 14% (3 of 22) of the control patients and in 43% (12 of 28) of the BCG-treated patients. In the control group 5 patients had stage I disease versus 9 in the treatment group. Thirty-two patients had Hodgkin's disease, 8 of 15 with favorable histology (LP or NS) in the control group and 13 of 16 in the treatment group. The median time to relapse after entering into the study was 10 months in the control and 32 months in the treated group, a difference statistically significant but totally invalidated by the inappropriate study design.

Another trial still in progress is evaluating BCG maintenance therapy in complete responders to combination chemotherapy (2), but only interim and coded results are available.

## DISCUSSION

Hodgkin's disease has generated a large number of randomized clinical trials, but most of them are characterized by inconsistent staging, small patient numbers, short periods of observation, and/or limited information regarding the criteria of selection and stratification. Although the available data must be interpreted with caution, some important facts have become apparent.

In nodal disease, radiotherapy has been a common initial therapeutic approach. Randomized trials have rapidly confirmed the previously stated benefit of wide-field radiotherapy in clinical stages I–II with the suggestion of an overall superiority of TN irradiation in an unselected population. However, the most appropriate treatment fields for more accurately defined prognostic categories of patients have not been ascertained. Nevertheless, the 70% relapse-free survival that may be achieved at 8 years in all the pathologic stages from IA through IIIA indicates that current radiotherapeutic techniques are likely to be curative in a substantial proportion of these patients. The analysis of survival data in relation to the type of initial treatment is obscured by the effectiveness of subsequent therapy given upon relapse.

The respective roles of radiotherapy and chemotherapy in nodal presentations has not been fully elucidated. Ongoing trials are exploring the usefulness of these combined modalities by comparing intensive irradiation followed by intensive chemotherapy, either immediately after radiotherapy or at disease progression. Presently available data in pathologic stage I-IIIA show a striking benefit in relapse-free survival with adjuvant combination chemotherapy, but this difference now is significant only in asymptomatic patients. No clear survival gain has resulted from adjuvant chemotherapy in any of these stages.

Survival rates of 85% are noted at 8 years without adjuvant chemotherapy in all pathologic stages from I through IIIA, emphasizing the need for a large number of patients and prolonged follow-up periods to detect further therapeutic improvement. The combined use of aggressive radiotherapy and chemotherapy is endowed with significant morbidity and appears to favor the occurrence of second malignancies (10). The risk cannot yet be actually quantified insofar as the proportion of patients cured by radiotherapy alone still remains hypothetical. Perhaps future trials should attempt to define more optimal integration of radiotherapy and chemotherapy, especially in patients who might be presently overtreated.

Comparative single-agent studies have provided minimal, if any, contribution to our ability to define effectiveness of these drugs. Interest in these trials has progressively disappeared with the development of highly effective combination chemotherapy. The MOPP regimen has achieved striking results in a nonrandomized study involving stage III-IV disease. None of the combinations subsequently compared to the MOPP combination have shown a clear improvement in therapeutic effectiveness. At present, there is no evidence indicating that maintenance therapy can prolong the complete remission induced by intensive combination chemotherapy given at least during 6 months or beyond the time it takes to achieve a complete remission. However, larger experience with these combinations should sharpen our knowledge of clinical factors of prognostic significance for the duration of these remissions. Maintenance treatment should then be further investigated in a well-defined, poor-risk population.

It usually appears that a trial *only* has to be controlled to be believed, whereas uncontrolled trials are dismissed as a source of data. The reverse is true in Hodgkin's disease. Randomized clinical trials have added little to the major improvements in therapeutic results obtained in nonrandomized trials. The treatment of Hodgkin's disease is now so effective, whatever the stage, that a considerable number of patients and long periods of observation will be required in future randomized studies of primary therapy, unless restricted to patients with unfavorable prognosis. Future randomized trials in Hodgkin's disease with favorable prognosis should be undertaken with extreme reservation.

## ACKNOWLEDGMENTS

The authors gratefully acknowledge the help of Drs. J. R. Durant, G. B. Hutchinson, A. M. Jelliffe, L. Lev, S. A. Rosenberg, Mr. W. T. Soper, Mrs. H. Lever, and Mrs. L. Edge in the preparation of this chapter.

# REFERENCES

1. Alison, R. E., and Whitelaw, D. M., (1970): A comparison of nitrogen mustard and vinblastine sulfate in the treatment of patients with Hodgkin's disease. *Can. Med. Assoc. J.,* 102:278–280.
2. Bakemeier, R., Costello, W., Horton, J., and De Vita, V. (1978): BCG immunotherapy following chemotherapy-induced remissions of stage III and IV Hodgkin's disease. In: *Immunotherapy of Cancer: Present Status of Trials in Man,* edited by W. D. Terry and D. Windhorst, pp. 513–517. Raven Press, New York.
3. Bennett, J. M., Bakemeier, R. F., Carbone, P. P., Ezdinli, E., and Lenhard, R. E., Jr. (1976): Clinical trials with BCNU (NSC-409962) in malignant lymphomas by the Eastern Cooperative Oncology Group. *Cancer Treat. Rev.,* 60:739–745.
4. Bonadonna, G., Uslenghi, C., and Zucali, R. (1975): Recent trends in the medical treatment of Hodgkin's disease. *Eur. J. Cancer,* 11:251–266.
5. Bonadonna, G., Zucali, R., De Lena, M., and Valagussa, P. (1977): Combined chemotherapy (MOPP or ABVD)—Radiotherapy approach in advanced Hodgkin's disease. *Cancer Treat. Rev.,* 61:769–777.
6. Brindley, C. O., Salvin, L. G., Potee, K. G., Lipowska, B., Shnider, B. I., Regelson, W., and Colsky, J. (1964): Further comparative trial of triethylene thiophosphoramide and mechlorethamine in patients with melanoma and Hodgkin's disease. *J. Chron. Dis.,* 17:19–30.
7. British National Lymphoma Investigation (1975): Value of prednisone in combination chemotherapy of stage IV Hodgkin's disease. *Br. Med. J.,* 3:413–414.
8. British National Lymphoma Investigation (1976): Initial treatment of stage III A Hodgkin's disease. Comparison of radiotherapy with combined chemotherapy. *Lancet,* II:991–995.
9. Brook, J., Clough, R. G., Schreiber, W., Mass, R., and Gocka, E. (1970): Hodgkin's disease: Survival with single agent induction and remission maintenance versus combination chemotherapy. *Proc. Am. Assoc. Cancer Res.,* 11:12.
10. Canellos, G. P., DeVita, V. T., Arseneau, J. C., Whang-Peng, J., and Johnson, R. E. C. (1975): Second malignancies complicating Hodgkin's disease in remission. *Lancet,* I:947–949.
11. Carbone, P. P., Kaplan, H. S., Musshoff, K., Smithers, D. W., and Tubiana, M. (1971): Report of the committee on Hodgkin's disease staging classification. *Cancer Res.,* 31:1860–1861.
12. Carbone, P. P., Spurr, C., Schneiderman, M., Scotto, J., Holland, J. F., and Shnider, B. (1968): Management of patients with malignant lymphoma: A comparative study with cyclophosphamide and vinca alkaloids. *Cancer Res.,* 28:811–822.
13. Carey, R. W., Hall, T. C., and Finkel, H. E. (1963): A comparison of two dosage regimens for vincristine. *Cancer Chemother. Rep.,* 27:91–96.
14. Carter, S. K., and Livingston, R. B. (1973): Single-agent therapy for Hodgkin's disease. *Arch. Intern. Med.,* 131:377–387.
15. Coltman, C. A., Jr., and Delaney, F. C. (1973): Five drug combination chemotherapy for advanced Hodgkin's disease. *Clin. Res.,* 21:876.
16. Coltman, C. A., Jr., Frei, E., III, and Delaney, F. C. (1973): Effectiveness of actinomycin D (A), methotrexate (MTX) and vinblastine (V) in prolonging the duration of combination chemotherapy (MOPP) induced remission in advanced Hodgkin's disease (HD). *Cancer Chemother. Rep.,* 57:109.
17. Coltman, C. A., Jr., Hall, W., Frei, E., III, and Moon, T. E. (1976): MOPP maintenance (MM) vs unmaintained remission (UMR) for MOPP induced complete remission (CR) of advanced Hodgkin's disease (HD): 7.2 year follow-up. *Proc. Am. Soc. Clin. Oncol.,* 17:289.
18. Cooper, I. A., Rana, C., Madigan, J. P., Motteram, R., Maritz, J. S., and Turner, C. N. (1972): Combination chemotherapy (MOPP) in the management of advanced Hodgkin's disease. A progress report on 55 patients. *Med. J. Aust.,* 1:41–49.
19. Cooper, M. R., Spurr, C. L., Glidewell, O., and Holland, J. F. (1975): The superiority of a nitrosourea (CCNU) containing four-drug combination over MOPP in the treatment of stage III and IV Hodgkin's disease. *Proc. Am. Soc. Hematol.,* p. 60.
20. De Lena, M., Monfardini, S., Beretta, G., Fossati-Bellani, F., and Bonadonna, G. (1973): Clinical trials with intensive chemotherapy and radiotherapy in Hodgkin's disease. *Natl. Cancer Inst. Monogr.,* 36:403–420.
21. De Vita, V., Canellos, G., Hubbard, S., Chabner, B., and Young, R. (1976): Chemotherapy

of Hodgkin's disease (HD) with MOPP: A 10 year progress report. *Proc. Am. Soc. Clin. Oncol.,* 17:269.

22. De Vita, V. T., and Serpick, A. (1967): Combination chemotherapy in the treatment of advanced Hodgkin's disease (HD). *Proc. Am. Assoc. Cancer Res.,* 8:13.

23. De Vita, V. T., Jr., Serpick, A. A., and Carbone, P. P. (1970): Combination chemotherapy in the treatment of advanced Hodgkin's disease. *Ann. Intern. Med.,* 73:881–895.

24. Diggs, C. H., Wiernik, P. H., Levi, J. A., and Kvols, L. K. (1977): Cyclophosphamide, vinblastine, procarbazine and prednisone with CCNU and vinblastine maintenance for advanced Hodgkin's disease. *Cancer,* 39:1949–1954.

25. Durant, J. R., Gams, R. A., Velez-Garcior, E., Bartolucci, A., Wirtschafter, D., and Dorfman, R. F. (1978): BCNU, cyclophosphamide, Velban, procarbazine and prednisone in advanced Hodgkin's disease. *Cancer (in press).*

26. E.O.R.T.C. Radiochemotherapy Cooperative Group (1977): Adjuvant chemotherapy after radiotherapy in stage I and II Hodgkin's disease. In: *Adjuvant Therapy of Cancer,* edited by S. E. Salmon and S. E. Jones, pp. 517–528. Elsevier/North-Holland Biomedical Press, Amsterdam.

27. Ezdinli, E. Z., and Stutzman, L. (1968): Vinblastine vs. nitrogen mustard therapy of Hodgkin's disease. *Cancer,* 22:473–479.

28. Fortuny, I. E., Theologides, A., and Kennedy, B. J. (1972): Single, combined and sequential use of uracil mustard and prednisone in the treatment of lymphoreticular tumors. *Minn. Med.,* 55:715–716, 728.

29. Frei, E., III, Luce, J. K., Gamble, J. F., Coltman, C. A., Jr., Constanzi, J. J., Talley, R. W., Monto, R. W., Wilson, H. E., Hewlett, J. S., Delaney, F. C., and Gehan, E. A. (1973): Combination chemotherapy in advanced Hodgkin's disease: Induction and maintenance of remission. *Ann. Intern. Med.,* 79:376–382.

30. Gilbert, R. (1939): Radiotherapy in Hodgkin's disease (malignant granulomatosis). Anatomic and clinical foundations; governing principles; results. *Am. J. Roentgenol. Radium Ther. Nucl. Med.,* 41:198–241.

31. Glatstein, E. (1977): Radiotherapy in Hodgkin's disease. Past achievements and future progress. *Cancer,* 39:837–842.

32. Gold, G. L., Shnider, B. I., Salvin, L. G., Schneiderman, M. A., Colsky, J., Owens, A. H., Jr., Krant, M. J., Miller, S. P., Frei, E., III, Hall, T. C., Spurr, C. L., McIntyre, O. R., Hoogstraten, B., and Holland, J. F. (1970): The use of mechlorethamine, cyclophosphamide, and uracil mustard in neoplastic disease: A cooperative study. *J. Clin. Pharmacol.,* 10:110–120.

33. Grasso, J. A., Panahon, A., Kaufman, J. H., Friedman, M., Moore, R., and Stutzman, L. (1977): A randomized study of radiation therapy (RT) vs RT and chemotherapy (CT) in stage IA-IIIB Hodgkin's disease. *Proc. Am. Assoc. Cancer Res.,* 18:173.

34. Greenberg, L. H., Wong, Y. S., Richardson, A. P., Jr., and Dollinger, M. R. (1972): Combination chemotherapy of Hodgkin's disease in private practice. *JAMA,* 221:261–263.

35. Hoogstraten, B., and Glidewell, O. (1974): Chemotherapy-radiotherapy for stage III Hodgkin's diease. *Proc. Am. Soc. Clin. Oncol.,* 15:160.

36. Hoogstraten, B., Holland, J. F., Kramer, S., and Glidewell, O. J. (1973): Combination chemotherapy-radiotherapy for stage III Hodgkin's disease. An Acute Leukemia Group B study. *Arch. Intern. Med.,* 131:424–428.

37. Huguley, C. M., Jr., Durant, J. R., Moores, R. R., Chan, Y. K., Dorfman, R. F., and Johnson, L. (1975): A comparison of nitrogen mustard, vincristine, procarbazine, and prednisone (MOPP) vs. nitrogen mustard in advanced Hodgkin's disease. *Cancer,* 36:1227–1240.

38. Hum, G. J., Sribour, L. M., and Bateman, J. R. (1976): A randomized phase III study for adult advanced Hodgkin's disease, MOPP vs CCNU, Velban, prednisone. *Proc. Am. Soc. Clin. Oncol.,* 17:310.

39. Jacobs, E. M., Peters, F. C., Luce, J. K., Zippin, C., and Wood, D. A. (1968): Mechlorethamine HCL and cyclophosphamide in the treatment of Hodgkin's disease and the lymphomas. *JAMA,* 203:392–398.

40. Jelliffe, A. M. (1973): The British National Lymphoma Investigation. *Natl. Cancer Inst. Monogr.,* 36:427–428.

41. Johnson, R. E., Glover, M. K., and Marshall, S. K. (1971): Results of radiation therapy and implications for the clinical staging of Hodgkin's disease. *Cancer Res.,* 31:1834–1837.

42. Johnson, R. E., Thomas, L. B., Schneiderman, M., Glenn, D. W., Faw, F., and Hafermann, M. D. (1970): Preliminary experience with total nodal irradiation in Hodgkin's disease. *Radiology*, 96:603–608.
43. Kaplan, H. S. (1962): The radical radiotherapy of regionally localized Hodgkin's disease. *Radiology*, 78:553–569.
44. Kaplan, H. S. (1966): Evidence for a tumoricidal dose level in the radiotherapy of Hodgkin's disease. *Cancer Res.*, 26:1221–1224.
45. Kaplan, H. S. (1971): Contiguity and progression in Hodgkin's disease. *Cancer Res.*, 31:1811–1813.
46. Kaplan, H. S., and Rosenberg, S. A. (1966): Extended-field radical radiotherapy in advanced Hodgkin's disease: Short-term results of 2 randomized clinical trials. *Cancer Res.*, 26:1268–1276.
47. Kaplan, H. S., and Rosenberg, S. A. (1973): Current status of clinical trials: Stanford experience, 1962–72. *Natl. Cancer Inst. Monogr.*, 36:363–371.
48. Kaung, D. T., Wittington, R. M., Spencer, H., and Patno, M. E. (1969): Comparison of chlorambucil and streptonigrin (NSC-45383) in the treatment of malignant lymphomas. *Cancer*, 23:1280–1283.
49. Laszlo, J., Grizzle, J., Jonsson, U., and Rundles, R. W. (1962): Comparative study of mannitol mustard, cyclophosphamide, and nitrogen mustard in malignant lymphomas. *Cancer Chemother. Rep.*, 16:247–250.
50. Lenhard, R. E., Jr. (1973): Eastern Cooperative Oncology Group Studies. *Arch. Intern. Med.*, 131:418–420.
51. Lowenbraun, S. DeVita, V. T., and Serpick, A. A. (1970): Combination chemotherapy with nitrogen mustard, vincristine, procarbazine, and prednisone in previously treated patients with Hodgkin's disease. *Blood*, 36:704–717.
52. Luce, J. K., Gamble, J. F., Wilson, H. E., Monto, R. W., Isaacs, B. L., Palmer, R. L., Coltman, C. A., Jr., Hewlett, J. S., Gehan, E. A., and Frei, E., III (1971): Combined cyclophosphamide, vincristine, and prednisone therapy of malignant lymphoma. *Cancer*, 28:306–317.
53. Lukes, R. J., Craver, L. F., Hall, T. C., Rappaport, H., and Ruben, P. (1966): Report of the Nomenclature Committee. *Cancer Res.*, 26:1311.
54. Moore, M. R., Jones, S. E., Bull, J. M., William, L. A., and Rosenberg, S. A. (1973): MOPP chemotherapy for advanced Hodgkin's disease. Prognostic factors in 81 patients. *Cancer*, 32:52–60.
55. Nissen, N. I., Stutzman, L., Holland, J. F., and Glidewell, O. J. (1973): Chemotherapy of Hodgkin's disease in studies by Acute Leukemia Group B. *Arch. Intern. Med.*, 131:396–401.
56. Nixon, D. W., and Aisenberg, A. C. (1974): Combination chemotherapy of Hodgkin's disease. *Cancer*, 33:1499–1504.
57. O'Connell, M. J., Wiernik, P. H., Brace, K. C., Byhardt, R. W., and Greene, W. H. (1975): A combined modality approach to the treatment of Hodgkin's disease. Preliminary results of a prospectively randomized clinical trial. *Cancer*, 35:1055–1065.
58. Olweny, C. L. M., Ziegler, J. L., Bernard, C. W., and Templeton, A. C. (1971): Adult Hodgkin's disease in Uganda. *Cancer*, 27:1295–1301.
59. Papac, R. J., and Wood, D. A. (1964): Long term results achieved with the use of alkylating agents in malignant lymphoma and Hodgkin's disease. *Acta Union Int. Cancer*, 20:377–379.
60. Pavlovsky, S., Morgenfeld, M., Somoza, H., Cavagnaro, F., and Bonesana, H. (1977): Combined chemotherapy cyclophosphamide, vinblastine, procarbazine and prednisone (CVPP) vs. CVPP plus CCNU (CCVPP) in Hodgkin's disease (HD). *Proc. Am. Assoc. Cancer Res.*, 18:218.
61. Peters, M. V. (1966): Prophylactic treatment of adjacent areas in Hodgkin's disease. *Cancer Res.*, 26:1232–1243.
62. Radiotherapy Hodgkin's Disease Group (1976): Survival and complications of radiotherapy following involved and extended field therapy of Hodgkin's disease, stages I and II. *Cancer*, 38:288–305.
63. Raich, P. C., Korst, D. R., and Dessel, B. H. (1975): Randomized study of lymphoma therapy. *Proc. Am. Assoc. Cancer Res.*, 16:182.
64. Rege, V. B., and Owens, A. H., Jr. (1974): BCNU (NSC-409962) in the treatment of advanced Hodgkin's disease, lymphosarcoma, and reticulum cell sarcoma. *Cancer Chemother. Rep.*, 58:383–392.
65. Rosenberg, S. A. (1966): Report of the committee on the staging of Hodgkin's disease. *Cancer Res.*, 26:1310.

66. Rosenberg, S. A., and Kaplan, H. S. (1970): Hodgkin's disease and other malignant lymphomas. *Calif. Med.,* 113(4):23–38.

67. Rosenberg, S. A., and Kaplan, H. S. (1975): The management of stages I, II, and III Hodgkin's disease with combined radiotherapy and chemotherapy. *Cancer,* 35:55–63.

68. Rosenberg, S. A., Kaplan, H. S., Glatstein, E., and Portlock, C. S. (1977): The role of adjuvant MOPP in the radiation therapy of Hodgkin's disease: A progress report after eight years on the Stanford trials. In: *Adjuvant Therapy of Cancer,* edited by S. S. Salmon and S. E. Jones, pp. 505–515. Elsevier/North-Holland Biomedical Press, Amsterdam.

69. Rozencweig, M., Kenis, Y., and Staquet, M. (1975): Hodgkin's disease: Prognostic factors and clinical evaluation. In: *Cancer Therapy: Prognostic Factors and Criteria of Response,* edited by M. J. Staquet, pp. 49–72. Raven Press, New York.

70. Scott, J. L. (1963): The effect of nitrogen mustard and maintenance chlorambucil in the treatment of advanced Hodgkin's disease. *Cancer Chemother. Rep.,* 27:27–32.

71. Selawry, O. S., and Hansen, H. H. (1972): Superiority of CCNU (1-(2-chloroethyl)-3-cyclohexyl-1-nitrosourea; NSC 79037) over BCNU (1,3-bis(2-chloroethyl)-1-nitrosourea; NSC 409962) in treatment of advanced Hodgkin's disease. *Proc. Am. Assoc. Cancer Res.,* 13:46.

72. Sokal, J. E., Aungst, C. W., and Snyderman, M. (1974): Delay in progression of malignant lymphoma after BCG vaccination. *N. Engl. J. Med.,* 291:1226–1230.

73. Solomon, J., Jacobs, E. M., Bateman, J. R., Lukes, R. J., Weiner, J. M., and Donohue, D. M. (1973): Chemotherapy of lymphoma with mechlorethamine and vinblastine. *Arch. Intern. Med.,* 131:407–417.

74. Spear, P. W., and Patno, M. E. (1962): A comparative study of the effectiveness of HN2 and cyclophosphamide in bronchogenic carcinoma, Hodgkin's disease, and lymphosarcoma. *Cancer Chemother. Rep.,* 16:413–415.

75. Stolinsky, D. C. (1970): Cytosine arabinoside (Ara-C) combined with either cyclophosphamide (CTX), vincristine (VCR), or trimethylcolchicinic acid (TMCA) in therapy for advanced cancer. In: *Oncology 1970. Abstracts of the Tenth International Cancer Congress,* edited by R. L. Clark, R. W. Cumley, J. E. McCay, and M. M. Copeland, p. 495. Medical Arts Publishing Co., Houston, Texas.

76. Stutzman, L. (1971): Combined radiotherapy and chemotherapy of lymphomas and other cancers. *Cancer Res.,* 31:1845–1850.

77. Stutzman, L., Ezdinli, E. Z., and Stutzman, M. A. (1966): Vinblastine sulfate vs cyclophosphamide in the therapy for lymphoma. *JAMA,* 195:173–178.

78. Stutzman, L., and Glidewell, O. (1973): Multiple chemotherapeutic agents for Hodgkin disease. Comparison of three routines: A cooperative study by Acute Leukemia Group B. *JAMA,* 225:1202–1211.

79. Stutzman, L., and Stutzman, M. (1969): Protection against hematologic depression of radiotherapy by corticosteroids. *Proc. Am. Assoc. Cancer Res.,* 10:89.

80. Sullivan, M. P. (1967): Cyclophosphamide (NSC-26271) therapy for children with generalized lymphoma and Hodgkin's disease. *Cancer Chemother. Rep.,* 51:393–397.

81. Thompson, E., Smith, K. L., Wilimas, J., and Kumar, M. (1977): Radiation, chemotherapy, or both in childhood and adolescent Hodgkin's disease (HD). *Proc. Am. Assoc. Cancer Res.,* 18:221.

82. Thompson Hancock, P. E., Austin, D. E., and Smith, P. G. (1973): Treatment of early Hodgkin's disease. *Lancet,* I:832–833.

83. Tubiana, M., and Mathe, G. (1973): Combined radiotherapy and chemotherapy in the treatment of Hodgkin's disease. *Ser. Haemat.,* 6:202–243.

84. Veterans Administration Cancer Chemotherapy Study Group (1959): A clinical study of the comparative effect of nitrogen mustard and DON in patients with bronchogenic carcinoma, Hodgkin's disease, lymphosarcoma, and melanoma. *J. Natl. Cancer Inst.,* 22:433–439.

85. Wasserman, T. H., Slavik, M., and Carter, S. K. (1975): Clinical comparison of the nitrosoureas. *Cancer,* 36:1258–1268.

86. Wiernik, P. H., and Lichtenfeld, J. L. (1975): Combined modality therapy for localized Hodgkin's disease. A seven-year update of an early study. *Oncology,* 32:208–213.

87. Young, R. C., Canellos, G. P., Chabner, B. A., Schein, P. S., and DeVita, V. T. (1973): Maintenance chemotherapy for advanced Hodgkin's disease in remission. *Lancet,* I:1339–1343.

88. Ziegler, J. L., Bluming, A. Z., Fass, L., Magrath, I. T., and Templeton, A. C. (1972): Chemotherapy of childhood Hodgkin's disease in Uganda. *Lancet,* II:679–682.

89. Zubrod, C. G., Schneiderman, M., Frei, E., III, Brindley, C., Gold, G. L., Shnider, B., Oviedo, R., Gorman, J., Jones, R., Jr., Jonsson, U., Colsky, J., Chalmers, T., Ferguson, B., Dederick, M., Holland, J., Selawry, O., Regelson, W., Lasagna, L., and Owens, A. H., Jr. (1960): Appraisal of methods for the study of chemotherapy of cancer in man: Comparative therapeutic trial of nitrogen mustard and triethylene thiophosphoramide. *J. Chron. Dis.,* 11:7–33.

*Randomized Trials in Cancer: A Critical Review by Sites,* edited by Maurice J. Staquet, Raven Press, New York © 1978.

# Solid Tumors in Children

## Renée Maurus and Jacques Otten

*Service de Médecine Infantile, Hôpital Universitaire Saint-Pierre, 1000 Bruxelles, Belgium*

The most frequent, nonlymphoid cancers of childhood are reviewed here: neuroblastoma, nephroblastoma, and rhabdomyosarcoma. Brain tumors, which are discussed elsewhere in this volume, are not considered.

Even the most prevalent malignant tumors of children are rare. Hence it comes as no surprise that all randomized clinical trials have been carried out by cooperative groups, which are the only sources of a large enough sample within a reasonable time. In spite of these cooperative efforts, however, some of the studies lack clear-cut conclusions because of the rather small number of evaluable patients who could be assembled in each subgroup of a stratified population.

These tumors are usually treated by multimodal therapy combining surgery, radiation therapy, and/or chemotherapy. The trials to be reviewed here have tested the role and modalities of radiation therapy and/or chemotherapy.

The purpose of cancer treatment in childhood is cure without long-term untoward sequelae. Accordingly, the main criteria used to evaluate the therapeutic efficiency are duration of disease-free survival and, accessorily, the survival rate. Partial responses such as 50% reduction of tumor volume have no meaningful value. Late complications of the treatment might become an important problem for this particular age group because of the long survival time during which they will have the opportunity to develop possible delayed effects of radiation therapy and chemotherapy on growth and pubertal development, etc. Such late effects have not been described yet in the published reports of randomized trials, but some of the groups have foreseen a long-term follow-up of their patients in order to uncover possible late effects of the various treatment arms.

### NEUROBLASTOMA

Neuroblastoma has a rather gloomy prognosis. But for patients under 1 year of age, truly localized (stage I) disease is rare and the addition of chemotherapy to surgery and radiation therapy in more advanced stages does not seem to have significantly increased the survival rate. Comparison of results from treat-

---

Received June 30, 1977.

ments given at various times since 1959, first without and later with chemotherapy, barely shows any trend toward better prognosis. This lack of any evident breakthrough might explain why all but one clinical trial have been single-arm studies comparing the results of a new therapy with those of historical controls. The only randomized trial for which conclusions have been published has been conducted by the Children's Cancer Study Group (CCSG) (5). Its purpose was to evaluate the effect of cyclophosphamide (CPM) given during 1 year after the treatment of the primary in stages I, II, and III neuroblastoma.

Primary treatment consisted of surgery, which was to be as complete as possible; use of postoperative radiation therapy was left to the discretion of each participating investigator.

The patients were stratified according to the known prognostic factors: age (0 to 11 months, 12 to 23 months, and over), site of the primary (above or below the diaphragm), and stage.

### Treatment Protocol and Randomization

Local tumor control was a prerequisite for entry into the study. No detail is given in the report as to how local control was ascertained when surgical removal was incomplete (by return to normal of V.M.A. excretion?).

Patients were randomized at the end of the primary treatment to receive either cyclophosphamide (CPM) in regimen 1 or nothing in regimen 2. CPM was given in courses of 10 mg/kg orally for 7 to 10 days every 28 days for 1 year. The trial began in May 1970, and within 4 years, 134 patients from 24 participating institutions were randomized. 113 patients were considered evaluable, 49 in regimen 1 and 64 in regimen 2. Patients were discarded from evaluation because of wrong diagnosis, wrong staging, and violation of protocol. Actual relapse-free survival was evaluated at 2 years for all patients.

### Results

For stages I, II, and III combined, there was no difference in 24-month relapse-free survival between the two regimens: The proportion of disease-free patients was 39/49 (80%) for regimen 1 and 53/64 for regimen 2.

More stage I patients were allocated to regimen 2 (19 versus 8) because randomization was discontinued for this subgroup during the last year of the trial and all stage I patients were henceforth allocated to the control arm.

As no relapse occurred in stage I patients, this could have biased the results in favor of the control group.

However, when stages II and III patients only are considered, relapse-free survival remains similar in both arms: In stage II, 31/41 or 76% in regimen 1 and 34/45 or 76% in regimen 2; in stage III, 10/18 or 56% in regimen 1 and 11/16 or 69% in regimen 2 are disease-free.

All relapses occurred during the first year of follow-up.

## Conclusions and Comments

The absence of relapse in stage I patients suggests that these have truly localized disease and need no adjuvant chemotherapy. For stage II and III patients, the chemotherapy chosen has failed to influence the relapse rate of the disease. The overall results are much better than those of previous studies, which gave a 2-year survival rate of 50% for comparable patients.

Because of stratification of the patients at randomization, the most important known prognostic factors were satisfactorily balanced in both arms of the trial.

As the decision to give radiation therapy was left to each participant, it should have been stated whether radiation therapy also was comparably given in the two groups, but this is not mentioned in the report.

Perhaps the most important observation is that the overall results in this trial are much better than those obtained previously by some of the same investigators (1). As the authors themselves stress, use of historical controls only would have led to the wrong conclusion that CPM as it was used was responsible for the increased survival rate. This unexpected finding emphasizes the need for controlled trials even when previous results have hitherto been disappointing. The authors give no satisfactory explanation for this discrepancy in the prognosis of two different groups of patients. One possible reason could be the prerequisite of local tumor control for entry into the trial. This condition might have selected a group of patients with more favorable prognoses.

The conclusion that adjuvant chemotherapy is superfluous in stage I patients is based on the 100% 24-month disease-free survival in 19 control patients, 7 of whom were older than 1 year. As these excellent results are discordant with previously reported data, they should be ascertained on a greater number of patients, in particular for those over 1 year of age. CPM was chosen because it had induced the highest proportion of remission when used as a single agent. As toxicity was rather mild, one could certainly try a more aggressive schedule, and nowadays a multiple-agent chemotherapy should have preference.

The CCSG is currently engaged in a study testing the combination of CPM, vincristine, and dimethyl-triazeno imidazole carboxamide (DTIC) for stage II and III patients.

## NEPHROBLASTOMA

Four randomized trials have been designed to answer this same question: What is the best adjuvant chemotherapy for patients with localized nephroblastoma? The rationale for the use of chemotherapy is the possibility that it will eradicate eventual microscopic metastatic foci. In all four trials, different drugs or schedules have been compared, but curiously enough none of the studies has included a group of patients given no chemotherapy. The advantage of adjuvant chemotherapy was considered established by previous reports that actinomycin D or vincristine impressively improved the remission rate of neph-

TABLE 1. *Staging of nephroblastoma patients*

---

In the NWTS, SIOP, and MRC trials, the patients were staged according to the system proposed by D'Angio (3).

In the CCSG trial, staging for selection of eligible patients was done according to Garcia et al. (7). In their second report (13), the authors mentioned that their randomized cases corresponded to groups I and II of D'Angio's classification. This staging system is given here in summarized form:

Group I:　Tumor limited to the kidney and completely excised
Group II:　Tumor extending beyond the kidney but completely resected
Group III:　Tumor not completely resected but without hematogenous spread; this group includes tumors that have been biopsied or ruptured before or after surgery
Group IV:　Presence of hematogenous metastases, including cases with liver metastases
Group V:　Bilateral renal tumor

---

roblastoma patients when compared to historical controls (6,11). Two of the trials also included questions about the role of radiation therapy as a preoperative treatment or as an adjuvant postoperative therapy. The staging system used for all four trials is given in Table 1.

## Single Versus Multiple Courses of Actinomycin D (Children's Cancer Study Group A, CCSGA) (12,13)

The purpose of the trial was to compare the efficacy of a single versus multiple courses of actinomycin D given after primary treatment of the tumor for the prevention of local or distant relapses.

Patients over 12 months of age were eligible for the trial if the tumor, whatever its local extension, had been totally removed and if no metastases were present.

According to the currently used staging classification of D'Angio et al. (7), these cases correspond to groups I and II.

For primary treatment, after surgical excision, all patients received radiation therapy which was given in "as standardized a regimen as possible."

### Randomization and Treatment Protocol

No stratification was applied. All patients received a first course of actinomycin D consisting of five consecutive doses (15 $\mu$g/kg/day) and beginning on the day of surgery. On the same day, they were randomized to receive either no further treatment (group 1) or multiple courses of actinomycin D at 6 weeks and 3 months and every 3 months for the first 15 months after operation.

From November 1964 through March 1969, 36 patients were enrolled in group 1 (28 evaluable) and 37 patients in group 2 (25 evaluable).

Reasons for exclusion from evaluation were mostly larger extension of the tumor than allowed for eligibility because of operative spillage and violation of protocol.

*Results*

Preliminary results were published in 1968 (12), and long-term evaluation was reported on in 1974 (13). At the time of the second report, all patients except one had been off chemotherapy for at least 2¾ years. The one exception was a patient who had relapsed after 6 years, had been treated again, and was disease-free.

In 1968, the relapse rate was significantly different between the two groups: 12 of 23 evaluable patients (52%) had relapsed in group 1 (single course), as compared to 3 of 22 (14%) in group 2 (multiple courses) ($p < 0.05$).

The second report confirmed the difference in relapse rate. Although smaller (57% relapse in group 1 versus 28% in group 2), the difference remained statistically significant at the 5% level.

At this time, survival was also analyzed. No significant difference was observed. Survival was 71% (20 of 28) in group 1 and 80% (20 of 25) in group 2.

The location of metastases was different in the two groups as evidenced by 12 of 16 relapses in the lung alone in group 1, and 1 of 7 in the lung alone in the second, indicating that maintenance chemotherapy was mostly effective is suppressing pulmonary metastases.

*Conclusions and Comments*

Multiple courses of actinomycin D prevent relapses of nephroblastoma. In the long run, they do not increase the survival rate because among the patients who relapse, those who received a single course of the drug are more often rescued into remission by subsequent therapy than those who received maintenance chemotherapy.

The toxic cost of the treatment needed for the relapse (surgical excision of lung metastases, radiation therapy of the lungs, chemotherapy, etc.) is prohibitive when compared to the complications of maintenance chemotherapy.

Results of randomized trials are not often analyzed after such a long follow-up. The discrepancy between unequal relapse rate and equivalent long-term survival rate is the most interesting fact brought up by this study.

It is generally admitted that 90% of the patients who have been disease-free for 2 years after treatment restricted to surgery and radiation therapy are expected to be cured (2). As all patients except one had been off therapy for more than 2¾ years at the time the long-term results were analyzed, one should accept the survival figures as grossly definitive. The balance of cost and benefit of each therapeutic arm is well analyzed. In summary, it appears that the sole but important advantage of maintenance chemotherapy is to spare some patients the high morbidity related to subsequent therapy needed for relapse.

Although 12 different institutions contributed cases to the trial over more than 4 years, the accrual rate was rather small. One feels uneasy to accept without reticence conclusions based on such a restricted number of patients

(28 in group 1, and 25 in group 2) even when statistically significant, when no stratification is applied. Several prognostic factors are now known or suspected, for instance, those related to histology, which could be unequally distributed between the 2 groups and bias the results.

Another variable that could possibly bias the results is the nonuniform radiotherapy, which was given according to prevailing usage at each participating institution.

All these possible sources of heterogeneity between the two arms of the trial and the small number of patients cast some doubt on the conclusion of the authors.

### Preoperative Versus Postoperative Radiotherapy, Single Versus Multiple Courses of Actinomycin D, in the Treatment of Wilms' Tumor (International Society of Paediatric Oncology, SIOP)

The purpose of this trial was twofold:

1. To compare two strategies for the primary treatment of nephroblastoma: pre- and postoperative radiation therapy versus postoperative radiation therapy alone.
2. To repeat the CCSGA trial (discussed above) comparing single and multiple courses of actinomycin D on a larger scale.

All patients between 1 and 15 years of age with group I, II, or III nephroblastoma were eligible for the trial. The eligible population is thus broader than in the CCSGA trial, as it includes tumors that could not be completely resected (group III).

Recruitment of patients started in September 1971 and was closed in October 1974. A preliminary report of the data collected before August 1975 has been published (9).

A total of 169 patients were eligible for the radiation therapy trial and 161 patients for the chemotherapy trial. The institutions could choose to participate in either one only or in the two parts of the trial.

#### Randomization and Treatment Protocol

*Radiation therapy trial:* Randomization was done at the time preoperative diagnosis was established. Patients were either allocated to preoperative irradiation (2,000 rads in 15 to 18 days) (arm A) or to immediate nephrectomy (arm B). After operation, group I patients received no further radiation in arm A and received 2,000 rads in arm B. Group II and III patients received a complement of 1.500 rads in arm A and 3,000 rads in arm B. Overall, the patients in the two arms received approximately the same number of RETS.

*Chemotherapy trial:* The protocol was that used in the CCSGA study. Comparison was made between a single postoperative course of actinomycin D and multiple courses given over a 15-month period. Before the second randomization, the patients were matched by pairs according to stage, type of irradiation, and, when possible, according to age and treatment center. Criteria for evaluation were disease-free survival 3 years after nephrectomy and complications of treatment at surgery or later.

## Results

*Radiation therapy trial:* 137 patients out of 169 were considered as evaluable. 23 patients were discarded from evaluation because of wrong diagnosis and 5 because of error in staging. 73 were evaluated in arm A (preoperative radiation therapy) and 64 in arm B (immediate nephrectomy).

For this part of the trial, the patients were not matched according to the criteria taken into account at the second randomization, but *a posteriori* comparison of the two arms showed no significant difference in age, size of the tumor, subsequent chemotherapy, or histology.

Stage distribution was different, but this was expected as a consequence of the difference in primary treatment. Patients in group A had more often staging group I disease and less staging group III.

No significant difference between the two arms was observed in actuarial disease-free survival nor in overall survival. The probability of remaining disease free at 36 months from diagnosis was 52% for arm A and 44% for arm B.

A great difference was observed in the number of tumor ruptures at surgery: This occurred in 3 patients out of 72 in arm A and in 20 patients out of 60 in arm B.

*Chemotherapy trial:* 160 patients were evaluable, 80 in each arm. Adherence to the protocol was good, although some courses of actinomycin D were omitted at 45 days and 3 months because of lack of tolerance.

No significant difference was observed in actuarial disease-free survival at 36 months from diagnosis: This was 58% for the patients who received a single course and 54% for those who received multiple courses. Actuarial overall survival was also similar in the two groups: 86% and 82% for single versus multiple course group.

## Conclusions and Comments

Control of disease was similarly achieved in the two arms of the radiation therapy trial. In the "surgery first" group, because of the high incidence of operative tumor rupture and spillage, abdominal irradiation often had to be given on a more extended field. This should have increased the risk of radiation-related morbidity. For this reason, this part of the study was prematurely stopped and the authors recommended systematic use of preoperative radiation therapy in patients over 1 year of age unless the tumor appeared so small that an easy and nontraumatic resection could be predicted.

In the chemotherapy trial, the conclusions of the CCSGA study were not confirmed, as no advantage in favor of iterative courses of actinomycin D was observed.

For the radiation therapy trial, the recommendations of the authors are based on the high risk of operative spillage when the patient is first operated on. At first sight, the number of tumor ruptures in the "surgery first" group is surprisingly high. Data from the literature about this risk are scanty and only incidentally reported, so comparison with results from other groups is difficult. We think that the great frequency with which this complication occurred is what should be expected and is not due to lack of surgical skill. It should first be stressed that for the first time this trial was specifically designed to investigate the relation, if any, between treatment strategy and such kinds of untoward consequences. The participants could choose not to randomize the small tumors which could be predicted to be easily resectable, so that the cases entered into this part of the trial were selected for their problematic resectability. Further, a comparison can be made with the results of the CCSGA study reviewed above. That trial excluded staging group III, that is, also the cases with operative tumor rupture. Nevertheless, 10% of the patients first entered into this study were later discarded from evaluation because operative spillage had occurred. For all these reasons, we should accept that the risk of surgical rupture of the tumor was correctly evaluated in the SIOP study. As discussed by the authors themselves, preoperative radiation therapy has its own drawback, that is, the possibility of wrong diagnosis and of irradiating benign lesions. This occurred in 4% of the patients allocated to the "radiation first" group.

After comparison of the disadvantages bound to each strategy, the SIOP concluded in favor of preoperative radiation. It should be noted that the risks of either strategy may be different in individual centers or could change with time. Diagnostic accuracy probably will be improved by better interpretation of i.v. pyelography and by use of new diagnostic tools and so will reduce the percentage of wrong diagnosis. On the other hand, the risk of traumatic manipulation of the tumor depends on surgical skill and preoperative evaluation of operability by the surgeon. Therefore, in this particular case, conclusions based on the results of a large cooperative trial should be adjusted to the particular conditions prevailing in each institution.

The results of the chemotherapy trial contradict those obtained by the CCSGA study. The population of eligible patients was different in the two trials: It included staging group I and II in the CCSGA trial, whereas the SIOP trial also accepted staging group III. This should, however, not explain the discrepancy between the results of the two studies. A likely explanation is that the two arms of the SIOP trial were really comparable for the known prognostic factors and for the type of radiation therapy because of the careful pair-matching of the patients before randomization. By contrast, as already discussed, the absence of stratification and the rather small number of patients in the CCSGA study could have introduced an important bias.

## Actinomycin D Versus Vincristine as Adjuvant Therapy for Nephroblastoma (Medical Research Council's Working Party on Embryonal Tumors in Childhood) (10)

The objective of this trial was to compare actinomycin D and vincristine, either drug being given alone in multiple courses after the primary treatment of nephroblastoma. The trial was initiated in August 1970 and was closed in March 1974 after a preliminary report of the NWTS trial (to be reviewed next) showed the superiority of the two-drug combination over single-agent chemotherapy.

### Randomization and Treatment Protocol

Any child between 1 and 14 years with nephroblastoma staged group I to III was eligible. All patients received one course of actinomycin D (15 μg/ kg/day for 4 days), which was started on the day of operation). Surgery was followed by radiation therapy as soon as possible and always before the 15th postoperative day.

Doses and schedule of irradiation varied according to age: 3,000 to 3,500 rads were given to the whole abdomen in 4 to 6 weeks. For staging group I, the participating institutions were allowed to irradiate only the affected side if this practice had previously prevailed. The pelvis was included in the field when operative spillage had occurred or when the tumor extended so far.

Six weeks after completion of radiation therapy, that is, 11 to 14 weeks after surgery, adjuvant chemotherapy was started. Patients were randomly allocated to one of two regimens: (a) iterative 4-day courses of actinomycin D (15 μg/ kg/day) at 12-week intervals for a total of 8 courses; and (b) vincristine (1.5 mg/m²) weekly for 6 weeks and then every other week until 2 years from surgery.

Of 114 patients entered into the study, 108 were randomized: 55 received actinomycin D and 53 vincristine. The proportion of stages I, II, and III was the same in each arm. Except for stage, the patients were not stratified. The results were assessed 2 years after randomization of the last patients. Criteria for evaluation were actuarial disease-free survival and overall survival at 1, 2, and 3 years from diagnosis.

### Results

In the actinomycin D group, the survival rate was 88.9%, 79.4%, and 66.2% at 1, 2, and 3 years, respectively. Disease-free survival was 66.1%, 53.6%, and 53.6%. In the vincristine group, the survival rate was 93, 87.6, and 83%, and disease-free survival 82%, 79.4%, and 75%. The difference in disease-free survival at 3 years, after adjustment is made for tumor stage, is statistically significant ($p = 0.031$ by the log-rank test). The difference in overall survival is not ($p = 0.097$).

Toxic complications seem to have been more important in the vincristine arm. Eleven children developed metastases before maintenance chemotherapy was started.

### Conclusions and Comments

After a primary treatment consisting of surgical excision, a paraoperative course of actinomycin D, and radiation therapy, the vincristine regimen prevents metastatic recurrence more efficiently than the actinomycin D regimen.

As in the CCSGA trial, a discrepancy is found between the effect of the best regimen in terms of disease-free survival and of overall survival. In this case, the results reported should be considered as preliminary. As the chemotherapy was pursued during 2 years, evaluation at 3 years from diagnosis, that is, 1 year after chemotherapy was stopped, need confirmation at a later date.

A weak point in the design of the protocol, which is also stressed by the authors, is the long interval before maintenance chemotherapy was started (11 to 14 weeks after surgery). Even after whole abdominal irradiation, chemotherapy could probably be initiated sooner without undue toxic risk for the patient. Earlier treatment could have prevented some of the metastatic recurrences which were observed in 11 of the randomized patients before maintenance treatment was started.

### Postoperative Radiation Therapy Versus No Radiation in Group I Nephroblastoma: Actinomycin D Versus Vincristine Versus Actinomycin D Plus Vincristine in Group II and III Nephroblastoma (National Wilms' Tumor Study, NWTS[1]) (4)

This study comprised three randomized trials with the following objectives:

1. To establish if postoperative radiation therapy is necessary in staging group I.
2. To compare the efficacy of three different adjuvant chemotherapy regimens in staging groups II and III: actinomycin D alone, vincristine alone, or both.
3. To evaluate the efficacy of preoperative vincristine in stage IV disease.

Very few patients were eligible for entering the third part of the study, and the first two parts only will be reviewed here.

### Randomization and Treatment Protocol

All patients under 14 years of age were eligible, infants under 1 year included. The study started in October 1969 and was closed in December 1973. Patients

---

[1] The NWTS has been conducted by three cooperative groups (Acute Leukemia Group B, Children's Cancer Study Group, and Southwest Oncology Group) and unaffiliated institutions which joined together.

were stratified in two categories according to age: less than 2 years and over 2 years. There was no stratification according to other criteria.

In the chemotherapy trial, groups II and III were pooled. Staging group was assigned by the surgeon and the pathologist within 2 days of operation.

The NWTS committee reviewed the grouping of all patients and considered that 16% had been incorrectly staged. In spite of this, the original grouping only was taken into account for the evaluation of the data.

Criteria for evaluation were actuarial proportion of relapse-free survivors at 2 years from surgery ("relapse-free survival") and of survivors.

*Radiation therapy trial for group I patients:* As soon as group I was ascertained, patients were randomized to receive or not to receive radiation therapy on the tumor bed. Doses and portals were precisely specified in the protocol. Doses varied according to age from 1,800 to 4,000 rads. All patients received actinomycin D in 5-day courses of 15 μg/kg/day after surgery, at 6 weeks, 3 months, and every 3 months thereafter until 15 months from surgery.

*Chemotherapy trial for group II and III patients:* All group II and III patients received postoperative radiation therapy. Portal recommendations for group II were the same as for group I. Initially, group III patients were given whole abdominal irradiation. Later in the trial, the field was adapted to the extent of the disease as appreciated at surgery.

The patients were randomly allocated to one of following regimens:

1. Actinomycin D alone, given according to the schedule described for group I.
2. Vincristine alone: 1.5 mg/m$^2$ given at diagnosis, then every week for 7 weeks. Thereafter, 2 injections at days 1 and 5 are given at 3-month intervals until 15 months from diagnosis.
3. Both regimens A and B are given in combination, except for the first postoperative vincristine injection which is omitted.

Some patients who at first had been incorrectly staged group I and who accordingly had already received actinomycin D, could no longer be allocated to regimen B, so that a relative excess of regimen A and C patients appear in the results.

## Results

With one exception, all relapses so far occurred during the first 2 years from surgery.

*Radiation therapy trial:* 154 group I patients were randomized, 77 in each arm. For children under 2 years of age (74 patients), 2-year relapse-free survival rate was 90% in the radiation therapy arm and 88% in the control group. For children older than 2 years (80 patients), relapse-free survival was 77% in the radiation-therapy arm and 58% for the controls.

The difference between the two age categories is statistically significant

($p = 0.002$). For children over 2 years, the difference between treated and control patients is just barely significant ($p = 0.04$ according to Kaplan and Meier's nonparametric estimation and $p = 0.07$ by the chi-square test). Five of 41 nonirradiated children over 2 years had abdominal recurrence versus 1 of 29 irradiated patients. The difference is not significant ($p = 0.11$). Three nonirradiated children had recurrence in the operative site, none in the radiation therapy group. There was no difference in overall survival between the two arms.

*Chemotherapy trial:* 166 patients were randomized. Of these, 63 were allocated to A (AMD), 44 to B (VCR), and 59 to C (AMD + VCR). Relapse-free survival at 2 years was significantly higher in C (81%) than in A (57%) or in B (55%) ($p = 0.002$). This significant difference holds true even if the patients first wrongly staged group I and afterwards randomized to A or C are deleted from the analysis.

There was no significant difference according to age categories nor according to group, except in regimen A where group III patients did worse (relapse-free survival = 44%) than group II patients (72%) ($p = 0.02$).

There was a trend for higher overall survival rate in the C arm.

## Conclusions and Comments

Radiation therapy offers no advantage for the control of disease in patients less than 2 years of age with staging group I nephroblastoma who receive actinomycin D as adjuvant chemotherapy. This observation is all the more important as radiation therapy may induce more deleterious side effects in very young children.

For older children, the conclusions of the authors do not appear clear-cut.

Combination therapy with actinomycin D and vincristine is better than either drug alone.

Results were evaluated at 2 years from diagnosis. This duration of follow-up is rather short for patients who were given chemotherapy during 15 months, even if we take into account that all relapses except one till now occurred during these 2 years.

With this reservation in mind, the results establish that radiation therapy has no place in the treatment of the youngest group I patients when they also receive iterative actinomycin D courses.

Children over 2 years with group I disease probably benefited from radiation therapy. From the results of the chemotherapy trial on group II and III, it is clear that the group I patients did not receive the optimal chemotherapy. The advantage, if any, afforded by radiation therapy should need confirmation if better adjuvant chemotherapy is to be used.

The chemotherapy trial has demonstrated the superiority of combined actinomycin D and vincristine over the single-drug regimens. The vincristine-alone regimen seems to have been designed so as to closely copy the actinomycin D regimen, 2 vincristine injections being given every 3 months in lieu of a 5-day actinomycin D course. This may sound logical as an attempt to make the two schedules quantitatively comparable. However, they probably do not evenly match as far as toxicity is concerned. Two vincristine injections at 3-month intervals seems a very modest regime, even after the first 7 postoperative doses. For these reasons, one may doubt whether vincristine as a single drug was given a fair trial.

This quantitative aspect of the chemotherapy study explains the difference with the results of the MRC trial. The British group showed that vincristine, when given for a total of 50 injections during 2 years, was superior to actinomycin D given in 4-day courses at 3-month intervals during the same lapse of time. By contrast, NWTS patients only received 18 vincristine injections over 15 months.

Actuarial relapse-free rate at 2 years in the vincristine arm of the MRC trial was 70.7% for group II and 61.9% for group III (patients under 1 year of age being excluded). In the NWTS, for both group II and III combined, infants under 1 year of age included, it was 55% in the vincristine arm and 81% in the combination chemotherapy arm. The advantage of the double drug regimen is thus less striking when compared to a more intensive single-drug schedule. On the whole, however, the combination therapy as devised by the NWTS seems to have provided the best results in terms of disease control at the lowest cost in toxicity.

## RHABDOMYOSARCOMAS

Rhabdomyosarcoma in children has a poor prognosis: About 80% develop local or distant recurrence by 1 year from primary treatment with surgery and radiation therapy. In recent years, several uncontrolled clinical trials have shown improved prognosis when patients received adjuvant chemotherapy. The usually bad outcome of children given only local therapy did not seem to warrant the comparison with untreated control patients to assess the possible efficiency of chemotherapy. Hitherto, the results of only one randomized trial have been reported.

### Actinomycin D plus Vincristine Versus No Chemotherapy (8)
### (Children's Cancer Study Group A, CCSGA)

The objective of this study was to evaluate the effect of combined chemotherapy given after surgery and radiation therapy on disease control.

#### Randomization and Treatment Protocol

The study was randomized for stage I patients only. Stage I was defined as cases where the tumor had been completely removed, both grossly and microscopically, and without evidence of metastatic disease. All patients with other stages received adjuvant chemotherapy. Patients under 21 years of age with histologically proven rhabdomyosarcoma (including embryonal, alveolar, pleomorphic and botryoid types) were eligible.

Primary treatment consisted of surgical removal followed by radiation therapy (6,000 rads in 6 weeks whenever feasible). Stage I patients were then randomly allocated to two groups:

1. A control group receiving no further treatment.

2. A treated group receiving 6 cycles of chemotherapy every 9 weeks for 1 year. Each cycle consisted of actinomycin D (15 μg/kg/day for 5 days) and of vincristine (75 μg/kg/week for 6 weeks beginning on day 21).

The patients other than stage I all received regimen B.

The study started in February 1967 and was closed in March 1971. Results were reported after at least 2 years of follow-up for all the patients.

Thirty-two patients with stage I disease were randomized: 15 were allocated to the control group and 17 to the treated group. The patients were not stratified. There was yet no great difference between the two arms in the distribution of sites of the primary tumor.

### Results

Eight of 15 control patients (53%) developed local recurrence or metastases, and 6 of these 8 died. Of the 17 treated patients, 3 (17.6%) developed a relapse, and 1 of these died of his disease. The difference between the two arms in the duration of the disease-free interval is statistically significant: $p = 0.03$. If adjustments are made for the slight difference in site distribution, $p = 0.02$. The authors do not state how the adjustments were made.

In the nonrandomized part of the study, 11 patients had microscopic residual disease (stage IIA) after surgery and received the same treatment as stage I patients allocated to adjuvant chemotherapy. None of these 11 patients relapsed. If they are pooled with the 17 randomized patients who received chemotherapy and compared with the control patients for duration of the disease-free survival, the difference becomes even more significant: $p = 0.002$.

The difference between the two arms in overall survival is not statistically significant ($p = 0.07$), but that between the controls and the pooled stage I and IIA treated patients is: $p = 0.002$.

### Conclusions and Comments

These results support the use of prolonged chemotherapy in those children who have a localized tumor that can be completely resected or can be reduced by surgery to microscopic residues.

It is not ethically comfortable to initiate a controlled trial when one copes with a tumor that is rare, that has a very bad prognosis when treated conventionally, and when some evidence already exists, based on comparison with historical controls, that a new kind of treatment has markedly improved the outcome of the patients. This was the situation of the authors at the time they designed this trial. They resolved the dilemma by restricting the randomization to the most favorable cases, that is, stage I patients.

Although the patients were not stratified prior to randomization, which was hardly possible owing to the very small accrual rate of patients eligible for the randomized trial, the two groups were not very different as far as distribution of sites and histology are concerned. Statistical comparison in favor of the adjuvant chemotherapy used is thus quite convincing. If, then, the most favorable cases benefit from it, one should be entitled to extrapolate this conclusion to the treatment of more advanced disease.

## REFERENCES

1. Breslow, N., and McCann, B. (1971): Statistical estimation of prognosis for children with neuroblastoma. *Cancer Res.,* 31:2098–2103.
2. Cassady, J. R., Tefft, M., Filler, R. M., Jaffe, N., Paed, D., and Hellman, S. (1973): Considerations in the radiation therapy of Wilms' tumor. *Cancer,* 32:598–608.
3. D'Angio, G. L. (1972): Management of children with Wilms' tumor. *Cancer,* 30:1528–1533.
4. D'Angio, G. L., Evans, A. E., Breslow, N., Beckwith, B., Bishop, H., Feigl, P., Goodwin, W., Leape, L. L., Sinks, L. F., Sutow, W., Tefft, M., and Wolff, J. (1976): The treatment of Wilms' tumor. *Cancer,* 38:633–646.
5. Evans, A. E., Albo, V., D'Angio, G. L., Finklestein, J. Z., Leiken, S., Santulli, T., Weiner, J., and Hammond, D. (1976): Cyclophosphamide treatment of patients with localized and regional neuroblastoma. *Cancer,* 38:655–660.
6. Farber, S. (1966): Chemotherapy in the treatment of leukemia and Wilms' tumor. *JAMA,* 198:826–836.
7. Garcia, M., Douglass, C., and Schlosser, J. V. (1963): Classification and prognosis in Wilms' tumor. *Radiology,* 80:574–580.
8. Heyn, R. M., Holland, R., Newton, W. A., Jr., Tefft, M., and Hartman, J. R. (1974). The role of combined chemotherapy in the treatment of rhabdomyosarcoma in children. *Cancer,* 34:2151–2165.
9. Lemerle, J., Voute, P. A., Tournade, M. F., Delemarre, J. F. M., Jereb, B., Ahstrom, L., Flamant, R., and Gerard-Marchant, R. (1976): Preoperative versus postoperative radiotherapy, single versus multiple courses of actinomycin D, in the treatment of Wilms' tumor. *Cancer,* 38:647–654.
10. Medical Research Council's Working Party on Embryonal Tumors in Childhood (Report prepared by Johnson, A., Morris Jones, P. H., and Pearson, D.) (1977): The management of nephroblastoma in childhood. A clinical study of two forms of maintenance chemotherapy. *Arch. Dis. Child. (in press).*
11. Sullivan, M. P., Sutow, W. W., Cangir, A., and Taylor, G. (1967): Vincristine sulfate in management of Wilms' tumor. *JAMA,* 202:381–384.
12. Wolff, J. A., Krivit, W., Newton, W. A., Jr., and D'Angio, G. L. (1968). Single versus multiple dose dactinomycin therapy of Wilms' tumor. *N. Engl. J. Med.,* 279:290–294.
13. Wolff, J. A., D'Angio, G., Hartmann, J., Krivit, W., and Newton, W. A., Jr. (1974): Long-term evaluation of single versus multiple courses of actinomycin D therapy of Wilms' tumor. *N. Engl. J. Med,* 290:84–86.

*Randomized Trials in Cancer: A Critical Review by Sites,* edited by Maurice J. Staquet, Raven Press, New York © 1978.

# Gastrointestinal Cancer: Esophagus, Stomach, Small Bowel, Colorectum, Pancreas, Liver, Gallbladder, and Extrahepatic Ducts*

Hugh L. Davis, Jr., Daniel D. Von Hoff, Marcel Rozencweig, Harry Handelsman, William T. Soper, and Franco M. Muggia

*Cancer Therapy Evaluation Program, Division of Cancer Treatment, National Cancer Institute, Bethesda, Maryland 20014*

This chapter reviews the published and unpublished data for controlled randomized trials in gastrointestinal cancer, including completed studies and those still in progress. "Controlled" trials are defined as those in which patients are randomly allocated to treatment groups. In some instances, uncontrolled trials are cited when they provide data important to the design of future controlled studies.

Each clinical trial was evaluated in terms of the study design criteria listed in Fig. 1, with particular attention to the stratification of patients (Fig. 1, part 4) according to the prognostic factors known to influence response to therapy (173). It is very important that proper stratification be accomplished before patients are randomized to the treatment arms of a study. This will assure a fair trial that does not, for example, assign all of the good- or poor-risk patients to any single treatment group, even though randomization alone does help to eliminate this occurrence (173). However, as noted elsewhere (91), randomization guarantees only average comparability of patients, and care must be taken to ensure that they are comparable with respect to known characteristics influencing prognosis. Failure to consider these prognostic variables may cause fluctuations within and between treatment groups that make comparisons of therapy relatively imprecise (205).

This chapter first considers the major tumor types and then proceeds to less common neoplasms at other sites in the gastrointestinal system. For the major tumors, and to a lesser extent in the miscellaneous types, the important prognostic factors are briefly discussed, followed by a consideration of the published and unpublished randomized trials within each therapeutic modality (i.e., surgery, radiotherapy, chemotherapy, immunotherapy, and combinations of

---

Received April 4, 1977.

* Abbreviations, chemical nomenclature, and NSC numbers for the chemotherapeutic agents cited are shown in the *List of Compounds* at the end of the text.

### 1. PATIENT ENTRY CRITERIA
A. Surgical Proof of Disease
B. Limited Local Disease
C. Locally Unresectable

### 2. PARTICIPATING INSTITUTIONS
A. Single Institution
B. Multiinstitutional

### 3. TRIAL CHARACTERISTICS
A. Double-Blind
B. Broad Phase II
C. All GI Tumors
D. Adjuvant Trial
E. Measurable Disease
F. Nonmeasurable Disease
G. Advanced Disease
H. Colon and Rectum
I. Colon Only

### 4. STRATIFICATION OF PROGNOSTIC VARIABLES
A. Prospective Analysis

1. Histology

2. Site of indicator lesion

3. Good risk/poor risk

4. Performance status

5. Site of primary tumor

6. Prior therapy

7. Age

8. Disease-free interval

9. Measurable/nonmeasurable disease

10. Type of surgery

11. Institution

12. Heart disease

13. Liver metastases

14. Disease stage or extent

15. Interval between histologic diagnosis and randomization

16. Residual tumor location

17. Patients refusing therapy

18. Geographic region

19. Jaundice, cirrhosis

20. Sex

21. Vascular invasion

22. Obstruction/perforation

23. Preoperative CEA

24. Dominant Site of disease

25. Tumor burden

26. Number positive nodes

27. Skin test reaction

28. Circumferential involvement

B. Retrospective Analysis

### 5. STRATIFICATION PROCEDURE
A. Random Number Selection
B. 3:1 Randomization to Combination Regimen
C. Sealed Envelope
D. Chance
E. By Institution

### 6. STATISTICAL ANALYSIS OF RESULTS
A. Chi-Square
B. Fisher's Exact Test

FIG. 1. Criteria for evaluating the design of randomized controlled trials in gastrointestinal malignancies.

these approaches). Discussion of each trial is centered, as appropriate, on the study design factors outlined in Fig. 1 in an attempt to determine if the conclusions are valid. Finally, the overall status of randomized trials in each tumor type is summarized and suggestions offered for future investigations.

## GASTRIC CANCER

The death rate for stomach carcinoma in the United States has declined from an age-adjusted mortality of 28.9 per 100,000 population in 1930 to 9.7 in 1967 (21,62,76). However, the incidence of the neoplasm and the death rate are not diminishing in other nations such as Japan and the Soviet Union (125, 153,190). Since the median survival time after diagnosis of unresectable gastric cancer without treatment is only 4 months (118), this is obviously an important area for intensive investigation.

### Prognostic Factors

Examination of the gross pathology of the primary tumor has shown that scirrhous lesions are associated with slightly better survival rates than ulcerative or polypoid lesions (21). Patients with tumors classified at a lower Broder's grade of malignancy have a higher response rate and longer survival with 5-FU therapy than do those having tumors exhibiting a higher degree of anaplasia (125).

According to Moertel et al. (125,132), the location of the indicator lesion is the most striking determinant of response to 5-FU. The response rates in patients with lesions in the abdominal cavity, cutaneous and subcutaneous lesions, and malignant hepatomegaly are significantly superior to those obtained in cases of more distant pulmonary and peripheral lymph node involvement. Survival time becomes shorter as the interval decreases between diagnosis of the primary lesion and recurrent metastatic disease. Likewise, patients with more indolent disease have responded better to 5-FU (125). There is a decrease in survival as the disease advances from regional node involvement to metastases in the peripheral nodes, liver, and lung (125,132).

According to Moertel et al. (125,132), median survival is not influenced by the sex of the patient. However, the larger number of long-term male survivors is reflected in a longer mean survival time for males. When the response rate with 5-FU is considered, males have a slight but not statistically significant advantage over females. As far as the influence of age is concerned, Moertel's retrospective study (125) of 307 patients showed a steady increase in median survival time with increasing age among those below 80 years of age. This probably reflects a smaller number of long-term survivors among young patients. However, older patients have less favorable response rates with 5-FU therapy (125,132). Performance status is a significant prognostic factor in the response obtained with 5-FU and other chemotherapeutic regimens (125,132).

Moertel's retrospective study (125), which was not randomized, shows that patients having palliative resection or bypass achieve significantly longer survival than those without any palliative surgery. The study emphasizes that the choice of surgery was frequently governed by whether or not a palliative procedure was technically possible. Patients who underwent resection of the primary gastric lesion responded more favorably to 5-FU than those without resection of the primary gastric lesion.

Of the many prognostic factors of possible importance for the stratification of patients (Fig. 1), seven were chosen for particular consideration in this analysis: histology, age, extent of disease at diagnosis, disease-free interval after resection, type of surgery, site of indicator lesion, and performance status. Obviously, each study would require a very large number of patients in order to consider all of these variables, and this practical limitation was considered in evaluating the individual trials.

### Randomized Surgical Trials

There have been no randomized surgical trials in gastric cancer. The tumor site usually dictates the type of curative surgery performed, with a high subtotal gastrectomy for tumors involving the antrum or corpus of the stomach and a proximal subtotal gastrectomy and esophogastrostomy for tumor at the cardiac end. Total gastrectomy is employed for extensive and diffuse tumors. This need for individualized approaches makes it difficult to envision a randomized trial of the three different procedures.

Nevertheless, one provocative possibility would be a randomization between splenic resection and no splenic resection. This would help clarify the V.A. Surgical Adjuvant Group (VASAG) findings of increased early postoperative mortality in splenectomized patients who are receiving thiotepa (46). With the proliferation of adjuvant trials it may be important to know the effect of splenectomy on operative mortality among patients undergoing gastric cancer surgery. Although retrospective analysis indicates that resection or bypass seems to produce longer survival, this has not been tested in a prospective randomized trial.

### Randomized Radiotherapy Trials

There are no "pure" randomized trials of radiotherapeutic regimens. Five published or ongoing trials employing radiotherapy in one of the treatment arms will be discussed in a later section concerning combined modality therapy.

### Randomized Chemotherapy Trials

Table 1 summarizes the published reports of eight trials of chemotherapy and cites the study design criteria in Fig. 1 that were employed in each instance. The study of Kovach et al. (99) at the Mayo Clinic compared 5-FU to BCNU

TABLE 1. *Published randomized trials of chemotherapy in gastric cancer*

| Investigators (reference) and treatment arms | Evaluation criteria[a] | No. responses/ no. patients | Response rate (%) |
|---|---|---|---|
| Kovach et al. (99) | 1A, 2A, 3E, 4A(1, 2, 5), 4B | | |
| A. 5-FU (13.5 mg/kg/d × 5, q. 5 wks i. v.) | | 8/28 | 29 |
| B. BCNU (50 mg/m²/d × 5, q. 8 wks i. v.) | | 4/23 | 17 |
| C. 5-FU (10 mg/kg/d × 5, q. 8 wks i. v.) BCNU (40 mg/m²/d × 5, q. 8 wks i. v.) | | 14/34 | 41 |
| Reitemeier et al. (165) | 2A, 3C, 4A(2) 5A | | |
| A. Fluorometholone (25 mg, q. 12 hr p. o.) | | 1/13 | 8 |
| B. 5-FU (15 mg/kg/d × 5; then q.o.d. × 4 i. v.) | | 1/11 | 9 |
| C. Fluorometholone (as in A) 5-FU (as in B) | | 2/10 | 20 |
| Moertel et al. (126,130,132) | 2B, 3E 4A(1, 4, 6, 15) | | |
| A. MeCCNU (200 mg/m² q. 7 wks p. o.) | | 3/37 | 8 |
| B. MeCCNU (175 mg/m² q. 7 wks p. o.) 5-FU (300 mg/m²/d × 5, q. 7 wks i. v.) | | 12/30 | 40 |
| C. CTX (1,200 mg/m² single dose i. v.) MeCCNU (200 mg/m² d22, then q. 7 wks p. o.) | | 2/30 | 7 |
| D. CTX (as in C) MeCCNU (175 mg/m² d22; then q. 7 wks p. o.) 5-FU (300 mg/m²/d × 5, d22–26; then q. 7 wks i. v.) | | 6/30 | 20 |
| Baker et al. (12,13) A. 5-FU (400 mg/m²/wk i. v.) B. 5-FU (as in A) MeCCNU (175 mg/m² q. 6 wks p. o.) | 2B, 3C, 4B, 5B | 2/9 6/29 | 22 21 |
| Rossi et al. (168) | 2A, 3C, 3E, 4A(2, 5, 15) | | |
| A. MeCCNU (200 mg/m² q. 6 wks p. o.) | | 1/5 | 20 |
| B. MeCCNU (120 mg/m² q. 6 wks p. o.) CTX (600 mg/m² q. 3 wks i. v.) | | 0/3 | — |
| Baker et al. (11) | 2A, 3B 4A(3), 5A | | |
| A. Mitomycin C (22.5 mg/m² q. 6–8 wks i. v.) | | 2/3 | 66 |

TABLE 1—*Cont.*

| Investigators (reference) and treatment arms | Evaluation criteria[a] | No. responses/ no. patients | Response rate (%) |
|---|---|---|---|
| B. Porfiromycin (75 mg/m² q. 6– 8 wks i. v.) | | 1/2 | 50 |
| Gailani et al. (65) | 2B, 3A, 3C | | |
| A. 5-FU (15 mg/kg/wk i. v.) Placebo (mannitol s. c.) | | 2/9 | 22 |
| B. 5-FU (as in A) Ara-C (30 mg/m²/wk s. c.) | | 3/15 | 20 |
| C. 5-FU (as in A) Ara-C (100 mg/m² wk i. v.) | | 0/3 | — |
| Bateman et al. (15) | 2B, 4B | | |
| A. 5-FU (15 mg/kg/wk i. v.) | | 2/6 | 33 |
| B. 5-FU (15 mg/kg/wk p. o.) | | 0/4 | — |
| Reitemeier et al. (164) | 2A, 3C 4A(1, 2) | | |
| A. 5-FU (13.5 mg/kg/d × 5, q. 4 wks i. v.) | | 0/4 | — |
| B. Mitomycin C (150 µg/kg/ d × 5, q. 8 wks i. v.) | | 1/2 | 50 |
| C. BCNU (50 mg/m²/d × 5, q. 8 wks i. v.) | | 1/4 | 25 |
| D. 5-FU (9 mg/kg/d × 5, q. 8 wks i. v.) Mitomycin C (110 µg/kg/ d × 5, q. 8 wks i. v. | | 2/5 | 40 |
| E. 5-FU (as in D) BCNU (37.5 mg/m²/d × 5, q. 8 wks i. v.) | | 4/6 | 66 |
| F. Mitomycin C (75 µg/kg/d × 5, q. 8 wks i. v.) BCNU (25 mg/m²/d × 5, q. 8 wks i. v.) | | 2/4 | 50 |
| G. 5-FU (8 mg/kg/d × 5, q. 8 wks i. v.) Mitomycin C (60 µg/kg/d × 5, q. 8 wks i. v.) BCNU (20 mg/m²/d × 5, q. 8 wks i. v.) | | 0/1 | — |

[a]See the criteria defined in Fig. 1.

and to a combination of both agents. Although the study stratified patients for only two (grade of anaplasia and site of indicator lesion) of the seven major prognostic variables, the authors did retrospectively find all treatment groups "similar" in sex, age, and risk. It was concluded that the 5-FU-treated patients showed significant superiority over the BCNU group in both response rate and survival. Also, the response rate and survival achieved with 5-FU + BCNU was significantly superior to BCNU alone. However, 5-FU + BCNU was not superior to 5-FU alone in response rate or overall survival, although at 18 months the combination drug regimen did show a statistically significant survival advantage. As a result of these observations, the authors concluded that the 5-FU + BCNU combination failed to produce enough survival advantage to warrant routine use.

The second study (165) found that fluorometholone added nothing to the response rate of 5-FU and did not reduce its toxicity. The study included only a few patients with gastric cancer and stratified for only one prognostic variable without even a retrospective review of others. Therefore, the findings apppear to be inconclusive.

Moertel et al. (126,130,132) reported the third study in Table 1, a well-designed protocol of the Eastern Cooperative Oncology Group (ECOG). The study was informative in showing that cyclophosphamide induction increased toxicity and detracted from responsiveness to subsequent treatment. It also showed that MeCCNU alone was relatively ineffective but that 5-FU + MeCCNU gave a significantly superior response rate compared to the other regimens. The 5-FU + MeCCNU also produced a survival time superior to that of MeCCNU-treated patients. The chief problem in the study design was that patients were not stratified for indicator lesions, even though the authors retrospectively found that this was an important factor in the response to 5-FU + MeCCNU. However, it seems reasonable to conclude that the observations in this study represent solid data.

None of the remaining studies outlined in Table 1 accrued enough patients to reach meaningful conclusions.

Table 2 outlines several published adjuvant trials in gastric cancer. The VASAG trial of thiotepa at a total dose of 0.8 mg/kg revealed a significant increase in early postoperative mortality in the treated group (195). As a result, the dose was reduced to 0.6 mg/kg by omitting the i. v. dose on the day of surgery as the study continued. The only prerandomization stratification was for type of surgery, but retrospective analysis showed that the patients in both arms were essentially similar in race, duration of symptoms, weight loss, and concomitant diseases. Thiotepa at both levels of total dose (0.6 or 0.8 mg/kg) increased the postoperative mortality rate in patients who had a splenectomy. The 2-year survival rates showed no difference between the treatment and control groups.

A Surgical Adjuvant Gastric Cancer Chemotherapy Study (46,107) used thiotepa as an adjuvant to surgical resection, but the results of a 10-year follow-up showed no difference between the survival figures of the treated and the control groups. The fact that the only stratification was for type of surgery detracts somewhat from the conclusions. However, retrospective analysis showed that age, extent of disease, type of surgery, and concomitant diseases were equally distributed. The sex distribution was unequal, that is, with more males than females in the group treated by curative surgery alone. The results obtained in the lengthy follow-up period make it rather certain that the thiotepa doses employed do not lend any survival advantage in the adjuvant setting.

The VASAG also conducted a trial of 5-FUDR versus an untreated control

TABLE 2. *Published randomized trials of adjuvant chemotherapy in gastric cancer*

| Investigators (reference) and treatment arms[a] | Evaluation criteria[b] |
|---|---|
| VASAG (84,195)[c] | 1A, 2B,[d] 3D, 4A(10) 4B, 5C |
|   A. Thiotepa (0.2 mg/kg i. p. and 0.2 mg/kg i. v. d0; 0.2 mg/kg i. v. d1 and 2)[e] | |
|   B. No chemotherapy | |
| Dixon et al. (46), Longmire et al. (107)[f] | |
|     Part I | 1A, 2B, 3D, 4A(10), 4B |
|   A. Thiotepa (0.2 mg/kg i. p. and 0.2 mg/kg i. v. d 0; 0.2 mg/kg i. v. d1 and 2; total dose 0.8 mg/kg)[g] | |
|   B. No chemotherapy | |
|     Part II | 1A, 2B, 3A, 3D, 4A(10), 5C |
|   A. Thiotepa (0.2 mg/kg i. p. d0; 0.2 mg/kg i. v. d1 and 2; total dose 0.6 mg/kg) | |
|   B. Placebo | |
| Serlin et al. (176), VASAG (196) | 1A, 2B,[d] 3D, 4A(10), 5C |
|   A. 5-FUDR (20 mg/kg/d X 3 i. v.; then 30 mg/kg/d X 5, d35–45; then, 15 mg/kg q.o.d. X 4) | |
|   B. No chemotherapy | |
| Blokhina et al. (20) | 2B, 3D, 4B |
|   A. 5-FU (15 mg/kg q.o.d. i. v. beginning d30 to total 3 g; then, 15 mg/kg q.o.d. i. v. beginning d90 to total 3 g) | |
|   B. No chemotherapy | |

[a] Day 0 = day of surgery.
[b] See the criteria defined in Fig. 1.
[c] Veterans Administration Surgical Adjuvant Cancer Chemotherapy Group.
[d] Males only.
[e] Intravenous dose on day 0 was later discontinued.
[f] Ten-year follow-up.
[g] Intravenous dose on day 0 into the portal vein.

group, but the trial suffered from the design problem of stratifying only for the type of surgery. With the exception of age, which was comparably represented in both arms of the study, a retrospective analysis of other prognostic factors was not done. The results at 3 years showed no better or worse survival in the treated group. This study is not as reliable as the thiotepa studies because of the lack of prerandomization stratification and absence of retrospective analysis of prognostic factors.

Blokhina et al. (20) of the Soviet Union have conducted a multiinstitutional study of adjuvant 5-FU. The trial had no stratification before randomization, but the prognostic factors were apparently balanced as shown by a limited retrospective analysis. Unfortunately, a large number of patients (20%) were

TABLE 3. *Ongoing or unpublished randomized trials of chemotherapy in gastric cancer*

| Investigators (reference)[a] and treatment arms | Evaluation criteria[b] |
|---|---|
| ECOG 4274 (47) | 2B, 3F, 3G, 4A(1, 4, 10, 15) |
| A. 5-FU (450 mg/m²/d × 5, q. 5 wks i. v.) | |
| B. 5-FU (as in A) Testolactone (50 mg t.i.d. p. o.) | |
| C. 5-FU (325 mg/m²/d × 5, d1–5, 375 mg/m²/d × 5, d36–40 i. v.) MeCCNU (150 mg/m²/d1, q. 10 wks p. o.) | |
| D. 5-FU (as in C) MeCCNU (as in C) Testolactone (as in B) | |
| ECOG 3275 (47) | 2B, 3D, 4A(1, 10, 14) |
| A. 5-FU (as in ECOG 4274, arm C, above) MeCCNU (as in ECOG 4274, arm C, above) | |
| B. No treatment | |
| ECOG 3274 (188) | 2B, 3E, 3G, 4A(1, 4, 6, 10, 12) |
| A. Adriamycin (60 mg/m², q. 3 wks i. v.) | |
| B. 5-FU (325 mg/m²/d × 5, q. 5 wks i. v.) Mitomycin C (3.75 mg/m²/d ×5, q. 5 wks i. v.) | |
| C. 5-FU (as in ECOG 4274, arm C, above) MeCCNU (as in ECOG 4274, arm C, above) | |
| GITSG 8174 (188)[c] | 2B, 3D, 4A(1, 5, 14, 15) |
| A. 5-FU (as in ECOG 4274, arm C, above) MeCCNU (as in ECOG 4274, arm C, above) | |
| B. No treatment | |
| GITSG 8375 (188) | 2B, 3E, 3F, 3G 4A(4, 6, 9, 10, 12) |
| A. Adriamycin (60 mg/m², q. 3 wks i. v.) | |
| B. 5-FU (350 mg/m²/d × 5, q. 5 wks i. v.) MeCCNU (150 mg/m² d1, q. 10 wks p. o.) Adriamycin (40 mg/m², q. 5 wks i. v.) | |
| C. 5-FU (300 mg/m²/d × 5, q. 5 wks i. v.) Mitomycin C (1 mg/m²/d × 5, q. 5 wks i. v.) Ara-C (50 mg/m²/d × 5, q. 5 wks s. c.) | |
| GITSG 8376 (188) | 2B, 3E, 3F, 3G, 4A(4, 6, 9, 10, 12) |
| A. 5-FU (325 mg/m²/d × 5, q. 5 wks i. v.) ICRF-159 (500 mg/m² d2–4 and d36–38, p. o.) MeCCNU (110 mg/m², q. 10 wks p. o.) | |

TABLE 3—*Cont.*

| Investigators (reference)[a] and treatment arms | Evaluation criteria[b] |
|---|---|
| B. 5-FU (275 mg/m²/d × 5, q. 5 wks i. v.)<br>Adriamycin (30 mg/m², q. 5 wks i. v.)<br>Mitomycin C (10 mg/m², q. 10 wks i. v.)<br>C. 5-FU (as in A)<br>MeCCNU (as in A)<br>Adriamycin (40 mg/m², q. 5 wks i. v.) | |
| VASAG 30 (188)<br>A. 5-FU (9 mg/kg/d × 5, q. 7 wks i. v.)<br>MeCCNU (4 mg/kg/d × 5, q. 7 wks p. o.)<br>B. No treatment | 2B, 3D, 4A(10) |
| SWOG 7434 (188)<br><br>A. 5-FU (1 g/m²/d × 4, q. 4 wks i. v.)[d]<br>Mitomycin C (20 mg/m² q. 3 wks i. v.)<br>B. 5-FU (as in A)<br>MeCCNU (175 mg/m² q. 8 wks p. o.) | 2B, 3C,<br>4A(3, 5, 9, 13) |
| SEG 347 (188,198)<br><br>A. MTX (125 mg/m² q. 6 hr × 4, wkly × 12 p. o.)<br>Leucovorin (5 mg q. 6 hr × 6 p. o.)<br>B. MTX (15 mg/m² q. 6 hr × 4, wkly × 12 p. o.)<br>C. MTX (60 mg/m²/wk × 12 i. v.) | 2B, 3C,<br>4A(1, 5, 7, 8) |
| CALGB 7383 (188)<br>A. VP–16 (60–70 mg/m²/wk i. v.)<br>B. VP–16 (90–130 mg/m²/wk i. v.) | 2B, 3B |
| CALGB 7282 (188)<br>A. CCNU (100 mg/m² q. 6 wks p. o.)<br>B. MeCCNU (150 mg/m² q. 6 wks p. o.) | 2B, 3B |
| WCG 114 (188)<br><br>A. Bleomycin (10 mg/m² 2 × wkly i. v.)<br>B. Bleomycin (10 mg/m² 2 × wkly i. m.) | 2B, 3B,<br>4A(1, 5, 6, 14) |
| WCG 124 (188)<br>A. 5-FU (15 mg/kg/wk i. v.)<br>B. 5-FU (as in A)<br>CTX (to be determined) | 2B, 3B, 4A(5) |
| Yorkshire Regional Chemotherapy Group (188)<br>A. 5-FU (500 mg/m²/d × 5, q. 6 wks i. v.)<br>B. L-PAM (6 mg/m²/d × 5, q. 6 wks p. o.) | 2B, 3C, 4A(2, 4, 5) |
| Yorkshire Regional Chemotherapy Group (188)<br>A. BCNU (40 mg/m²/d × 5, q. 8 wks i. v.)<br>5-FU (400 mg/m²/d × 5, q. 8 wks p. o.)<br>B. No treatment | 1A, 3D, 4A(5, 16) |
| Mayo Clinic (188)<br>A. 5-FU (13.5 mg/kg/d × 5 i. v.)<br>B. 5-FU (35 mg/kg, q. 7 d i. v.) | 2A, 3C, 4A(5, 6) |

[a] Abbreviations: ECOG (Eastern Cooperative Oncology Group); GITSG (Gastrointestinal Tumor Study Group); SWOG (Southwest Oncology Group); SEG (Southeastern Cancer Study Group); CALGB (Cancer and Leukemia Group B); WCG (Western Cancer Study Group).

[b] See the criteria defined in Fig. 1.

[c] Two-year program.

[d] Intravenous infusion.

excluded from evaluation because of protocol violations. The investigators concluded that the 5-FU therapy in the first 18 months after surgery decreased the incidence of metastases and prolonged the time to disease recurrence when compared to the untreated control group. However, this advantage had vanished at the 2- and 3-year points in the analysis. Like the 5-FUDR study of the VASAG, this investigation suffers from the lack of prerandomization stratification, and the results can only be considered as possibly reliable data.

Table 3 summarizes 16 randomized trials that have not been published or are in progress.

Nine of these trials are gastric cancer-oriented studies of large cooperative clinical oncology groups, which should accrue a large number of patients who can be stratified before randomization. A review of the prerandomization stratification for the most important variables shows the following: four studies stratified for degree of anaplasia, one for extent of disease at diagnosis, six for type of surgery, one for site of the indicator lesion, and one for performance status. In addition, three studies were stratified for prior therapy, four for location of the primary lesion, and two for measurable/unmeasurable disease. Four of the ongoing trials are adjuvant studies, including three (ECOG 3275, GITSG 8174, and VASAG 30) employing MeCCNU + 5-FU versus no treatment and one by the Yorkshire Group that compares BCNU + 5-FU and an untreated group.

Surprisingly, few new agents are being tested against gastric cancer. This is an area of investigation that certainly should be worthy of further interest.

### Randomized Immunotherapy Trials

There have been no randomized trials exclusively devoted to immunotherapy. The trials that do employ immunotherapy will be discussed in the next section.

### Randomized Combined Modality Trials

The published randomized trials of combined modalities are listed in Table 4.

The first study (37,129) concluded that 5-FU + radiotherapy gave statistically significant improvement in survival compared to radiotherapy alone. The chief merit of the study design lies in its double-blind nature and the stratification of patients according to the grade of malignancy. However, it did select out for study patients with better prognosis (limited disease), and the conclusions are not applicable to disseminated gastric malignancies.

The study by Falkson et al. (60) compares 5-FU + radiotherapy versus a four-drug combination plus radiotherapy. Unfortunately, the study was not stratified. The authors concluded that a larger group of patients, which would permit adequate stratification, might show an advantage for the four-drug regimen. The study suggests that there is no difference between the treatments but it is by no means definitive.

TABLE 4. Published combined modality trials in gastric cancer

| Treatment arms | Modality | | Chemotherapy | Evaluation criteria[a] | Survival time | Investigators (reference) |
|---|---|---|---|---|---|---|
| | Surgery | Radiotherapy | | | | |
| A. | Unspecified | 900–1,200 rads/wk (3,500–4,000 rads total) | Saline placebo | 1B, 2A, 3B, 3C, 4A(1) | 5.9 mos. | Moertel et al. (129), Childs et al. (37,38) |
| B. | Unspecified | As in A | 5-FU (15 mg/kg/d ×3) | | 13 mos. | |
| A. | Unknown | 2,000 rads/12 days (10 treatments starting d1 of 1st 5-FU course); then, 1,200 rads with 2nd and 5th course of chemotherapy | 5-FU (12.5 mg/kg/d ×5, q. 5 wks i. v.) | 4B | 220 days | Falkson et al. (60) |
| B. | Unknown | As in A | 5-FU (10 mg/kg/d ×5, q. 5 wks i. v.) DTIC (3 mg/kg/d ×2, q. 5 wks i. v.) VCR (0.025 mg/kg/ d ×1, q. 5 wks i. v.) BCNU (1.5 mg/kg/d ×1, q. 5 wks i. v.) | | 199 days | |

[a]See the criteria defined in Fig. 1.

A number of combined modality trials in gastric cancer are still in progress (Table 5). There are two surgical adjuvant studies (Mayo Clinic and W. W. Cross Cancer Institute), three trials combining radiotherapy and chemotherapy (ECOG 1274B, GITSG 8274, and Mayo Clinic), and three studies of drugs and immunotherapy (M. D. Anderson, NCI of Canada, and Sloan-Kettering). All of these trials, except GITSG 8274, suffer from a lack of prerandomization stratification and probably will yield uninterpretable data. In spite of the lack of bona fide phase II trials of immunotherapy, this modality is still being used in combined modality regimens.

## Conclusions

This review of randomized trials in gastric cancer is enlightening for a number of reasons. Seven prognostic factors of particular importance in the prerandomization stratification of patients were identified. Also, the review showed that no randomized trials devoted exclusively to surgery, radiotherapy, or immunotherapy have been performed, although radiotherapy or immunotherapy are used with chemotherapy in some combined modality studies.

The 13 published trials of chemotherapy (Tables 1 and 2) yielded a fair amount of information. However, improper experimental designs and an insufficient number of patients detract greatly from the conclusions in many studies. The apparently valid data include the following:

1. 5-FU or 5-FU + BCNU produce statistically better response rate and longer survival than BCNU alone. However, 5-FU + BCNU does not provide an advantage in survivorship over 5-FU alone except at 18 months, where it barely reaches statistical significance.

2. Cyclophosphamide detracts from the response rate obtained by induction therapy with 5-FU + MeCCNU or MeCCNU alone.

3. 5-FU + MeCCNU is superior to MeCCNU alone in terms of response rate and survival.

4. The thiotepa regimens used by the two major group studies (Table 2) do not prolong survival in an adjuvant situation.

Less definite results indicate that 5-FUDR or 5-FU, in the doses used, do not afford any survival advantage as surgical adjuvants.

All of the chemotherapy studies now in progress show poor prerandomization stratification (Table 3). Very few of the trials are evaluating new antitumor agents, which should provide fertile ground for further studies.

Although the published accounts (Table 4) of combined modality studies reveal some design problems, the results are probably firm enough to conclude that 5-FU plus radiotherapy is superior to radiotherapy alone in limited local disease. The data indicating that 5-FU + radiotherapy is as effective as 5-FU + DTIC + vincristine + BCNU and radiotherapy are not as convincing because of protocol design problems (60).

TABLE 5. Ongoing or unpublished combined modality trials in gastric cancer

| Treatment arms | Modality | | | | Evaluation criteria[a] | Investigators (references)[b] |
|---|---|---|---|---|---|---|
| | Surgery | Radiotherapy | Chemotherapy | Immunotherapy | | |
| A. | Unspecified | — | 5-FU (600 mg/m²/wk i. v.) | — | 1C, 2B, 4A(1) | ECOG 1274B (188) |
| B. | As in A | 4,000 rads | 5-FU (600 mg/m² i. v., 1st 3 days of RT) | — | | |
| A. | Unspecified | — | MeCCNU (150 mg/m² q. 10 wks p. o.) 5-FU (325 mg/m²/d ×5, q. 10 wks, begin d1 of MeCCNU; then 375 mg/m²/d ×5, q. 10 wks, begin d36–40) | — | 1C, 2B, 4A(1, 10, 16) | GITSG 8274 (188) |
| B. | As in A | 5,000 rads, split course in 8 wks | 5-FU (500 mg/m²/ d ×3 i. v. with each RT course) 5-FU (325 mg/m²/ d ×5, d71–76; 375 mg/m²/d ×5, d106–111) MeCCNU (150 mg/m² q. 10 wks) | — | | |
| A. | Unspecified | — | Ftorafur (2 gm/m²/ d ×5) Baker's Antifol (250 mg/m²/d ×3, q. 4 wks) | — | 2A, 3C | M. D. Anderson Hospital (188) |
| B. | As in A | — | As in A | C. parvum (5 mg/m² i. v. over 1 hr, monthly | | |

| | | | | | | |
|---|---|---|---|---|---|---|
| A. | Curative or palliative | — | 5-FU (15 mg/kg/d × 4; then wkly ×3, q. 4 wks) | — | 2B, 3C, 4A(5) | NCI, Canada (188) |
| B. | As in A | — | As in A | BCG (2 mg i. p.; then 120 mg p. o. q. 4 wks) | | |
| A. | Unspecified | Unspecified | Mitomycin C (10 mg/m² d1 i. v.) 5-FU (400 mg/m² d1–3; repeat d22) Adriamycin (40 mg/m² d2 i. v.; repeat d22) Repeat cycle q. 6 wks | C. parvum (0.1 ml s. c. wkly) | 2A, 3G | Memorial Sloan-Kettering Cancer Center (188) |
| B. | As in A | As in A | As in A | — | | |
| A. | Curative | — | — | — | 2A, 3D, 4A(17) | Mayo Clinic (188) |
| B. | As in A | 3,000 rads/ 28 days | 5-FU (15 mg/kg/d ×3 i. v., 1st 3 days of RT) | — | | |
| A. | Curative | — | — | — | 2A, 3D | W. W. Cross Cancer Institute (40) |
| B. | As in A | — | 5-FU + MeCCNU[c] | — | | |
| C. | As in A | — | — | BCG (120 mg p. o., ? interval × 5 yrs) | | |

[a] See the criteria defined in Fig. 1.
[b] Abbreviations: See previous tables.
[c] Dosage unspecified.

Randomized trials in gastric cancer have provided some basic information for building further investigations, but major design problems limited some of the more important trials. As in the case with all of the major solid tumors, more basic therapeutic tools are needed to attack gastric cancer. Further well-designed randomized phase II trials with new drugs, new techniques of radiotherapy, and old and new immunotherapeutic agents should help to fill those needs.

## PANCREATIC CANCER

The rising prevalence of pancreatic carcinoma in the United States is marked by a rate of increase in reported cases that is second only to lung cancer. It is now the fourth leading cause of cancer deaths, exceeded only by cancer of the lung, large bowel, and breast (2,101). In 1973, it was estimated that 19,000 Americans would develop pancreatic carcinomas and essentially the same number would die of this neoplasm (124). The usually brief course of the disease, whether treated or not, is characterized by a mean survival of 3.5 to 6 months and a 5-year survival rate of 0 to 5% (74,118,124,146).

### Prognostic Factors

Not all of the important prognostic factors in pancreatic cancer are entirely clear, but they have been the topic of several studies and discussions (30,118,124).

Histologically, pancreatic adenocarcinoma most frequently has ductal or acinar architecture. Ductal adenocarcinoma is the most common histologic type and is found in 80 to 90% of reported cases (114,178). Squamous cell histology originating from metaplasia of the major ducts is observed in rare instances (124). Pancreatic adenocarcinomas may exhibit varying degrees of differentiation within the same tumor, but a review of the natural history of the disease by Moertel et al. (30,118,124) has noted that these variations (Broder's grade of malignancy) affect survival, with longer survival occurring in patients with more well-differentiated tumors.

Conclusions regarding the prognostic significance of age and sex have been contradictory. The review of Moertel et al. (30,118,124) noted that the sex of the patient has little or no influence on survival. On the other hand, Baylor and Berg (16) reviewed end-result registries and found that females have a slight but persistent survival advantage over males. Moertel et al. (30,118,124) found that among patients under 80 years of age, survival rose steadily with increasing age, reflecting a smaller proportion of long-term survivors among younger patients. Again, Baylor and Berg reached the opposite conclusion, finding decreased survival with increasing age at diagnosis.

Caucasians have shown a slight survival advantage during the first year after diagnosis but no significant difference thereafter (16).

A certain diagnosis of pancreatic cancer must be obtained, usually at laparotomy. It is important to distinguish cancer of the head of the pancreas from other tumors in the intrapancreatic portion of the common bile duct, the ampulla of Vater, and the duodenal mucosa, which may be resectable with a more favorable prognosis (31). Patients with a primary lesion in the head of the pancreas have a more favorable outlook for survival than those with lesions in the body or tail (30,31). This may be related to earlier diagnosis of the lesions having a greater propensity for obstructing the common bile duct.

The extent of disease at the time of diagnosis also has important implications for survival. Tumors disseminated at the time of diagnosis have a significantly poorer prognosis than local or regional disease (16,118,124). As would be expected, it appears that a longer duration of symptoms favors better survival (118,124).

As far as the influence of surgery is concerned, biliary diversion and gastroenterostomy can provide palliation and moderately increase survival when the tumor is not amenable to an attempt at curative resection (43). Moertel (118), in a nonrandomized retrospective study, has found that patients who have a palliative bypass procedure have a median survival of 4.5 months versus only 2 months for exploratory surgery only.

Several other factors, such as performance status (131), liver involvement, prior therapy, and disease-free interval after surgery, may influence prognosis, but their significance is poorly understood because of the lack of adequate study. Some of the clinical trials reviewed in this section deal with these prognostic factors, but the data still are not clear. Thus, assessment of the trials centers on six of the prognostic variables (Fig. 1) that are of major importance to the stratification of patients with this disease, that is, age, histology, location of the primary lesion, extent of disease at diagnosis, type of surgery, and duration of symptoms.

### Randomized Surgical Trials

Several surgical procedures may be undertaken for cancer of the pancreas, including pancreatoduodenectomy (Whipple's procedure), radical distal pancreatectomy, total pancreatectomy, and extended resection of the pancreas. Most of these approaches are directed to tumors in the head region of the gland because the vast majority of body and tail lesions are diagnosed too late for surgery (90). In spite of the various methods of resection, no controlled trials randomizing patients to these procedures have been conducted.

It is unclear whether a definitive resection gives overall better results than a bypass procedure (30). Some investigators have reported a 14.3% survival rate at 5 years among patients with ductal adenocarcinoma undergoing the Whipple procedure (143). Moertel et al. (118) have shown by retrospective analysis that palliative bypass results in longer survival than an exploratory procedure. At the present time there is little support for conducting studies employing randomization between the various surgical procedures or between palliative surgery and no treatment, and the choice of procedure must depend on the individual surgeon's evaluation.

## Randomized Radiotherapy Trials

"Pure" randomized trials confined strictly to comparing various radiotherapy regimens are completely lacking. Instead, most randomized studies of radiotherapy are really combined modality trials with irradiation as one treatment arm and radiotherapy plus chemotherapy as the other. These will be discussed in a later section.

On the other hand, there certainly have been a few studies that provide data that could be used for designing randomized radiotherapy trials. A retrospective study by Childs (36) at the Mayo Clinic has shown that survival curves for 62 patients with locally unresectable tumors treated with a total dose of 3,500 rads are identical to those of matched untreated patients. In addition, the treated patients experienced little palliation of symptoms. One approach to improving these poor results was made by Cavanaugh (34), who proposed use of high-dose split-course radiotherapy. Pancreatic cancer represents a rather slow-growing radioresistant tumor in close anatomic relationship to the rapidly proliferating, highly radiosensitive epithelium of the small bowel. Fractionation schedules might be one approach allowing recovery of radiosensitive tissues and retention of antitumor effect. Haslam et al. (78) obtained some potentially positive results using 6,000 rads fractionated in three series of 2,000 rads given in 10 fractions over 2 weeks (2-week rest intervals), but concomitant 5-FU was given to most patients. Another recently proposed concept (117) is implantation of [222]Rn, [192]Ir, and [198]Au, but no controlled trials have been attempted.

## Randomized Chemotherapy Trials

Table 6 summarizes the published reports of randomized trials of chemotherapy and cites the study design criteria from Fig. 1 that were employed in each trial.

The first study (128) was a provocative comparison of analgesics, concluding that aspirin was significantly more effective than placebo and "superior" to oral codeine sulfate. Although the prognostic factors for pain relief in pancreatic cancer are uncertain, extent of disease would appear to be a logical one since certain types of spread would cause different types of pain or make it more refractory. The study did not deal with this important factor. In addition, only a small number of patients were studied, but they did serve as their own controls through rerandomization to one of the other treatment arms at an unspecified time. The study has merit because of its originality, the double-blind procedure, and the laparotomy proof of disease. However, the authors failed to mention any differences in the toxic effects of the treatment arms.

The small number of patients and lack of prior stratification for any prognostic

TABLE 6. *Published randomized trials of chemotherapy in pancreatic cancer*

| Investigators (reference) and treatment arms | Evaluation criteria[a] | No. responses/ no. patients | Response rate (%) |
|---|---|---|---|
| Moertel et al. (128) | 1A, 2A, 3A, 6A | | |
| A. Aspirin (650 mg, p. r. n., p. o.) | | 7/13 | 54 |
| B. Codeine (60 mg, p. r. n., p. o.) | | 5/13 | 38 |
| C. Placebo (lactose, p. r. n., p. o.) | | 3/13 | 23 |
| Stolinsky et al. (187) | 2B, 4B, 6B | | |
| A. 5-FU (15 mg/kg/wk p. o.) | | 0/16 | — |
| B. 5-FU (15 mg/kg/wk i. v.) | | 3/14 | 21 |
| Kovach et al. (99) | 1A, 2A, 4A(1, 2), 4B | | |
| A. 5-FU (13.5 mg/kg/d × 5, q. 5 wks i. v.) | | 5/31 | 16 |
| B. BCNU (50 mg/m²/d × 5, q. 8 wks i. v.) | | 0/21 | — |
| C. 5-FU (10 mg/kg/d × 5, q. 8 wks i. v.) BCNU (40 mg/m²/d × 5, q. 8 wks i. v.) | | 10/30 | 33 |
| Reitemeier et al. (165) | 2A, 3C, 4A(2), 5A | | |
| A. Fluorometholone (25 mg, q. 12 hr p. o.) | | 0/6 | — |
| B. 5-FU (15 mg/kg/d × 5; then q.o.d. × 4 i. v.) | | 1/7 | 14 |
| C. Fluorometholone (as in A) 5-FU (as in B) | | 0/8 | — |
| Baker et al. (11) | 2A, 3B, 4A(3), 5A | | |
| A. Mitomycin C (22.5 mg/m², q. 6–8 wks i. v.) | | 1/4 | 25 |
| B. Porfiromycin (75 mg/m², q. 6–8 wks i. v.) | | 1/3 | 33 |
| Gailani et al. (65) | 2B, 3A, 3C | | |
| A. 5-FU (15 mg/kg/wk i. v.) Placebo (mannitol s. c.) | | 0/6 | — |
| B. 5-FU (as in A) Ara-C (30 mg/m²/wk s. c.) | | 1/1 | 100 |
| Reitemeier et al. (164) | 2A, 3C, 4A(1, 2) | | |
| A. 5-FU (13.5 mg/kg/d × 5, q. 4 wks i. v.) | | 1/2 | 50 |
| B. Mitomycin C (150 µg/kg/d × 5, q. 8 wks i. v.) | | 1/2 | 50 |
| C. BCNU (50 mg/m²/d × 5, q. 8 wks i. v.) | | 0/1 | — |
| D. 5-FU (9 mg/kg/d × 5, q. 8 wks i. v.) Mitomycin C (110 µg/kg/d × 5, q. 8 wks i. v.) | | 0/2 | — |
| E. 5-FU (as in D) BCNU (37.5 mg/m²/d × 5, q. 8 wks i. v.) | | 2/3 | 66 |
| F. Mitomycin C (75 µg/kg/d × 5, q. 8 wks i. v.) BCNU (25 mg/m²/d × 5, q. 8 wks i. v.) | | 0/1 | — |
| G. 5-FU (8 mg/kg/d × 5, q. 8 wks i. v.) | | 1/3 | 33 |

TABLE 6—*Cont.*

| Investigators (reference) and treatment arms | Evaluation criteria[a] | No. responses/ no. patients | Response rate (%) |
|---|---|---|---|
| Mitomycin C (60 µg/kg/d X 5, q. 8 wks i. v.) BCNU (20 mg/m²/d X 5, q. 8 wks i. v.) | | | |
| Baker et al. (12,13) | 2B, 3C, 4B, 5B | | |
| A. 5-FU (400 mg/m²/wk i. v.) | | 1/6 | 16 |
| B. 5-FU (as in A) | | 3/15 | 20 |
| MeCCNU (175 mg/m², q. 6 wks p. o.) | | | |

[a] See the categories defined in Fig. 1.

variable, except that diagnosis was confirmed in most patients at laparotomy, hinder evaluation of the second study (187). Retrospectively, performance status and serum bilirubin levels were similar in both treatment arms, but these are not clearly established prognostic factors. These problems detract from the authors' conclusion that intravenous 5-FU was superior to oral 5-FU in both response rate and survival. A previous study by the same group had too few patients in each arm of therapy to permit interpretation (15).

The third study outlined in Table 6 is an interesting single institution trial of 5-FU versus BCNU versus 5-FU + BCNU (99). A major problem is that 49 of the 82 patients had a primary pancreatic lesion established at surgery, whereas 33 cases were presumed to be pancreatic cancer based on histology of a metastatic lesion, negative barium studies, and a "convincing clinical presentation." Obviously, the study could have included other tumors with different prognoses, such as ampullary carcinoma. The only real prognostic factor for which patients were stratified was grade of anaplasia, but the authors noted that the patients in each arm were similar in age, sex, and estimated risk (i.e., good, fair, or poor) of treatment. The conclusions were that 5-FU + BCNU or 5-FU alone produced statistically significant superiority in response rates over that obtained with BCNU alone. Of course, these findings must be tempered by the above discussion of the study design. Therapy with 5-FU + BCNU was not statistically better than therapy with 5-FU alone, nor was there any difference among the three treatment arms insofar as survival was concerned. The authors did not recommend routine use of the combination regimen because overall improvement in survival was not statistically significant.

The fourth study in Table 6 concluded that the steroid fluorometholone added nothing to the response rate with 5-FU nor did it alter the toxicity of the drug. Unfortunately, the study included only a few patients with pancreatic cancer, and there was only one stratification factor without even a retrospective review of other prognostic factors. Therefore the findings of the study appear to be inconclusive.

Unfortunately, the other published studies included too few pancreatic cancer patients for any meaningful conclusions.

Fourteen randomized studies of chemotherapy in pancreatic cancer have not been published or are still in progress. These are summarized in Table 7 in order to note some important factors that merit the attention of readers interested in further trials. Most of the studies will soon yield results and be published, so it is interesting to speculate on the data that may be expected in terms of the study designs.

Seven of the trials are pancreatic cancer-oriented studies of cooperative clinical oncology groups and, for this reason, should accrue a large number of patients who can be stratified appropriately before randomization. However, a review of prerandomization stratification in these seven studies shows the following: three protocols stratified for histology, three for location of the primary lesion, two for type of surgery performed, five for performance status, one for institution, three for prior therapy (RT and/or CT), one for measurable/nonmeasurable disease, and one for heart disease. Considering the rather limited stratification in each trial, the outlook for obtaining meaningful data in the ongoing trials is not very bright.

In the seven major pancreatic cancer studies in Table 7 it is interesting to note the anticancer agents being used. Fifteen different drugs are involved, the most common being 5-FU (six studies) and streptozotocin (five studies). The use of newer agents by the Gastrointestinal Tumor Study Group (GITSG) is an encouraging approach. One study by the V.A. Surgical Adjuvant Cancer Chemotherapy group (VASAG) is employing an untreated control arm.

### Randomized Immunotherapy Trials

At present there are no pure randomized trials of immunotherapy. The trials that do include immunotherapeutic agents will be discussed in the next section.

### Randomized Combined Modality Trials

Table 8 cites the published randomized trials of combined modalities. The Mayo Clinic Group (37,129) has compared radiotherapy alone and combined with 5-FU, concluding that mean survival was significantly improved with the combined modalities. The study excluded patients with distant metastases and those having regional disease with dimensions greater than 20 cm × 20 cm. The only parameter of stratification was Broder's degree of anaplasia. Although the relative lack of stratification detracts from the conclusions, the trial did have merit in the double-blind administration of the chemotherapy. The results do provide fair to good evidence that the combination was more effective than radiotherapy alone.

A recently published GITSG trial compared radiotherapy (4,000 rads) + 5-FU, radiotherapy (6,000 rads) + 5-FU, and radiotherapy (6,000 rads) alone.

TABLE 7. *Ongoing or unpublished randomized trials of chemotherapy in pancreatic cancer*

| Investigators (reference)[a] and treatment arms | Evaluation criteria[b] |
| --- | --- |
| GITSG 9374 (31,188) | 2B, 4A(4, 6, 12) |
|   A. Actinomycin D (0.4 mg/m² /d × 5, q. 4 wks i. v.) | |
|   B. MTX (40 mg/m² /wk i. v.) | |
|   C. Adriamycin (60 mg/m², q. 3 wks i. v.)[c] | |
| Mayo Clinic (188) | 2A, 3C, 4A(5, 6) |
|   A. 5-FU (13.5 mg/kg/d × 5 i. v.) | |
|   B. 5-FU (35 mg/kg, q. 7 d i. v.) | |
| SEG 347 (188,198) | 2B, 3C, 4A(1, 5, 7, 8) |
|   A. MTX (125 mg/m² q. 6h × 4, wkly p. o.) | |
|     Leucovorin (5 mg q. 6h × 6, wkly p. o.) | |
|   B. MTX (15 mg/m² q. 6h × 4, wkly p. o.) | |
|   C. MTX (60 mg/m² /wk i. v.) | |
| CALGB 7383 (188) | 2B, 3B |
|   A. VP–16 (60–70 mg/m² /wk i. v.) | |
|   B. VP–16 (90–130 mg/m² /wk i. v.) | |
| CALGB 7282 (188) | 2B |
|   A. CCNU (100 mg/m² q. 6 wks p. o.) | |
|   B. MeCCNU (150 mg/m² q. 6 wks p. o.) | |
| WCG 114 (188) | 2B, 3B, 4A(1, 5, 6) |
|   A. Bleomycin (10 mg/m² 2 × wkly i. v.) | |
|   B. Bleomycin (10 mg/m² 2 × wkly i. m.) | |
| COG 7230 (30,31,102) | 2B, 4A(9) |
|   A. 5-FU (12.5 mg/kg/d × 5; then q. wk × 6 i. v.) | |
|   B. 5-FU (12.5 mg/kg, d1–3, 17, 31, 45 i. v.) | |
|     Tubercidin (1,500 γ/kg/d1 i. v. infusion) | |
|     Streptozotocin (12.5 mg/kg d10, 24, 38 i. v.) | |
| WCG 124 (188) | 2B, 3B, 4A(5) |
|   A. 5-FU (15 mg/kg/wk i. v.) | |
|   B. 5-FU (as in A) | |
|     CTX (to be determined) | |
| ECOG 2272 (47) | 2B, 4A(1, 4, 5) |
|   A. MeCCNU (200 mg/m², single dose p. o.) | |
|   B. Streptozotocin (500 mg/m² /d × 5 i. v.) | |
|     5-FU (400 mg/m² /d × 5 i. v.) | |
|   C. Streptozotocin (as in B) | |
|     CTX 1 g/m² d1 and 21 i. v.) | |
| ECOG 2275 (47) | 2B, 3E, 4A(1, 4–6) |
|   A. 5-FU (350 mg/m² /d × 5 i. v.; then 400 mg/ m² /d × 5 on d36–40) | |
|     Streptozotocin (400 mg/m² /d × 5 i. v.) | |
|     MeCCNU (150 mg/m² d1 p. o.) | |
|   B. L-PAM (6 mg/m² /d × 5, wkly p. o.) | |
| ECOG 5274 (188) | 2B, 3F, 3G, 4A(1, 4, 5) |
|   A. 5-FU (450 mg/m² /d × 5, q. 5 wks i. v.) | |
|   B. 5-FU (as in A) | |
|     Spironolactone (50 mg t.i.d. p. o.) | |
|   C. 5-FU (400 mg/m² /d × 5, q. 5 wks i. v.) | |
|     Streptozotocin (500 mg/m² /d × 5, q. 5 wks i. v.) | |
|   D. 5-FU (as in C) | |
|     Streptozotocin (as in C) | |
|     Spironolactone (as in B) | |

TABLE 7—*Cont.*

| Investigators (reference)[a] and treatment arms | Evaluation criteria[b] |
|---|---|
| VASAG 25 (30,31,188) | 1A, 2B, 4A(10) |
|   A. 5-FU (9 mg/kg/d X 5, q. 6 wks i. v.)[d] | |
|     CCNU (70 mg/m² q. 6 wks p. o.) | |
|   B. No postoperative therapy | |
| SWOG 7414 (188) | 2B, 3C, 4A(3, 5, 9, 13)[e] |
|   A. 5-FU (1 g/m²/d X 4, q. 4 wks i. v. infusion) | |
|     Mitomycin C (20 mg/m², q. 7 wks i. v. infusion) | |
|   B. 5-FU (as in A) | |
|     MeCCNU (175 mg/m² q. 8 wks p. o.) | |
| GITSG 9376 (188) | 2B, 4A(4, 6, 10, 11) |
|   A. Streptozotocin (1 g/m² d1, 8, 29, 36 i. v.) | |
|     Mitomycin C (10 mg/m² q. 8 wks i. v.) | |
|     5-FU (600 mg/m² d1, 8, 29, 36 i. v.) | |
|   B. Hexamethylmelamine (320 mg/m²/d p. o.) | |
|   C. Galactitol (25 mg/m²/d X 5, q. 2 wks i. v.) | |
|   D. ICRF–159 (850 mg/m²/d X 3, q. 4 wks p. o.) | |
|   E. β-2-TGdR (100 mg/m²/d X 5, q. 3 wks i. v.) | |
|   F. Streptozotocin (350 mg/m² q. 5 wks i. v.) | |
|     Mitomycin C (10 mg/m² q. 10 wks i. v.) | |
|     5-FU (500 mg/m²/d X 5 i. v.) | |

[a] Abbreviations: COG (Central Oncology Group); see others in previous tables.
[b] See the categories defined in Fig. 1.
[c] 5-FU maintenance after total adriamycin dose of 500 mg/m².
[d] Combination regimen for eight courses; then, 5-FU for life.
[e] Poor-risk patients received reduced drug dose.

This was a well-designed study with good stratification for four prognostic variables, including performance status. There were no statistical differences in median survival produced by the three arms, but the combination arms consistently yielded longer survival times than radiotherapy alone. The study selected out ambulatory patients and showed that they fared significantly better in terms of survival after treatment with the combined modalities, thus bolstering the importance of performance status as a bonafide prognostic factor. The higher dose of radiotherapy added nothing to patient survival.

The first study in Table 9 represents the only ongoing combined modality adjuvant trial in pancreatic cancer, which is an extension of the GITSG trial discussed above (Table 8). Stratification is fairly good, including four of the six major prognostic factors, and the final results should be meaningful when they become available.

The remainder of Table 9 outlines four other unpublished or ongoing combined modality trials. Two of these combine radiotherapy and chemotherapy and two employ chemotherapy and immunotherapy. Only one study (ECOG 1274B) stratified patients according to a minimal number of prognostic factors. Therefore, three of the trials may yield interesting but uninterpretable data.

TABLE 8. *Published combined modality trials in pancreatic cancer*

| Treatment arms | Modality | | Chemotherapy | Evaluation criteria [a] | Survival time | Investigators (reference) [b] |
|---|---|---|---|---|---|---|
| | Surgery | Radiotherapy | | | | |
| A. | Unspecified | 900–1,200 rads/wk (3,500–4,000 rads total) | Saline placebo | 1A, 2A, 3B, 3C, 4A(1) | 6.3 mos. [c] | Moertel et al. (129), Childs et al. (37) |
| B. | Unspecified | As in A | 5-FU (15 mg/kg/d × 3) | | 10.4 mos. [c] | |
| A. | Variable | 4,000 rads (split course, 2,000 rads beginning d1 and 29) | 5-FU (500 mg/m² i. v. d1–3, 29–31, 71, 78, and wkly thereafter) | 1C, 2B, 3C, 4A(1, 4, 5, 10) | 35 wks [d] | GITSG (30,31,131) |
| B. | Variable | 6,000 rads (3 courses, beginning d1, 29, and 57) | 5-FU (500 mg/m² i. v. d1–3, 29–31, 57–59, 99, 106, and wkly thereafter) | | 28 wks [d] | |
| C. | Variable | As in B | None | | 17 wks [d] | |

[a] See the categories defined in Fig. 1.
[b] See abbreviations in previous tables.
[c] Mean survival.
[d] Median survival.

TABLE 9. Ongoing or unpublished combined modality trials in pancreatic cancer

| Treatment arms | Surgery | Radiotherapy | Chemotherapy | Immunotherapy | Evaluation criteria [a] | Investigators (reference) [b] |
|---|---|---|---|---|---|---|
| | | | Modality | | | |
| A. | Curative (Whipple or total) | — | — | — | 3D, 4A(1, 5, 10, 14) | GITSG 9173 (30,31) |
| B. | As in A | Split course, wks 1–2 and 4–6, 2,000 rads each course | 5-FU (500 mg/m² d1–3, 29–31, 71, 78, wkly thereafter) | — | | |
| A. | Curative or palliative | — | 5-FU (15 mg/kg/d × 4; then wkly × 3, q. 4 wks) | — | 2B, 3C, 4A(5) | NCI, Canada (188) |
| B. | As in A | — | As in A | BCG (2 mg i. p.; then 120 mg p. o. q. 4 wks) | | |
| A. | Unspecified | — | Ftorafur (2 g/m²/d × 5); Baker's antifol (250 mg/m²/d × 3, q. 4 wks) | — | 2A, 3C | M. D. Anderson Hospital (188) |
| B. | As in A | — | As in A | C. parvum (5 mg/m² i. v. over 1 hr, monthly | | |
| A. | Unspecified | — | 5-FU (600 mg/m²/wk i. v.) | — | 1A, 2B, 4A(1, 5) | ECOG 1274B (188) |
| B. | As in A | 4,000 rads | 5-FU (600 mg/m² i. v., first 3 days of RT; then wkly after RT) | — | | |
| A. | Variable | 2,000 rads/5 days | MeCCNU (125 mg/m² q. 6 wks p. o.) 5-FU (400 mg/m²/wk i. v.) Testolactone (200 mg/d) | — | 2B, 4A(10) | SWOG 7509 (188) |
| B. | As in A | As in A | As in A, but without testolactone | — | | |

[a] See the categories defined in Fig. 1.
[b] See abbreviations in previous tables.

Immunotherapy has not been tested in Phase II trials against pancreatic cancer, but still appears in combined modality studies. In the single study where BCG is given intraperitoneally, even the route of administration has not been evaluated individually.

## Conclusions

The review of randomized studies of treatment in pancreatic cancer reveals a marked need for understanding the prognostic factors influencing the course of the disease. Six specific prognostic indicators, and one or two others of possible importance, were considered in the analysis of all trials. The overall conclusion is that there is a need for better study designs that carefully stratify patients according to these prognostic factors and provide the data that will determine their role in the outcome of treatment.

There have been no randomized trials of surgery. Although there are differences of opinion as to whether or not a palliative procedure is better than no surgery at all, there is probably little interest in performing controlled trials that might answer the questions. Since the type of surgery is dictated by the findings at exploratory laparotomy, there seems to be little chance for performing a randomized trial of the Whipple procedure versus total pancreatectomy versus partial pancreatectomy.

The absence of pure randomized trials of radiotherapy does not preclude the existence of several possible leads. Split-course irradiation versus conventional radiotherapy or implantation of radioactive isotopes might provide fertile areas for investigation. In addition, trials with radiosensitizers certainly offer a potential approach.

The eight published accounts of randomized trials of chemotherapy share a surprising paucity of useful information, largely because of poor study design with improper stratification and insufficient numbers of patients for adequate comparison of treatments. The only really firm information is that aspirin is probably better than placebo or codeine sulfate in the relief of pain. Less conclusive data show that the response rate with 5-FU + BCNU is probably better than with BCNU alone, but no better than with 5-FU alone. The borderline difference in response rate does not produce any advantage in survival time.

The trials still in progress also offer little prospect of useful results. Seven of the 14 studies lack the stratification that could yield meaningful data. The remaining studies being conducted by large clinical groups may fare better because they have some prerandomization stratification. It is also encouraging that some of these groups are exploring the activity of single agents in pancreatic cancer.

The only published combined modality studies have some design problems but are probably sufficient to conclude that 5-FU + radiotherapy is superior to radiotherapy alone in limited local disease. However, no trials have included a 5-FU alone arm. There also is reasonable evidence that an increase of irradiation from 4,000 to 6,000 rads adds nothing to patient survival. The future of combined modality therapy seems to lie with adjuvant studies, but only one such trial has been started in pancreatic cancer. Of course, the major problem is the lack of the proper therapeutic tools for use in the combined modality approach.

In summary, randomized trials have made very little impact on response or survival in pancreatic cancer and have yielded very little useful information. Clearly, more basic and well-designed randomized trials are needed in the separate areas of chemotherapy, surgery, radiotherapy, and immunotherapy to provide the basic tools for building more complicated phase III or combined modality trials.

## COLORECTAL CANCER

Cancer of the colon and rectum is among the leading causes of morbidity and mortality in the Western World. In the United States, it ranks second only to lung cancer in males and breast cancer in females as a cause of cancer deaths (179). The significant advances in diagnostic and surgical techniques, which have improved overall survival, have reached a plateau. Combined modality therapy now seems to offer the greatest potential for the future (9,29).

About 98% of the large bowel malignancies are adenocarcinomas, whereas the remainder include squamous carcinoma, carcinoid tumors, malignant lymphomas, and leiomyosarcomas (119). The overall 5-year survival for colorectal cancer was reported in 1973 as 41% for males and 46% for females (179).

### Prognostic Factors in Primary Treatment

The most widely accepted prognostic factors influencing the outcome of primary treatment in colorectal cancer are included in Fig. 1. Mortality rates tend to be higher with advancing age (9,179) as a result of multiple factors that include coexistent illness and the potential for increased postoperative morbidity and mortality. Occurrence under the age of 30 years has also been associated with a poor prognosis (116). The overall prognosis is slightly more favorable in women than in men, regardless of the disease stage (9,179). This advantage is most marked in women having rectal and rectosigmoid lesions with regional lymph node involvement (181).

A significant difference in survival may be associated with the location of the primary tumor; that is, overall survival rates in rectal carcinomas are purported to be 10 to 15% lower than in colon carcinomas (29). This difference has been supported (61) or denied (18) in other series. Carcinoma of the right colon, especially the cecum, may also have a less favorable prognosis (61).

As in other malignancies, the disease stage at presentation influences prognosis (18,79,201). The most widely used staging classifications are outlined in Table 10. Of course, the prognostic influence of disease stage, as reported in the vast surgical literature, varies widely because of a complex interplay of patient charac-

TABLE 10. *The most widely used staging classifications in colorectal cancer*

| Numeric classification (94) | ASC end results (9,179) | Dukes (50) rectal cancer | Astler and Coller (8) | Copeland et al. (42) |
|---|---|---|---|---|
| I Confined within bowel wall | Localized | A. Limited to rectal wall | A. Confined to mucosa | |
| | | | B₁. Penetration into muscularis mucosae | |
| II Penetration through serosa | | B. Extension through wall into perirectal tissues | B₂. Penetration into muscularis | |
| III With regional node involvement | Regional (lymph node involvement) | C. Metastases in regional lymph nodes | C₁. B₁ or B₂ with regional node metastases | C₁. Positive regional nodes |
| IV Distant metastases | Metastatic | | C₂. Penetration through bowel wall with regional node metastases | C₂. Positive nodes at point of ligature of vessels <5 positive nodes ≥5 positive nodes |
| | | | D. Unresectable or metastatic | |

TABLE 11. *Overall survival in colorectal cancer by disease stage*

| Stage | 5-year survival (%) | Reference |
|---|---|---|
| I | 80.3 | |
| II | 70.6 | (94) |
| III | 31.9 | |
| Localized | 69–72 | |
| Regional | 35–47 | (28) |
| Dukes A | 61–81 | |
| Dukes B | 25–64 | (119) |
| Dukes C | 6–28 | |
| <5 Positive nodes | 15–29 | |
| ≥5 Positive nodes | 9.1 | (42) |

teristics, differences in the time periods covered by the studies, and variations from one institution to another. The effect of disease stage on overall survival is summarized in Table 11. These data emphasize the need for stratification by disease stage in randomized trials.

The histologic classification of gastrointestinal adenocarcinoma shows that well-differentiated tumors fare better than those that are progressively less differentiated (24). Obviously, histologic grade is more easily determined postoperatively when the entire specimen is available (67). The presence of vascular invasion adversely influences survival without regard to disease stage (45,46). In one large surgical adjuvant trial stratified for this prognostic factor, it was recorded in approximately 15% of the patients (46). Complications of obstruction or perforation indicate the presence of advanced disease, adding to postoperative morbidity and mortality and reducing the possibility of surgical cure (18,61).

Since the initial interest in the carcinoembryonic antigen (CEA) discovered by Gold and Freedman in 1965 (69), enthusiasm for its screening potential has waned (19). However, recent reviews concerning the utility of CEA testing suggest a correlation of high levels with advanced disease, particularly the presence of metastases (68,111). Increasing postoperative CEA levels have been identified as an early sign of recurrent disease. However, even when they are metastatic, not all tumors produce measurable CEA levels and only serial changes in levels are useful.

In addition to the prognostic factors generally used, the overall poor prognosis of colorectal carcinomas associated with ulcerative colitis and multiple intestinal polyposis has been repeatedly emphasized (67,119).

### Prognostic Factors in Secondary Treatment

Cure is rarely achieved in locally unresectable or recurrent disease and essentially never occurs in metastatic disease, but there are some well-defined prognostic factors (Fig. 1) that influence the probability and length of response to treatment (119,134,138,205). These factors are widely accepted and used to varying degrees in both prospective and retrospective stratification of randomized studies.

The histologic grade of malignancy has been used as a stratification parameter in many of the trials. Careful stratification of the extent of metastases (tumor burden) is also an important consideration, but it is difficult to achieve and may be approximated by evaluating performance status as a measure of general physical condition. For example, patients with liver metastases have a median survival of about 5 months (93,119,134), but this could be influenced by other factors such as histologic grade, extent of liver involvement, and the type of prior surgery (26,93). Patients with moderately to well-differentiated tumors survive twice as long as those having poorly differentiated tumors; those who have one or "a few" metastatic sites survive 12 to 17 months, whereas survival is only 3 to 9 months with multiple metastases. Jaundice and/or ascites are particularly ominous signs (119). Patients with unresectable primary tumors have a much poorer prognosis than those in whom the primary can be resected, an observation that correlates well with the effects of the total tumor burden.

The influence of prior treatment is an extremely critical factor in assessing the activity of new single agents or combination chemotherapy. Extensive radiotherapy may impair the bone marrow reserve, rendering the patient a poor risk for chemotherapy trials (6). In patients with progressive disease the inevitable decline in performance status also unfavorably influences the outcome of therapy (138). All of three factors must be appreciated, as well as the probability of cross-resistance among drugs within the same or in different classes of antitumor agents.

## Randomized Trials of Primary Therapy

This section reviews and analyzes the completed and ongoing randomized trials in local, potentially curable colorectal cancer. A few uncontrolled studies are cited, as appropriate, when they exhibit some potential for significantly improving therapy. Some of the results in these trials may be provocative and, at times, definitive when carefully compared to historical series (66).

### Surgery

Variations in the type of surgery and surgical technique potentially influence the outcome of primary treatment. However, randomized surgical trials are conspicuously lacking, and their usefulness in refining standard surgical therapy remains a point of continuing controversy.

In colon cancer, Turnbull et al. (191) developed the "no touch isolation" technique involving early high ligation of the vascular pedicle, isolation and transection of the surgical margins of the bowel followed by mobilization of the involved area and, finally, resection of the specimen. Among 460 patients resected for cure, the overall 5-year survival rate was 68.8% versus 52.1% in patients at the same institution undergoing "conventional" surgery in which ligation of the vessels was the last step before resection. In a group of 153 patients staged as Dukes C, the "no touch" technique yielded a particularly striking 5-year survival rate of 57.8% compared to 28% for "conventional" surgery.

The value of early vascular ligation noted by Turnbull has been challenged by Stearns and Schottenfeld (186), who reported on a large uncontrolled surgical series differing in the time sequence of ligation but comparable in the extent of resection and patient selection. They felt that the extent of resection was the common factor accounting for nearly identical results in the two series (68.8% in Turnbull's study and 69.2% by Stearns and Schottenfeld for Dukes A-C; 57.8% in Turnbull's versus 52.2% by Stearns and Schottenfeld for Dukes C). Both of these studies, although neither was randomized, have set standards for future surgical trials in colon cancer.

In rectal cancers originating <18 cm above the anal verge, the surgeon has the choice of abdominoperineal resection, anterior resection, or the "pull-through" operation, depending on anatomic considerations and surgical preference. Prospective randomized trials are not available in the literature, and the principal controversies revolve around anterior versus abdominoperineal resection and the roles of cryosurgery or fulguration in small lesions.

Anterior resection is often technically feasible in tumors 6 to 8 cm above the anal verge but is rarely feasible below this level. An analysis of two large series (181,184) using anterior resection indicates that the morbidity and mortality, rate of local recurrence, and disease-free survival are comparable to abdominoperineal resection. Thus, for tumors 6 to 8 cm above the anal verge either type of surgery would be comparable if the prognostic factors were similar. Relatively few reports have been published on patients treated by the "pull-through" operation, but results in selected cases have been similar (184).

The selection of patients for fulguration or cryosurgery depends on the tumor size, degree of infiltration, and the presence of well-differentiated histology (17). These procedures generally are not recommended when an anterior resection or "pull-through" operation can be performed. However, they offer potentially excellent treatment for a patient with medical contraindications to abdominoperineal resection and a small, favorable cancer. When these factors are considered, the survival rate compares favorably with radical surgery, but these procedures are still selective approaches for a small subset of patients and have no place in the routine management of rectal cancer (109).

## Radiotherapy

Primary treatment with irradiation is limited to rectal cancer, where it has a well-established role in palliative management of inoperable or recurrent disease. In fact, a few patients achieve surprisingly long survival (97). Thus, primary radiotherapy could conceivably play a role in definitive treatment of operable disease.

Rider (167) recently reviewed the experience with radiotherapy and concluded that the overall results were superior to a concurrent group treated by abdomino-perineal resection. The series included inoperable patients and others who refused abdominoperineal resection; the radiotherapy was not standardized. This contro-versy might be settled by a prospective randomized trial, but the participation of the surgical community is highly unlikely in view of the excellent survival with resection in patients with early disease.

Papillion (154) has obtained remarkable results in rectal cancer treated with endocavitary irradiation. The criteria of patient selection were similar to those advocated by proponents of fulguration and cryosurgery, that is, well-differenti-ated adenocarcinoma $\lesssim 5 \times 3$ cm and confined to the rectal wall (Dukes A) $< 12$ cm above the anal verge. Treatment was provided by contact irradiation, with interstitial irradiation of very small lesions, at an overall dose of 10,000 to 15,000 rads given in 4 weeks. Of 133 patients treated between 1951 and 1968, 78% (104) survived disease-free for 5 years or longer; there were 11 local failures, of which three underwent radical surgery. These results had the additional benefits of preserving the rectum with a virtual absence of morbidity. The method seems promising enough to merit a controlled trial, but this would probably meet the same resistance cited above.

## Combined Modalities in Colorectal Cancer

The published and unpublished combined modality trials employing chemo-therapy, immunotherapy, and chemoimmunotherapy in localized colorectal can-cer are summarized in Tables 12 and 13. In addition, there have been a number of unpublished studies at individual institutions for which no results are available (40,41). The 11 published trials (Table 12) have some interesting features in common, including (a) untreated control arms in all but one study (112,113), (b) separate analysis of colon and rectal patients, and (c) prospective stratification of "palliative resections" when these were eligible for study.

With one exception, the randomized trials of short-term therapy showed no difference in disease-free or total survival. In the single exception, women treated with short-term thiotepa experienced superior survival compared to concurrent controls and this persisted throughout the 10-year follow-up period (46). Only minor benefit, or none at all, has been obtained by prolonged therapy. Although these controlled adjuvant chemotherapy trials seem "negative," some proponents of short-term therapy have reported spectacular results in uncontrolled trials (96,108). The controlled studies that show "benefit" simply do not have enough patients to demonstrate statistical superiority for treatment.

It can only be regretfully concluded that, as Moertel (127) pointed out, 5-FU has been "the breakthrough that never was." The single attempt to improve the efficacy of 5-FU was by the addition of BCG (112,113). However, the princi-pal comparisons were with historical controls and there was no control arm of chemotherapy alone. Thus, the study cannot be readily interpreted. Final

TABLE 12. *Published randomized trials of combined modality therapy in localized colorectal cancer*

| Treatment arms | Modality | | Evaluation criteria [b] | Investigators (reference) |
| | Surgery | Chemotherapy [a] | | |
| --- | --- | --- | --- | --- |
| A. | Conventional | Nitrogen mustard (0.1 mg/kg i. p. and 0.1 mg/kg i. v. on d0; 0.1 mg/kg i. v. d1 and 2; 0.4 mg/kg i. v. q. 4 mos.) | 3D | Mrazek et al. (144) |
| B.<br>IA. | As in A<br>Conventional | —<br>Thiotepa (0.2 mg/kg i. v. portal vein and 0.2 mg/kg i. p. on d0; 0.2 mg/kg i. v. d1 and 2) | 3D, 4A(11) | Dwight et al. (52), Higgins et al. (84) |
| IB.<br>IIA. | As in I A<br>Conventional | —<br>Thiotepa (0.2 mg/kg i. p. on d0; 0.2 mg/kg i. v. d1 and 2) | | |
| IIB.<br>A. | As in II A<br>Conventional | —<br>Thiotepa (0.2 mg/kg i. p. on d0; 0.2 mg/kg i. v. d1 and 2) | 3A, D | Dixon et al. (46), Holden et al. (85) |
| B.<br>A. | As in A<br>Conventional | —<br>FUDR (20 mg/kg i. v. d1–3; 30 mg/kg/d × 3–5, d35–39; then 15 mg/kg i. v. on alternate days × 4 if no toxicity) | 3D, 4A(10, 11) | Dwight et al. (53) |
| B.<br>IA. | As in A<br>Curative (no evidence of residual disease) | —<br>5-FU (14–30 days postop; 12 mg/kg/d × 3–5, repeat twice at 6–8 wk intervals) | 3D, 4A(10) | Higgins et al. (80,82,83) |
| IB.<br>IIA. | As in I A<br>Curative or palliative (histologic evidence of residual disease) | —<br>5-FU (dose as in I A, q. 6 wks to progression) | | |
| IIB.<br>IIIA. | As in II A<br>Curative or palliative (only clinical evidence of residual disease) | —<br>5-FU (as in I A) | | |

TABLE 12—Cont.

| Treatment arms | Modality Surgery | Chemotherapy[a] | Evaluation criteria[b] | Investigators (reference) |
|---|---|---|---|---|
| IIIB. | | — | | |
| IA. | As in III A Curative | *14–30 days postop.* 5-FU (12 mg/kg/d × 5, q. 6 wks/18 mos.) | 3D, 4A(10, 14, 21) | Higgins et al. (80,83) |
| IB. | As in I A Palliative | — | | |
| IIA. | | CT as in IA, until progression or death | | |
| IIB. | | — | | |
| A. | As in II A Radical | 5-FU (2 courses, 1 and 3 mos. postop.) | 3D | Blokhina et al. (19) |
| B. | | — | | |
| A. | As in A Radical | *30 days postop.* 5-FU (12 mg/kg/d × 4 i. v.; then 6 mg/kg q.o.d. × 5; then 12 mg/kg/wk × 1 yr.) | 3D, 4A(10) | Grage et al. (72) |
| B. | | — | | |
| A. | As in A Radical | 5-FU (30 mg/kg intraluminal at surgery) 5-FU (10 mg/kg d1 and 2 i. v. postoperatively) | 3D, 4A(14) | Grossi et al. (73) |
| B. | As in A | Intraluminal placebo at surgery + no further therapy | | |
| A. | Radical[c] | 5-FU (30 mg/kg intraluminal at surgery; 10 mg/kg d1 and 2 i. v. in 1,000 cc saline) Maintenance—5 courses at 2 mo. intervals, 5-FU (12 mg/kg p. o., 6 mg/kg p. o. on alternate days × 7 doses) | 3D, 4A(14) | Lawrence et al. (105) |
| B. | As in A | — | | |

| | | | |
|---|---|---|---|
| A. | Conventional | 5-FU (150 mg/m² q.i.d., d × 5, p. o., q. mo. × 2 yrs.) BCG [(Pasteur) $6 \times 10^8$/wk × 3 mo.; then d7 and 21 each course × 2 yrs.] | 3D, 4A(26) | Mavligit et al. (112, 113) |
| B. | As in A | BCG [(Pasteur) $6 \times 10^8$/wk × 3 mo.; then q. o. wk × 2 yrs.] | | |

[a]Day 0 = day of surgery.
[b]See the categories listed in Fig. 1.
[c]Surgery identical to that in study of Grossi et al. (73).

TABLE 13. *Ongoing or unpublished combined modality trials in colorectal cancer*

| Treatment arms | Modality | | | Evaluation criteria[a] | Investigators (reference)[b] |
|---|---|---|---|---|---|
| | Surgery | Chemotherapy | Immunotherapy | | |
| A. | Radical; no touch isolation recommended | *14–30 days postop* MeCCNU (120 mg/m² d1, p. o.) 5-FU (9 mg/kg d1–5, i. v.) Repeat q. 7 wks/1 yr | — | 2B, 3D, 3H, 4A(14) | VASAG 27A (188) |
| B. | | — | | | |
| A. | Resection possible but not curative | *2 wks postop* MeCCNU (120 mg/m² d1, p. o.) 5-FU (9 mg/kg d1–5, i. v.) Repeat q. 6 wks | — | 2B, 3D, 3H, 4A(25) | VASAG 27B (188) |
| B. | As in A | As in A | MER-BCG (0.4 mg i. d. in each of 5 sites 7–10 days postop; then, 2 wks postop, repeat on d1 of each CT course.) Repeat q. 6 wks | | |
| A. | Conventional | *21–49 days postop* 5-FU (450 mg/m² d1–5 i. v., q. 5 wks 15 cycles) | — | 2B, 3D, 4A(5, 14, 26, 27) | ECOG 2276 (188) |
| B. | As in A | *21–49 days postop* 5-FU (325 mg/m² d1–5 i. v.; 375 mg/m² d36–40) MeCCNU (130 mg/m² d1, p. o.) | — | | |

| | Intent | Chemotherapy | Immunotherapy | Response codes | Study |
|---|---|---|---|---|---|
| A. | Curative | Repeat q. 10 wks 15 cycles of 5 wks each | — | 2B, 3D, 4A(5, 14, 26) | GITSG 6175 (188) |
| B. | As in A | 5-FU + MeCCNU; As in ECOG 2276 above | — | | |
| C. | As in A | — | MER–BCG (1 mg over 5 sites on d1 and 8; then 2 mg over 5 sites q. 5 wks × 5, then q. 15 wks) | | |
| D. | As in A | As in B | As in C | | |
| A. | Conventional | MeCCNU (175 mg/m² q. 8 wks p. o.) 5-FU (400 mg/m²/wk × 3 i. v.; repeat q. 8 wks × 1 yr) | — | 2B, 3D, 3H, 4A(14, 26) | SWOG 7510 (188) |
| B. | As in A | As in A | BCG (Connaught) 6 × 10$^8$ p. o. q. 2 wks × 1 yr. | | |
| A. | Palliative | 5-FU (450 mg/m²/ d1–5 i. v., q. 5 wks) | — | 2B, 3G, 4A(1, 4, 16) | ECOG 1276 (188) |
| B. | As in A | 5-FU (325 mg/m² d1–5 i. v.; 375 mg/m² d36–40) MeCCNU (150 mg/m² d1) Repeat q. 10 wks to progression | — | | |
| A. | Palliative | — | | 2B, 3G, 4A(16, 25) | Yorkshire 3 (University Hospital, Leeds) (188) |
| B. | As in A | 5-FU (400 mg/m² d1–5 i. v., q. 8 wks) | — | | |

TABLE 13—*Cont.*

| Treatment arms | Modality | | | Evaluation criteria[a] | Investigators (reference)[b] |
| | Surgery | Chemotherapy | Immunotherapy | | |
| --- | --- | --- | --- | --- | --- |
| A. | Palliative | MeCCNU (200 mg/m² d1, q. 16 wks) 5-FU (15 mg/kg/d × 4 i. v.; then wkly to progression) | — | 2A, 3G, 3H, 4A(27) | Toronto General Hospital 7501 (40) |
| B. | As in A | As in A | BCG (Connaught) 2 mg i. p. by catheter within 1 mo. postop.; then, 120 mg p. o. in 1 wk; then, 120 mg p. o. on week 4 of each 5-FU cycle | | |

[a] See the criteria defined in Fig. 1.
[b] Abbreviations: See previous tables.

conclusions have not been made in three adjuvant trials (72,73,105), and final judgment awaits further publication.

The ongoing adjuvant trials (Table 13) are also susceptible to some general concerns and comments. Only three of these studies have untreated control arms (VASAG 27A, GITSG 6175, and Yorkshire 3). Fortunately, two of these (VASAG 27A and GITSG 6175) deal with curative resection and another study (ECOG 2276) will have a common analysis with one of the studies (GITSG 6175) having an untreated arm (188). Separate protocols are being developed for patients with curative and palliative resections, which should better define the results. The extent of surgery and definition of surgical technique were prospectively considered in only one study (VASAG 27A). It must be concluded that surgery was not standardized in the remaining trials.

5-Fluorouracil alone was used as a treatment arm in three studies (ECOG 2276, ECOG 1276, and Toronto General Hospital 7501), but published articles suggest it has only minimal or no benefit in conjunction with both curative and palliative resections. Presumably, 5-FU was included in the studies with the hope that further follow-up would reveal benefits, as yet unrealized, for the use of this agent. The survival benefits and therapeutic index of 5-FU + MeCCNU have not been conclusively established. The use of intraperitoneal and oral BCG is a noteworthy addition in adjuvant trials, but there is nonuniformity of stage classification with considerable modification of the original Dukes classification in many of the studies.

## Combined Modalities in Rectal Cancer

Analysis of the combined modality trials strictly for rectal cancer can be divided into preoperative radiotherapy, postoperative radiotherapy, and other modalities following curative resection, studies involving palliative resection, and those involving unresectable or recurrent local disease.

Most of the published trials of preoperative radiotherapy (Table 14) have shown an advantage for low-dose irradiation, but this has statistical significance only in the VASAG study (81). These trials require large numbers of patients and standardized techniques of irradiation and surgery. These requirements are not met in all the trials, which probably explains the variable results in an approach that, at best, can only be expected to show modest improvement.

The ongoing trials of preoperative radiotherapy in rectal cancer (Table 15) generally use higher irradiation doses and require supervoltage equipment; preoperative chemotherapy has been added in some studies. The results of preoperative radiotherapy are unproven, and final results in current trials will not appear for years. There has also been considerable reluctance on the part of some surgeons to participate in these randomized trials. For example, case accrual in the COG-RTOG study (188) has been such a problem that the trial probably will not be completed.

No controlled trials involving only postoperative radiotherapy have been pub-

TABLE 14. *Published trials of preoperative radiotherapy in rectal cancer*

| Treatment arms | Modality | | Surgery | Evaluation criteria[a] | Investigators (reference) |
| --- | --- | --- | --- | --- | --- |
| | Radiotherapy | | | | |
| A. | 2,000 rads/10 fractions | | Usually abdominoperineal, 2 days–6 wks post-RT | 5D | Stearns et al. (185) |
| B. | — | | As in A, immediately | | |
| A. | 4.500 rads/4.5 wks | | Mainly abdominoperineal, some anterior resections, 4–6 wks post-RT | 5D | Kligerman et al. (98) |
| B. | — | | As in A, immediately | | |
| A. | 2,000 rads/2 wks; booster dose 500 rads for low-lying lesions through perineal port. | | Abdominoperineal or anterior resection | 2B, 4A(10), 5E | Higgins et al. (81) |
| B. | — | | As in A, immediately | | |
| A. | 3,000 rads | | "Radical" surgery 5–10 days post-RT | Unknown | Simbirtseva (180) |
| B. | — | | As in A, immediately | | |
| A. | 500 rads $^{60}$CO | | Abdominoperineal or anterior resection on day of RT | 2A, 3A | Rider (167) |
| B. | "Sham" RT | | As in A, immediately | | |

[a]See the criteria defined in Fig. 1.

TABLE 15. Ongoing or unpublished trials of preoperative radiotherapy in rectal cancer[a]

| Treatment arms | Modality | | Evaluation criteria[b] | Investigators (reference)[c] |
| | Radiotherapy | Surgery | | |
| --- | --- | --- | --- | --- |
| A. | 3,150 rads/18 fractions in 24 days | Abdominoperineal resection within 10 days | 1A, 2B, 3D, 4A(10), 5E | VASAG 28 (188) |
| B. | — | As in A | | |
| A. | 4,500 rads/4.5 wks | Abdominoperineal resection 3–5 wks post-RT | 2B, 3D, 4A(5, 14, 28) | COG 7240-RTOG 72-3 (188) |
| B. | 2,000 rads/2 wks 500 rads perineal boost if needed | As in A, as soon as possible but no later than 1 wk post-RT | | |
| C. | — | As in A, within 1 wk | | |
| A. | 500 rads single fraction | Abdominoperineal and anterior resections | 3D, 4A(5, 7, 14, 28) | Duncan and Smith (51) |
| B. | 2,000 rads/10 fractions over 2 wks | As in A | | |
| A. | 3,450 rads/15 fractions over 18 days | Radical "no touch" 4–15 days post-RT | 2B, 4A(14) | European Organization for Research on the Treatment of Cancer (170) |
| B. | — | As in A | | |
| A. | 3,450 rads/15 fractions over 18 days | Radical 2 wks after RT | 2B, 4A(14) | European Organization for Research on the Treatment of Cancer (170); Wassif (200) |
| B. | As in A, with 5-FU (375 mg/m² /d i. v., d1–4) | As in A | | |
| A. | 2,000 rads/10 fractions over 2 wks | Abdominoperineal resections 6–8 wks post-RT | 3D | SWOG 7618 (188) |
| B. | As in A, with mitomycin C (10 mg/m² i. v. d1) and 5-FU (1 g/m² 24-hr infusion d1–4 and d28–31) | As in A | | |

[a] Some studies include chemotherapeutic agents with the preoperative radiotherapy.
[b] See the criteria defined in Fig. 1.
[c] Abbreviations: See previous tables.

lished. The extensive experience with postoperative adjuvant chemotherapy in rectal cancer is included in Tables 12 and 13.

The three current investigations of postoperative combined modality therapy following curative resection in rectal cancer are summarized in Table 16. In these studies, curative resection is mandatory and early-stage lesions (Dukes A) are excluded; precise staging is ensured by placing surgery first. Two of the trials have an untreated control arm. The treatment arms of radiotherapy, chemotherapy, and chemotherapy + radiotherapy are uniformly applied with a resultant well-balanced randomization. The irradiation techniques, dosage, and fields are standardized and comparable; likewise, the drug regimens are well standardized. It is not possible to comment on toxic effects or projected results, but answers to these questions should be forthcoming. A particular concern will be the tolerance to radiotherapy after resection when loops of bowel may be fixed and a fresh anastomosis is included in the irradiation field.

Several ongoing trials of postoperative combined modality therapy in patients with residual, recurrent, or unresectable disease are presented in Table 17. These studies have a rather solid basis in a randomized trial conducted at the Mayo Clinic (52,129). In this investigation, 65 patients were treated with 4,000 rads/ 4 weeks and given either i. v. placebo or 5-FU (15 mg/kg) on the first 3 days of radiotherapy; no further chemotherapy was used. The median and mean survival times were 10.5 and 16.8 months, respectively, with placebo and 16 and 23 months with 5-FU ($p < 0.05$). There were at least 3 long-term survivors and 2 possible cures. The current studies are designed to conform and extend the observations by including higher irradiation doses, additional chemotherapy, and immunotherapy in randomized trials.

## Randomized Trials of Secondary Therapy

The therapeutic strategy in studies targeted toward advanced and metastatic colorectal cancer has been designed to evaluate treatment programs in terms of remission rate and duration. Survival observations after therapy have been a secondary goal. The basic design considerations common to these trials include patient eligibility criteria, stratification and randomization techniques, and criteria of response and disease progression.

The patients eligible for these studies have been those with advanced and/ or metastatic cancer unsuitable for treatment with local modalities. They have measurable indicator lesions, unless otherwise specified, and usually have a life expectancy of 6 to 12 weeks. The extent of allowable prior therapy has been dependent on the purpose of the trial. Phase III studies usually permit no prior chemotherapy, whereas phase II studies require a definition of previous therapy including explanation of any exclusions. Acceptable risk is also defined and, for the most part, the trials specify the age limits, the amount of permissible prior irradiation (especially to pelvic marrow), and definitions of normal and impaired marrow reserve.

TABLE 16. *Ongoing postoperative combined modality trials in rectal cancer after curative resections*

| Treatment arms | Modality | | Evaluation criteria [a] | Investigators (reference) [b] |
| | Radiotherapy | Chemotherapy | | |
|---|---|---|---|---|
| A. | — | *8 cycles (10 wks each)* 5-FU (325 mg/m²/d i. v., d1–5; 375 mg/m²/d i. v., d36–40) MeCCNU (130 mg/m² p. o. d1) | 3D, 4A(4, 7, 14) | ECOG 4276 (188) |
| B. | 21–42 days postop. (4,500–5,100 rads/5–6 wks) | — | | |
| C. | As in B | 4 wks after RT complete; CT as in A | | |
| A. | — | *Every 10 wks for 18 mos.* 5-FU + MeCCNU as in ECOG 4276 above | 2B, 3D, 4A(10, 14) | RTOG 76-04 (188) |
| B. | 4,500–5,100 rads/5–6 wks | — | | |
| C. | As in B | 4–8 wks after RT complete; CT as in A | | |
| D. | — | — | | |
| A. | — | *Every 10 wks for 18 mos.* 5-FU and MeCCNU as in ECOG 4276 above. | 2B, 4A(10, 14) | GITSG 7175 (188) |
| B. | 4,000 *or* 4,800 rads/ 4.5–5.5 wks | — | | |
| C. | As in B | 5-FU (500 mg/m²/d i. v., d1–3 of RT and last 3 days of RT) Then, 5 wks later, CT used as in ECOG 4276 for 18 mos. | | |
| D. | — | — | | |

[a]See the criteria defined in Fig. 1.
[b]RTOG = Radiation Therapy Oncology Group; see other abbreviations in previous tables.

TABLE 17. Ongoing postoperative combined modality trials in residual, recurrent, or unresectable rectal cancer

| Treatment arms | Modality | | | Evaluation criteria [a] | Investigators (reference)[b] |
| --- | --- | --- | --- | --- | --- |
| | Radiotherapy | Chemotherapy | Immunotherapy | | |
| A. | 4,000–5,000 rads/ 4–5 wks | 5-FU (600 mg/m² d1–3 of RT; then 600 mg/ m²/wk after RT) | — | 1B, 1C, 2B | ECOG 1274A (188) |
| B. | As in A | | — | | |
| A. | 4,500–5,100 rads/ 5–6 wks Boost to 5,000– 6,000/6–6½ wks | 5-FU (500 mg/m² d1–3 of RT) | — | 1C, 2B, 4A(4, 10, 14) | ECOG 3276 (188) |
| B. | Split course, 6,000 rads/10 wks (2-wk courses; 2-wk rest intervals) Maintenance for both arms (5 wks after complet- ing RT): 1st course: 5-FU (300 mg/m² d1–5, 36–40 i. v.) MeCCNU (100 mg/m² d1) Then, 5-FU (325 mg/m² d1–5, 375 mg/m² d36–40) MeCCNU (130 mg/m² d1) q. 10 wks to progression) | 5-FU (500 mg/m² d1–3 of each RT course) | — | | |
| A. | Split course, 6,000 rads/10 wks (2-wk courses; 2-wk rest intervals) | 5-FU (500 mg/m² d1–3 of each RT course) 5-FU + MeCCNU (as in ECOG 3276; 6 courses) | — | 1C, 2B, 4A(4, 10, 14) | GITSG 7276 (188) |
| B. | As in A | 5-FU (500 mg/m² d1–3 of each RT course) | BCG (Tice) 10⁸ organisms i. d. q. 2 wks × 5; then q. 5 wks | | |

| | | | | |
|---|---|---|---|---|
| A. | 2,500 rads/2 wks × 2 with 2-wk rest interval | — | MER-BCG (2 mg d1 and 7 of 1st RT course; 2 mg d1 and 14 of 2nd course) | 1B, 1C, 2A, 4A(1, 4, 10, 14) | Mayo 70–18–72 (188) |
| B. | | | | | |
| A.[c] | 3,450 rads/18 days | 5-FU (375 mg/m²/d, d1–4 of RT)[d] | — | 2B, 4A(10, 13) | EORTC PR-2 and PR-3 (170) |
| | As in A | *or* | | | |
| | No RT | 5-FU (500 mg/m²/wk i. v. *or* 600 mg/m²/wk p. o.) | | | |
| B.[e] | — | 5-FU (500 mg/m²/wk i. v. *or* 600 mg/m²/wk p. o.) | — | | |

[a] See the criteria defined in Fig. 1.

[b] Abbreviations: See previous tables.

[c] Study PR-2: Patients had preop. RT ± 5-FU in an earlier study (PR-1). They were inoperable or had residual tumor after surgery; the physicians' choice of the two therapies was based on the condition of the patient.

[d] Following RT + 5-FU, patients randomized to (1) no further treatment or (2) 5-FU (500 mg/m²/wk i. v. *or* 600 mg/m²/wk p. o.).

[e] Study PR-3: Patients had preop. RT ± 5-FU in study PR-1. At surgery they had liver metastases.

Stratification has been accomplished either prospectively or retrospectively for the following parameters: site of indicator lesions; histologic grade of primary or metastatic lesions; performance status (e.g., ECOG 0–4, Karnofsky 100% to 0); prior therapy, if allowable; sex; and, institution. Various randomization techniques have included digits in the hospital identification number, selection of alternate consecutive patients, and random numbers by closed envelopes or central telephone assignment.

Three criteria of responses have been most commonly used. *Objective remission* has been defined as 50% reduction in the products of two largest diameters of one or more indicator lesions plus stability of other lesions without the appearance of new ones. The additional indicators of performance status and weight are often used. *Progressive disease* has meant an increase of 25% in the products of the diameters of the indicator lesions or development of new lesions. Decreased performance status or a specified weight loss have also been used. *Stable disease* has been marked by disease improvement without meeting the criteria of response or by a degree of progression below the criteria set for progressive disease.

Remission of disease has been further subdivided into *complete response* (CR), with objective and subjective evidence of complete disappearance of tumor, and *partial response* (PR) as defined by the 50% reduction required in objective remission. The accepted *duration of response* varies from a low of 2 weeks to the most frequent figure of 8 to 10 weeks.

There has been great variability in reporting the categories of *entered* and *evaluable* patients. Most of the studies have reported results in terms of evaluable patients, but in the following review of trials any exceptions will be noted.

### Single-Agent Trials

Nine trials (3,4,14,15,77,89,140,161,162,175) involving 930 evaluable patients have been conducted to determine the optimum dose, schedule, and route of administration of 5-FU (Table 18). These studies have included comparisons of i. v. and oral loading courses, prolonged i. v. infusions versus i. v. push schedules, and weekly i. v. or oral schedules as substitutes for more toxic regimens. All of the trials suffered from an intrinsically low response rate with 5-FU, making it difficult to show definite superiority for any particular regimen. Response rates have varied from only 4% for a 7.5 mg/kg weekly i. v. regimen (89) to 44% with a 120-hr infusion at 30 mg/kg daily (175). The average overall response rate of 19% (176 CR + PR) closely resembles the 21% rate in 2,000 patients reviewed by Carter and Friedman (32).

Loading courses by i. v. push produced an average 22% response rate in 277 patients when the induction regimen was followed by either monthly reinduction or weekly maintenance (3,4,77,140, 161,162,175). Oral loading courses induced remission in 15 (16%) of 96 patients (3,4,77). Weekly i. v. administration produced a response rate of 19% (45/231) or 21% (44/206) if a nontoxic schedule of 7.5 mg/kg weekly (89) is eliminated from consideration; oral weekly adminis-

TABLE 18. *Published randomized trials of single-agent chemotherapy in colorectal cancer*

| Investigators (reference) and treatment arms | Evaluation criteria[a] | No. responses/ no. patients | Response rate (%) |
|---|---|---|---|
| Moertel et al. (140) | 2A, 3A, 3E, 4A(6) | | |
| A. 5-FU (20 mg/kg/d as a 2-hr infusion X 5, q. 5 wks) | | 9/75 | 12 |
| B. 5-FU (13.5 mg/kg/d X 5 i. v., q. 5 wks) | | 9/74 | 12 |
| Reitemeier and Moertel (162) | 2A, 3E, 4A(6) | | |
| A. 5-FU (22.5 mg/kg/d as an 8-hr infusion X 5, q. 5 wks) | | 5/45 | 11 |
| B. 5-FU (15 mg/kg/d X 5 i. v.; 7.5 mg/kg q.o.d. X 4, q. 5 wks) | | 9/45 | 20 |
| Seifert et al. (175) | 2A, 3E, 4A(6), 5D | | |
| A. 5-FU (12 mg/kg/d X 4–5 i. v., q. 4 wks) | | 8/36 | 22 |
| B. 5-FU (30 mg/kg, 24-hr infusion X 5, q. 4 wks) | | 15/34 | 44 |
| Ramirez et al. (161) | 2A, 3E, 4A(6), 5D | | |
| A. 5-FU (12 mg/kg/d X 4–5 i. v., 6 mg/kg q.o.d. to toxicity, repeat monthly) | | 3/15 | 20 |
| B. 5-FU (loading course; then 500–1,000 mg weekly maintenance) | | 4/20 | 20 |
| Hahn et al. (77) | 2A, 3A, 3E, 4A(1, 4, 5, 6) | | |
| A. 5-FU (13.5 mg/kg/d X 5 i. v., q. 5 wks) | | 14/53 | 26 |
| B. 5-FU (20 mg/kg/d X 5 p. o., q. 5 wks) | | 9/47 | 19 |
| Horton et al. (89) | 2B, 3E, 4A(6), 5C | | |
| A. 5-FU (7.5 mg/kg/wk i. v.) | | 1/25 | 4 |
| B. 5-FU (15 mg/kg/wk i. v.) | | 5/25 | 20 |
| C. 5-FU (20 mg/kg/wk i. v.) | | 5/17 | 29 |
| Bateman et al. (15) | 2B, 3E, 4A(6) | | |
| A. 5-FU (15 mg/kg/wk i. v.) | | 3/12 | 25 |
| B. 5-FU (15 mg/kg/wk p. o.) | | 4/10 | 40 |
| Bateman et al. (14) | 2B, 3E, 4A(6) | | |
| A. 5-FU (15 mg/kg/wk i. v.) | | 23/97 | 24 |
| B. 5-FU (15 mg/kg/wk p. o.) | | 12/93 | 13 |
| Ansfield et al. (3,4) | 2B, 3E, 3H, 4A(6) | | |
| A. 5-FU (12 mg/kg/d X 4–5 i. v.; 6 mg/kg q.o.d. to toxicity or 11 doses; maintenance 15 mg/kg i. v. wkly) | | 16/18 | 33 |
| B. 5-FU (15–20 mg/kg/wk i. v.) | | 7/52 | 13 |
| C. 5-FU (500 mg/d X 4 i. v.; 500 mg wkly maintenance) | | 7/50 | 14 |
| D. 5-FU (15 mg/kg/d X 5–6 p. o.; 15 mg/kg/wk p. o.) | | 6/48 | 13 |

TABLE 18—*Cont.*

| Investigators (reference) and treatment arms | Evaluation criteria[a] | No. responses/ no. patients | Response rate (%) |
|---|---|---|---|
| Reitemeier et al. (163) | 2A, 3E, 4A(6), 4B | | |
| A. 5-FU (15 mg/kg/d ✕ 5 i. v.; 7.5 mg/kg q.o.d. ✕ 4, q. 5 wks) | | 10/84 | 12 |
| B. 5-FUDR (40 mg/kg/d ✕ 5 i. v.; 20 mg/kg q.o.d. ✕ 4) | | 19/84 | 22 |
| Moertel et al. (135) | 2A, 3A, 3E, 4A(6), 4B | | |
| A. 5-FUDR (40 mg/kg/d ✕ 5 i. v.) | | 17/98 | 17 |
| B. 5-FUDR (1.5–2.5 mg/kg/ d ✕ 5, 24-hr continuous infusion) | | 6/98 | 6 |
| Moertel et al. (141) | 2A, 3E, 4A(6) | | |
| A. 5-FU (13.5 mg/kg/d ✕ 5 i. v., q. 5 wks) | | 11/74 | 15 |
| B. As in A, with 100% oxygen | | 13/75 | 19 |
| ECOG (54) | 2B, 3A, 3E, 4A(6) | | |
| A. 5-FU (15 mg/kg/d ✕ 4 i. v.; 7.5 mg/kg q.o.d. ✕ 4, q. 4 wks) | | 13/48 | 27 |
| B. 5-FUDR (30 mg/kg/d ✕ 4 i. v.; 15 mg/kg q.o.d. ✕ 4, q. 4 wks) | | 2/46 | 4 |
| C. MTX (0.4 mg/kg/d ✕ 4 i. v.; 0.2 mg/kg q.o.d. ✕ 4, q. 4 wks) | | 4/40 | 10 |
| Gold et al. (70) | 2B, 3E | | |
| A. CTX (15 mg/kg wkly i. v.) | | 0/7 | — |
| B. Uracil mustard (0.15 mg/kg wkly p. o.) | | 0/5 | — |
| C. Nitrogen mustard (0.2 mg/ kg/d ✕ 2 i. v., q. 2 wks ✕ 2; then 0.1 mg/kg wkly) | | 1/8 | 12 |
| Bullen et al. (25) | 2B, 3E, 4A(6) | | |
| A. L-PAM (6 mg/m² /d ✕ 5 p. o. q. 6 wks) | | 2/13 | 15 |
| B. 5-FU (500 mg/m²/d ✕ 5 i. v., q. 6 wks) | | 4/20 | 20 |
| Baker et al. (11) | 2A, 4A(6) | | |
| A. Mitomycin C (17.5–22.5 mg/m² q. 6–8 wks i. v.) | | 4/12 | 33 |
| B. Porfiromycin (55–75 mg/ m² q. 6–8 wks i. v.) | | 2/12 | 17 |
| Moertel et al. (122,142) | 2A, 4A(6) | | |
| A. BCNU (50 mg/m²/d ✕ 5 i. v., q. 8 wks) | | 3/24 | 12 |
| B. 5-FU (13.5 mg/kg/d ✕ 5 i. v., q. 6 wks) | | 8/25 | 32 |
| Moertel (122) | 2A, 4A(6) | | |
| A. MeCCNU (200–250 mg/m² q. 8 wks) | | 5/19 | 24 |

TABLE 18—*Cont.*

| Investigators (reference) and treatment arms | Evaluation criteria[a] | No. responses/ no. patients | Response rate (%) |
|---|---|---|---|
| B. 5-FU (13.5 mg/kg/d × 5 i. v., q. 5 wks) | | 3/21 | 16 |
| Frytak et al. (64) | 2A, 3E, 4A(6) | | |
| A. Adriamycin (40–75 mg/m² q. 3 wks) | | 3/23 | 13 |
| B. 5-FU (13.5 mg/kg/d × 5 i. v., q. 5 wks; *or* 20 mg/ kg/d × 5 p. o., q. 5 wks) | | 5/25 | 24 |
| Kovach et al. (100) | 3E, 4A(6) | | |
| A. Cis-platinum (50 mg/m² i. v., q. 5 wks) | | 0/19 | — |
| B. 5-FU (13.5 mg/kg/d × 5 i. v., q. 5 wks *or* 20 mg/ kg/d × 5 p. o., q. 5 wks) | | 4/23 | 17 |
| Horton et al. (87) | 2B, 3E, 4A(4, 6) | | |
| A. Streptozoticin (0.5 g/m² i. v. wkly) | | 5/50 | 10 |
| B. CCNU (130 mg/m² p. o., q. 6 wks) | | 6/55 | 10 |
| C. 6-Thioguanine (1 mg/kg/d p. o.) | | 4/54 | 8 |
| D. Procarbazine (3 mg/kg/d p. o.) | | 1/38 | 2 |
| Vogler and Jacobs (198) | 2B, 3E, 4A(6) | | |
| A. MTX (125 mg/m² q. 6 hr wkly p. o.) Leucovorin (36 hr after MTX 6 mg p. o. q. 6 hr × 6) | | 2/19 | 10 |
| B. MTX (15 mg/m² q. 6 hr wkly p. o.) | | 1/18 | 6 |
| C. MTX (60 mg/m²/wk i. v.) | | 3/23 | 13 |
| Douglass and Moertel (48) | 2B, 3E, 4A(4, 6) | | |
| A. MeCCNU (175 mg/m² p. o., q. 8 wks) | | 3/78 | 4 |
| B. β-2-TGdR (100 mg/m²/ d × 5 i. v., q. 3 wks) | | 2/84 | 2 |

[a]See the criteria defined in Fig. 1.

tration gave a 15% (16/103) response rate (14,15). A schedule consisting of a nontoxic loading course followed by weekly doses (3,4) was about as successful, giving a 13% (7/54) response rate (4,5). Prolonged infusion therapy of 2-, 8-, and 120-hr duration has received limited study, with an overall response rate of 25% in 154 patients.

In the individual series, remission induction was most successful in the i. v. loading course of COG 7030 (3,4) which gave a 33% response rate (16/48) in colorectal cancer, compared to poorer results by weekly, nontoxic, and oral doses. In addition, the i. v. loading course employed by the Mayo Clinic was superior to the same schedule given orally (77). These two series also produced longer response durations by the i. v. loading schedules.

The optimum i. v. weekly dose, which produced the best overall therapeutic index, was 15 mg/kg in the ECOG randomized dose-response study (89). Weekly oral 5-FU was decidedly inferior to i. v. administration in the WCG series (14). THe use of a nontoxic loading course followed by weekly maintenance in COG 7030 (4,5) was interesting in that activity was observed, although it was to a lesser extent than more aggressive schedules. Prolonged i. v. infusion therapy was consistently less toxic but more troublesome to administer (140, 162,175). The response rates were lower with 2- and 8-hr infusions and higher with a 120-hr infusion, but the latter study (175) was not stratified and had the fewest cases that could be evaluated.

Overall, these studies showed that the effects of dose, schedule, and route of administration of 5-FU varied with the selection of patients and their numbers. The results tended to be clustered around the overall average response rate for 5-FU that is reported in the literature (32). It appears that the most consistent response rates were obtained by loading courses or aggressive weekly maintenance with or without loading.

A number of the studies in Table 18 have compared loading courses of 5-FU as "standard" therapy versus other single agents including 5-FUDR, methotrexate, melphalan, nitrosoureas (BCNU and MeCCNU), adriamycin, and cisplatinum diamminedichloride (25,54,64,100,122,135,142,163). MeCCNU and 5-FUDR were the most active of the test agents, but none have shown definite superiority over 5-FU. These inconclusive findings indicate that randomized phase II trials should be conducted to rank the activity of other agents and make crossover comparisons.

Some of the other trials in Table 18 involved drugs other than the fluoropyrimidines (11,48,70,87,198). However, most of the patients had prior fluoropyrimidine therapy and the trials were designed to test other agents in 5-FU refractory patients. The minimal drug activity found in these trials showed that second trials after 5-FU failure are usually unsuccessful, or of only marginal value, and have only slight application to predicting the agents likely to be additive in combination chemotherapy programs.

A separate chemotherapeutic approach with single agents administered by prolonged infusion into the hepatic artery has been taken in patients with liver metastases (Table 19) (10,63,188). Although the published trials have been uncontrolled, the literature indicates some advocacy for this route of administration (5,27). Two of the trials in Table 19 are currently in progress and no results are available. There have been no published studies of 5-FU or 5-FUDR by systemic administration versus intraarterial infusion.

### Combination Chemotherapy

The published trials of combination drug regimens are outlined in Table 20. The earliest trials at the Mayo Clinic (164) evaluated 5-FU, mitomycin C,

TABLE 19. *Published and unpublished randomized trials of hepatic artery infusion (HAI) in colorectal cancer*

| Investigators (reference) and treatment arms | Evaluation criteria[a] | No. responses/ no. patients |
|---|---|---|
| Fortuny et al. (63) | 2A, 4A(6, 9, 13) | |
| A. 5-FU (25 mg/kg HAI to total 12 g; i. v. wkly maintenance 1 g) | | 10/12 |
| B. Mitomycin C (1 mg/kg, 2–3 day HAI) | | 6/13 |
| Infusions may be repeated q. 8–10 wks | | |
| COG 7032 (188) | 2B, 4A(13, 25) | In progress |
| A. 5-FU (12 mg/kg/d X 4 i. v.; 6 mg/kg q.o.d. X 6; 15 mg/kg wkly) | | |
| B. 5-FU (20 mg/kg HAI X 14 days; 10 mg/kg X 7 days; wkly i. v. 5-FU maintenance) | | |
| Reinfuse if progression occurs | | |
| Baker (10) | 4A(13) | In progress |
| A. 5-FUDR (0.1–0.4 mg/kg HAI) | | |
| B. 5-FUDR (as in A) | | |
| 5-FU (1 g/m² d1–5, q. 4 wks) | | |
| Mitomycin C (22.5 mg/m² q. 8 wks) | | |
| C. 5-FU + mitomycin C (as in B) | | |

[a] See the criteria defined in Fig. 1.

and BCNU as single agents, two-drug combinations, and as a three-drug regimen. In the doses and schedules tested, 5-FU alone was only slightly superior to the other single agents and the combinations.

An early study by the South African Group (59) indicated an advantage for 5-FU + BCNU + DTIC + vincristine versus 5-FU even though it included only half as many patients as the more recent trials (57,139). The most exciting results of combination chemotherapy were obtained in comparisons of 5-FU versus 5-FU + MeCCNU + vincristine by the Mayo Clinic (139) and Falkson and Falkson (57) in South Africa. These remarkably similar studies had comparable patients, and the results suggested the superiority of the combination regimen over 5-FU alone.

Major evidence establishing the superiority of 5-FU + MeCCNU over 5-FU alone was provided in a study of the Southwest Oncology Group (SWOG) (13). This study was prospectively stratified to separately analyze patients with liver metastases and the results demonstrated a significant difference; that is, patients with liver metastases had a 30% response rate (13/43) with the combination versus no response (0/11) to 5-FU alone. The overall response to 5-FU, regardless of metastatic sites, was only 9.5% (4/42) compared to 31% (48/152) with 5-FU + MeCCNU. Interestingly, this response rate with 5-FU was much lower than any recorded in the single-agent trials (Table 18).

The trials performed by Wayne State University and Providence Hospital (192,194) can be viewed as feasibility studies because of the few patients involved.

TABLE 20. *Published randomized trials of combination chemotherapy in colorectal cancer*

| Investigators (reference) and treatment arms | Evaluation criteria[a] | No. responses/ no. patients | Response rate (%) |
|---|---|---|---|
| Reitemeier et al. (164) | 2A, 3E, 4A(6), 4B | | |
|   A. 5-FU (13.5 mg/kg/d × 5, q. 5 wks i. v.) | | 5/20 | 25 |
|   B. Mitomycin C (150 μg/kg/ d × 5, q. 6–8 wks i. v.) | | 3/21 | 14 |
|   C. BCNU (50 mg/m² /d × 5, q. 8 wks i. v.) | | 3/17 | 18 |
|   D. 5-FU (9 mg/kg/d × 5, q. 8 wks i. v.) Mitomycin C (110 μg/kg/ d × 5, q. 8 wks i. v.) | | 3/17 | 18 |
|   E. 5-FU (as in D) BCNU (37.5 mg/m² /d × 5, q. 8 wks i. v.) | | 1/20 | 5 |
|   F. Mitomycin C (75 μg/kg/ d × 5, q. 8 wks i. v.) BCNU (25 mg/m² /d × 5, q. 8 wks i. v.) | | 2/19 | 10 |
|   G. 5-FU (8 mg/kg/d × 5, q. 8 wks i. v.) Mitomycin C (60 μg/kg/ d × 5, q. 8 wks i. v.) BCNU (20 mg/m² /d × 5, q. 8 wks i. v.) | | 1/18 | 5 |
| Vaitkevicius et al. (192) | 2A, 3E | | |
|   A. 5-FU (1 g/m² 24-hr infusion × 5, q. 4 wks) Mitomycin C (22.5 mg/m² q. 8 wks i. v.) | | 3/6 | 50 |
|   B. Mitomycin C (as in A) | | 1/6 | 17 |
| Vaughn et al. (194) | 2A, 3C, 3G | | |
|   A. 5-FU (1 g/m² 24-hr infusion × 5, q. 4 wks) MeCCNU (175 mg/m² q. 8 wks p. o.) | | ? | 55 |
|   B. 5-FU (as in A) Mitomycin C (20 mg/m² q. 8 wks i. v.) | | ? | 68 |
| Baker et al. (13) | 2B, 3E, 3H, 4A(6, 13), 5B | | |
|   A. 5-FU (400 mg/m² /wk i. v.) | | 4/42[b] | 9.5 |
|   B. 5-FU (as in A) MeCCNU (175 mg/m² q. 6 wks p. o.) | | 48/152[c] | 31 |
| Rossi et al. (168) | 3G, 4A(6) | | |
|   A. MeCCNU (200 mg/m² q. 6 wks p. o.) | | 1/19 | 5 |
|   B. MeCCNU (120 mg/m² q. 6 wks p. o.) CTX (600 mg/m² q. 3 wks i. v.) | | 3/14 | 21 |

TABLE 20—*Cont.*

| Investigators (reference) and treatment arms | Evaluation criteria[a] | No. responses/ no. patients | Response rate (%) |
|---|---|---|---|
| Moertel et al. (139) | 2A, 3G, 4A(6), 4B | | |
| A. 5-FU (13.5 mg/kg/d × 5, q. 5 wks i. v.; 20 mg/kg/ d × 5, q. 5 wks p. o.) | | 8/41 | 20 |
| B. 5-FU (10 mg/kg d1–5, 36–40 i. v.) MeCCNU (175 mg/m² d1, q. 10 wks p. o.) VCR (1 mg/m² d1 and 36 i. v.) | | 17/39 | 43 |
| Falkson and Falkson (57) | 3G, 4A(6), 4B | | |
| A. 5-FU (15 mg/kg/d × 5, q. 4 wks i. v.) | | 10/45 | 22 |
| B. 5-FU (12 mg/kg/d × 5, q. 4 wks i. v.) MeCCNU (100 mg/m² d1, q. 4 wks p. o.) VCR (0.025 µg/kg/ d1, q. 4 wks i. v.) | | 17/46 | 37 |
| Falkson et al. (59) | 3G, 3I, 4A(6) | | |
| A. 5-FU (15 mg/kg d1–5, monthly i. v.) | | 6/24 | 25 |
| B. 5-FU (10 mg/kg d1–5, monthly i. v.) DTIC (3 mg/kg d1–2, monthly i. v.) BCNU (1.5 mg/kg d1, i. v.) VCR (0.025 µg/kg d1, i. v.) | | 12/28 | 43 |
| Gailani et al. (65) | 2B, 3A, 3G, 4A(6) | | |
| A. 5-FU (15 mg/kg/wk i. v.) Placebo (mannitol s. c.) | | 6/29 | 20 |
| B. 5-FU (as in A) Ara-C (30 mg/m²/wk s. c.) | | 3/38 | 8 |
| C. 5-FU (as in A) Ara-C (100 mg/m²/wk s. c.) | | 2/5 | 40 |
| Richards et al. (166) | 2A, 3E, 3G, 4A(6) | | |
| A. 5-FU (12 mg/kg d1–5 i. v.; 12 mg/kg/wk i. v.) | | 8/38 | 21 |
| B. 5-FU (12 mg/kg d1–5 i. v., wkly) CTX (10 mg/kg d1 i. v., wkly) MTX (0.1 mg/kg d1 i. v., wkly) | | 7/38 | 18 |
| Horton et al. (88) | 2A, 3E, 3G, 4A(6) | | |
| A. 5-FU (10 mg/kg/wk i. v.) | | 1/22 | 4 |
| B. 5-FU (as in A) | | 1/26 | 4 |

TABLE 20—*Cont.*

| Investigators (reference) and treatment arms | Evaluation criteria[a] | No. responses/ no. patients | Response rate (%) |
|---|---|---|---|
| Mitomycin C (0.075 mg/kg/ wk i. v.) Thiotepa (0.15 mg/kg/wk i. v.) Fluoxymesterone (20 mg/d p. o.) | | | |

[a] See the criteria defined in Fig. 1.
[b] Among 11 patients with liver metastases 5-FU gave no responses.
[c] Among 43 patients with liver metastases 5-FU + MeCCNU gave 13 (30%) responses.

Similarly, the investigations of the Istituto Nazionale Tumori in Milan (168) and Cancer and Leukemia Group B (CALGB) (65) included too few patients for any meaningful analysis of combination regimens versus single-agent therapy.

In substance, the published trials of combination chemotherapy show that the response rate obtained with MeCCNU + 5-FU is superior to that of 5-FU alone. The results also suggest that DTIC may have an additive effect in the BCNU + 5-FU regimen. Vincristine, which has been inactive as a single agent (32), was added in three of the trials that produced the highest response rates.

The successes of the completed trials are reflected in the designs of current studies outlined in Table 21. For example, one of the studies (ECOG 4275) is attempting to define the roles of vincristine and DTIC in combination with 5-FU + MeCCNU (188). Ongoing trials are investigating commercially available antitumor drugs (i.e., hydroxyurea) as well as investigational agents that have shown some activity in previous studies.

The activity shown by two combination regimens (96-hr infusion of 5-FU plus mitomycin C *or* MeCCNU) in an independent pilot study (192,194) is the basis of a current large-scale trial (SWOG 7434). This study stratifies patients according to liver involvement and randomly assigns them to the two regimens. Although no 5-FU control arm is included, a comparison can be made with a previous study (13) of weekly 5-FU versus weekly 5-FU + MeCCNU q. 8 wks showing response rates of 9.5% and 31%, respectively. The present study is showing rather low comparative response rates varying from 10 to 18% among stratified categories and suggests no improvement by the infusion method of 5-FU administration. Definitive measurements of the length of response and survival must await final analysis of the study.

### Immunotherapy and Chemoimmunotherapy

Trials of immunotherapy with or without antitumor agents (Table 22) have only been reported in a preliminary fashion (55,133,154,193) and final conclusions must await more comprehensive publications.

TABLE 21. *Ongoing or unpublished randomized trials of single-agent and combination chemotherapy in colorectal cancer (188)*

| Investigators[a] and treatment arms | Evaluation criteria[b] |
|---|---|
| CALGB 7282 | 2B, 3B, 3C, 3E, 3G |
|   A. CCNU (100–300 mg/m² q. 6 wks, p. o.) | |
|   B. MeCCNU (150–200 mg/m² q. 6 wks p. o.) | |
| Sidney Farber Cancer Center 75–30 | 3E, 3G, 4A(2, 4, 6) |
|   A. Chromomycin A₃ (0.9 mg/m²/d × 5, q. 5 wks i. v.) | |
|   B. Cytembena (200 mg/m² b.i.d. daily × 5, q. 5 wks i. v.) | |
|   C. ICRF–159 (1 g/m²/d × 3, q. 5 wks p. o.) | |
| Sidney Farber Cancer Center 75–30 | 3E, 3G, 3H |
|   A. 5-FU (12 mg/kg/d × 5, q. 4 wks i. v.) | |
|   B. 5-FU (as in A) + antibiotics[c] and low-bacterial diet | |
| Wayne State University 196–76 | 3E, 3G |
|   A. Ftorafur (2 g/m²/d × 5, q. 4 wks i. v.) | |
|     Mitomycin C (20 mg/m² d1, q. 8 wks i. v.) | |
|   B. Ftorafur (as in A) | |
|     MeCCNU (175 mg/m² d1, q. 8 wks p. o.) | |
| Memorial Sloan Kettering Cancer Center 75–88 | 3E, 3G |
|   A. 5-FU (300 mg/m² d1–5 and d36–40, q. 10 wks i. v.) | |
|     MeCCNU (150 mg/m² d1, q. 10 wks p. o.) | |
|     VCR (1 mg/m² d1 and 36, q. 10 wks i. v.) | |
|   B. 5-FU (as in A) | |
|     MeCCNU (30 mg d1–5 p. o.) | |
|     VCR (as in A) | |
| Sidney Farber Cancer Center 76–008 | 2A, 3E, 3G, 3H |
|   A. MTX (3 g/m²/wk i. v.) | |
|     Leucovorin (10 mg/m² d1 i. v.; then 10 mg/m² q. 6 hr × 12 p. o.) | |
|   B. MTX (3 g/m² i. v. 1st wk; then 7.5 g/m²/wk i. v.) | |
|     Leucovorin (as in A) | |
| WCG 124 | 3E, 3H |
|   A. CTX (20 mg/kg/wk × 1 i. v.) | |
|     5-FU (15 mg/kg wks 2–6 i. v.) | |
|   B. 5-FU (15 mg/kg/wk i. v.) | |
| SWOG 7434 | 3E, 3G, 4A(9, 13) |
|   A. 5-FU (1 g/m² 24-hr infusion d1–4, q. 4 wks i. v.) | |
|     Mitomycin C (20 mg/m² d1, q. 8 wks i. v.) | |
|   B. 5-FU (as in A) | |
|     MeCCNU (175 mg/m² d1, q. 8 wks p. o.) | |
| ECOG 4273 | 3E, 3G, 4A(5, 6) |
|   *I. No Prior Chemotherapy* | |
|   A. 5-FU (600 mg/m²/wk i. v. *or* p. o.) | |
|   B. CTX (1 g/m² d1, q. 8 wks) | |
|     5-FU (600 mg/m² wks 2–5, q. 8 wks p. o.) | |
|   C. 5-FU (600 mg/m²/wk, q. 8 wks p. o.) | |
|     6-Thioguanine (40 mg/m²/d × 14, q. 8 wks) | |
|   D. MeCCNU (175 mg/m² q. 8 wks p. o.) | |
|   *II. Prior 5-FU, Nitrosoureas, or Progression* | |
|   A. β-2-TGdR (100 mg/m²/d × 5 i. v., q. 3 wks) | |
|   B. MeCCNU (as in ID) | |

TABLE 21—*Cont.*

| Investigators[a] and treatment arms | Evaluation criteria[b] |
|---|---|
| C. CTX + 5-FU (as in IB) | |
| D. 5-FU + 6-thioguanine (as in IC) | |
| ECOG 1275 | 3E, 3G, 4A(4–6) |
|   A. MeCCNU (130 mg/m², q. 8 wks p. o.) | |
|   β-2-TGdR (60 mg/m²/d X 5, q. 4 wks i. v.) | |
|   B. VP-16 (125 mg/m² d1, 3, and 5, q. 4 wks i. v.) | |
|   C. Diglycoaldehyde (1.5–2 g/m² d1–3, q. 4 wks i. v.) | |
| ECOG 4275 | 2B, 3E, 3G, 3H, 4A(2, 4–6), 5A |
| *I. No Prior Chemotherapy (Cycles q. 10 wks)* | |
|   A. 5-FU (325 mg/m² d1–5, d36–40 i. v.) | |
|     MeCCNU (150 mg/m² d1 p. o.) | |
|   B. 5-FU (as in A) | |
|     MeCCNU (as in A) | |
|     VCR (1 mg/m² d1 and 36 i. v.) | |
|   C. 5-FU (250 mg/m² d1–5, 36–40 i. v.) | |
|     MeCCNU (100 mg/m² d1 p. o.) | |
|     DTIC (100 mg/m² d1, 2, 36, 37 i. v.) | |
|   D. 5-FU + MeCCNU + DTIC (as in C) | |
|     VCR (1 mg/m² d1 and 36 i. v.) | |
|   E. 5-FU (600 mg/m² d1, 8, 15, 22; then wkly i. v.) | |
|     Hydroxyurea (800 mg/m² q. 8 hr on d4, 11, 18, and 25 p. o.; then wkly) | |
| *II. Prior 5-FU (Cycles q. 8 wks)* | |
|   A. MeCCNU (175 mg/m² d1, p. o.) | |
|     VCR (1 mg/m² q. 2 wks i. v.) | |
|   B. MeCCNU (130 mg/m² d1, p. o.) | |
|     DTIC (150 mg/m² d1–5, d29–32, i. v.) | |
|   C. MeCCNU (as in B) | |
|     DTIC (as in B) | |
|     VCR (as in A) | |
|   D. MeCCNU (as in B) | |
|     β-2-TGdR (60 mg/m² d1–5, d29–33 i. v.) | |

[a] Abbreviations: See previous tables.
[b] See the criteria defined in Fig. 1.
[c] Vancomycin (1 g p. o. 3X daily); Tobramycin (400 mg p. o. 3X daily).

One particularly interesting study compared two dose levels of the methanol extraction residue of BCG (MER–BCG) versus saline placebo (150). However, there were no objective responses and changes in skin reactivity were similar in the high-dose MER–BCG and placebo groups. No advantage for added immunostimulants (BCG, MER–BCG, or Levamisole) has yet been demonstrated, and the studies have been considerable and continued use of randomized therapeutic trials in colorectal cancer appears mandatory for now and the immediate future.

TABLE 22. *Published and unpublished trials of chemoimmunotherapy in advanced colorectal cancer*

| Investigators (reference) and treatment arms | Evaluation criteria[a] | No. responses/ no. patients | Response rate (%) |
|---|---|---|---|
| O'Connell et al. (150) | 3A, 3G | | |
| A. MER-BCG (0.4 mg in each of 5 sites wkly X 5, then monthly) | | 0/17 | — |
| B. MER-BCG (0.1 mg in each of 5 sites wkly X 5, then monthly) | | 0/14 | — |
| C. Saline (same schedule) | | 0/17 | — |
| Valdivieso et al. (193) | 2A, 3E, 3G, 4A(6) | | |
| A. Ftorafur (2 g/m² d2–6, q. 4 wks i. v.) MeCCNU (100 mg/m² d1, q. 4 wks p. o.) MTX (30 mg/m² d1, 8, and 15, q. 4 wks i. v.) BCG (6 X 10⁸ cells scarification d11, 18, and 25 each course) | | 14/32 | 43 |
| B. 5-FU (800 mg/m² d2–6, q. 4 wks i. v.) MeCCNU, MTX, BCG (as in A) | | 1/12 | 8 |
| Engstrom et al. (55) | 2A, 3E, 3G | | |
| A. 5-FU (600 mg/m²/wk X 8, then q. 2 wks i. v.) | | 5/24 | 20 |
| B. 5-FU (as in A) BCG (Glaxo) (0.1 ml i. d. in each of 5 sites, q. 2 wks X 4, then monthly) | | 8/23 | 35 |
| Moertel et al. (133) | 2A, 3E, 4A(2, 4, 6) | | |
| A. 5-FU (400 mg/m²/d X 5, q. 5 wks i. v.) Cis-platinum (20 mg/m² d1 i. v.) | | 7/28 | 25 |
| B. 5-FU + cis-platinum (as in A) MER-BCG (0.4 mg in each of 5 sites i. d. d1, 7, 21, and 36, q. 5 wks *or* d21 and 36, q. 5 wks) | | 7/28 | 25 |
| C. 5-FU (300 mg/m² d1–5; 400 mg/m² d36–40, q. 10 wks i. v.) MeCCNU (175 mg/m² d1, q. 10 wks p. o.) | | 7/33 | 21 |
| D. 5-FU + MeCCNU (as in C) MER-BCG (as in B) | | 3/29 | 10 |
| E. 5-FU + MeCCNU (as in C) VCR (1 mg/m² d1 and 36 i. v.) | | 6/31 | 20 |

TABLE 22—*Cont.*

| Investigators (reference) and treatment arms | Evaluation criteria[a] | No. responses/ no. patients | Response rate (%) |
|---|---|---|---|
| F. 5-FU + MeCCNU (as in C) MER-BCG (as in B) | | 9/32 | 28 |
| M. D. Anderson 7548 (188) | 3E, 3G | Unpublished | |
|   A. Ftorafur (2g/m² d1–5 i. v.) MTX (15 mg/m² d22–25 i. m.) Levamisole (150 mg/m² d7 and 8, 14, and 15) | | | |
|   B. Ftorafur (as in A) Baker's Antifol (250 mg/m² d22–25 i. v.) Levamisole (as in A) | | | |

[a] See the categories defined in Fig. 1.

## TUMORS OF THE LARGE INTESTINE OTHER THAN ADENOCARCINOMA

Melanomas and sarcomas of the colon, rectum, and anus are too rare to have been the subject of controlled investigations.

Squamous cell carcinoma of the anus and lower part of the rectum is a relatively infrequent neoplasm that is generally treated by surgery alone or combined with radiotherapy. Overall survival ranges from 40% to 50% (171). No controlled trials are being performed, although chemotherapy has been used in selected cases of advanced disease (149).

## LIVER CANCER (HEPATOCELLULAR AND CHOLANGIOCELLULAR HEPATOMA)

Although there are some difficulties in determining the precise number of deaths, estimates are that each year approximately 2,500 persons in the United States die of this disease (39). Thus, liver cancer is relatively uncommon in the United States but is the most common cause of cancer deaths in many areas of the world.

### Prognostic Factors

The factors of prognostic significance in this disease are only beginning to be defined.

There is some evidence that in the United States the disease is less aggressive and more responsive to chemotherapy than is the African variety of hepatoma (110,126,152,159). A staging system for hepatocellular carcinoma devised in 1971 (197) was applied to 72 untreated African patients whose median survival was 1 month. Then, the historical clinical and laboratory aspects of the staging system were quite negative to date (55,133). In addition, the previously observed high response rates were combination chemotherapy seem less firm (133).

## Conclusions

5-Fluorouracil is the best single agent by a narrow margin. In fact, no single agent induces a response rate much greater than 20%. Slightly higher overall response rates are produced by intensive loading courses of 5-FU in comparison to aggressive weekly administration, but the difference is of slight, if any, overall clinical significance. Oral 5-FU is less effective than the i. v. route by either schedule. Intraarterial infusion of fluoropyrimidines in patients with liver metastases still cannot be evaluated in controlled trials (10,63,188).

There is suggestive evidence of an additive effect, albeit a small one, in the 5-FU + MeCCNU combination but it is of marginal clinical benefit in terms of survival, particularly in view of the increased toxicity of the two agents. No definitive evidence exists that will support an additive effect for mitomycin C combined with 5-FU. The possibility of increased effectiveness with the addition of vincristine and/or DTIC to 5-FU + MeCCNU must be subjected to further study.

The addition of nonspecific immunotherapy has produced no clinical benefits in controlled trials to date.

In general, it must be concluded that the published literature reflects only the results of selected studies and overall clinical benefits remain speculative. Probably the major obstacle to the successful application of controlled trials is the lack of highly effective drugs. When truly effective agents appear they will surely be obvious in comparison to the marginal agents now being investigated, regardless of the controls used. However, the value of controlled observations remains examined for prognostic significance (159). It was found that age and sex seemed to have no effect on prognosis. A serum bilirubin concentration of $> 2$ mg% or a loss of $> 25\%$ of body weight heralded the poorest prognosis for survival. Other factors of prognostic significance included the duration of symptoms before diagnosis, visible abdominal collateral circulation, ascites, tumor differentiation, and serum levels of SGOT, alkaline phosphatase, $\alpha$-fetoprotein, and proline hydroxylase. The study defined the important stratification groups in Ugandan patients, but this has not been done for the U.S. population.

Other investigators have concluded that performance status has no significant impact on survival and patients with metastases have no different prognosis than those without metastases (183). These prognostic factors must be defined for each population in order to properly design randomized trials.

## Therapeutic Trials

The few randomized trials that have been completed or are in progress are summarized in Table 23, without any attempt to subdivide them into modalities.

TABLE 23. *Randomized trials of chemotherapy in liver cancer*[a]

| Investigators (reference) and treatment arms | Evaluation criteria[b] | No. responses/ no. patients | Response rate (%) | Survival |
|---|---|---|---|---|
| Gailani et al. (65) | 2B, 3A, 3C | | | |
|   A. 5-FU (15 mg/kg/wk i. v.) Placebo (mannitol s. c.) | | 0/16 | — | |
|   B. 5-FU (as in A) Ara-C (30 mg/m²/wk s. c.) | | 1/16 | 6 | |
|   C. 5-FU (as in A) Ara-C (100 mg/m²/wk i. v.) | | 0/6 | — | |
| South African Primary Liver Cancer Research Group (183) | 2B, 4A(4, 14, 18) 5C | | | |
|   A. 2,800–3,000 rads/21–28 days | | 0/8 | — | 30 days–6 + mos. |
|   B. RT (as in A) Procarbazine (150–300 mg/d p. o., 4 days before RT and q. d until leucopenia) | | 0/7 | — | 34–78 days |
| Ong and Chan (152) | 4A(18) | | | |
|   A. Surgery with hepatic dearterialization | | ?/18 | | 15.4 wks[c] |
|   B. Hepatic artery ligation 5-FU infusion into portal vein | | ?/18 | | 15 wks[c] |
|   C. 5-FU infusion into hepatic artery | | ?/19 | | 10.4 wks[c] |
|   D. Radiotherapy | | ?/11 | | 8–13 wks[c] |
|   E. No treatment | | ?/15 | | 10 wks[c] |
| ECOG 2273—Part I (47,58,126,188) | 2B, 4A(4, –6, 12, 19) | | | |
|   A. Adriamycin (60 mg/m², d1, 22, 43, i. v.) | | 7/41 | 17 | 19 wks[d] |
|   B. 5-FU (600 mg/m²/d × 5, d1–5 and d36–40 p. o.) | | 0/40 | — | 9 wks[d] |
|   C. 5-FU (500 mg/m²/d × 5, d1–5 and d36–40 p. o.) MeCCNU (150 mg/m², d1, p. o.) | | 2/36 | 6 | 17 wks[d] |
|   D. 5-FU (as in B) Streptozotocin (500 mg/m²/ d × 5, d1–5 i. v.) | | 3/18 | 17 | 21 wks[d] |
| ECOG 2273—Part II (47,126,188) | 2B, 4A(4–6, 12, 19) | | | |
|   A. Adriamycin (60 mg/m², d1, 22, 43 i. v.) | | | | |
|   B. 5-FU (325 mg/m²/d × 5, d1–5 i. v., 375 mg/m²/d × 5, d36–40) MeCCNU (150 mg/m², d1, p. o.) | | | | |
|   C. 5-FU (400 mg/m²/d × 5, d1–5, d36–40, i. v.) Streptozotocin (500 mg/m²/ d × 5, d1–5, d36–40 i. v.) | | | | |
|   D. 5-FU (275 mg/m²/d × 5, d1–5, d36–40, i. v.) | | | | |

TABLE 23—*Cont.*

| Investigators (reference) and treatment arms | Evaluation criteria [b] | No. responses/ no. patients | Response rate (%) | Survival |
|---|---|---|---|---|
| MeCCNU (110 mg/m², d1, p. o.) Adriamycin (40 mg/m² d1 and 36, i. v.) | | | | |

[a] All trials have been published except presently ongoing Part II of ECOG 2273.
[b] See the criteria defined in Fig. 1.
[c] Mean survival.
[d] Median survival.

The first study (65) was a pure chemotherapy trial in gastrointestinal tumors that did not include enough hepatoma patients and lacked the stratification of prognostic variables needed to assess the drug regimens. The number of patients was also insufficient in the second trial, which compared radiotherapy and radiotherapy + procarbazine in an African population (183). Patients treated by radiotherapy alone survived longer than those who also received procarbazine, but the difference was not significant.

The third study, which compares five arms of therapy, is still in progress without significant differences at this time (152). This is an Oriental population unstratified for risk factors, which will certainly limit the interpretation of results when the study is completed.

The recent activity of adriamycin reported by Olweny et al. (151) in unrandomized trials among Ugandan patients has stimulated studies in the Eastern Cooperative Oncology Group (ECOG). These joint African-American efforts are currently evaluating adriamycin alone and combined in various regimens with 5-FU, MeCCNU, and streptozotocin (ECOG 2273, Table 23). Preliminary results in Part I of these studies indicate fewer responses in the Bantu population of patients (58), but only a small number of patients is included in each treatment group. The survival data indicate that adriamycin alone and the two combination regimens are each significantly superior to oral 5-FU alone ($p < 0.05$). Part II of the study is continuing and new treatment arms have been added.

The important prognostic factors in hepatocellular carcinoma are only beginning to be recognized and may vary with the geographic location and race. Hepatic dearterialization and radiotherapy are being explored and a few randomized chemotherapy trials are being performed. However, more effective therapeutic tools will be needed before more complex studies can be designed. Future studies should have a few well-stratified arms of therapy that can answer basic questions and determine if new drugs are effective in the disease. Immunotherapy may be an intriguing approach in view of the association of $\alpha$-fetoprotein with this tumor.

## ESOPHAGEAL CANCER

Evaluation of primary and secondary treatment for this lethal neoplasm has been extremely difficult. The notable lack of effective therapy for all disease stages has engendered little enthusiasm for performing controlled therapeutic trials. As a result, any analysis of treatment methods is almost universally based on retrospective comparisons of patients treated during different time periods, frequently at different institutions in diverse geographic locations.

Attempts at curative treatment have been frustrated by the insiduous onset of symptoms and the anatomic location of the primary tumor. Few patients have truly localized lesions amenable to local treatment modalities and, as a corollary, there is a high incidence of occult metastases associated with the clinical presentation at diagnosis. Attempts at local eradication are beset by complications, morbidity, and potential mortality.

Therefore, efforts at combined modality treatment are hampered by the basic biology of the disease and the fact that relatively few patients are diagnosed at a suitably early stage. The integration of systemic therapy into local treatment is sorely needed but, unfortunately, the results of chemotherapy in advanced disease have not been noteworthy. An excellent response to a chemotherapeutic agent is rare; thus, investigators lack the most important clue for selecting potentially active agents. By the time the disease recurs following primary treatment, or has been classified unsuitable for attempting cure by primary treatment, the patient is usually a poor candidate for palliative chemotherapy. The combination of inanition and local and systemic effects of an uncontrolled primary tumor are disastrous.

However, in spite of the generally unfavorable clinical picture, controlled studies are in progress to define and refine some of the therapeutic possibilities found in the extensive literature on this disease.

### Comparative Uncontrolled Trials

#### *Surgery*

Surgical therapy of esophageal carcinoma involves subtotal esophagectomy with wide margins and restoration of gastrointestinal continuity by anastomosis of the stomach or interposition of a segment of the colon or jejunum. Curative resection depends on finding local cancer without invasion of mediastinal structures. An analysis of large series (106,157) has shown that approximately 35% of patients have clinical dissemination, 65% have clinically localized disease, and only 20% of cases are pathologically localized.

In the period 1944–1966, analysis of the Memorial Hospital statistics (155) revealed that operability rate increased from 18% to 34%, whereas the resectability rate rose from 34.2% (14 of 41 patients explored) to 61% (260/426). This series was complicated by the fact that 41 of the 260 patients had preoperative or postoperative irradiation and three separate surgical procedures were used (esophagectomy, esophagectomy and esophagogastrostomy, and esophagectomy with subsequent colon transplant). The overall 5-year survival rate was 6% (16/260); half of the survivors had received either pre- or postoperative irradiation. During the period analyzed, the surgical mortality rate steadily declined from 30% to 13%, for an overall rate of 23%. This decreased surgical mortality paralleled improvement in surgical technique and intensive care, and has been substantiated by other authors (155,204).

The experience of Nakayama et al. (145) was even more favorable, with an overall surgical mortality rate of 6% in 725 patients. In fact, the rate was only 3.9% among 303 patients who were treated by a three-stage procedure involving esophagectomy and eventual antethoracic esophagogastrostomy (145).

A detailed analysis of the success of surgery alone reveals a number of problems in determining its true value as a single therapeutic modality. Many of the surgical series include patients with carcinoma of all sites and histologic types. The precision of staging procedures also varies with the series. The situation is further complicated by the fact that combined modality treatment with pre- or postoperative irradiation has been included in surgical series. The state of the surgical art as primary treatment for esophageal carcinoma has been summarized by Moertel (121), using 17 series involving 4,008 resected patients. In this analysis, the average operative mortality was 22% (range 6 to 40%) and overall 5-year survival was 9.5% (range 3 to 20%). Clearly, surgery has reached a plateau as the sole modality of treatment.

## Radiotherapy

Palliative radiotherapy is clearly established as a valuable method for temporary control and symptomatic benefit. In fact, curative radiation therapy is not only possible but also preferable to surgery in the management of carcinoma of the cervical esophagus (Table 24). Pearson (156–158) has also made a strong case for irradiation as the primary modality for carcinoma of the esophagus in all sites. His conclusions are based on the lesser morbidity and mortality of aggressive radiotherapy, as well as comparative statistics (Table 25). This analysis suggests that irradiation is the better choice for carcinoma of the cervical and upper half of the thoracic esophagus, whereas there is no therapeutic preference for lesions in the lower half. However, as in all uncontrolled nonrandomized trials, there is dissent about these conclusions.

TABLE 24. *Results of radiotherapy in carcinoma of the upper esophagus*

| Investigator | No. of patients | 5-year survival rate (%) |
|---|---|---|
| Jacobsson (92) | 56 | 17 |
| Pearson (156) | 31 | 23 |
| Gunnlaugsson et al. (75) | 45 | 13 |

TABLE 25. *Radiotherapy versus surgery in treatment of esophageal cancer of all sites (158)*

| Tumor site | | 5-year survival (%) | |
|---|---|---|---|
| | | Surgery | Radiotherapy |
| Cervical | | 4/19   (2%) | 14/46   (30%) |
| Thoracic–upper half | | 11/135 (8%) | 12/73   (16%) |
| Thoracic–lower half | | 31/275 (11%) | 6/50   (12%) |
| | Total | 46/429 (11%) | 32/169 (19%) |

Wilson et al. (203) have reported a retrospective comparison of resection versus radiotherapy in 20 pairs of patients. The analysis showed short-term survival favoring the resected group. Parker et al. (155) found intermediate results with nine 2-year survivors among 166 patients treated with radiotherapy alone. However, these authors were distressed by findings in a subset of 17 patients with small tumors who experienced only temporary tumor arrest.

Supervoltage irradiation (4,500 to 5,000 rads/4 weeks to 6,000 rads/6 weeks) is the optimum technique at this time. It is clearly superior to orthovoltage irradiation (103).

## Combined Modality Treatment

The largest world experience with planned preoperative radiotherapy is summarized in Tables 26 and 27.

Nakayama et al. (145) developed a multistage treatment program beginning with staging abdominal laparotomy and gastrostomy. Stabilized nutrition by gastrostomy feeding was usually obtained 7 to 10 days after surgery. Preoperative irradiation was then given (2,000 to 2,500 rads in 4 or 5 fractions) using megavoltage therapy with a linear accelerator or Cobalt-60 source. Then, 3 to 5 days after the completion of radiotherapy, the entire thoracic esophagus was resected. An external cervical esophagostomy was performed and connected to the gastrostomy by a rubber tube, making oral alimentation possible. The final stage of therapy, performed 6 to 12 months later, involved antethoracic mobilization

TABLE 26. *Experience of Nakayama et al. (145) with combined radiotherapy and surgery*

| Therapy | Survival rate (%) | |
|---|---|---|
| | 3-year | 5-year |
| Radiotherapy + surgery | 11/40   (27%) | 3/8   (37%) |
| Surgery | 7/32   (22%) | 4/21   (19%) |
| Radiotherapy | 8/123  (6%) | 6/77   (8%) |

TABLE 27. *Experience of Akakura et al. (1) with combined radiotherapy and surgery*

| Therapy | No. of patients | Resectability rate (%) | 5-year survival rate |
|---|---|---|---|
| Radiotherapy + surgery | 117 | 65% | 25% |
| Surgery | 229 | 26% | 14% |

of the stomach with anastomosis to the cervical esophagus. The experience with this procedure is outlined in Table 26.

The approach of Akakura et al. (1) consisted of preoperative megavoltage therapy (5,000 to 6,000 rads in 5 to 6 weeks) followed by a 2- to 4-week rest and a one-stage esophageal resection with a substernal colon transplant or esophagogastric anastomosis (Table 27).

The results in both of these series suggest improvement over historical surgical controls in the same institutions. However, it is debatable whether these results would be achieved in other countries and multiple institutions; conflicting reports have appeared (71,155,160,182). Nevertheless, randomized trials have been proposed and are in progress, as will be discussed in a later section.

## Chemotherapy

As discussed earlier, chemotherapeutic agents have not been studied extensively in carcinoma of the esophagus. A recent analysis by Wasserman et al. (199) of activity of 30 "standard" anticancer agents and investigational drugs

TABLE 28. *Miscellaneous trials of chemotherapy in esophageal cancer*

| Drug regimen | No. responses/ evaluable patients | Investigator |
|---|---|---|
| Methyl GAG (5 mg/kg/d X 2) | 5/21[a] | Falkson (56) |
| Bleomycin (10–30 mg/m² biwk) | 15/29[b] | Tancini et al. (189) |
| Bleomycin (10 mg/m² biwk) Methotrexate (40 mg/m² biwk) | 4/5[c] | |
| L-PAM Colchamine | 73/75[d] | Larionov and Chudahova (104) |
| Cyclophosphamide (variable dosage by i. v., intratumor, and p. o. routes) | 32/32[e] | Nelson (147) |

[a]Partial responses; 5 others had improvement.
[b]One was a complete response; duration of responses 1–2 mos.
[c]One was a complete response; duration of responses 2–7 mos.
[d]Response = "clinical improvement."
[e]Response = "clinical improvement"; rapid improvement in swallowing; average survival 9 mos., with one of 15 mos.

demonstrated that only blomycin (7 responses in 42 patients) has received adequate evaluation in phase II trials. In addition, there have been scattered trials of other agents and somewhat favorable anecdotal reports in some instances (Table 28).

The overall medical value of chemotherapy for esophageal carcinoma remains undetermined. Reports of clinical improvement with alkylating agents (104,147), bleomycin (189,199), 5-fluorouracil (199), and bleomycin plus methotrexate (189) suggest possibilities for combined modality trials. Methyl-GAG (56) demonstrates significant activity, but the responses are brief and the acute toxicity of this agent is devastating. Trials of combined chemotherapy and irradiation have been reported by Japanese and French investigators but defy definitive analysis (7,169).

## Randomized Trials

With rare exceptions, there are no definitive results available for the controlled trials in progress at this time. Thus, they can only be presented and analyzed from the standpoint of the general experience with uncontrolled studies.

There are two ongoing trials that are comparing surgery alone versus radiotherapy followed by surgery. These protocols, one by the Veterans Administration Surgical Adjuvant Group and the other by the EORTC, are outlined in Figs. 2 and 3.

Two other studies have been designed to evaluate irradiation as a single modality. Holsti (86) has reported on the efficacy and patient tolerance in a comparison

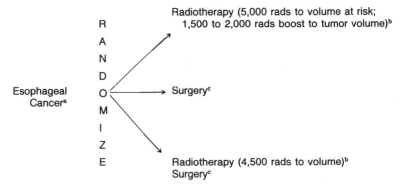

**FIG. 2.** Veterans Administration Surgical Adjuvant Group Protocol 32: Comparison of surgery, radiotherapy, and preoperative radiotherapy in esophageal cancer.

[a] Minimum of 250 patients for analysis of any treatment differences. Eligibility: histologically confirmed squamous cancer; medically operable and clinically resectable; tumor < 8 cm length, below thoracic inlet; performance status > 40; informed consent.
[b] Supravoltage equipment.
[c] Surgery alone—as soon as feasible; postirradiation surgery 3 to 6 wks after RT.

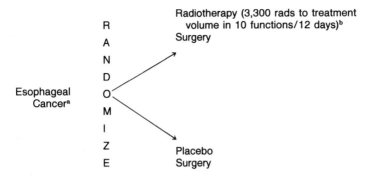

Esophageal
Cancer[a]

R
A
N
D
O
M
I
Z
E

Radiotherapy (3,300 rads to treatment
volume in 10 functions/12 days)[b]
Surgery

Placebo
Surgery

**FIG. 3.** European Organization for Research on the Treatment of Cancer Protocol 40762: Surgery versus preoperative radiotherapy in esophageal cancer.

[a] Clinically operable; 26 patients per arm for statistical analysis. Staging workup: esophagoscopy, laryngoscopy, and bronchoscopy; mediastinoscopy; azygography; chest x-ray and liver scans; routine blood counts and chemistries.
[b] Megavoltage equipment.

of split-course versus continuous radiotherapy in patients judged unresectable or medically inoperable. The continuous therapy was applied at 5,700 to 6,300 rads/6 to 7 weeks, whereas the split-course consisted of 2,700 to 3,000 rads/2 weeks, a 2- to 3-week rest, and a repeat course in a total elapsed time of 8 to 9 weeks. The patients were randomized by birth dates, a technique that is subject to misuse since the investigator may know in advance what the patient will receive. Although in a trial of this nature such knowledge is certainly not critical, it could bias patient selection in more aggressive or controversial treatment options. The results of split-course irradiation in 58 patients showed 41% 1-year survival and 21% at 2 years; continuous radiotherapy in 74 patients gave a 1-year survival rate of 23% and 16% at 2 years. The trial did demonstrate better patient tolerance and short-term survival for the split-course technique. The purpose of the trial was well accomplished in terms of palliation.

The Radiation Therapy Oncology Group (RTOG) also has an ongoing trial of radiotherapy as a single modality (Fig. 4). The investigation is comparing the efficacy of adjunctive oxygen breathing versus air breathing in radiotherapy of tumors of the upper digestive tract and esophagus. The general objectives include comparisons of patient tolerance, local tumor control, lymph node clearance, and survival. At this time 40 patients have been entered in the study, but no conclusions have been reached.

Radiotherapy is also being studied in combined modality approaches employing chemotherapy. Roussel et al. (169) have published a preliminary report of radiotherapy versus preirradiation methotrexate (Fig. 5) showing that the combined therapies increase short-term survival. In addition, the wide-field irradiation gave superior results. They plan to continue the trial with increased emphasis on nutritional support before therapy.

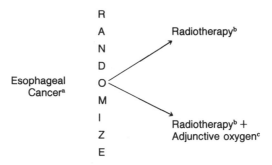

**FIG. 4.** Radiation Therapy Oncology Group Protocol 9171: Adjunctive oxygen versus air breathing in conjunction with radiotherapy for esophageal cancer.

[a] All stages; no distant metastases; performance status > 40; age < 75.

[b] Megavoltage equipment; technique in accord with institutional preference; 6000 rads/5 to 7 wk, opposed fields in first half of RT supplemented by oblique wedge or rotational fields in remaining RT; margin of 5 cm from lesion required.

[c] By mouthpiece or face mask; pure $O_2$ for 10 min before RT, 95% $O_2$ + 5% $CO_2$ at start and during RT.

The Eastern Cooperative Oncology Group (ECOG) has in progress an evaluation of bleomycin as an adjuvant to radiotherapy (Fig. 6). This study will require 100 patients to determine the quality and quantity of survival. Since January 1974, 57 patients have been entered and an estimated 2 years will be required to complete the investigation.

The ECOG is also investigating chemotherapy as the sole modality in advanced esophageal carcinoma (Fig. 7). Patients are first randomized to adriamycin,

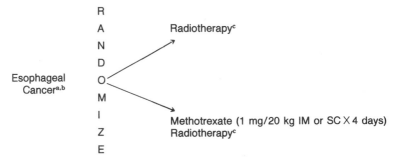

**FIG. 5.** Centre Francois (Baclesse, France) protocol for preirradiation methotrexate therapy in esophageal cancer.

[a] Patient eligibility: age < 75, no distant metastases, inoperable/unresectable.

[b] Laparotomy and gastrostomy with stratification by positive or negative celiac nodes before randomization.

[c] 4,500 rads supervoltage to include primary tumor with wide margins and any involved nodes.

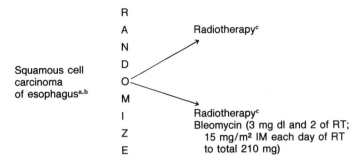

**FIG. 6.** Eastern Cooperative Oncology Group Protocol 1273: Adjuvant bleomycin in the radiotherapy of squamous cell carcinoma of the esophagus.

[a] Eligibility: Unresectable at any site; carcinoma in region of aortic arch; postpalliative resection; confirmed local recurrence after resection; no evident distant metastases; absence of infection and tracheoesophageal fistula; no prior RT or bleomycin.

[b] Stratification: Tumor site (above or below aortic arch); surgical status (no resection, palliative resection, local recurrence after resection); performance status according to ECOG scale.

[c] 6,000 rads/6 wks, megavoltage equipment, individualized technique allowed.

methotrexate, or 5-FU on the basis of prior therapy, performance status, and the presence or absence of active heart disease. Patients showing disease progression after 6 weeks are randomized again as shown in Fig. 7; the third crossover in therapy is assigned automatically. This study is the first randomized phase II trial of chemotherapy for esophageal cancer in the United States. Ineffective therapies will be discontinued as they appear and untested and/or promising drugs will be substituted.

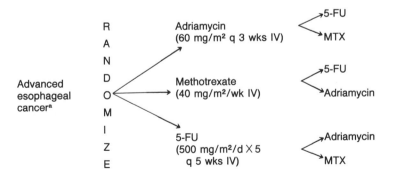

**FIG. 7.** Eastern Cooperative Oncology Group Protocol 2274: Chemotherapy in advanced esophageal cancer.

[a] Patient eligibility: not eligible for curative radiotherapy or surgery; measurable disease; histologic proof of disease; no prior chemotherapy with study agents; medically suitable for treatment (includes no active heart disease for adriamycin).

## Conclusions

Therapeutic progress in esophageal cancer will be slow and definition of optimum primary therapy will be difficult, even with the well-designed EORTC and VASAG trials (Figs. 2 and 3). These studies are important because of the previous observations of the value of radiotherapy alone (158) or before surgery (145). The role of chemotherapeutic agents with or without radiotherapy is still unknown. The ECOG studies (1273 and 2274) shown in Figs. 6 and 7, as well as the French study (Fig. 5), are initial steps toward an orderly evaluation of these approaches. Immunotherapy has not been studied in esophageal cancer.

## CARCINOMA OF THE GALLBLADDER AND EXTRAHEPATIC BILE DUCTS

These malignancies are usually reported together with carcinoma of the liver, and it is difficult to establish their exact incidence. Carcinoma of the gallbladder is a virulent tumor with a median survival of 2 to 5 months (median 2.5 months) after histologic proof of unresectable malignant disease. The prognostic factors have only recently been explored by Nevin et al. (148), who developed five pathologic stages of disease and correlated them with prognosis. Their findings should be helpful in stratifying patients in future studies.

Surgery, even when extensive, provides a very low (6%) 5-year survival rate, but further investigation of radical approaches seems justified (49). Of course, surgical palliation by diversion may provide some relief and, although the impact on survival is unknown, this procedure seems worthy of further study.

A number of clinical studies include cases of gallbladder carcinoma, but generally the number of such patients is too few (12,13). One study of great interest was performed by the Western Cancer Study Group (WCG), which randomized between oral and i. v. weekly 5-FU (15). Unfortunately, the 3 patients in one arm and 5 in the other provided no insight into which route of administration was most active.

Table 29 details two ECOG studies that may provide more information on the important prognostic variables and the therapeutic role of radiotherapy, single agents, and combination chemotherapy. Immunotherapy has never been investigated in gallbladder cancer.

Cancer of the extrahepatic bile ducts has been estimated to be only one-half as common as gallbladder cancer (123). A median survival of 5 months (mean 7.2 months) after proof of unresectable disease has been reported in 59 patients (134). The prognostic factors are not well defined, but the location of the tumor within the bile duct system is of great importance to the ease of surgical approach and resectability (31). The best potential for cure lies in tumors of the distal common duct where the procedure of choice is pancreatoduodenectomy. It is still unclear whether or not palliative surgery offers any survival advantage over no procedure, although evidence from uncontrolled studies suggests a considerable extension of survival (202).

TABLE 29. *Ongoing or unpublished trials in gallbladder and bile duct cancer*

| Investigators (reference) and treatment arms | Evaluation criteria[a] |
|---|---|
| ECOG 2273 (47,188) | 2B, 4A(4–6, 19) |
| A. 5-FU (600 mg/m²/d $\times$ 5, d1–5, d36–40 p. o.) | |
| B. 5-FU (as in A) | |
| Streptozotocin (500 mg/m²/d $\times$ 5, d1–5, i. v.) | |
| C. 5-FU (500 mg/m²/d $\times$ 5, d1–5, d36–40 p. o.) | |
| MeCCNU (150 mg/m², d1, p. o.) | |
| ECOG 1274A (188) | 1C, 2B, 4A(1, 5) |
| A. Radiotherapy (4,000 rads) | |
| B. Radiotherapy (4,000 rads) | |
| 5-FU (600 mg/m² i. v., first 3 days of RT; then wkly after RT) | |

[a]See the criteria defined in Fig. 1.

The ECOG studies in Table 29 also include tumors in the extrahepatic bile ducts. Immunotherapy has not been studied.

## MALIGNANT CARCINOID

Nearly 4,000 cases of carcinoid tumors found in many organs have been reported (35). Although these tumors represent only 0.05 to 0.2% of all neoplasms, they account for 0.4 to 1% of all tumors in the gastrointestinal tract (115), where the most common site is the small bowel. The neoplasm is usually indolent and patients have a prolonged course of disease before experiencing real disability (44). The carcinoid syndrome occasionally accompanying this tumor consists of cutaneous flushing, hypotension, intestinal hypermotility, bronchial constriction, and development of endocardial lesions.

The prognostic factors influencing this disease are just beginning to be defined. It is also difficult to differentiate between benign and malignant lesions (115). The likelihood of metastasis appears to be proportional to the size of the primary lesions, with 80% of tumors $\geq$ 2 cm in diameter having metastatic spread compared to only 2% incidence of metastasis in those $<$ 2 cm (137). It is unusual for carcinoid to occur in the absence of liver involvement and with that constellation of symptoms the patient usually has metastatic disease. However, the 5-year survival rate is 57% in patients with inoperable nodal or peritoneal metastases and 31% in those with hepatic metastases (137).

Thus far, surgery is the only curative therapy, but no randomized trials have been performed. In fact, the indolent nature of the disease would require that such trials have a prolonged follow-up to cover the interval between resection and recurrent disease (137). Palliative surgery with bypass of obstructing lesions or resection of hepatic metastases may provide benefit but have not been evaluated in a prospective controlled manner.

Since many patients live a long time after diagnosis, it is difficult to select a time for beginning chemotherapy. However, drug therapy should be withheld until the tumor mass or the carcinoid syndrome begins to cause significant disability or symptoms that cannot be controlled by other means. Both 5-FU (126) and streptozotocin (126,136) have shown some activity in uncontrolled studies and these agents are in use in two nearly completed ECOG studies of carcinoid tumors. The first trial (ECOG 3272) is in advanced carcinoid tumors and randomizes patients to streptozotocin (500 mg/m$^2$/day $\times$ 5 i. v.) plus cyclophosphamide (1 gm/m$^2$ day 1 and 21 i. v.) versus streptozotocin (500 mg/m$^2$/day $\times$ 5 i. v.) plus 5-FU (400 mg/m$^2$/day $\times$ 5 i. v.). The stratification is for prior therapy, functional status of the tumor, site of indicator lesion, and performance status. The second study (ECOG 5272) randomizes previously untreated patients to adriamycin (60 mg/m$^2$ day 1, 22, and 43 i. v.; then q. 4 weeks) versus streptozotocin (500 mg/m$^2$/day $\times$ 5 i. v.) plus 5-FU (400 mg/m$^2$/day $\times$ 5, day 1–5 and day 36–40 i. v., q. 10 weeks). The trial is stratified for prior therapy, functional status of tumor, site of indicator lesion, and performance status.

Neither radiotherapy nor immunotherapy has been tested in a controlled fashion. Obviously, the small number of cases with this tumor type precludes many major studies. However, one chemotherapy trial that is needed would be a comparison of either streptozotocin or 5-FU and the best regimen developed by the ECOG.

## ADENOCARCINOMA OF THE SMALL BOWEL

In contrast to the carcinoid tumors, this uncommon neoplasm occurs most commonly in the proximal small bowel (120). Carcinomas of the duodenum tend to follow a more virulent course than those of the jejunum or ileum. Median survival in duodenal carcinoma is 5 months (mean 5.8 months) compared to 9 months (mean 10.4 months) for carcinomas of the lower small bowel (134). Thus, the site of the tumor would seem an important prognostic factor in designing controlled trials.

There have been no randomized trials in small bowel carcinomas. A few randomized trials in gastrointestinal cancer have included one or two cases that are insufficient to obtain meaningful data (12,13).

## ISLET CELL TUMORS

Neoplasms of the islets of Langerhans are uncommon (22). Most of them are nonfunctional, but they may be active and produce systemic effects ranging from hypoglycemia to uncontrollable diarrhea (22). The prognostic factors have not been identified but should be important because of the variety of diseases and symptoms in this tumor category.

These tumors are usually classified according to cell type, hormone secretion, and associated clinical syndrome. The β-cell tumors or insulinomas, of which 90% are benign adenomas and 10% show metastases, are the most common functional islet cell tumors (174). The α-cell tumors have been associated with secretion of a glucagon-like substance; patients may also have a chronic generalized bullous and eczematoid skin eruption (33). The other non-β-cell tumors have produced the Zollinger–Ellison syndrome, pancreatic cholera, and other endocrine syndromes.

There have been no randomized surgical trials, and none utilizing radiotherapy or immunotherapy. The pharmacologic therapy of these tumors is interesting but will not be discussed. Cytotoxic chemotherapy is a burgeoning area of investigation, particularly since streptozotocin has been found active in these tumors (22,23,95,172,177). The ECOG has an ongoing trial randomized between streptozotocin (500 mg/m²/day × 5, q. 6 weeks) and the same dose of streptozotocin plus 5-FU (400 mg/m²/day × 5, q. 6 wks). Patients are stratified for prior therapy, functional status of the tumor, site of indicator lesion, and performance status.

## CONCLUSIONS

Several issues are apparent in this analysis of randomized trials in gastrointestinal cancer, a heterogeneous group of neoplasms with widely differing natural histories:

1. Therapeutic modalities employed are frequently of a low order of effectiveness.

2. The natural history of some of the tumors (e.g., stomach, pancreas, liver, esophagus, and gallbladder) is so unfavorable that results are marginal in all trials, whether testing single or combined modalities.

3. Conclusions are derived from studies employing small numbers of patients with tumors in several sites of the gastrointestinal tract. When coupled with patient population heterogeneity, they cannot be definitive.

4. Even in common tumors (e.g., colon and rectum), variability of prognostic factors and surgical techniques, and the need for very large test populations, have led to conclusions subject to nonuniform interpretation.

5. It follows that large-scale trials often stop short of statistically significant results because the need for adequate sample size cannot be met. Thus, modest treatment benefit may not be apparent.

6. In the ongoing adjuvant studies there is apparent progressive difficulty in incorporating a control arm of standard treatment. More and more frequently, reliance is being placed on historical controls, which can be expected to introduce severe difficulties in the analysis of results.

In summary, these trials are beset by difficulties—refractory diseases, inadequate therapeutic modalities, and lack of attention to adequate sample size and known prognostic factors. It would seem that future generations of trials in the adjuvant setting should be based on adequate stratification and sample size estimations. Furthermore, the trials should persevere toward adequate accrual so that conclusions can be definitive even when they are negative. Controlled trials in advanced disease also should address these issues or else should be replaced by single activity-seeking trials with realistic analysis. When promising leads are established, definitive comparative trials can then be designed.

## LIST OF COMPOUNDS

*Actinomycin D:* NSC–3053

*Adriamycin:* NSC–123127

*Ara-C:* Cytosine arabinoside, NSC–63878; cytosine, 1-β-D-arabinofuranosyl-, monohydrochloride

*β-2-TGdR:* NSC–71261; 9H-purine-6-thiol, 2-amino-9-(2-deoxy-β-D-erythro-pentofuranosyl)-, monohydrate.

*Baker's Antifol:* NSC–139105

*BCG:* Bacillus Calmette-Guerin (various strains, i.e., Pasteur, Connaught, Glaxo, Tice)

*BCNU:* NSC–409962; urea, 1,3-bis(2-chloroethyl)-1-nitroso-

*Bleomycin:* NSC–125066; [2,4'-bithiazole]-4-carboxylic acid, 2'-(2-aminoethyl)-, monohydrate

*CCNU:* NSC–79037; urea, 1-(2-chloroethyl)-3-cyclohexyl-1-nitroso-

*Chromomycin $A_3$:* NSC–58514

*Colchamine:* NSC–403147; Colchicine, N-deacetyl-N-methyl-

*C. parvum;* Corynebacterium parvum (various strains, i.e., Merieux, Burroughs–Wellcome)

*CTX:* Cyclophosphamide; NSC–26271; 2H-1,3,2-oxazaphosphorine, 2-[bis(2-chloroethyl)amino]tetrahydro-, 2-oxide, monohydrate

*Cytembena:* NSC–104801; acrylic acid, 3-p-anisoyl-3-bromo-, sodium salt

*Diglycoaldehyde:* NSC–118994

*DTIC:* NSC–45388; imidazole-4-carboxamide, 5-(3,3-dimethyl-1-triazeno)-

*Fluorometholone:* NSC–33001; Pregna-1,4-diene-3, 20-dione, 9-fluoro-11β, 17-dihydroxy-6α methyl-

*Fluoxymesterone:* NSC–12165; androst-4-en-3-one, 9-fluoro-11β,17β-dihydroxy-17-methyl-

*Ftorafur:* NSC–148958; uracil, 5-fluoro-1(tetrahydro-2-furyl)-

*5-FU:* 5-fluorouracil, NSC–19893

*5-FUDR:* NSC–27640; uridine, 5-fluoro-2'-deoxy-

*Galactitol:* Diannhydrogalactitol, NSC–132313

*Hexamethylmelamine:* NSC–13875

*Hydroxyurea:* NSC–32065

*ICRF-159:* NSC–129943; 2,6-piperazinedione, 4,4'-propylenedi-, (±)-

*Leucovorin:* Citrovorum factor; folinic acid; glutamic acid, N-[p-[[(2-amino-5-formyl-5, 6, 7, 8-tetrahydro-4-hydroxy-6-pteridinyl)-methyl]amino]benzoyl]-, calcium salt

*Levamisole:* NSC–177023; imidazo [2,1-6] thiazole, 2,3,5,6-tetrahydro-6-phenyl-, monohydrochloride

L-*PAM:* Melphalan, NSC–8806; alanine, 3-[p-[bis(2-chloroethyl)amino]phenyl]-, monohydrochloride, L-

*MeCCNU:* Methyl CCNU, NSC–95441; urea, 1-(2-chloroethyl)-3-(4-methyl-cyclohexyl)-1-nitroso-

*MER-BCG:* NSC–143769, Methanol Extraction residue of BCG

*Methyl GAG:* NSC–32946; guanidine, 1,1'-[(methylethanediylidene)dinitrilo]di-, dihydrochloride, monohydrate

*Mitomycin C:* NSC–26980

*MTX:* Methotrexate, NSC–740; glutamic acid, N-[p-[[(2,4-diamino-6-pteridinyl)methyl]methylamino]benzoyl]-

*Nitrogen mustard:* Mechlorethamine, NSC–762; diethylamine, 2,-2'-dichloro-N-methyl-, hydrochloride

*Porfiromycin:* NSC–56410; methyl mitomycin C

*Procarbazine:* NSC–77213; p-toluamide, N-isopropyl-α-(2-methylhydrazino)-, monohydrochloride

*Spironolactone:* NSC–150399; 17α-pregn-4-ene-21-carboxylic acid, 17-hydroxy-7α-mercapto-3-oxo-, γ-lactone, acetate

*Streptozotocin:* NSC–85998

*Testolactone:* NSC–23759; 1-phenanthrenepropionic acid, 1,2,3,4,4a,4b,7,9,10 α-decahydro-2-hydroxy-2,4b-dimethyl-7-oxo, δ-lactone

*6-Thioguanine:* NSC–752; purine-6-thiol, 2-amino-

*Thiotepa:* NSC–6396; phosphine sulfide, tris(1-aziridinyl)-

*Tubercidin:* NSC–56408

*Uracil mustard:* NSC–34462; 5[bis-(2-chlorethyl)amino] uracil

*VCR:* Vincristine, NSC–67574

*VP-16:* VP 16–213, NSC–141540; 4'-demethylpipodophyllotoxin 9-(4,6-O-ethylidene-β-D-glucopyranoside)

## REFERENCES

1. Akakura, I., Nakamura, Y., Kakegawa, T., Nakayama, R., Watanabe, H., and Yamashita, H. (1970): Surgery of carcinoma of the esophagus with preoperative radiation. *Chest,* 57:47–57.
2. American Cancer Society (1920): *Cancer Facts and Figures.* ACS, New York.
3. Ansfield, F. J. (1975): A randomized phase III study of four dosage regimens of 5-fluorouracil: A preliminary report. *Proc. Am. Assoc. Cancer Res.,* 16:224 (Abst. 1014).
4. Ansfield, F. J., Klotz, J., Nealon, T., Ramirez, G., Minton, J., Hill, G., Wilson, W., Davis, H., and Cornell, G. (1977): A phase III study comparing the clinical utility of four regimens of 5-fluorouracil: A preliminary report. *Cancer,* 39:34–40.
5. Ansfield, F. J., Ramirez, G., Davis, H. L., Jr., Wirtanen, G. W., Johnson, R. O., Bryan, G. T., Manalo, F. B., Borden, E. C., Davis, T. E., and Esmaili, M. (1975): Further clinical studies with intrahepatic arterial infusion with 5-fluorouracil. *Cancer,* 36:2413–2417.
6. Ansfield, F. J., Schroeder, J. M., and Curreri, A. R. (1962): Five years clinical experience with 5-fluorouracil. *JAMA,* 181:295–299.
7. Asakawa, H., Gtawa, K., and Watarai, J. (1972): Treatment of cancer of the esophagus with a combination of radiation and bleomycin. *Gan No Rinsho Jap. J. Cancer Clin.,* 18:311–316.

8. Astler, V. B., and Coller, F. A. (1954): The prognostic significance of direct extension of carcinoma of the colon and rectum. *Ann. Surg.*, 139:846–852.
9. Axtell, L. M., Cutler, S. J., and Meyers, M. H. (1972): End Results in Cancer, Report No. 4. *DHEW Publication NIH 73–272.* National Institutes of Health, Bethesda, Md.
10. Baker, L. H. (1977): Personal communication.
11. Baker, L. H., Izbicki, R. M., and Vaitkevicius, V. K. (1976): Phase II study of porfiromycin vs. mitomycin C utilizing acute intermittent schedules. *Med. Ped. Oncol.*, 2:207–213.
12. Baker, L. H., Talley, R. W., Matter, R., Lehane, D. E., Ruffner, B. W., Jones, S. E., Morrison, F. S., Stephens, R. L., Gehan, E. A., and Vaitkevicius, V. K. (1976): Phase II comparison of the treatment of advanced gastrointestinal cancer with bolus weekly 5-FU vs. methyl-CCNU plus bolus weekly 5-FU. *Cancer*, 38:1–7.
13. Baker, L. H., Vaitkevicius, V. K., Gehan, E., and the Gastrointestinal Committee of the Southwest Oncology Group (1976): Randomized prospective trial comparing 5-fluorouracil (NSC 19893) to 5-fluorouracil and methyl-CCNU (NSC 95441) in advanced gastrointestinal cancer. *Cancer Treatment Rep.*, 60:733–737.
14. Bateman, J., Irwin, L., Pugh, R., Cassidy, F., and Weiner, J. (1975): Comparison of intravenous (IV) and oral (PO) administration of 5-fluorouracil for colorectal carcinoma. *Proc. Am. Soc. Clin. Oncol.*, 16:242 (Abst. 1087).
15. Bateman, J. R., Pugh, R. P., Cassidy, F. R., Marshall, G. J., and Irwin, L. E. (1971): 5-Fluorouracil given once weekly: Comparison of intravenous and oral administration. *Cancer*, 28:907–913.
16. Baylor, S. M., and Berg, J. W. (1973): Cross-classification and survival characteristics of 5,000 cases of cancer of the pancreas. *J. Surg. Oncology*, 5:335–358.
17. Beahrs, O. H. (1974): Status of fulguration and cryosurgery in the management of colonic and rectal cancer and polyps. *Cancer*, 34:965–968.
18. Beahrs, O. H., and Sanfelippo, P. M. (1971): Factors in prognosis of colon and rectal cancer. *Cancer*, 28:213–218.
19. Blokhina, N. G., Garin, A. M., Lipatov, A. M., Karev, N. I., Voznysi, E. K., Bousion, V. I., Koralchuk, V. P., Kuchharw, P. N., Scharenhov, V. A., and Sokolov, V. N. (1974): Results of 5 yr. observations of patients receiving 5-fluorouracil after radical surgery for carcinoma of colon and rectum. *Proc. Second All-Union Cancer Chemother. Conf. Kiev.* pp. 243–244.
20. Blokhina, N. G., Garin, A. M., Moroz, L. V., Pershin, M. P., Chumakina, S. I., Gunka, Iu. I., Pantophel, A. M., Steklenev, N. A., Zirin, M. A., Grjaznova, I. N., Shain, A. A., Pecherskaja, B. G., Saveliev, N. P., Bashirova, N. G., Kuzmin, V. P., Budarina, E. M., Svedencov, E. P., Phateeva, K. V., Iunusmetov, I. R., Silitrin, N. P., Shklovskii, G. S., Balas, A. N., and Ushivoeva, A. E. (1972): Treatment with 5-fluorouracil in prophylaxis of relapses and metastases of stomach cancer. *Neoplasma*, 19:351–356.
21. Boles, R. L. (1958): Cancer of the stomach. *Gastroenterology*, 34:847–858.
22. Broder, L. E., and Carter, S. K. (1973): Pancreatic islet cell carcinoma. I. Clinical features of 52 patients. *Ann. Intern. Med.*, 79:101–107.
23. Broder, L. E., and Carter, S. K. (1973): Pancreatic islet cell carcinoma. II. Results of treatment with streptozotocin in 52 patients. *Ann. Intern. Med.*, 79:108–118.
24. Buckwalter, J. A., Jr., and Kent, T. H. (1973): Prognosis and surgical pathology of carcinoma of the colon. *Surg. Gynec. Obstet.*, 136:465–472.
25. Bullen, B. R., Giles, G. R., Malhotra, A., Bird, G. G., Hall, R., Bunch, G. A., and Brown, G. J. A. (1976): Randomized comparison of melphalan and 5-fluorouracil in the treatment of advanced gastrointestinal cancer. *Cancer Treatment Rep.*, 60:1267–1271.
26. Cady, B., Monson, D. O., and Swinton, N. W. (1970): Survival of patients after colonic resection for carcinoma with simultaneous liver metastases. *Surg. Gynec. Obstet.*, 131:697–700.
27. Cady, B., and Oberfield, R. A. (1974): Regional infusion chemotherapy of hepatic metastases from carcinoma of the colon. *Am. J. Surg.*, 127:220–227.
28. Cancer Statistics 1976 (1976): *CA, A Journal for Clinicians*, 26:14–29.
29. Carter, S. K. (1976): Large bowel cancer—The current status of treatment. *J. Natl. Cancer Inst.*, 56:3–10.
30. Carter, S. K., and Comis, R. L. (1975): Adenocarcinoma of the pancreas: Current therapeutic approaches, prognostic variables, and criteria of response. In: *Cancer Therapy: Prognostic Factors and Criteria of Response*, edited by M. J. Staquet, pp. 237–253. Raven Press, New York.

31. Carter, S. K., and Comis, R. L. (1975): The integration of chemotherapy into a combined modality approach for cancer treatment. VI. Pancreatic adenocarcinoma. *Cancer. Treatment Rev.*, 2:193–214.
32. Carter, S. K., and Friedman, M. (1974): Integration of chemotherapy into combined modality treatment of solid tumors. II. Large bowel carcinoma. *Cancer Treatment Rev.*, 1:111–129.
33. Case Records of the Massachusetts General Hospital (1975): 292:1117–1123.
34. Cavanaugh, P. J. (1975): Considerations appropriate to a clinical trial of definitive radiation therapy in adenocarcinoma of the pancreas. *J. Surg. Oncology*, 7:135–137.
35. Cheek, R. C., and Wilson, H. (1970): Carcinoid tumors. *Curr. Probl. Surg.*, Nov.:4–31.
36. Childs, D. S., Jr. (1969): Role of the radiation therapist in palliative management. In: *Advanced Gastrointestinal Cancer/Clinical Management and Chemotherapy*, edited by C. G. Moertel, and R. J. Reitemeier, pp. 58–62. Hoeber Medical Division, Harper & Row, New York.
37. Childs, D. S., Jr., Moertel, C. G., Holbrook, M. A., Reitemeier, R. J., and Colby, M. Y., Jr. (1965): Treatment of malignant neoplasms of the gastrointestinal tract with a combination of 5-fluorouracil and radiation. *Radiology*, 84:843–845.
38. Childs, D. S., Jr., Moertel, C. G., Holbrook, M. A., Reitemeier, R. J., and Colby, M., Jr. (1968): Treatment of unresectable adenocarcinomas of the stomach with a combination of 5-fluorouracil and radiation. *Radiology*, 102:541–544.
39. Clinical Biometry Section, National Cancer Institute. (1964): *End Results in Cancer, Report No. 2.* U.S. Public Health Service, National Institutes of Health, Bethesda, Md.
40. Compendium of Tumor Immunotherapy Protocols. International Registry of Tumor Immunotherapy, August 1976.
41. Controlled Therapeutic Trials in Cancer (1974): *IUCC Technical Report Series*, Geneva, 14:69–72.
42. Copeland, E. M., Miller, L. D., and Jones, R. S. (1968): Prognostic factors in carcinoma of the colon and rectum. *Am. J. Surg.*, 116:875–881.
43. Crile, G., Jr. (1970): The advantages of bypass operation over radical pancreaticoduodenectomy in the treatment of pancreatic carcinoma. *Surg. Gynec. Obstet.*, 130:1049–1053.
44. Davis, Z., Moertel, C. G., McIlrath, D. C., and Adson, M. A. (1973): The malignant carcinoid syndrome. *Surg. Gynecol. Obstet.*, 137:637–644.
45. Depeyster, F. A., and Gilchrist, R. K. (1969): Pathology and manifestations of cancer of the colon and rectum. In: *Diseases of the Colon and Anorectum*, edited by R. Turrel, pp. 428–452. W. B. Saunders Co., Philadelphia.
46. Dixon, W. J., Longmire, W. P., and Holden, W. (1971): Use of triethylenethiophosphamide as an adjuvant to the surgical treatment of gastric and colorectal carcinoma—ten-year follow-up. *Ann. Surg.*, 173:26–39.
47. Douglass, H. O., Jr., Lavin, P. T., and Moertel, C. G. (1976): Nitrosoureas: Useful agents for the treatment of advanced gastrointestinal cancer. *Cancer Treatment Rep.*, 60:769–770.
48. Douglass, H. O., Jr., and Moertel, C. (1976): Chemotherapy of previously treated colorectal adenocarcinoma with Methyl CCNU or Beta-2'-deoxythioguanosine (BTGdR). A phase II-III study of ECOG. *Proc. Am. Soc. Clin. Oncol.*, 17:306 (Abst. C278).
49. Dowdy, G. S., Jr. (1969): *The Biliary Tract*, pp. 165–169. Lea & Febiger, Philadelphia.
50. Dukes, C. E. (1932): The classification of cancer of the rectum. *J. Pathol. Bacteriol.*, 35:323–332.
51. Duncan, W., and Smith, A. N. (1976): Preoperative radiotherapy in rectal cancer. *Lancet*, 2:364–365.
52. Dwight, R. W., Higgins, G. A., and Keehn, R. J. (1969): Factors influencing survival after resection in cancer of the colon and rectum. *Am. J. Surg.*, 117:512–522.
53. Dwight, R. W., Humphrey, E. W., Higgins, G. A., and Keehn, R. J. (1973): FUDR as an adjuvant to surgery in cancer of the large bowel. *J. Surg. Oncol.*, 5:243–249.
54. Eastern Cooperative Group in Solid Tumor Chemotherapy (1967): Comparison of antimetabolites in the treatment of breast and colon cancer. *JAMA* 200:770–780.
55. Engstrom, P. F., Paul, A. R., Cutalano, R. B., Mastrangelo, M. J., and Creech, R. J. (1978): Fluoracil vs fluorouracil + Bacillus Calmette-Guerin in colorectal adenocarcinoma. In: *Immunotherapy of Cancer: Present Status of Trials in Man*, edited by W. D. Terry and D. Windhorst, pp. 587–596. Raven Press, New York.
56. Falkson, G. (1971): Methyl-CAG (NSC 32946) in the treatment of esophagus cancer. *Cancer Chemother. Rep.*, 55:209–212.
57. Falkson, G., and Falkson, H. C. (1976): Fluorouracil, methyl-CCNU and vincristine in cancer of the colon. *Cancer*, 38:1468–1470.

58. Falkson, G., Moertel, C. G., and Lavin, P. J. (1976): Chemotherapy of primary liver carcinoma, a parallel study in American and African Bantu patients. *Proc. Am. Assoc. Cancer Res.,* 17:21.
59. Falkson, G., Van Eden, E. B., and Falkson, H. C. (1974): Fluorouracil, imidazole carboxamide dimethyl triageno, vincristine and bis-chloroethyl nitrosourea in colon cancer. *Cancer,* 33:1207–1209.
60. Falkson, G., Van Eden, E. B., and Sandison, A. G. (1976): A controlled clinical trial of fluorouracil plus imidazole carboxamide dimethyl triazeno plus vincristine plus bis-choroethyl nitrosourea plus radiotherapy in stomach cancer. *Med. Pediatr. Oncol.,* 2:111–117.
61. Falterman, K. W., Hill, C. B., Markey, J. C., Fox, J. W., and Cohn, I., Jr. (1974): Cancer of the colon, rectum and anus: A review of 2313 cases. *Cancer,* 34:951–959.
62. Forrest, A. P. M., and Buchan, R. (1972): Advances in surgery. *Practitioner,* 209:424–436.
63. Fortuny, I. E., Theologides, A., and Kennedy, B. J. (1975): Hepatic arterial infusion for liver metastases from colon cancer: Comparison of mitomycin C (NSC 26980) and 5-fluorouracil (NSC 19893). *Cancer Chemother. Rep.,* 59:401–404.
64. Frytak, S., Moertel, C. G., Schutt, A. J., Hahn, R. G., and Reitemeier, R. G. (1975): Adriamycin (NSC 123127) therapy for advanced gastrointestinal cancer. *Cancer Chemother. Rep.,* 59:405–409.
65. Gailani, S., Holland, J. F., Falkson, G., Leone, L., Burningham, R., and Larsen, V. (1972): Comparison of treatment of metastatic gastrointestinal cancer with 5-fluorouracil (5-FU) to a combination of 5-FU with cytosine arabinoside. *Cancer,* 29:1308–1313.
66. Gehan, E. A., and Freireich, E. J. (1974): Nonrandomized controls in cancer clinical trials. *N. Engl. J. Med.,* 290:198–203.
67. Gerard, A. (1975): Carcinoma of the colon and rectum: Prognostic factors and criteria of response. In: *Cancer Therapy: Prognostic Factors and Criteria of Response,* edited by M. J. Staquet, pp. 199–227. Raven Press, New York.
68. Go, V. L. W. (1976): Carcinoembryonic antigen-clinical application. *Cancer,* 37:562–566.
69. Gold, P., and Freedman, S. O. (1965): Demonstration of tumor specific antigens in human colonic carcinoma by immunological tolerance and absorption techniques. *J. Exp. Med.,* 121:439–462.
70. Gold, G. L., Shnider, B. I., Salvin, L. G., Schneiderman, M. A., Colsky, J., Owens, A. H., Jr., Krant, M. J., Miller, S. P., Frei, E., III, Hall, T. C., Spurr, C. L., McIntyre, O. R., Hoogstraten, B., and Holland, J. F. (1970): The use of mechlorethamine, cyclophosphamide and uracil mustard in neoplastic disease: A cooperative study. *J. Clin. Pharm.,* 10:110–120.
71. Goodner, J. T. (1974): Surgical principles of resection and reconstruction in current concepts in cancer number 42 cancer of the gastrointestial tract II esophagus treatment—localized and advanced. *JAMA,* 227:176–178.
72. Grage, T., Cornell, G., Strawitz, J., Jonas, K., Frelick, R., and Metter, G. (1975): Adjuvant therapy 5-FU after surgical resection of colorectal cancer. *Proc. Am. Soc. Clin. Oncol.,* 16:258 (Abst. 1149).
73. Grossi, G. F., Wolff, W., Nealon, T. F., Jr., Pasternack, B., Ginzburg, L., and Rousselot, L. M. (1975): Intraluminal and intravenous 5-FU chemotherapy adjuvant to surgery for resectable colorectal cancer: A clinical cooperative multihospital project. *Chir. Gastroenterol.,* 9:61–68.
74. Gullick, H. D. (1959): Carcinoma of the pancreas: A review and clinical study of 100 cases. *Medicine* (Baltimore), 38:47–84.
75. Gunnlaugsson, G. H., Wychulis, A. R., Roland, C., and Ellis, F. H., Jr. (1970): Analysis of the records of 1657 patients with carcinoma of the esophagus and cardia of the stomach. *Surg. Gynec. Obstet.,* 130:997–1005.
76. Haenszel, W. (1958): Variation in incidence of and mortality from stomach cancer, with particular reference to the United States. *J. Natl. Cancer Inst.,* 21:213–262.
77. Hahn, R. G., Moertel, C. G., Schutt, A. J., and Bruckner, H. W. (1975): A double blind comparison of intensive course 5-fluorouracil by oral vs intravenous route in the treatment of colorectal carcinoma. *Cancer,* 35:1031–1035.
78. Haslam, T. B., Cavanaugh, P. J., and Stroup, S. L. (1973): Radiation therapy in the treatment of irresectable adenocarcinoma of the pancreas. *Cancer,* 32:1341–1345.
79. Hertz, R. F. L., Deddish, M. R., and Day, E. (1960): Value of periodic examinations in detecting cancer of the rectum and colon. *Postgrad. Med.,* 27:290–294.
80. Higgins, G. A. (1976): Chemotherapy. Adjuvant to surgery for gastrointestinal cancer. *Clin. Gastroenterol.,* 5:795–808.

81. Higgins, G. A., Jr., Conn, J. H., Jordan, P. H., Jr., Humphrey, E. W., Roswit, B., and Keehn, R. J. (1975): Preoperative radiotherapy for colorectal cancer. *Ann. Surg.,* 181:624–631.
82. Higgins, G. A., Dwight, R. W., Smith, J. V., and Keehn, R. J. (1971): Fluorouracil as an adjuvant to surgery in carcinoma of the colon. *Arch. Surg.,* 102:339–343.
83. Higgins, G. A., Jr., Humphrey, E., Juler, G. L., LaVeen, H. H., McCaughan, J., and Keehn, R. J. (1976): Adjuvant chemotherapy in the surgical treatment of large bowel cancer. *Cancer,* 38:1461–1467.
84. Higgins, G. A., Serlin, O., Hughes, F., and Dwight, R. W. (1962): The Veterans Administration Surgical Adjuvant Group-Interim Report. *Cancer Chemother. Rep.,* 16:141–148.
85. Holden, W. D., Dixon, W. J., and Kuzma, J. W. (1967): The use of triethylene-thiophosphoramide as an adjuvant to the surgical treatment of colorectal carcinoma. *Ann. Surg.,* 165:481–503.
86. Holsti, L. R. (1969): Clinical experience with split-course radiotherapy. A randomized clinical trial. *Radiology,* 92:591–596.
87. Horton, J., Mittelman, A., Taylor, S. G. III, Jurkowitz, L., Bennett, J. M., Ezdinli, E., Colsky, J., and Hanley, J. A. (1975): Phase II trials with procarbazine (NSC 77213), streptozotocin (NSC 85998), 6-thioguanine (NSC 752) and CCNU (NSC 79037) in patients with metastatic cancer of the large bowel. *Cancer Chemother. Rep.,* 59:333–340.
88. Horton, J., Olson, K. B., Cunningham, T., and Sullivan, J. (1968): Comparison of a combination of 5-fluorouracil (NSC 19893), mitomycin C (NSC 26980), triethylenethiophosphoramide (NSC 6396) and fluoxymesterone (NSC 12165) with 5-fluorouracil alone in patients with advanced cancer. *Cancer Chemother. Rep.,* 52:597–600.
89. Horton, J., Olson, K. B., Sullivan, J., Reilly, C., Shnider, B., and the Eastern Cooperative Oncology Group. (1970): Fluorouracil in cancer: An improved regimen. *Ann. Intern. Med.,* 73:897–900.
90. Howard, J. M., and Jordan, G. L. (1960): *Surgical Diseases of the Pancreas,* p. 449. J. B. Lippencott Co., Philadelphia and Montreal.
91. International Union Against Cancer Controlled Therapeutic Trials in Cancer. Geneva, 1974.
92. Jacobsson, F. (1951): Carcinoma of hypopharynx. A clinical study of 332 cases treated at Radiumhemmet from 1939 to 1947. *Acta Radiol.,* 35:1–21.
93. Jaffe, B. M., Donegan, W. L., Watson, F., and Spratt, J. S., Jr., (1968): Factors influencing survival in patients with untreated hepatic metastases. *Surg. Gynec. Obstet.,* 127:1–11.
94. James, A. G. (1966): *Cancer Prognosis Manual,* 2nd ed., p. 53. American Cancer Society, New York.
95. Kahn, C. R., Levy, A. G., Gardner, J. D., Miller, J. V., Gordon, P., and Schein, P. S. (1975): Pancreatic cholera: Beneficial effects of treatment with streptozotocin. *N. Engl. J. Med.,* 292:941–945.
96. Kim, R. H., Ross, S. T., Li, M. C. (1975): Chemoprophylaxis for patients with colorectal cancer. Prospective study with 5-year follow-up. *Proc. Am. Assoc. Cancer Res.,* 16:231 (Abst. 1040).
97. Kligerman, M. M. (1975): Irradiation of the primary lesion of the rectum and rectosigmoid. *JAMA,* 231:1381–1384.
98. Kligerman, M. M., Urdaneta, N., Knowlton, A., Vidone, R., Hartman, P. V., and Vera, R. (1972): Preoperative irradiation of rectosigmoid carcinoma including its regional lymph nodes. *Am. J. Roetgenol. Radium Ther. Nucl. Med.,* 114:498–503.
99. Kovach, J. S., Moertel, C. G., Schutt, A. J., Hahn, R. G., and Reitemeier, R. J. (1974): A controlled study of combined 1,3-bis-(2-chloroethyl)-1-nitrosourea and 5-fluorouracil therapy for advanced gastric and pancreatic cancer. *Cancer,* 33:563–567.
100. Kovach, J. S., Moertel, C. G., Schutt, A. J., Reitemeier, R. G., and Hahn, R. G. (1973): Phase II study of cis-diaminedichloroplatinum (NSC 119875) in advanced carcinoma of the large bowel. *Cancer Chemother. Rep.,* 57:357–359.
101. Krain, L. S. (1970): The rising incidence of carcinoma of the pancreas. *Am. J. Gastroenterol.,* 54:500–506.
102. Krayhill, W. G., Jr., Anderson, D. D., Lindell, T. D., and Fletcher, W. S. (1976): Effective therapy with 5-fluorouracil, streptozotocin, and tubercidin. *Amer. Surg.,* 42:467–470.
103. Kuttig, H., and Sunaric, D. (1966): Vergleich der ergebisse nach strahlentherapie des osophaguskarzinoms mit konventioneelen rontgen and $Co^{60}$ gammastrahlen. *Strahlentherapie,* 129:341–347.

104. Larionov, L. F., and Chudakova, M. A. (1963): The use of sarcolysin in combination with colchamine in the treatment of esophageal cancer. *Vop. Onkol.,* 9:3.
105. Lawrence, W., Jr., Terz, J. J., Horsley, S., III, Donaldson, M., Lovett, W. L., Brown, P. W., Ruffner, B. W., Regelson, W. (1975): Chemotherapy as an adjuvant to surgery for colorectal cancer. *Ann. Surg.,* 181:616–623.
106. Le Roux, B. T. (1962): The influence of resection on the natural history of carcinoma of the hypopharynx esophagus and proximal stomach. *Surg. Gynecol. Obstet.,* 115:162–170.
107. Longmire, W. P., Jr., Kuzma, J. W., and Dixon, W. J. (1968): The use of triethylene-thiophosphoramide as an adjuvant to the surgical treatment of gastric carcinoma. *Ann. Surg.,* 167:293–312.
108. Mackman, S., Ansfield, F. J., Ramirez, G., and Curreri, A. R. (1974): A second look at the second look operation in colonic cancer after the administration of fluorouracil. *Am. J. Surg.,* 128:763–766.
109. MacLennan, G., Stogryn, R. D., and Voitk, A. J. (1976): Abdominoperineal resection: Treatment of choice for carcinoma of the rectum. *Cancer,* 38:953–956.
110. Malt, R. A., Van Vroonhoven, T. J., and Kakumoto, Y. (1972): Manifestations and prognosis of carcinoma of the liver. *Surg. Gynecol. Obstet.,* 35:361–364.
111. Martin, E. W., Jr., Kibbey, W. E., DiVecchia, L., Anderson, G., Catalano, P., and Minton, J. P. (1976): Carcinoembryonic antigen-clinical and historical aspects. *Cancer,* 37:62–81.
112. Mavligit, G. M., Burgess, M. A., Siebert, G. B., Jubert, A. V., McBride, C. M., Gehan, E. A., Gutterman, J. U., Khankhanian, N., Speer, J. F., Martin, R. C., Copeland, E. M., and Hersh, E. M. (1976): Prolongation of postoperative disease-free interval and survival in human colorectal cancer by BCG or BCG plus 5-fluorouracil. *Lancet,* 1:871–876.
113. Mavligit, G. M., Gutterman, J. V., Malahy, M. A., Burgess, M. A., McBride, C. M., Jubert, A., and Hersh, E. M. (1976): Systemic adjuvant immunotherapy and chemoimmunotherapy in patients with colorectal cancer (Dukes' C class). Prolongation of disease-free interval and survival. In: *Immunotherapy of Cancer: Present Status of Trials in Man,* edited by W. D. Terry and D. Windhorst, pp. 597–603. Raven Press, New York.
114. McDermott, W. V., Jr., and Bartlett, M. K. (1953): Pancreaticoduodenal cancer. *New Engl. J. Med.* 248:927–931.
115. Mengel, C. E., and Shaffer, R. D. (1973): The carcinoid syndrome. In: *Cancer Medicine,* edited by J. F. Holland, and E. Frei, pp. 1584–1594. Lea & Febiger, Philadelphia.
116. Miller, F. E., and Liechty, R. D. (1967): Adenocarcinoma of the colon and rectum in persons under thirty years of age. *Am. J. Surg.,* 113:507–510.
117. Miller, L. S. (1973): In: *Textbook of Radiotherapy,* edited by G. H. Fletcher, p. 606. Lea & Febiger, Philadelphia.
118. Moertel, C. G. (1969): In: *Advanced Gastrointestinal Cancer/Clinical Management and Chemotherapy,* edited by C. G. Moertel and R. J. Reitemeier, pp. 3–14. Hoeber Medical Division, Harper & Row Publishers, New York.
119. Moertel, C. G. (1973): Cancer of the large bowel. In: *Cancer Medicine,* edited by J. F. Holland, and E. Frei, pp. 1597–1627. Lea & Febiger, Philadelphia.
120. Moertel, C. G. (1973): Small intestine. In: *Cancer Medicine,* edited by J. F. Holland and E. Frei, pp. 1579–1580. Lea & Febiger, Philadelphia.
121. Moertel, C. G., (1973): The esophagus. In: *Cancer Medicine,* edited by J. F. Holland, and E. Frei, pp. 1519–1526. Lea & Febiger, Philadelphia.
122. Moertel, C. G. (1973): Therapy of advanced gastrointestinal cancer with the nitrosoureas. *Cancer Chemother. Rep.,* 4(3):27–34.
123. Moertel, C. G. (1974): In: *Cancer Medicine,* edited by J. F. Holland and E. Frei, p. 1549. Lea & Febiger, Philadelphia.
124. Moertel, C. G. (1974): In: *Cancer Medicine,* edited by J. F. Holland and E. Frei, pp. 1559–1590. Lea & Febiger, Philadelphia.
125. Moertel, C. G. (1975): Carcinoma of the stomach: Prognostic factors and criteria of response to therapy. In: *Cancer Therapy: Prognostic Factors and Criteria of Response,* edited by M. J. Staquet. Raven Press, New York.
126. Moertel, C. G. (1975): Clinical management of advanced gastrointestinal cancer. *Cancer,* 36:675–682.
127. Moertel, C. G. (1976): Fluorouracil as an adjuvant to colorectal cancer surgery: The breakthrough that never was. *JAMA,* 236:1935–1936.

128. Moertel, C. G., Ahmann, D. L., Taylor, W. F., and Schwartau, N. (1971): Aspirin and pancreatic cancer pain. *Gastroenterology,* 60:552–553.
129. Moertel, C. G., Childs, D. S., Jr., Reitemeier, R. J., Colby, M. Y., Jr., and Holbrook, M. A. (1969): Combined 5-fluorouracil and supervoltage radiation therapy of locally unresectable gastrointestinal cancer. *Lancet,* 2:865–867.
130. Moertel, C. G., and Hanley, J. A. (1965): Phase II-III studies in chemotherapy of advanced gastric cancer. *Proc. Am. Assoc. Cancer Res.,* 16:260.
131. Moertel, C. G., Lokich, J. J., Childs, D. S., Jr., and Lavin, P. T. (1976): An evaluation of high dose radiation and combined radiation and 5-fluorouracil (5-FU) therapy for locally unresectable pancreatic carcinoma. *Proc. Am. Assoc. Cancer Res.,* 17:244.
132. Moertel, C. G., Mittleman, J. A., Bakemeier, R. F., Engstrom, P., and Hanley, J. (1976): Sequential and combination chemotherapy of advanced gastric cancer. *Cancer,* 38:678–682.
133. Moertel, C. G., O'Connell, M. J., Ritts, R. E., Jr., Schut, A. J., Reitemeier, R. J., Hahn, R. G., and Frytak, S. K. (1976): A controlled evaluation of combined immunotherapy (MER-BCG) and chemotherapy for advanced colorectal cancer. In: *Immunotherapy of Cancer: Present Status of Trials in Man,* edited by W. D. Terry and D. Windhorst, pp. 573–586. Raven Press, New York.
134. Moertel, C. G., and Reitemeier, R. J. (1969): *Advanced Gastrointestinal Cancer/Clinical Management and Chemotherapy.* Harper & Row, New York.
135. Moertel, C. G., Reitemeier, R. J., and Hahn, R. G. (1967): A controlled comparison of 5-fluoro-2'-deoxyuridine therapy administered by rapid intravenous injection and by continuous intravenous infusion. *Cancer Res.,* 27:549–552.
136. Moertel, C. G., Reitemeier, R. J., Schutt, A. J., and Hahn, R. G. (1971): Phase II study of streptozotocin (NSC-85998) in the treatment of advanced gastrointestinal cancer. *Cancer Chemother. Rep.,* 55:303–307.
137. Moertel, C. G., Sayer, W. G., Dockerty, M. B., and Baggenstoss, A. H. (1961): Life history of the carcinoid tumor of the small intestine. *Cancer,* 14:901–912.
138. Moertel, C. G., Schutt, A. J., Hahn, R. G., and Reitemeier, R. J. (1974): Effects of patient selection on results of phase II chemotherapy trials in gastrointestinal cancer. *Cancer Chemother. Rep.,* 58:257–259.
139. Moertel, C. G., Schutt, A. J., Hahn, R. G., and Reitemeier, R. J. (1975): Therapy of advanced colorectal cancer with a combination of 5-fluorouracil, methyl-1,3-cis(2 chlorethyl)-1-nitrosourea and vincristine. *J. Natl. Cancer Inst.,* 54:69–71.
140. Moertel, C. G., Schutt, A. J., Reitemeier, R. J., and Hahn, R. G. (1972): A comparison of 5-fluorouracil administered by slow infusion and rapid injection. *Cancer Res.,* 32:2717–2719.
141. Moertel, C. G., Schutt, A. J., Reitemeier, R. J., and Hahn, R. G. (1974): 100% oxygen inhalation and 5-fluorouracil (NSC 19893). Therapy for large bowel carcinoma. *Cancer Chemother. Rep.,* 58:951–952.
142. Moertel, C. G., Schutt, A. J., Reitemeier, R. J., and Hahn, R. G. (1976): Therapy for gastrointestinal cancer with the nitrosoureas alone and in drug combination. *Cancer Treatment Rep.,* 60:729–732.
143. Monge, J. J., Judd, E. S., and Gage, R. P. (1964): Radical pancreaticoduodenectomy: A 22-year experience with the complications, mortality rate, and survival rate. *Ann. Surg.,* 160:711–722.
144. Mrazek, R., Economou, S., McDonald, G. O., Slaughter, D. P., and Cole, W. H. (1959): Prophylactic and adjuvant use of nitrogen mustard in the surgical treatment of cancer. *Ann. Surg.,* 150:745–755.
145. Nakayama, K., Orihata, H., and Yamaguchi, K. (1967): Surgical treatment combined with preoperative concentrated irradiation for esophageal cancer. *Cancer,* 20:778–788.
146. Nayera, M. E., and White, R. R., III (1973): Carcinoma of the pancreas. *Arch. Surg.,* 106:293–294.
147. Nelson, C. S. (1972): Chemotherapy as the definitive form of therapy in esophageal carcinoma. *J. Thoracic Cardiovasc. Surg.,* 63:827–837.
148. Nevin, J. E., Moran, T. J., Kay, S., and King, R. (1976): Carcinoma of the gallbladder. Staging, treatment, and prognosis. *Cancer,* 37:141–148.
149. Newman, H. K., and Quan, S. H. Q. (1976): Multi-modality therapy for epidermoid carcinoma of the anus. *Cancer,* 37:12–19.
150. O'Connell, M. J., Ritts, R. E., Jr., Moertel, C. G. (1976): Immunologic assessment of MER

and placebo in advanced cancer: A double blind study. *Proc. Am. Assoc. Cancer Res.*, 17:214 (Abst. 854).

151. Olweny, C. L., Toya, T., Katongole-Mbidde, Mugerwa, J., Kyalwazi, S. K., and Cohen, H. (1975): Treatment of hepatocellular carcinoma with adriamycin. *Cancer*, 36:1250–1257.
152. Ong, G. B., and Chan, P. K. W. (1976): Primary carcinoma of the liver. *Surg. Gynecol. Obstet.*, 143:31–38.
153. Pack, G. T. (1965): Tumors of the stomach. *Geriatrics*, 20:699–706.
154. Papillon, J. (1975): Resectable rectal cancers: Treatment by curative endocavity irradiation. *JAMA*, 231:1385–1387.
155. Parker, E. F., Gregorie, H. B. (1976): Carcinoma of the esophagus, long term results. *JAMA*, 235:1018–1020.
156. Pearson, J. G. (1969): The value of radiotherapy in the management of esophageal cancer. *Am. J. Roentgenol.*, 105:500–514.
157. Pearson, J. G. (1971): The value of radiotherapy in the management of squamous oesophageal cancer. *Br. J. Surg.*, 58:794–798.
158. Pearson, J. G. (1974): Value of radiation therapy in current concepts in cancer number 42— cancer of the gastrointestinal tract II esophagus: treatment—localized and advanced. *JAMA*, 227:181–183.
159. Primack, A., Vogel, G. L., Kyalwazi, S. K., Ziegler, J. L., Simon, R., and Anthony, P. P. (1975): A staging system for hepatocellular carcinoma: Prognostic factors in Ugandan patients. *Cancer*, 35:1357–1364.
160. Rambo, V. B., O'Brien, P. H., Miller, M. C., III, Stroud, M. R., and Parker, E. F. (1975): Carcinoma of the esophagus. *J. Surg. Oncol.*, 7:355–365.
161. Ramirez, G., Korbitz, B. C., Davis, H. L., Jr., and Ansfield, F. J. (1969): Comparative study of monthly courses versus weekly doses of 5-fluorouracil (NSC 19893). *Cancer Chemother. Rep.*, 53:243–247.
162. Reitemeier, R. J., and Moertel, C. G. (1962): Comparison of rapid and slow intravenous administration of 5-fluorouracil in treating patients with advanced carcinoma of the large intestine. *Cancer Chemother. Rep.*, 25:87–89.
163. Reitemeier, R. J., Moertel, C. G., and Hahn, R. G. (1965): Comparison of 5-fluorouracil (NSC 19893) and 2'-deoxy-5-fluorouridine (NSC 27640) in treatment of patients with advanced adenocarcinoma of colon or rectum. *Cancer Chemother. Rep.*, 44:39–43.
164. Reitemeier, R. J., Moertel, C. G., and Hahn, R. G. (1970): Combination chemotherapy in gastrointestinal cancer. *Cancer Res.*, 30:1425–1428.
165. Reitemeier, R. J., Moertel, C. G., and Hahn, R. G. (1976): Comparative evaluation of palliation with fluorometholone (NSC 33001), 5-fluorouracil (NSC 19893), and combined fluorometholone and 5-fluorouracil in advanced gastrointestinal cancer. *Cancer Chemother. Rep.*, 51:77–80.
166. Richards, F., II, Pajak, T. L., Cooper, M. R., and Spurr, C. L. (1975): Comparison of 5-fluorouracil with 5-fluorouracil, cyclophosphamide, and methotrexate in metastatic colorectal carcinoma. *Cancer*, 36:1589–1592.
167. Rider, W. D. (1975): Is the Miles operation really necessary for the treatment of rectal cancer? *J. Can. Assoc. Radiol.*, 26:167–175.
168. Rossi, A., Riva, A., and Bonadonna, G. (1975): Methyl-CCNU (NSC 95441) versus methyl-CCNU plus cyclophosphamide (NSC-26271) in advanced gastrointestinal cancer. *Cancer Chemother. Rep.*, 59:1161–1162.
169. Roussel, A., Robillard, J., Souloy, J., Fourre, D., and Abbatucci, J. S. (1974): Results in 600 cases of oesophageal cancer treated at the Francois-Baclesse Center between 1964 and 1971. *J. Radiol. Electrol.*, 55:485–489.
170. Rozencweig, M. (1977): Personal communication.
171. Rubin, P. (1975): Comment: Carcinoma of the anus. *JAMA*, 232:187–188.
172. Schein, P. S. (1972): Chemotherapeutic management of the hormone secreting endocrine malignancies. *Cancer*, 30:1616–1626.
173. Schneiderman, M. A. (1975): How do you know you've done any better? *Cancer*, 35:64–69.
174. Scholz, D. A., Remine, W. H., and Priestly, J. T. (1960): Hyperinsulinism: Review of 95 cases of functioning pancreatic islet cell tumors. *Proc. Staff Meet. Mayo Clinic*, 35:545–550.
175. Seifert, P., Baker, L. H., Reed, M. L., and Vaitkevicius, V. K. (1975): Comparison of continuously infused 5-fluorouracil with bolus injection in treatment of patients with colorectal adenocarcinoma. *Cancer*, 36:123–128.
176. Serlin, O., Wolkoft, T. S., Amadeo, J. M., and Keehn, R. J. (1969): Use of 5-fluorodeoxyuridine

(FUDR) as an adjuvant to the surgical management of carcinoma of the stomach. *Cancer,* 24:223–228.

177. Siegel, S. R., and Muggia, F. M. (1975): Treatment of "pancreatic cholera." *N. Engl. J. Med.,* 293:198.
178. Silen, W. (1969): In: *Principles of Surgery,* edited by S. I. Schwartz, p. 1112. McGraw-Hill, New York.
179. Silverberg, E., and Holleb, A. I. (1973): Cancer statistics 1973. *CA-A Journal for Clinicians,* 23:2–27.
180. Simbirtseva, L. P., Sneshko, L. I., and Smirnov, N. M. (1975): Results of intensive combined therapy for carcinoma of the rectum. *Vopr. Onkol.,* 21:7–12.
181. Slanetz, C. A., Jr., Herter, F. P., and Grinnell, R. S. (1972): Anterior resection versus abdominoperineal resection for cancer of the rectum and rectosigmoid—an analysis of 524 cases. *Am. J. Surg.,* 123:110–117.
182. Smith, F. S., Gibson, P., and Nicholls, T. T. (1975): Carcinoma of the oesophagus: Preoperative irradiation followed by planned resection for lesions in the middle and lower thirds. An interim report. *Aust. NZ. J. Surg.,* 45:176–178.
183. South African Primary Liver Cancer Research Group (1967): Malignant hepatoma—controlled therapeutic trials. *S.A. Med. J.,* 25:309–314.
184. Stearns, M. W., Jr. (1974): The choice among anterior resection, the pull-through and abdominoperineal resection of the rectum. *Cancer,* 34:969–971.
185. Stearns, M. W., Jr., Deddish, M. R., Quan, S. H. Q., and Leaming, R. H. (1974): Preoperative roentgen therapy for cancer of the rectum and rectosigmoid. *Surg. Gynecol. Obstet.,* 138:584–586.
186. Stearns, M. W. Jr., and Schottenfeld, D. (1971): Techniques for the surgical management of colon cancer. *Cancer,* 28:165–169.
187. Stolinsky, D. C., Pugh, R. P., and Bateman, T. R. (1975): 5-Fluorouracil (NSC 19893) therapy for pancreatic carcinoma: Comparison of oral and intravenous routes. *Cancer Chemother. Rep.,* 59:1031–1033.
188. *Summaries of Clinical Protocols for Tumors of the Gastrointestinal System.* Prepared by International Cancer Research Data Bank Progam, National Cancer Institute, Bethesda, Md.
189. Tancini, G., Bajetta, E., and Bonadonna, G. (1974): Terapia con bleomi cina da sola o in associazone con methotrexate nel carcinoma epidermoide dell'esofago. *Tumori,* 60:65–71.
190. Trapezhikov, N. N. (1959): Results of surgical treatment of cancer of the stomach. *Br. Med. J.,* 2:857–859.
191. Turnbull, R. B., Jr., Kyle, K., Watson, F. R., and Spratt, J. (1967): Cancer of the colon: The influence of the no-touch isolation technique on survival rates. *Ann. Surg.,* 166:420–425.
192. Vaitkevicius, V. K., Baker, L. H., Buroker, T. R., Kun, P. N., and Reed, M. L. (1975): Chemotherapy of gastrointestinal adenocarcinoma. In: *Cancer Chemotherapy—Fundamental Concepts and Recent Advances,* pp. 263–278. Yearbook Medical Publishers, Chicago.
193. Valdivieso, M., Mavligit, G. M., Burgess, A., and Bodey, G. P. (1976): Chemoimmunotherapy of gastrointestinal (GI) malignancies, Ftorafur (FTOR) or 5-fluorouracil (FU) plus methyl CCNU (Me), methotrexate (M) and BCG (B) (FTORMeM+B vs FUMeM+B). *Proc. Am. Soc. Clin. Oncol.,* 17:281 (Abst. C178).
194. Vaughn, C. B., Chinn, B. J., Daverson, G., and Parzuchowski, J. (1975): Comparison of combination chemotherapy in advanced gastrointestinal malignancy. 5-Fluorouracil plus mitomycin C versus 5-fluorouracil plus 1(2-choroethyl) 3-(4 methycyclohexyl)-1-nitrosourea. *Proc. Am. Assoc. Cancer. Res.,* 16:252 (Abst. 1126).
195. Veterans Administration Cooperative Surgical Adjuvant Study Group (1965): Use of thiotepa as an adjuvant to the surgical management of carcinoma of the stomach. *Cancer,* 18:291–297.
196. Veterans Administration Surgical Adjuvant Cancer Chemotherapy Study Group (1962): The use of 5-fluoro-2'-deoxyuridine as a surgical adjuvant in carcinoma of the stomach and colon-rectum. *Cancer Chemother. Rep.,* 24:35–38.
197. Vogel, C. L., and Linsell, C. A. (1972): International Symposium on Hepatocellular Carcinoma, Kampala, Uganda (July 1971). *J. Natl. Cancer Inst.,* 48:567–571.
198 Vogler, W. R., and Jacobs, J. (1975): High divided dose methotrexate (MTX) with leucovorin (LCV) rescue vs low oral divided dose MTX vs single dose IV MTX in advanced carcinoma of head, neck, breast, and colon. *Proc. Am. Assoc. Cancer Res.,* 16:266.
199. Wasserman, T. H., Comis, R. L., Goldsmith, M., Handelsman, H., Penta, J. S., Slavik, M.,

Soper, W. T., and Carter, S. K. (1975): Tabular analysis of the clinical chemotherapy of solid tumors. *Cancer Chemother. Rep. Part 3,* 6:399–419.

200. Wassif, S. B. (1974): A pilot study for the evaluation of a new regimen of combined therapy for the radical treatment of marginally operable rectal (or colo-rectal) cancer. *Eur. J. Cancer,* 10:615–619.

201. Welch, C. E., and Burke, J. F. (1962): Carcinoma of the colon and rectum. *N. Engl. J. Med.,* 266:211–219.

202. Welton, M. J., Petrelli, M., George, P., Young, W. B., and Sherlock, S. (1969): Carcinoma of the function of the main hepatic ducts. *Quart. J. Med.,* 38:211–230.

203. Wilson, S. E., Plested, W. G., and Carey, J. S. (1970): Esophagogastrectomy versus radiation therapy for mid esophageal carcinoma. *Ann. Thorac. Surg.,* 10:195–202.

204. Younghusband, J. D., and Aluwihare, A. P. R. (1970): Carcinoma of the oesophagus: Factors influencing survival. *Br. J. Surg.,* 57:422–430.

205. Zelen, M. (1975): Importance of prognostic factors in planning therapeutic trials. In: *Cancer Therapy: Prognostic Factors and Criteria of Response,* edited by M. J. Staquet. Raven Press, New York.

Randomized Trials in Cancer: A Critical
Review by Sites, edited by Maurice J.
Staquet, Raven Press, New York © 1978.

# Breast Cancer

*M. Rozencweig, **J. C. Heuson, *D. D. Von Hoff, **W. H.
Mattheiem, *H. L. Davis, and *F. M. Muggia

*Cancer Therapy Evaluation Program, Division of Cancer Treatment, National Cancer
Institute, Bethesda, Maryland 20014
**Institut Jules Bordet, 1000 Bruxelles, Belgium

Breast cancer is the most frequent malignancy among women in the Western hemisphere (37,132). The duration of its clinical evolution may vary from weeks to several decades, and various treatment modalities have succeeded in temporarily controlling its clinical course. It is also noteworthy that the disseminated stage of the disease relatively often presents measurable criteria that can be used to assess the effectiveness of therapy.

All these features have led to numerous clinical studies that, in fact, have perpetuated the controversies over the adequacy of various therapeutic approaches for managing both early and advanced disease. This chapter considers the contributions of randomized clinical trials reported up to December 1976.

## RANDOMIZED TRIALS IN EARLY BREAST CANCER

Recurrence and survival rates following treatment of primary breast cancer have been correlated with various parameters of prognostic significance (129). The status of regional lymph nodes has been the most prominent predictive factor in operable disease. According to Urban and Castro (144), the 10-year survival rates after extended radical mastectomy were 75% when the axillary and internal mammary nodes were disease-free, 52 to 53% if one of these nodal areas was involved, and 21% when both areas were invaded. If the status of the internal mammary nodes is not considered, the strongest prognostic indicator is the extent of axillary involvement as measured by the anatomic level of axillary invasion (125) or, more usually, by the number of invaded nodes (64). As reported by Fisher et al. (64), the 10-year relapse rates after radical mastectomy were 24% in patients with negative axillary lymph nodes, 65% when less than 4

---

Received December 31, 1976.
Abbreviations, chemical nomenclature, and NSC numbers for chemotherapeutic agents cited are shown in the List of Compounds at the end of the text.

axillary nodes were invaded, and 86% with 4 or more positive nodes. The corresponding 10-year survival rates were 65%, 38%, and 13%.

Several clinical staging systems have been proposed for selecting therapeutic modalities (Table 1). All of them are characterized by the same inaccuracies (35), especially with regard to the clinical assessment of the axilla. The large discrepancy between clinical and histologic examination of the axillary content precludes an accurate interpretation of therapeutic results in early disease when they are expressed in terms of the initial clinical staging. Thus, in the absence of pathologic staging, comparisons between treatment modalities should be undertaken with extreme reservation.

TABLE 1. *Comparison of common clinical staging systems*[a]

| Element to be assigned | Staging system[b] | | | |
|---|---|---|---|---|
| | Columbia[c] | Manchester | American TNM | International TNM[d] |
| Breast involvement | | | | |
| Tumor size | — | — | — | ≤2 cm: I >5 cm: III |
| Nipple inversion | — | — | I | I |
| Paget's disease | — | — | I | — |
| Skin "involvement" | — | "Small": I "Large": III | — | III |
| Skin fixation | — | "Large": III | — | incompl. compl., III |
| Skin retraction | — | — | I | I |
| Skin infiltration or invasion | — | III | III | III |
| Skin edema | <⅓ of breast: C ≥ ⅓ of breast: D | — | III | III |
| Ulceration | C | — | III | III |
| Inflammation | D | — | — | — |
| Vicinal involvement | | | | |
| Fixation to pectoralis | — | III | III | I |
| Fixation to chest wall | C | IV | III | III |
| Regional involvement | | | | |
| Parasternal metastases | D | — | — | — |
| Infraclavicular metastases | — | "Fixed": III | III | III |
| Supraclavicular metastases | D | IV | IV | III |
| Axillary metastases | <2.5 cm: B ≥2.5 cm: C | II | II | II |
| Axillary fixation | C | IV | III | III |
| Edema of arm | D | — | — | III |
| Satellite skin nodules | D | IV | — | III |
| Distant involvement | | | | |
| Beyond cited locations | D | IV | IV | IV |

[a] Based on Charlson and Feinstein (35).
[b] "—" = Omitted from staging *or* assigned to lowest category (A or I) if no "higher" elements are present.
[c] Patients with two stage C characteristics are cited as stage D.
[d] Modified according to the 1975 TNM classification.

## Surgical Trials

Various surgical techniques have been used in breast cancer, the most common procedures being those briefly depicted in Table 2. *Segmental* mastectomy (lumpectomy, extended tylectomy) removes the primary tumor and surrounding breast tissue. *Simple* (total) mastectomy removes the entire breast and, in the *extended* procedure, an additional resection of the axillary lymph nodes is performed. *Radical* mastectomy removes *en bloc* the entire breast, axillary lymph nodes, and the major and minor pectoralis muscles. The so-called *modified radical* mastectomy is similar but does not involve the pectoralis major, whereas the *extended radical* mastectomy includes a resection of the internal mammary node chain. *Super radical* mastectomy consists of a resection of supraclavicular nodes, with or without dissecting the mediastinal nodes, in addition to the extended radical surgery.

Four randomized trials restricted to the study of surgical procedures have been reported (Table 3). Only incomplete or partial data are available for all of the trials except that of Lacour et al. (102), which compared radical mastectomy with extended radical mastectomy. In this study, subsequent treatment for local or distant recurrence was standardized for both treatment groups. The criteria for patient eligibility required a primary tumor <7 cm in diameter, without complete pectoral muscle fixation, skin involvement, and inflammatory signs. The clinical presence of homolateral axillary lymph nodes that were palpable, but movable, was acceptable for entry in the trial. Invasion of internal mammary lymph nodes was encountered in less than 10% of the patients without axillary involvement. In these patients, no therapeutic difference was noted between the two surgical techniques. However, a retrospective rearrangement of the data showed that, in tumors of the outer quadrants of the breast, the 5-year survival rate was significantly greater with radical mastectomy (88%) than with the extended radical procedure (79%). In the presence of axillary involvement, both treatment groups also achieved similar results when the location of the primary was not taken into consideration. Invasion of internal mammary nodes was found in 37% of the primaries located in the inner or medial quadrants of the breast with involved axillary nodes. In these patients the 5-year survival rate was significantly higher for $T_1$ and $T_2$ tumors with the extended mastectomy (71%) as compared to radical mastectomy (52%) but this difference disappeared in $T_3$ tumors. In the TNM classification, the T value depends on clinical estimation of the size of the primary tumor and its degree of fixation to the skin or underlying structures. The general lack of accuracy of this T value and the retrospective nature of the analysis cast some doubt on the validity of these findings.

In the trial performed by Yonemoto et al. (148), all patients fulfilled Haagensen's criteria of operability but the recommended triple biopsy was not performed. Standard radical mastectomy, with and without intraarterial chemotherapy, was compared to extended radical mastectomy. Chemotherapy given during the early

TABLE 2. Surgical techniques in breast cancer (34)

| Type of mastectomy | Primary tumor | Breast tissue | Pectoralis major | Pectoralis minor | Nodes | | |
|---|---|---|---|---|---|---|---|
| | | | | | Axillary | Internal mammary | Supraclavicular |
| Segmental | + | 0 | 0 | 0 | 0 | 0 | 0 |
| Simple | + | + | 0 | 0 | 0 | 0 | 0 |
| Extended simple | + | + | 0 | 0 | + | 0 | 0 |
| Modified radical | + | + | 0 | ± | + | 0 | 0 |
| Radical | + | + | + | + | + | 0 | 0 |
| Extended radical | + | + | + | + | + | + | 0 |
| Super radical | + | + | + | + | + | + | + |

TABLE 3. *Randomized surgical trials in early breast cancer*

| Investigators and treatment arms[a] | 5-year survival | |
| --- | --- | --- |
| | No. of evaluable patients | Rate (%) |
| Lacour et al. (102) | | |
| A. Radical mastectomy | 746 | 69 |
| B. Extended radical mastectomy | 697 | 72 |
| Yonemoto et al. (148) | | |
| A. Radical mastectomy | 55 | 60 |
| B. Extended radical mastectomy | 54 | 69 |
| C. Radical mastectomy + intraarterial nitrogen mustard | 53 | 68 |
| Helman et al. (85)[b] | | |
| A. Radical mastectomy | 0 | — |
| B. Simple mastectomy | 0 | — |
| Fisher and Wolmark (65)[c] | | |
| A. Radical mastectomy | 0 | — |
| B. Total mastectomy | 0 | — |
| C. Total mastectomy + RT | 0 | — |

[a] Abbreviations: RT, radiotherapy.
[b] Trial discontinued after 3 years.
[c] Only preliminary results available.

phase of surgery consisted of nitrogen mustard infusion into the internal mammary artery, the lateral thoracic artery, or the pectoral branch of the achromiothoracic artery. Of the 272 patients randomized, 162 were followed for 5 years or more. No difference in 5-year survival could be found among the three treatment groups, whatever the histologic findings in the axilla. However, the number of patients followed for at least 5 years was too small to analyze these results according to the status of axillary nodes.

Helman et al. (85) compared simple and radical mastectomy in TNM stages I and II; in stage II the simple mastectomy was completed by limited excision of enlarged lymph nodes in the axilla, but not by extensive axillary dissection. This trial was discontinued after 3 years because of the high local and regional recurrence rates observed following simple mastectomy. Of the 51 patients subjected to that operation, 5 (9.8%) developed lymph node involvement in the ipsilateral axilla and 7 (13.7%) had skin-flap recurrences. Among 44 patients who had the radical surgery, there was one skin-flap recurrence but none in the axillary nodes. These findings were not detailed by initial clinical staging and length of follow-up and, as reported, they are not amenable to a proper analysis.

The final trial in Table 3 was reported by Fisher and Wolmark (65). In potentially curable patients having clinically negative axillary nodes, radical mastectomy was compared to total mastectomy plus regional irradiation, and to total mastectomy plus subsequent node removal if significant palpable nodes developed. Patients with clinically positive nodes were assigned to radical mastectomy or total mastectomy with regional irradiation. Preliminary results are available for 1,665 patients with a period of observation ranging from 26 to 62 months. No statistically significant difference in disease-free interval or in survival time has been detected between any treatment group within each of the clinical nodal categories.

To summarize, it may only be concluded that, as compared to radical mastectomy, the extended procedure does not improve the results obtained in patients without axillary involvement. However, it might prolong the survival in some subgroups of patients with axillary involvement. The respective value of the other surgical approaches used alone for the therapy of early breast cancer remains unsettled.

## Combined Surgery and Radiotherapy

The usefulness of postoperative radiotherapy remains a much debated matter (96) despite the large number of randomized trials involving both surgery and radiotherapy (Table 4). Some trials have specifically investigated the additional value of radiotherapy following simple or radical mastectomy. Most of the others have tested whether a simple or segmental mastectomy plus radiotherapy was equivalent to a more aggressive surgical procedure with or without subsequent radiotherapy.

All the randomized clinical studies specifically testing the role of postoperative radiotherapy have suggested that this adjuvant technique decreased the frequency of local and/or regional recurrence, particularly when axillary involvement was histologically demonstrated. However, this benefit did not seem to be translated in a prolongation of survival.

Patients in the trial of the Cancer Research Campaign (30) had Manchester clinical stage I or II disease. After simple mastectomy without axillary node dissection, they were randomized to either a watch policy, where further treatment was used only for recurrent disease, or to orthovoltage or supervoltage radiotherapy to the skin-flap, axilla, and supraclavicular and internal mammary areas. Large variations in dose fractionation of radiotherapy were allowed. Results were available for 2,268 evaluable patients in terms of standard life table probabilities of survival and freedom from recurrence, but two-thirds of the patients were not followed for a minimum of 5 years. No difference in the survival curves up to 5 years was detected between the two treatment regimens in stage I or stage II disease. In contrast, the incidence of local recurrence was significantly higher ($p < .001$) following surgery alone than after the combined modalities for both stage I and stage II patients. Nodes obtained from the axillary tail or pectoral regions in the simple mastectomy specimen were analyzed histologically in 350 patients (107). In the 167 lymph node-negative patients, standard life table probabilities showed that the two treatment groups

TABLE 4. *Randomized trials of surgery and postoperative radiotherapy in early breast cancer* [a]

| Investigators and treatment arms [b] | Initial disease stage | 5-year survival rate (%) (no. patients at risk) | Local and regional recurrence rate (%) (no. of evaluable patients) |
|---|---|---|---|
| Cancer Research Campaign (30) | Manchester I and II | | |
| A. Simple mastectomy | | 78 (354) | 15 (1152) |
| B. Simple mastectomy + RT | | 74 (348) | 5 (1116) |
| Easson (51) | | | |
| A. Radical mastectomy | Axilla − | 80[c] (283) | 16[d] (283) |
| | Axilla + | 50[c] (467) | 42[d] (467) |
| | | 61[c] (750) | 32[d] (750) |
| B. Radical mastectomy + RT | Axilla − | 77[c] (243) | 10[d] (243) |
| | Axilla + | 49[c] (464) | 25[d] (464) |
| | | 59[c] (707) | 19[d] (707) |
| Fisher et al. (63) | | | |
| A. Radical mastectomy | Axilla − | 80 (50) | 8 (52) |
| | Axilla + | 48 (63) | 28 (65) |
| | | 62 (113) | 19 (117) |
| B. Radical mastectomy + RT | Axilla − | 74 (62) | 9 (56) |
| | Axilla + | 47 (133) | 8 (124) |
| | | 56 (195) | 8 (180) |
| Høst and Brennhovd (90) | | | |
| A. Radical mastectomy | Axilla − | 90 (172) | See text |
| | Axilla + | 72 (92) | |
| | | 84 (264) | |
| B. Radical mastectomy + RT | Axilla − | 91 (173) | See text |
| | Axilla + | 71 (109) | |
| | | 83 (282) | |
| Hamilton et al. (78) | Manchester I-III | | |
| A. Radical Mastectomy | | 74[c] (203) | Unknown |
| B. Simple mastectomy + RT | | 70[c] (191) | Unknown |
| Kaae and Johansen (95) | | | |
| | Columbia A | 74 (134) | 20 (134) |
| | Columbia B | 47 (32) | 32 (32) |
| A. Super radical mastectomy | Columbia C | 50 (8) | 50 (8) |
| | Columbia D | 22 (9) | 33 (9) |
| | | 66 (183) | 24 (183) |
| | Columbia A | 70 (159) | 19 (159) |
| | Columbia B | 50 (28) | 29 (28) |
| B. Simple mastectomy + RT | Columbia C | 22 (9) | 33 (9) |
| | Columbia D | 0 (3) | 33 (3) |
| | | 64 (199) | 21 (199) |
| Brinkley and Haybittle (25) | TNM II | | |
| A. Radical mastectomy + RT | | 58 (91) | Unknown |
| B. Simple mastectomy + RT | | 63 (113) | Unknown |
| Hayward (83) | | | |
| A. Radical mastectomy + RT 1 | Manchester I | 77 (?) | 6 (108) |
| | Manchester II | 73 (?) | 18 (80) |

TABLE 4—*Cont.*

| Investigators and treatment arms [b] | Initial disease stage | 5-year survival rate (%) (no. patients at risk) | Local and regional recurrence rate (%) (no. of evaluable patients) |
|---|---|---|---|
| B. Lumpectomy + RT 2 | Manchester I | 80 (?) | 20 (112) |
| | Manchester II | 61 (?) | 43 (70) |
| Burn (29) | Unknown | | |
| A. Radical mastectomy + RT 1 | | 70 (?) | 13 (76) |
| B. Simple mastectomy + RT 2 | | 65 (?) | 14 (76) |
| Edland et al. (54) | Unknown | | |
| A. Radical mastectomy + RT 1 | | 48 (44) | 7 (44) |
| B. Simple or radical mastectomy + RT 2 | | 64 (42) | 5 (42) |

[a] Other trials without reports of 5-year survival include studies of various fractionation regimens (14,106,109), trials of radical RT after simple mastectomy (49,65), a study (66) of modified radical versus simple mastectomy (± RT in each case where nodal invasion is histologically demonstrated), and a study of pre- and postop. RT (47). See also Table 3 and (156).

[b] Abbreviations: RT, radiotherapy; RT 1 and RT 2, differing RT regimens.

[c] Estimated from survival curves.

[d] Local recurrence rate (%) by TNM clinical stages I and II after 10-year follow-up.

exhibited no difference in survival or freedom from recurrence up to 5 years. In 183 lymph node-positive patients, the same statistical analysis estimated that radiotherapy shortened the survival ($p < .05$) in spite of a decrease in the probability of local recurrence ($p < .001$). These data, based on a partial pathologic staging, should be interpreted with caution and should await confirmation of findings with a larger number of patients followed for at least 5 years.

Three trials have examined the potential of radiotherapy in combination with radical mastectomy. In the Manchester trial reported by Easson (51), patients were randomized on the basis of their birthdate to either immediate postoperative irradiation or radiotherapy delayed until the local recurrence. Two different techniques were employed. In the first half of patients, irradiation was directed to the anterior chest wall and apex of the axilla without exposing the supraclavicular fossa or, to any significant extent, the internal mammary lymph node chain. In the most recently entered patients, irradiation was directed to the internal mammary lymph node chain, the axilla, and the supraclavicular fossa in continuity; the skin flaps were not irradiated. Survival curves up to 10 years were similar for both methods of radiotherapy regardless of the pathological status of the axilla. There was also no difference between the survival rates obtained with immediate or delayed radiotherapy. The incidence of local recurrence within 10 years was greater in patients treated by surgery alone than in those given immediate postoperative radiotherapy, particularly in clinical stage

II disease. However, for both clinical stage I and II, the percentage of patients with uncontrolled local recurrence at the time of death was almost identical in both treatment groups. These results were not reported according to pathologic staging.

The National Surgical Adjuvant Breast Project (NSABP) study was reported by Fisher et al. (63) with a follow-up period of 5 years or more for slightly more than one-third of the patients. The irradiation fields included the internal mammary chain of nodes, the apex of the axilla, and the supraclavicular region; the chest wall and axilla as a whole were not irradiated. Of the radiotherapy patients, approximately 75% received supervoltage irradiation, and the type of equipment varied from one institution to another. At 5 years, the survival rates and disease-free rates were apparently not influenced by the choice of the treatment. No difference in recurrence rate was detected in patients with axilla free of disease at the time of radical mastectomy. However, in patients with axillary node invasion, the incidence of first sign of relapse within the area of operation or irradiation was significantly lower following postoperative radiotherapy than after surgery alone.

In their postoperative radiotherapy group, Høst and Brennhovd (90) irradiated the internal mammary lymph node chain, the ipsilateral axilla, supraclavicular fossa, and skin flaps. All locally irradiated patients, as well as control patients, also had ovarian irradiation as part of the initial treatment. The minimum follow-up time was 5 years. The irradiated group and the control group exhibited no difference in survival or freedom from relapse regardless of the histologic status of the axilla. The rates of local and regional recurrence were reported separately for the site of operation, the axilla, and the supraclavicular fossa regardless of simultaneous relapses in other areas. No difference was noted in patients without axillary involvement. In the presence of axillary involvement, the frequency of relapse was lower in all three sites with postoperative radiotherapy; however, the difference was significant only for the recurrence rate in homolateral supraclavicular lymph nodes. These findings are difficult to interpret because of the systematic ovarian irradiation and the lack of information regarding results by menopausal age.

Fisher and Wolmark (65), as discussed in the previous section, Hamilton et al. (78), as well as Kaae and Johansen (95), have attempted to determine whether or not an aggressive surgical procedure can be replaced by more conservative surgery followed by radiotherapy. This important question still remains unanswered in all of the early stages.

The study by Hamilton et al. investigated standard radical mastectomy versus simple mastectomy plus radical radiotherapy involving the chest wall, axilla, and supraclavicular region in patients with Manchester clinical stages I to III. Stratification was made according to clinical stage and age; patients under 60 years of age also underwent prophylactic oophorectomy. The crude 5-year survival curves were similar for both methods of treatment. There was also no difference in the disease-free survival rates obtained with the two therapies. Since the results were not detailed according to the initial stage of disease and age of the patients, no conclusion was possible.

Kaae and Johansen (95) compared super radical mastectomy versus simple mastectomy followed by irradiation of the axilla, supraclavicular region, and the chest wall including the internal mammary chain. The randomization procedure was not properly made, treatments being selected according to the number, odd or even, of the patient's case records. No difference was found in any of the Columbia clinical stages in terms of 5- and 10-year survival rates or incidence of local recurrence. However, it should be pointed out that the trial included a substantial number of patients with stage A disease but very few patients with other stages. Thus, this trial merely indicated that both therapeutic approaches probably achieved similar results in terms of recurrence or survival rate among patients without axillary involvement. It does not exclude the possibility of a significant therapeutic difference in more advanced but still early disease.

The remaining trials have randomized patients to different surgical approaches that were always followed by radiotherapy. None has greatly contributed to a definition of the most appropriate local treatment in early breast cancer. Brinkley and Haybittle (24,25) compared radical mastectomy, with occasional removal of internal mammary nodes, versus simple mastectomy that could include removal of accessible axillary glands but no *en bloc* dissection of the axilla. In both treatment groups, the surgical procedure was followed by standardized radiotherapy to the skin flaps and all the regional lymph node areas, including the pectoral area as well as the axillary, supraclavicular, and internal mammary nodes. A minimum of 3,250 rads was delivered over 18 days using a 250-kV unit. Entry into the trial was confined to clinical stage II patients according to the international TNM classification but regardless of the tumor size. Patients were randomized by drawing of an odd or an even number from a random number table. No significant difference was found in the crude 5-year recurrence or survival rates between the two treatment groups. However, the number of patients included in this trial was small insofar as, based on histologic findings at radical mastectomy, the patient selection apparently was quite favorable, almost half of them having no axillary involvement.

Hayward (83) has compared radical and conservative surgery, each followed by a different irradiation regimen. Patients with Manchester clinical stages I and II were randomized to radical mastectomy or to lumpectomy, which occasionally became a simple mastectomy in patients with large tumors and small breasts. The radical procedure was followed by radiotherapy to the axilla, supraclavicular triangle, and internal mammary chain (2,500 to 2,700 rads over 18 days). The second surgical approach was followed by irradiation of the axilla and supraclavicular region (2,500 to 2,700 rads over 12 days) as well as the internal mammary chains and the remaining breast tissue (3,500 to 3,800 rads over 3 weeks). At the beginning of the trial, all patients received intraoperative thiotepa, but this adjuvant chemotherapy was later abandoned completely. Accrual in the trial was closed in 1970, with 188 patients treated by radical mastectomy and 182 by lumpectomy. The latest results, published in 1974, showed that an unreported number of patients had not completed a minimum follow-up of 5 years. In clinical stage I patients, the statistical analysis estimated that the probability of local recurrence would be significantly higher 5 and 10 years after lumpectomy, whereas no difference would be found in the rate of distant recurrence or survival. In clinical stage II, estimates at 5 years indicated a higher local and distant recurrence rate following lumpectomy, whereas the probable 10-year survival rate after lumpectomy and radical mastectomy was 23% and 67%, respectively ($p < .01$). However, even if these results were to be confirmed by additional follow-up, radiotherapy might be regarded as too suboptimal to conclude definitively that radical surgery confers survival advantage over conservative surgery when both procedures are followed by irradiation.

Burn (29) compared radical versus simple mastectomy. Both techniques were also followed by radiotherapy. The system of paired stratification was adopted for allocating treatments; that is, patients were matched for age, menopausal status, childbearing history, and TNM clinical stage. Prophylactic oophorectomy was performed in all patients according to the menopausal status. In a follow-up period of at least 4 years there was no difference in terms of survival or recurrence rate, but results were not given by stage and menopausal status.

Finally, Edland et al. (54) randomized their patients to two different radiotherapeutic techniques, but without regard to surgical procedure and disease stage. The method of staging was not defined, and only a small number of patients were entered in the study.

## Adjuvant Systemic Treatment

All the studies involving surgery, with or without radiotherapy, have clearly indicated that the prognosis in early breast cancer is extremely severe when the regional lymph nodes are invaded, whatever the type of local therapy. This observation is consistent with a high frequency of clinically occult distant dissemination in these apparently still operable patients. Adjuvant systemic treatment using regimens effective in clinically disseminated disease should, in principle, be even more effective in the control of smaller tumor masses. The following sections summarize the current status of adjuvant hormone and antitumor drug therapy.

### *Adjuvant Hormonotherapy*

The vast majority of trials testing adjuvant hormonotherapy have used castration by irradiation or surgery (Table 5). Adjuvant castration has been routinely performed by several investigators as already mentioned in this chapter (29, 78,90), yet this procedure has actually not been properly tested.

Nissen-Meyer (116) studied in three randomized trials the value of adjuvant castration following radical mastectomy and radiotherapy to the primary. Pre-

TABLE 5. *Randomized trials of adjuvant hormonotherapy*[a]

| Investigators and treatment arms | Initial disease stage | 5-year crude survival rate (%) (no. patients at risk) |
|---|---|---|
| **Nissen-Meyer (116)** | | |
| I. Premenopausal patients | Unknown | |
| A. RT castration | | 70[b] (?) |
| B. Oophorectomy | | 66[b] (?) |
| II. Premenopausal patients | Unknown | |
| A. RT castration | | 90[b] (?) |
| B. No adjuvant therapy | | 95[b] (?) |
| III. Postmenopausal patients | | |
| A. RT castration | Axilla — | 88[b] (40) |
| | Axilla + | 58[b] (48) |
| B. No adjuvant therapy | Axilla — | 80[b] (40) |
| | Axilla + | 50[b] (46) |
| **Cole (39)** | | |
| A. RT castration | Axilla — | 80[c] (90) |
| | Axilla + | 44[c] (203) |
| | | 55[c] (293) |
| B. No adjuvant therapy | Axilla — | 69[c] (105) |
| | Axilla + | 37[c] (200) |
| | | 48[c] (305) |
| **Nevinny et al. (115)** | | |
| A. Oophorectomy | Axilla — | 85 (13) |
| | Axilla + | 72 (18) |
| | | 77 (31) |
| B. No adjuvant therapy | Axilla — | 79 (14) |
| | Axilla + | 83 (18) |
| | | 81 (32) |
| **Ravdin et al. (123)** | | |
| A. Oophorectomy | Axilla — | 77 (30) |
| | Axilla + | 39 (44) |
| | | 54 (74) |
| B. Placebo | Axilla — | 77 (17) |
| | Axilla + | 40 (20) |
| | | 57 (37) |
| **Bland et al. (16)** | Unknown | |
| A. Oophorectomy | | 54 (13) |
| B. Miscellaneous | | 38 (109) |

[a] Other trials include a study of adjuvant testosterone (108) and another of prophylactic RT castration ± prednisone (108,154).
[b] Estimated from crude survival curves.
[c] Ten-year survival rate.

menopausal patients were divided into good- and poor-risk categories according to the disease stage, the location of the primary, and the grade of malignancy. The first trial randomized 112 premenopausal patients, who had a poor prognosis, to prophylactic ovarian irradiation or prophylactic oophorectomy. In the second trial, 161 premenopausal patients with a good prognosis were randomized to prophylactic or therapeutic castration by radiotherapy. No difference was found in either trial in terms of disease-free or crude survival curves. In the third trial, 80 stage I and 95 stage II patients with a mean age of 60 years and at least 6 months beyond natural menopause were randomly allocated to prophylactic or therapeutic castration by radiotherapy. Comparative curves of disease-free survival and crude survival suggested a slight benefit by the prophylactic castration, especially for stage II patients. However, these differences were too narrow to reach statistical significance with the small number of patients selected for the study.

Another trial, reported by Cole (39), compared radical mastectomy alone or followed by radiotherapeutic castration in patients who were premenopausal or within 2 years of menopause. Treatments were allocated by the birthdate of the patients, most of whom were referred to the investigators for induction of artificial menopause after surgery had been performed elsewhere. Patients without invaded axillary nodes exhibited no difference in relapse rate or crude survival as a result of therapy. In patients with axillary involvement, the difference between the relapse rate for adjuvant versus no adjuvant therapy (18% at 1 year, 12% at 5 years, and 10% at 10 and 15 years) strongly favored prophylactic castration. No significant difference was detected in crude survival curves for as long as 15 years. However, various irradiation techniques were used and a return of the menstrual period in almost one-third of the cases suggested that the castration procedures lacked long-term effectiveness.

The effect of adjuvant oophorectomy after radical mastectomy has been studied in two trials (115,123). Preliminary results limited to patients observed for 5 years or more did not show any significant difference (Table 5), but both trials had an insufficient number of patients. Nevinny et al. (115) selected 143 pre- and postmenopausal women; at the initial radical mastectomy, 53 were free of disease in the axilla and 90 had node involvement. Ravdin et al. (123) assigned 331 patients to oöphorectomy and 161 to placebo before radical mastectomy. In the former group, 24% were excluded for refusal of adjuvant therapy or incompleteness of data, and 29% for various other reasons; corresponding figures in the placebo group were 6% and 43%. These exclusions cast serious doubt on the reliability of this study; moreover, the duration of patient accrual (nearly 7 years) also introduces additional problems in interpreting the data.

Bland et al. (16) treated 124 consecutive pre- and postmenopausal patients having clinical stage III tumors (international TNM classification) by radical mastectomy with or without radiotherapy, adjuvant chemotherapy, or hormonotherapy. Fifteen of the patients were "randomly" selected for oophoroadrenalectomy and their median survival was significantly longer as compared to the entire remaining group of patients. However, definite conclusions are not possible without specification regarding methods of patient selection and randomization.

### Adjuvant Chemotherapy

The apparently conflicting results obtained with adjuvant chemotherapy have been thoroughly analyzed in a recent review (142). Most of the trials have

TABLE 6. *Surgical adjuvant chemotherapy trials in breast cancer*[a]

| Investigator | Patient selection and stratification | Treatment arms (no. of patients) |
|---|---|---|
| Fisher et al. (64) | See text | A. Radical mastectomy + placebo (406)<br>B. Radical mastectomy + TTP daily × 3 (414) |
| Blokhina and Karev (17) | TNM I-IIb | A. Radical mastectomy (191)<br>B. As in A + TTP × 2 wks (246)<br>C. As in A + CTX × 2 wks (150) |
| Finney (59) | Tumor confined to breast and/or axilla | A. Simple or radical mastectomy + RT (40)<br>B. As in A + CTX pre- and postop. for 10 days (43) |
| Rieche et al. (124) | TNM stage I-III | A. Radical mastectomy (144)<br>B. As in A + CTX postop, 200 mg/day to total 100 mg/kg (143) |
| Nissen-Meyer (117) | Unknown | A. Surgery ± RT ± prophylactic castration (554)<br>B. As in A + CTX postop daily × 6 (534) |
| Fisher et al. (62) | See text, Fisher et al. (64) | A. Radical mastectomy + placebo (207)<br>B. Radical mastectomy + 5-FU postop daily × 4 (450) |
| Yoshida et al. (149) | Unknown | A. Radical mastectomy (?)<br>B. As in A + mitomycin C (?) |
| Mrazek (110) | Unknown | A. Radical mastectomy (78)<br>B. As in A + nitrogen mustard postop. daily × 3; then daily × 3, q. 3 mos for 1 yr (78) |
| Donegan (48) | Resectable tumors | A. Radical mastectomy (92)<br>B. As in A + TTP postop daily × 3, then wkly for 1 yr (125) |
| Fisher et al. (61) | Potentially curable tumors, axilla +<br>Stratification: age and extent of axillary involvement | A. Radical mastectomy (136)<br><br>B. As in A + L-PAM for 2 yrs (133) |
| Duncan et al. (49) | TNM I-III<br>Stratification: stage and menopausal status | A. Simple mastectomy and/or RT (?)<br>B. As in A + 5-FU/48 wks (?) |
| Fisher et al. (61) | Potentially curable tumors, axilla +<br>Stratification: age and extent of axillary involvement | A. Radical mastectomy + L-PAM/2 yrs (306)<br>B. Radical mastectomy + L-PAM, 5-FU, 2 yrs (299) |
| Bonadonna et al. (18) | Potentially curable tumors, axilla +<br>Stratification: age, type of mastectomy and extent of axillary involvement | A. Radical *or* extended radical mastectomy (179)<br>B. As in A + CTX, MTX, and 5-FU for 48 wks (207) |
| Tejada et al. (141) | Stage III | A. RT (8)<br>B. RT + radical mastectomy (11)<br>C. RT + CTX, MTX, and 5-FU (9) |

TABLE 6—*Cont.*

| Investigator | Patient selection and stratification | Treatment arms (no. of patients) |
|---|---|---|
| Haskell et al. (82) | Stage II | A. Radical or modified radical mastectomy + CTX, MTX, 5-FU and BCG (?) |
| | | B. As in A + tumor cell vaccine (?) |

[a]See also Table 3.

used single agents, especially alkylating agents, which were generally given over short periods of time (Table 6). With the exception of one NSABP trial (64), all of these trials are characterized by a lack of information on crude 5-year recurrence or survival rates in a sufficient number of patients.

The trial of the NSABP (Table 7) began in 1958 and patient entry continued until 1961; the 10-year follow-up results were recently published by Fisher et al. (64). Eligibility criteria included (a) tumor confined to the breast and axilla; (b) tumor movable in relation to the chest wall, without extensive skin involvement or ulceration; (c) axillary nodes, if present, movable in relation to chest wall and blood vessels, and (d) no evidence of edema in the arm.

After radical mastectomy, patients were randomized to thiotepa (TTP) or placebo. In most cases (636 patients), the total drug dose was 0.6 mg/kg (0.2 mg/kg on the day of surgery and on each of the next 2 days). The remaining patients each received a total 0.8 mg/kg with 0.4 mg/kg given at the time of operation and 0.2 mg/kg per day the first 2 postoperative days. Subsequent analysis of data showed no significant difference between patients treated by either dose level.

TABLE 7. *NSABP study of radical mastectomy plus adjuvant thiotepa: 5-year results (64)*

| Patients | Percent recurrence rate (no. of patients) | | Percent survival rate (no. of patients) | |
|---|---|---|---|---|
| | TTP | Placebo | TTP | Placebo |
| Premenopausal | | | | |
| Axilla − | 22 (54) | 21 (52) | 82 (55) | 83 (52) |
| Axilla + | 59 (44) | 70 (60) | 61 (44) | 41 (61) |
| Total | 39 (98) | 47 (112) | 73[a](99) | 60[a](113) |
| Postmenopausal | | | | |
| Axilla − | 19 (130) | 16 (146) | 74 (152) | 77 (167) |
| Axilla + | 56 (142) | 63 (112) | 51 (163) | 49 (126) |
| Total | 38 (272) | 36 (258) | 62 (315) | 65 (293) |

[a]$p < .01$.

Of the 826 women in the trial, 99.3% were followed for 5 years and 95.3% were observed for at least 10 years. No significant difference in treatment failure rates was detected 5 and 10 years after radical mastectomy. Among the premenopausal patients, the 5-year survival rate was significantly greater in the TTP-treated arm ($p < .01$), and this result was more specifically ascribed to the subgroup of patients with 4 or more invaded nodes at the time of surgery. However, the distinction between the categories of 1–3 and 4 or more nodes was apparently made during the data analysis. These differences were still apparent at 10 years but were no longer significant.

On completion of this study, the NSABP performed a second study designed to compare a placebo, TTP, 5-fluorouracil, radiotherapy, and oophorectomy following radical mastectomy (62,63,123). Results of the postoperative radiotherapy (63) or adjuvant oophorectomy (123) versus placebo have already been cited in this chapter. In patients with invaded axilla, radiotherapy significantly reduced the 5-year recurrence rate within the operated and irradiated areas as compared to both placebo and TTP. No difference was noted in the rate of relapse at distant sites. The number of patients reported with a follow-up time of at least 5 years was too small to analyze survival data by nodal and menopausal status (63). Results with adjuvant oophorectomy were similar to those obtained with placebo or TTP but, as discussed earlier, the study has some glaring flaws (123).

The expertise gained in all the NSABP trials resulted in the design of two trials that have dramatically affected the field of adjuvant therapy, although the results were first reported with only an average follow-up time of less than 2 years (18,61). Both studies involved patients with axillary disease stratified according to age ($<50$ and $\geq 50$) and nodal status (1–3 versus 4 or more axillary nodes). Fisher et al. (61) tested L-PAM versus placebo given for 2 years after radical mastectomy in 348 evaluable patients. No difference was noted in postmenopausal patients. A striking prolongation of disease-free interval was apparent in patients under 50 given L-PAM ($p < .007$). However, further analysis indicated that this difference was significant only in women with 1 to 3 positive axillary nodes ($p < .008$) and not in the other nodal category. Bonadonna et al. (18) administered twelve 4-week courses of a combination of cyclophosphamide (CTX), methotrexate (MTX), and 5-fluorouracil (5-FU). The study included 391 patients who underwent radical or extended radical mastectomy. At the time of the report, the 3-year relapse rate was 45.7% in the control group compared to 26.3% in patients given chemotherapy ($p < .0001$). In premenopausal women, the difference remained highly significant whatever the axillary nodal status, 1 to 3 and 4 or more positive axillary nodes. The recurrence rate among patients at risk at 36 months with and without drug-induced amenorrhea was 9.2 and 27.2%, but this difference did not reach statistical significance. In postmenopausal patients, a difference in relapse rate could be detected only during the first 12 months following mastectomy and was no longer apparent thereafter. Of note, the incidence of early recurrences in the control group was lower in postmenopausal than in premenopausal patients, whereas in patients given chemotherapy, this incidence was similar whatever the menopausal status.

Undoubtedly, in both trials, longer observation periods will be needed to confirm these extremely provocative but very preliminary results, with special emphasis on survival data.

## RANDOMIZED TRIALS IN ADVANCED BREAST CANCER

### Ablative Hormone Therapy

Only a few randomized trials have investigated the role of ablative hormonal therapy in advanced breast cancer (Table 8). In most of them, the selection of patients was not defined in terms of disease-free interval and sites of involvement, two parameters of apparently independent and marked prognostic significance (129). Results of prior oophorectomy, whenever it was performed, were usually not available in trials dealing with major ablative procedures. Finally, interpretation of these data are often further complicated by the use of inaccurate response criteria and methods of data reporting.

The trials reviewed in this section have investigated the relative value of various types of ablative hormone therapy and that of surgical versus medical hormone therapy with or without subsequent surgical treatment.

Two completed trials of hypophysectomy versus adrenalectomy have yielded somewhat conflicting results. The first trial was carried out by Hayward et al. (84) and compared transfrontal hypophysectomy with adrenalectomy plus oophorectomy in 147 patients who had failed to respond to previous conventional hormone treatment. Response to treatment was defined as improvement of all visible, palpable, or radiologic lesions for at least 6 months. The response rates (36% versus 23%) and the mean response durations (37 versus 26 months) suggested a greater efficacy of hypophysectomy. The mean survival was 20.2 months in the hypophysectomy group and 12.2 months in the other therapeutic group ($p < .01$). However, one patient, who was still alive in remission 12 years after hypophysectomy, accounted for 25% of this increase in mean survival.

Roberts (126) compared a yttrium–90 (Y–90) implant in the pituitary versus adrenalectomy in postmenopausal or castrated patients. The disease-free interval and percentage of postmenopausal patients were similar in both therapeutic groups. No difference was noted in the rate of "clear-cut" response. However, despite the small number of patients in the study, a significant difference in survival of the responders was detected with 153 weeks for the adrenalectomy group and 91 weeks for the Y–90 group. Since response was not defined, the actual significance of this difference is unclear. Another trial reported by the same investigator (126) randomly compared transethmoidal hypophysectomy and pituitary ablation by Y–90. The 101 patients who were entered in the study were matched for the presence or absence of primary disease, previous oophorectomy or postmenopausal status, local or generalized disease, and length

TABLE 8. *Randomized trials of ablative hormone therapy in advanced breast cancer*

| Investigators and treatment arms | No. responses/ no. patients | Response rate (%) |
|---|---|---|
| Hayward et al. (84) | | |
| A. Hypophysectomy | 25/70 | 36 |
| B. Adrenalectomy + oophorectomy | 18/77 | 23 |
| Roberts (126) | | |
| A. Y–90 pituitary implant | 8/37 | 22 |
| B. Adrenalectomy + oophorectomy | 9/39 | 24 |
| Oberfield et al. (118) | | |
| A. Hypophysectomy | Unknown | |
| B. Adrenalectomy | Unknown | |
| Roberts (126) | | |
| A. Hypophysectomy | 6/51 | 12 |
| B. Y–90 pituitary implant | 12/50 | 24 |
| Harvey et al. (80) | | |
| A. Hypophysectomy | 3/12 | 25 |
| B. Aminoglutethimide + dexamethasone | 10/21 | 50 |
| Stewart et al. (136) | | |
| A. Y–90 pituitary implant | Unknown | |
| B. "Conventional" therapy | Unknown | |
| Dao (45) | | |
| I | | |
| A. Adrenalectomy | 50/108 | 46 |
| B. Fluoxymesterone or testosterone | 17/106 | 16 |
| (subsequent adrenalectomy) | 14/40 | 35 |
| C. Experimental steroids | 3/105 | 3 |
| (subsequent adrenalectomy) | 20/71 | 28 |
| II | | |
| A. Adrenalectomy | 6/17 | 35 |
| B. Diethylstilbestrol | 3/18 | 17 |
| (subsequent adrenalectomy) | 3/8 | 38 |
| Atkins et al. (11) | | |
| A. Ablative hormonotherapy | 28/94 | 30 |
| B. Additive hormonotherapy | 15/97 | 16 |
| (subsequent ablative hormonotherapy) | 13/57 | 23 |
| Selwood et al. (133) | | |
| A. First-line Y–90 pituitary implantation | 13/54 | 22 |
| B. Third-line Y–90 pituitary implantation | 15/54 [b] | 27 |

[a] See also (157).
[b] Response to first-, second-, or third-line treatment.

of disease-free interval. No significant difference was found in terms of response or survival rate.

Transethmoidal hypophysectomy has also been compared to the transfrontal approach in a trial conducted by Hayward et al. (84). This trial was discontinued after treating 40 or 50 patients because, prior to its onset, little experience had accumulated on the transethmoidal resection and it appeared that the study would really point out this lack of expertise rather than compare two techniques.

Several investigators have addressed themselves to the respective merits of surgical ablative versus medical suppressive or additive hormone therapy. Harvey et al. (80) compared hypophysectomy and medical adrenalectomy using aminoglutethimide and dexamethasone, 3 mg daily. This latter therapeutic modality achieved encouraging results in 20 patients but must await further experience for full assessment.

The trial of Stewart et al. (136) attempted to establish whether implantation of Y–90 in the pituitary resulted in longer survival than initial use of conventional treatments in patients not previously treated with adequate systemic palliative therapy. However, the lack of well-defined treatment options precludes any clear conclusion in this study.

The comparative value of early and late ablative hormone therapy has been tested by Dao at Roswell Park Memorial Institute (45). Three hundred nineteen postmenopausal women, previously untreated with hormone therapy, were randomized by date of menopause and dominant site of involvement to immediate adrenalectomy without oophorectomy, standard androgen therapy (fluoxymesterone or testosterone), or to several experimental steroids. The study design called for eventual adrenalectomy in all patients who failed to respond to additive hormone therapy. Assessment of response was made by independent investigators according to the criteria of the Cooperative Breast Cancer Group (41). Significantly higher response rates were achieved with the primary surgical procedure than with primary administration of standard androgens (46% versus 16%). Fifty-three percent of the patients treated with hormones subsequently underwent adrenalectomy. The response rate for delayed adrenalectomy was significantly lower than that observed when this surgical treatment was performed initially (46% versus 31%). Crude or actuarial survival curves of each treatment group were not given.

This same report gave the results of a trial comparing adrenalectomy versus stilbestrol followed by adrenalectomy at failure or relapse. No difference in response or survival rate was noted, but this trial involved a small number of patients. Along the same line, it must be mentioned that sequential treatments using adrenalectomy and chemotherapy have also been investigated at the same institution (113). Results are quite preliminary (see Table 11).

Atkins et al. (11) compared ablative versus additive hormone therapy followed by ablative hormone therapy in patients with advanced disease not previously treated with hormones. The ablative measures were transfrontal hypophysectomy or bilateral adrenalectomy plus oophorectomy. Androgens or estrogens were given as first-line hormonotherapy in the other group of patients according to their menopausal status. Improvement for at least 6 months in all visible, palpable, and radiological lesions, without appearance of new lesions, was considered response to treatment. Using these criteria, the response rate was also significantly greater after ablative than after additive hormone therapy (30% versus 16%).

Results were not given by menopausal status. Over one-third of the patients originally assigned to the additive treatment did not subsequently undergo surgery; most of them died or became unfit during hormone administration. The survival curves were similar in both groups of patients.

The last trial considered in this section was performed by Selwood et al. (133) and also studied the impact of the timing of major endocrine ablation. After stratification for site of the disease and menopausal status, 113 patients were randomly allocated to first- or third-line Y–90 treatment of the pituitary. In the second treatment group, premenopausal patients were treated by oöphorectomy and then by fluoxymesterone when failure or relapse occurred. Postmenopausal patients received estrogens as first-line therapy and fluoxymesterone as second-line therapy. In the group of patients assigned to delayed pituitary suppression, 30% died before ablation could be accomplished. Response to treatment was defined as a clear objective evidence of regression of all lesions without appearance of any new ones. Response rates and survival curves up to 5 years were virtually identical for both groups of patients.

Thus, the survival of patients with advanced breast cancer appeared to be similar if ablative hormone therapy was performed either initially or after failure on additive hormone therapy, even when the surgical treatment achieved higher response rates than the medical approach.

## Additive Hormone Therapy

Randomized trials of additive hormone therapy have largely been devoted to clinical screening of new agents (15,32,36,41,42,55,56,70,74,93,99,131, 143,146) or to pharmacologic studies of standard compounds (58,76). Most of the large-scale comparative trials of standard compounds have been carried out by the Cooperative Breast Cancer Group (Tables 9,10). Their master study protocol (41) required postmenopausal patients that had not received prior hormone therapy with the exception of oophorectomy. Stratification was made according to menopausal age and location of dominant lesions, two prognostic parameters of major significance (129). Of note, the clinical and laboratory findings of all cases were reviewed by independent investigators of the group at the completion of studies.

Results of a study comparing testosterone propionate (100 mg/day, 3 times a week i.m.) to diethylstilbestrol (15 mg/day p.o.) have been reported separately for the several participating institutions of the Cooperative Breast Cancer Group (42,97). The cumulative results of all these studies, which are tabulated by menopausal status and predominant site of metastatic invasion in Table 9, showed a statistically significant superiority of the estrogen over the androgen in terms of response rate. However, it would be premature to conclude that estrogens are more effective than androgens as additive hormone therapy in advanced breast cancer. Other promising androgenic compounds have been more recently introduced into clinical trials, and their antitumor activity relative to diethylstil-

TABLE 9. *Cooperative Breast Cancer Group comparisons of testosterone propionate and diethylstilbestrol (42,97)*

| Hormone | Dominant lesion | Patients castrated[a] <1 year | Years postmenopausal[a] 1-5 | 5-10 | 10+ | Total |
|---|---|---|---|---|---|---|
| Testosterone propionate | Breast | 0/5 | 1/18 | 2/5 | 6/18 | 9/46 |
| | Osseous | 0/15 | 1/17 | 1/12 | 5/42 | 7/86 |
| | Visceral | 0/17 | 0/25 | 1/17 | 7/62 | 8/121 |
| | Total | 0/37 | 2/60 | 4/34 | 18/122 | 24/253 (10%) |
| Diethylstilbestrol | Breast | 0/6 | 2/7 | 2/5 | 10/23 | 14/41 |
| | Osseous | 1/12 | 0/13 | 4/12 | 5/41 | 10/78 |
| | Visceral | 1/19 | 1/23 | 6/19 | 12/60 | 20/121 |
| | Total | 2/37 | 3/43 | 12/36 | 27/124 | 44/240 (18%) |

[a]Number of objective regressions/total number of patients.

TABLE 10. *Large-scale randomized trials of additive hormonotherapy by the Cooperative Breast Cancer Group*[a]

| Investigators and treatment arms | Response | |
|---|---|---|
| | No. responses/total patients | Rate (%) |
| Goldenberg (69) | | |
|   A. Testolactone | 5/103 | 5 |
|   B. Medroxyprogesterone acetate | 10/108 | 9 |
|   C. Oxylone acetate | 21/108 | 19 |
| Volk et al. (145) | | |
|   A. Testolactone (200 mg/day p.o.) | 5/118 | 4 |
|   B. As in A, 1000 mg/day p.o. | 18/123 | 15 |
|   C. As in A, 2000 mg/day p.o. | 15/121 | 12 |
| Goldenberg et al. (73) | | |
|   A. Testolactone | 21/115 | 18 |
|   B. Calusterone | 30/109 | 28 |
| Talley et al. (138) | | |
|   A. 7-$\alpha$-methyl-19-nortestosterone | | |
|     1. 10 mg (3 × wkly i.m.) | 17/111 | 15 |
|     2. 33 mg (3 × wkly i.m.) | 27/121 | 22 |
|     3. 100 mg (3 × wkly i.m.) | 29/103 | 28 |
|   B. Dromostanolone propionate | | |
|     1. 100 mg (3 × wkly i.m.) | 19/85 | 22 |
|     2. 200 mg (3 × wkly i.m.) | 13/80 | 16 |
| O'Bryan et al. (119) | | |
|   A. Surgical castration + thyroid substance (U.S.P.) | 28/109 | 26 |
|   B. Surgical castration + placebo | 30/109 | 28 |

[a] See also (153).

bestrol or testosterone propionate remains unsettled. Additional studies of the Cooperative Breast Cancer Group have also pointed to the difficulties in assessing hormonal agents with insufficient knowledge of their optimal mode of administration (Table 10).

Oxylone acetate was found to yield a better response rate than delta-1-testololactone or medroxy progesterone acetate, but its toxicity at the dose schedule used was also much more severe (69). In that trial, delta-1-testololactone was given at a daily oral dose of 150 mg but, in a subsequent trial (145), a similar dose was significantly less active than a daily oral dose of 1,000 or 2,000 mg. This compound given at 1,000 mg/day (73) was then found to achieve lower response rates than calusterone, although not to a significant extent. The next trial (138) compared 7-alpha-methyl-19-nortestosterone versus dromostanolone, and included a simultaneous dose-response evaluation of both drugs. A significant dose-response relationship was found with the former compound, but there was no difference in response rates of both drugs given at optimal dose levels. In the last trial (119), thyroid substance (U.S.P.) which was never tested in a conventional phase II study, failed to enhance the response rate or survival time following surgical castration.

Other trials have compared hormonal treatments of proven efficacy but did not include substantial numbers of patients. In an E.O.R.T.C. study (86) involving 98 patients treated with nafoxidine or ethynylestradiol, response rates were 31% and 14%, respectively, a difference almost statistically significant. A British study compared an estrogen, androgens, and a progestational agent, but only preliminary results were available (94).

Finally, several trials have investigated the value of hormone combinations: androgens with estrogens (42,77,97), antiestrogens (143), or progestational agents (67) and estrogens with progestational agents (7,139). None of these combinations emerged as clearly superior to single hormonal agents, especially to the individual constituents of these combinations. However, these trials also included small numbers of patients.

### Hormonotherapy and Chemotherapy

Various studies have compared hormonal agents, chemotherapeutic drugs, and their combination in advanced breast cancer (Table 11). No clear conclusion can be drawn from the presently available data, mainly as a consequence of the small number of entries in most of these trials. Results of a study by the Cooperative Breast Cancer Group (71) suggested that a greater antitumor activity may be obtained with chlorambucil and prednisone as compared to chlorambucil alone. However, the difference in response rate (20% versus 10%) was not statistically significant.

### Chemotherapy

Cytotoxic agents have played an increasingly prominent role in the therapy of breast cancer. The prognostic factors predictive for response to these agents do not appear to be specific to that malignancy. Prior treatment with cytotoxic agents, far-advanced disease, and unsuitability for receiving full-dose therapy are major features that result in a lower probability of response to chemotherapy in breast cancer. In addition, osseous and visceral metastases appear to be more resistant than soft tissue lesions. A prognostic role of the disease-free interval and menopausal status has been suggested in chemotherapy but has not yet been as clearly demonstrated as in hormone therapy (129).

A large number of phase II and III trials have investigated various single agents in breast cancer (Table 12). Adriamycin, CTX, 5-FU, MTX, and vincristine (VCR) are currently the standard chemotherapeutic drugs used in the treatment of this disease. However, little information is available to establish their relative individual efficacy. One of the most informative trials was reported by Brennan and Talley (23) and compared CTX and 5-FU in postmenopausal women who had failed on prior hormone therapy. Treatments were allocated according to odd–even case numbers; in the event of failure or relapse with one agent, patients were subsequently treated with the other. Responses were reported according to criteria of the Cooperative Breast Cancer Group. The respective remission rates to CTX and 5-FU were 22% (7/32) versus 37%

TABLE 11. *Randomized trials of hormonotherapy and chemotherapy in advanced breast cancer*[a]

| Investigators and treatment arms | No. responses/ total patients |
|---|---|
| Firat and Olshin (60) | |
|   A. Ovariectomy | 2/7 |
|   B. CTX | 1/6 |
|   C. Ovariectomy + CTX | 3/5 |
| Nemoto et al. (113) | |
|   A. Adrenalectomy | 9/30 |
|   B. Adriamycin | 11/33 |
|   C. CTX, 5-FU, prednisone | 13/31 |
| Nevinny et al. (114) | |
|   A. Testosterone propionate | 4/10 |
|   B. MTX | 5/20 |
| Cole et al. (40) | |
|   A. Nandrolone decanoate | 0/26 |
|   B. CTX | 7/30 |
|   C. Nandrolone decanoate + CTX | 1/22 |
| Goldenberg et al. (72) | |
|   A. Testolactone | 8/40 |
|   B. 5-FU | 2/35 |
|   C. Testolactone + 5-FU | 5/36 |
| Kennedy (98) | |
|   A. Diethylstilbestrol | 5/21 |
|   B. Diethylstilbestrol + CTX | 8/23 |
| Firat and Olshin (60) | |
|   A. Diethylstilbestrol | 5/18 |
|   B. CTX | 3/14 |
|   C. Diethylstilbestrol + CTX | 4/14 |
| Sponzo et al. (135) | |
|   A. Diethylstilbestrol | 1/13 |
|   B. Chemotherapy (various) | 9/13 |
| Firat and Olshin (60) | |
|   A. Prednisone | 1/9 |
|   B. 5-FU | 0/4 |
|   C. Prednisone + 5-FU | 1/6 |
| Goldenberg et al. (71) | |
|   A. Hydrocortisone + T3 | 10/85 |
|   B. Chlorambucil | 8/82 |
|   C. Chlorambucil + prednisone | 18/87 |
| Wolff and Prahl (147) | |
|   A. Hormonotherapy (various) | ? |
|   B. As in A + CTX | ? |
| Taylor et al. (140) | |
|   A. 5-FU | ?/32 |
|   B. 5-FU + premarin | ?/28 |
| Lloyd et al. (105) | |
|   A. Adriamycin, CTX | 18/28 |
|   B. As in A + calusterone | 3/7 |
| Band et al. (13) | |
|   A. CTX, MTX, 5-FU[b] | — |
|   B. As in A + fluoxymesterone[b] | — |
| Eagan et al. (50) | |
|   A. CTX, 5-FU, prednisone | 9/17 |
|   B. As in A + calusterone | 8/17 |
|   C. Adriamycin, VCR, MTX | 11/30 |

TABLE 11—*Cont.*

| Investigators and treatment arms | No. responses/ total patients |
|---|---|
| Ahmann et al. (9) | |
| A. CTX, 5-FU, prednisone, ± calusterone | 11/21 |
| B. CTX, adriamycin | 13/24 |
| C. As in B + 5-FU | 10/23 |
| Falkson et al. (57) | |
| A. CTX + calusterone | 3/28 |
| B. CTX + fluoxymesterone | 10/31 |
| Stott et al. (137) | |
| A. CTX, MTX, 5-FU, VCR, prednisone | 5/10 |
| B. CTX, MTX, 5-FU, VCR, medroxypro- gesterone acetate | 11/16 |
| Irwin et al. (91) | |
| A. Alternating regimens of CTX + 5-FU *and* MTX, T3 + prednisone | ? |
| B. Drugs as in A, given sequentially | ? |
| Horton et al. (89) | |
| A. 5-FU | 0/9 |
| B. 5-FU, mitomycin C, TTP, fluoxymesterone | 3/20 |

[a] See also (151, 152).
[b] Maintenance regimens.

TABLE 12. *Randomized trials of single-agent chemotherapy in advanced breast cancer*[a]

| Investigators and treatment arms | No. responses/ total patients |
|---|---|
| Cunningham et al. (44) | |
| A. CTX (schedule 1) | 0/19 |
| B. CTX (schedule 2) | 2/16 |
| Coggins et al. (38) | |
| A. CTX (schedule 1) | 2/16 |
| B. CTX (schedule 2) | 5/17 |
| Ahmann et al. (3) | |
| A. 5-FU (schedule 1) | 0/15 |
| B. 5-FU (schedule 2) | 0/15 |
| Ansfield et al. (10) | |
| A. 5-FU (schedule 1) | 14/42 |
| B. 5-FU (schedule 2) | 9/38 |
| C. 5-FU (schedule 3) | 8/41 |
| D. 5-FU (schedule 4) | 8/42 |
| Carey et al. (33) | |
| A. VCR (schedule 1) | ?/1 |
| B. VCR (schedule 2) | ?/3 |
| Knight et al. (100) | |
| A. Adriamycin (schedule 1) | 7/18 |
| B. Adriamycin (schedule 2) | 9/21 |

TABLE 12—*Cont.*

| Investigators and treatment arms | No. responses/ total patients |
|---|---|
| Bonnet et al. (19) | |
|   A. BCNU (schedule 1) | 13/36 |
|   B. BCNU (schedule 2) | 6/30 |
| Ahmann et al. (8) | |
|   A. BCNU | |
|   B. BCNU, prednisone | 0/16[b] |
| Zubrod et al. (150) | |
|   A. Nitrogen mustard | 7/37 |
|   B. TTP | 3/39 |
| Gold et al. (68) | |
|   A. CTX | 4/9 |
|   B. Nitrogen mustard | 1/6 |
|   C. Uracil mustard | 2/6 |
| Brennan and Talley (23) | |
|   A. CTX | 14/62 |
|   B. 5-FU | 15/62 |
| Eastern Cooperative Group (52) | |
|   A. 5-FU | 8/30 |
|   B. 5-FUDR | 9/31 |
|   C. MTX | 5/35 |
| Papac et al. (120) | |
|   A. 5-FUDR | 1/3 |
|   B. IUdR | 1/5 |
|   C. 5-FUDR, IUdR | 3/5 |
| Gottlieb et al. (75) | |
|   A. Adriamycin | 15/40 |
|   B. CCNU | 4/20 |
|   C. MeCCNU | 1/31 |
| Ahmann et al. (3) | |
|   A. CCNU | 2/21 |
|   B. TIC-mustard | 2/20 |
| Cunningham et al. (44) | |
|   A. CCNU | 3/27 |
|   B. 5-Azacytidine | 2/27 |
| Ahmann et al. (2) | |
|   A. VP-16 | 0/28 |
|   B. Cytembena | 0/25 |

[a] See additional studies including hormone therapy in Table 11.
[b] Cumulative results for both regimens.

(11/30) when both drugs were given as primary treatment and 23% (7/30) versus 13% (4/32) after crossover therapy, with a similar overall remission rate of 23 to 24% for both agents. No difference was noted in the mean duration of remissions induced by either of these drugs.

The comparative value of single agent and combination chemotherapy has been investigated in several trials (Table 13). Only two of them will be discussed in this chapter (31,87). The remaining trials have used unclear criteria of response

TABLE 13. *Single agents and combination chemotherapy in advanced breast cancer*[a]

| Investigators and treatment arms | Patient selection and stratification | No. responses/ total patients (%) |
|---|---|---|
| Hoogstraten et al. (87) | No prior CT | |
| A. Adriamycin | | 31/79 (39) |
| B. CTX, MTX, 5-FU, VCR, pred- nisone (schedule 1)[b] | | 39/98 (40) |
| C. As in B (schedule 2)[c] | | 59/106 (59) |
| Canellos et al. (31) | No prior CT; stratified by prior hormone therapy and meno- pausal status | |
| A. L-PAM | | 18/91 (20) |
| B. CTX, MTX, 5-FU | | 49/93 (53) |
| Rubens et al. (130) | No prior CT | |
| A. CTX | | 27/49 (55)[d] |
| B. CTX, MTX, 5-FU, VLB | | 31/50 (62)[d] |
| Lemkin and Dollinger (103) | Unknown | |
| A. 5-FU | | 5/17[d] |
| B. 5-FU, MTX, VCR, CLB, prednisone | | 6/20[d] |
| Ahmann et al. | No prior CT; Stratified by disease-free in- terval, menopausal age, dominant | |
| I (1) | lesions | |
| A. Adriamycin | | 10/20 |
| B. CTX, 5-FU, prednisone, ± VCR | | 13/28 (46) |
| II (4) | | |
| A. MeCCNU | | 1/22 |
| B. As in IB | | 12/21 |
| III (5) | | |
| A. Iphosphamide | | 4/20 |
| B. As in IB and IIB | | 10/20 |
| Kuperminc et al. (101) | Unknown | |
| A. Tilorone | | 0/25 |
| B. 5-FUDR, ara-C | | — |

[a]See additional studies including hormone therapy in Table 11.
[b]CTX (120 mg/m$^2$/d $\times$ 5 i.v.), MTX (4 mg/m$^2$/d $\times$ 5 i.v.), 5-FU (180 mg/m$^2$/d $\times$ 5 i.v.), VCR (0.625 mg/m$^2$ d1 and 5 i.v.), prednisone (40 mg/m$^2$/d $\times$ 5 p.o.)—Repeat course q. 4 wks.
[c]CTX (60 mg/m$^2$/d p.o.), MTX (15 mg/m$^2$ wk i.v.), 5-FU (300 mg/m$^2$/wk i.v.), VCR (0.625 mg/m$^2$/wk i.v.), Prednisone (30–10 mg/m$^2$/d p.o.).
[d]Unclear criteria of response.

or studied a limited number of patients often as part of a clinical screening program (1,4,5,101).

The Southwest Oncology Group (87) compared adriamycin to a five-drug regimen given intermittently or weekly in patients not previously treated with chemotherapy. The method of stratification was not reported, but there was no difference in the incidence of visceral, osseous, and soft tissue involvement in the three treatment groups. A temporary shortage of adriamycin resulted in relatively fewer patients in that treatment group. The weekly combination achieved significantly higher response rate (59%) than the intermittent combination (40%) or adriamycin alone (39%). Adriamycin was given at 60 mg/m$^2$ every 3 weeks and one may argue that a higher dose might have achieved a higher response rate. It was noteworthy that the most active treatment was the least toxic combination. The median duration of remission was about 9 months with the most active combination and 4 months with adriamycin ($p < .01$). This difference could be related to the higher rate of complete remission observed among responders to the combination and to the longer duration of complete responses as compared to partial responses. In addition, in order to prevent cumulative cardiotoxicity, adriamycin was systematically discontinued at a total dose of 500 mg/m$^2$, another factor that might have contributed to shorter response durations with adriamycin.

The Eastern Cooperative Oncology Group (31) undertook a comparison of L-PAM and a combination of CTX, MTX, and 5-FU (CMF), the regimens that have been used respectively by Fisher et al. (61) and Bonadonna et al. (18) in the adjuvant situation. Patients entered in the study had no prior chemotherapy; stratification was made according to prior hormonal therapy and menopausal status. Distribution of patients was similar in both arms with respect to age, disease-free interval, and prior radiotherapy. The combination achieved a significantly higher response rate than L-PAM, that is, 53% versus 20% ($p < .001$). Nearly 30% of the responders to both treatments had a complete disappearance of all measurable disease for at least 4 weeks; the median duration of response was 25 weeks on CMF and 13 weeks on L-PAM, a difference statistically significant at the .05 level. The toxicity of the combination was noticeably more severe than that recorded with L-PAM. A comparison of equitoxic regimens might have led to more conclusive results. The actual importance of these data will have to be evaluated in the light of corresponding results obtained with these treatments in the adjuvant situation.

A large number of randomized clinical trials have been devoted to comparisons of combination chemotherapy (Table 14). Therapeutic differences in terms of response rates were noted in three of these trials.

Smalley et al. (134) reported results obtained by the Southeastern Cancer Study Group. Patients previously untreated with cytotoxic chemotherapy were randomly allocated without stratification to single-drug chemotherapy administered sequentially and to weekly or intermittent combination chemotherapy. CTX, MTX, 5-FU, VCR, and prednisone (CMFVP) were used in all three treatment arms. The sequential treatment was to start with 5-FU. Median free-interval and distribution of dominant sites of disease were similar in each group of patients. Response rates were 18% with 5-FU, 46% with the weekly, and 27% with the intermittent combination. Thus, this study appeared to confirm results reported by Hoogstraten et al. (87) (see above and Table 13); there was a trend favoring the weekly over the intermittent combination ($p > .05$)

TABLE 14. *Combination chemotherapy in advanced breast cancer*[a]

| Investigators and treatment arms[b] | No. responses/ total patients (%) |
|---|---|
| Horton et al. (88) | |
|   A. CA | 6/10 |
|   B. CAF | 3/11 |
|   C. CPF | 1/5 |
|   D. CPF/CA | 4/4 |
| Priestman (121) | |
|   A. CA | 11/25 (44) |
|   B. CAFV | 11/25 (44) |
| Boston et al. (20)[c] | |
|   A. CA | 12/20 |
|   B. CAFM | 10/22 |
| Brambilla et al. (21) | |
|   A. AV | 10/15 |
|   B. AVP | 12/21 |
| Brown and Ward (26)[d] | |
|   A. AV | 5/20 |
|   B. AVC | 8/27 (30) |
|   C. AVCF | 13/34 (38) |
| Brambilla et al. (22) | |
|   A. AV | 35/75 (47) |
|   B. CMF | 28/68 (42) |
| Band et al. (13) | |
|   A. AV | — |
|   B. CMF | — |
|   C. CMFP | — |
| Ahmann et al. (6) | |
|   A. AM | 11/34 (32) |
|   B. CFP | 12/25 (48) |
|   C. CFVP | 10/19 (53) |
| Rossi et al. (128) | |
|   A. SF[e] | 5/10 |
|   B. SF[f] | 3/7 |
|   C. SFP | 2/5 |
| Brunner et al. (27) | |
|   A. CM | 7/39 (18) |
|   B. LM | 5/23 (20) |
| Bull et al. (28) | |
|   A. CMF | 20/32 (63) |
|   B. CAF | 20/30 (66) |
| Creech et al. (43) | |
|   A. CMF | 22/40 (55) |
|   B. CMFA | 26/37 (70) |
| Muss (111)[c] | |
|   A. CMF | 14/57 (24) |
|   B. CMFVP | 26/81 (32) |
| Brunner et al. (27) | |
|     I | |
|   A. CMP | 21/49 (44) |
|   B. CMV | 15/46 (33) |
|     II[d] | |
|   A. CMP | 8/18 (43) |
|   B. CMPFV | 45/91 (49) |

TABLE 14—*Cont.*

| Investigators and treatment arms[b] | No. responses/ total patients (%) |
|---|---|
| Baker et al. (12) | |
|   A. CFV (sequential) | 9/30 (30)[g] |
|   B. CFV | 20/46 (44) |
| Hancock et al. (79) | |
|   A. CFV | 15/46 (33) |
|   B. CFVA | 15/45 (33) |
| Ahmann et al. (1, 4–6) | |
|   A. CFP | 41/86 (48) |
|   B. CFPV | 33/74 (45) |
| Leone and Rege (104)[c] | |
|   A. FVP | 27/64 (42) |
|   B. CMFVP | 40/64 (63) |
| Edelstyn et al. (53) | |
|   I | |
|   A. CMFV (schedule 1) | 23/39 (59) |
|   B. CMFV (schedule 2) | 20/41 (49) |
|   II | |
|   A. CMFV (schedule 1) | 27/51 (53) |
|   B. CMFV (schedule 3) | 34/49 (69) |
| Ramirez et al. (122) | |
|   A. CMFV | 23/52 (44) |
|   B. CMFVP | 30/48 (63) |
| Smalley et al. (134) | |
|   A. CMFVP (sequential) | 6/34 (18)[g] |
|   B. CMFVP (schedule 1) | 16/35 (46) |
|   C. CMFVP (schedule 2) | 9/33 (27) |
| Muss et al. (112) | |
|   A. CMFVP | 18/28 (64) |
|   B. CAFVP | 14/20 (70) |

[a] See additional studies including hormone therapy in Table 11 and (155).
[b] Abbreviations: A = Adriamycin; C = CTX; F = 5-FU; L = Chlorambucil; M = MTX; P = Prednisone; S = L-PAM; V = VCR.
[c] "Comparative" study.
[d] Partially randomized.
[e] F given i.v.
[f] F given p.o.
[g] Response to first agent (5-FU).

whereas the weekly treatment achieved a significantly higher response rate than a single agent ($p < .05$).

A weekly CMFVP regimen was compared with the same combination without prednisone in a Central Oncology Group study (122). Prior chemotherapy with one of these drugs excluded entry in the study. Patients were evenly distributed according to menopausal age and type of tumor involvement. A greater antitumor activity was achieved with the five-drug combination (63% versus 44%), this difference between response rates almost reaching statistical significance.

A CMFVP regimen was also found by Leone and Rege (104) to be more effective than a three-drug combination including 5-FU, VCR, and prednisone. Analysis of this trial must await additional information.

Significant increases in remission duration have been suggested in other investigations despite a lack of difference in response rates. Thus, Bull et al. (28) compared combination regimens consisting of CTX, MTX, and 5-FU (CMF) or CTX, adriamycin, and 5-FU (CAF) in previously untreated patients. Sites of dominant disease were similarly distributed in both treatment groups. Response rates were 63 and 66%, respectively, but the median duration on study was 24 weeks for CMF and 40 weeks for CAF ($p < .05$), indicating that CAF provided a longer duration of disease control. Only partial data are presently available for analysis of this study, and a definite assessment should await publication of the final report.

Edelstyn et al. (53) have compared various schedules of a combination including CTX, MTX, 5-FU, and VCR. Treatment courses were repeated after 3 clear weeks. Response rates following the 5-day and the 1-day regimen were 59% versus 49% after 3 months, 54% versus 27% after 6 months ($p < .05$), and 34% versus 8% after 15 months ($p < .01$). Unfortunately, a direct statistical analysis of remission duration was lacking. The population studied in this trial was not defined, results were not detailed by prognostic parameters, and the drug-related toxicity was minimally described, precluding a clear interpretation of these results.

The other trials summarized in Table 14 have failed to show significant therapeutic differences, but a substantial number of patients was studied only in trials performed at the Mayo Clinic and the Istituto Nazionale Tumori. In the former institution, a combination of CTX, 5-FU, and prednisone (with or without VCR) served as a control arm in four consecutive phase II-III evaluations, with subsequent crossover of treatment assignment (1,4–6). These trials involved postmenopausal patients not previously exposed to chemotherapy. Results were analyzed by site of dominant disease, disease-free interval, date of menopause, and performance status. No improvement in the response rate to the three-drug combination could be detected with the addition of vincristine.

In the Italian study (22), patients without prior chemotherapy were allocated to either CTX plus MTX and 5-FU or to adriamycin plus VCR with crossover at progression or relapse. Stratification was made according to menopausal status, disease-free interval, and site of dominant disease. The respective response rates were 47% versus 52% after primary treatment and 30% versus 35% following secondary treatment. These combinations also achieved similar median duration of remission and median survivals.

In summary, this review of randomized trials of chemotherapy in advanced breast cancer showed that the relative value of standard single agents remains unsettled, but combination chemotherapy appeared more effective than adriamycin, L-PAM, or 5-FU used alone. Comparisons of combination regimens including different drugs have not yet demonstrated a clear superiority of any of them, but combinations including the same drugs used at different schedules have yielded significant therapeutic differences. A possible role of prednisone in combination with chemotherapy (71,122) is being further explored (13). Finally, development of combinations with little or no cross-resistance presently allows sequential administration of highly effective regimens. Fixed crossover studies of these combinations are in progress.

## Immunotherapy

Randomized trials of immunotherapy in breast cancer have exclusively tested the value of immunostimulation combined with other cytotoxic modalities (Table 15). Clinical results reported to date are still too preliminary or insufficiently detailed to allow a proper analysis. Thus, for example, Rojas et al. (127) investigated the potential of levamisole following radiotherapy in stage III breast cancer (international TNM classification). The initial workup of patients was not mentioned. This study was not truly randomized, since the patients were alternately assigned to either program after completion of radiotherapy. The response to radiotherapy alone was not detailed for each treatment group. Five of the 48 patients entered in the study were lost to follow-up and were excluded from the analysis; their original treatment assignment was not specified. The remaining patients were followed for at least 21 months after irradiation therapy. Relapses occurred in 11 of the 20 treated patients and in 21 of the 23 control patients. A significant superiority ($p < .01$) of the levamisole group was reported in me-

TABLE 15. *Randomized trials of immunotherapy*[a]

| Investigators and treatment arms | Disease stage | No. of evaluable patients | Results | |
|---|---|---|---|---|
| Rojas et al. (127)[b] | TNM III | | Mean disease-free interval[c] | |
| A. RT + DNCB | | 23 | 9 mos. | |
| B. As in A + levamisole | | 20 | 25 mos. | |
| Israel (92) | Advanced | | Median survival by skin test[c] | |
| | | | − | + |
| A. CTX, MTX, 5-FU, VLB, and STG | | ? | 5 mos. | 15 mos. |
| B. As in A + *C. parvum* | | ? | 9 mos. | 24 mos. |
| Haskell et al. (81) | Advanced | | | |
| A. CTX, MTX, and 5-FU | | 8 | Similar myelosuppression in both groups[c] | |
| B. As in A + *C. parvum* | | 6 | | |
| DeJager et al. (46) | Advanced | | | |
| A. CTX, MTX, 5-FU, and adriamycin | | 32 | Similar myelosuppression in both groups[c] | |
| B. As in A + *C. parvum* | | ? | | |

[a] See also Table 6.
[b] Alternate allocation to treatment groups after RT.
[c] Details on study protocol and results are lacking.

dian disease-free interval (25 versus 9 months) and in survival rate (90 versus 35%) at 30 months. However, the actual significance of these data remains unsettled.

## CONCLUSIONS

A number of randomized clinical trials have been performed in breast cancer but, by current standards, few have been adequately designed or included a sufficient number of patients. In fact, after excluding studies devoted to clinical screening of new regimens, it appears that a little amount of information lends itself to a meaningful analysis.

In clinical stage I breast cancer, no difference in 5-year survival has been detected between simple mastectomy versus simple mastectomy plus radiotherapy (30), simple mastectomy plus radiotherapy versus super radical mastectomy (95), or wide excision of the primary plus radiotherapy versus radical mastectomy plus radiotherapy (83). These results suggest that conservative therapy should be preferable to more aggressive approaches in that stage of the disease. However, if this assessment is true for the clinical stage I population as a whole, it is quite obvious that a therapeutic strategy based on clinical staging may be completely inappropriate for patients whose surgical staging demonstrates the presence of more advanced disease. In clinical stage I, invaded axillary nodes are found in approximately one-third of the patients. This relatively high proportion of erroneous understaging through clinical diagnoses appears sufficiently large to consider that the evaluation of local treatments in clinical stage I should not be made without careful surgical exploration at least of the axilla.

Only a limited number of investigations have provided meaningful results in patients with histologic stage II disease. When postoperative irradiation is not given, extended mastectomy appears to possibly prolong the survival in comparison to radical mastectomy in some subgroups of patients (102). Immediate postoperative radiotherapy does not influence the survival rate after radical mastectomy but does appear to decrease the locoregional recurrence rate (51, 63,90). However, the rate of locoregional recurrence as first evidence of relapse is only about 28% within 5 years after radical mastectomy without radiotherapy (63) and, probably radiotherapy remains as effective in controlling local disease at the time of its recurrence. The delayed use of this modality would then prevent a large number of patients from receiving inappropriate cytotoxic and immunosuppressive treatment for purely local disease.

So far, only one trial of systemic adjuvant therapy has had a sufficient period of study for proper analysis (64). In that trial, thiotepa given during a short period of time achieved an apparent increase in survival in premenopausal patients having 4 or more invaded axillary nodes. These findings are encouraging in view of the minimal chemotherapy used. The difference in the results according to menopausal status suggested that the chemotherapy might, in part, have acted as a medical oophorectomy. This interpretation remains debatable since the adjuvant value of oophorectomy has not yet been adequately tested. Recently completed studies have employed more intensive regimens (18,61). Longer follow-up is still needed to confirm their initial promising results and to define further the potential of adjuvant chemotherapy.

In advanced disease, no clear difference has been found between the overall results of any type of hypophysectomy or adrenalectomy. Most of the studies investigating major ablative hormonotherapy failed to consider important prognostic factors and used outdated criteria of response. In postmenopausal women, adrenalectomy achieved higher response rates than fluoxymesterone or testosterone, or subsequent adrenalectomy performed when resistance to these androgens occurred (45). Testosterone has been shown less active than diethylstilbestrol, and the efficacy of the latter seems at least equal to that of several other hormonal compounds. Thus, the relative merit of optimal ablative versus optimal additive hormone therapy remains unsettled. The respective roles of hormone therapy and chemotherapy in advanced disease are still completely unknown and should be investigated further, particularly in subcategories of patients with clear prognostic features regarding response to hormone therapy or chemotherapy.

Adriamycin, CTX, 5-FU, MTX, and VCR are the five chemotherapeutic agents commonly used in breast cancer. Adriamycin is generally believed to induce the highest response rate but, in fact, only CTX and 5-FU have been significantly compared with each other and have shown the same efficacy. Various combinations of these five agents, with or without prednisone, have been investigated. They seem to produce higher response rates and longer remissions than the presently available agents used alone. Currently available data emphasize the importance of a proper scheduling. The effect of number and selection of drugs is being investigated.

Much emphasis has recently been placed on immunotherapy with or without other treatment modalities. These efforts have not yet produced meaningful results.

In summary, this analysis of randomized clinical trials indicates a striking lack of firm information in trials for which preliminary or final results have been published as recently as 1976. Larger accrual and/or longer follow-up is required in a number of these studies before a full analysis can be made. Results of numerous completed but still unpublished clinical trials are now accumulating and should answer a number of the important questions raised in this chapter.

## LIST OF COMPOUNDS

*Ara-C:* Cytosine arabinoside, NSC–63878; cytosine, 1-$\beta$-D-arabinofuranosyl-, monohydrochloride
*BCG:* Bacillus Calmette-Guerin
*BCNU:* NSC–409962; urea, 1,3-bis(2-chloroethyl)-1-nitroso-
*CCNU:* NSC–79037; urea, 1-(2-chloroethyl)-3-cyclohexyl-1-nitroso-

*C. parvum;* Corynebacterium parvum
*CTX:* Cyclophosphamide; NSC–26271; 2H-1,3,2-oxazaphosphorine, 2-[bis(2-chloroethyl)amino] tetrahydro-,2-oxide, monohydrate
*DNCB:* Dinitrochlorobenzene
*5-FU:* 5-fluorouracil, NSC–19893
*5-FUDR:* NSC–27640; uridine, 5-fluoro-2'-deoxy-
*IUdR:* NSC–39661; 5-iodo-2'-deoxyuridine
*L-PAM:* Melphalan, NSC–8806; alanine, 3-[*p*-[bis(2-chloroethyl)amino]phenyl]-, monohydrochloride, L-
*MeCCNU:* Methyl CCNU, NSC–95441; urea, 1-(2-chloroethyl)-3-(4-methylcyclohexyl)-1-nitroso-
*MTX:* Methotrexate, NSC–740; glutamic acid, N-[*p*-[[(2,4-diamino-6-pteridinyl)methyl]methylamino]benzoyl]-
*STG:* Streptonigrin; NSC–45383
*T3:* Triiodothyronine; liothyronine sodium
*TTP:* thiotepa; NSC–6396; phosphine sulfide, tris(1-aziridinyl)-
*VCR:* Vincristine, NSC–67574
*VLB:* Vincblastine, NSC–49842
*VP-16:* VP 16–213, NSC–141540; 4'-demethylpipodophyllotoxin 9-(4,6-O-ethylidene-β-D-glucopyranoside)

## REFERENCES

1. Ahmann, D. L., Bisel, H. F., Eagan, R. T., Edmonson, J. H., and Hahn, R. G. (1974): Controlled evaluation of adriamycin (NSC–123127) in patients with disseminated breast cancer. *Cancer Chemother. Rep.,* 58:877–882.
2. Ahmann, D. L., Bisel, H. F., Eagan, R. T., Edmonson, J. H., Hahn, R. G., O'Connell, M. J., and Frytak, S. (1976): Phase II evaluation of VP 16–213 (NSC–141540) and cytembena (NSC–104801) in patients with advanced breast cancer. *Cancer Treat. Rep.,* 60:633–635.
3. Ahmann, D. L., Bisel, H. F., and Hahn, R. G. (1973): Difficulties designing clinical trials as exemplified by a phase 2 drug evaluation of 5[3,3-bis(2-chloroethyl)-1-triazenol]-imidazole-4-carboxamide and 1-(2-chloroethyl)-3-cyclohexyl-1-nitrosourea in patients with disseminated breast cancer. *Cancer Res.,* 33:1707–1710.
4. Ahmann, D. L., Bisel, H. F., and Hahn, R. G. (1974): A phase 2 evaluation of 1-(2-chloroethyl)-3-(4-methylcyclohexyl)-1-nitrosourea (NSC–95441) in patients with advanced breast cancer. *Cancer Res.,* 34:27–30.
5. Ahmann, D. L., Bisel, H. F., and Hahn, R. G. (1974): Phase II clinical trial of isophosphamide (NSC–109724) in patients with advanced breast cancer. *Cancer Chemother. Rep.,* 58:861–865.
6. Ahmann, D. L., Eagan, R. T., Bisel, H. F., Hahn, R. G., O'Connell, M. J., and Edmonson, J. H. (1975): Evaluation of combination therapy with adriamycin (NSC–123127) and methotrexate (NSC–740) in patients with disseminated breast cancer. *Cancer Chemother. Rep. Part 3,* 6:335–338.
7. Ahmann, D. L., Hahn, R. G., and Bisel, H. F. (1972): Disseminated breast cancer: Evaluation of hormonal therapy utilizing stilbestrol and medrogestone (AY-62022) singly and in combination. *Cancer,* 30:651–653.
8. Ahmann, D. L., Hahn, R. G., and Bisel, H. F. (1972): Evaluation of 1,3-bis(2-chloroethyl)-1-nitrosourea (BCNU; NSC-409962) in the management of patients with advanced breast cancer. *Cancer Chemother. Rep.,* 56:93–94.
9. Ahmann, D. L., O'Connell, M. J., and Bisel, H. F. (1976): An evaluation of cytoxan/adriamycin (CA) vs. cytoxan/adriamycin/5-fluorouracil (CAF) vs cytoxan/5-fluorouracil/prednisone (CFP) in advanced breast cancer. *Proc. Am. Soc. Clin. Oncol.,* 17:278.

10. Ansfield, F., Klotz, J., Nealon, T., Ramirez, G., Minton, J., Hill, G., Wilson, W., Davis, H., Jr., and Cornell, G. (1977): A phase III study comparing the clinical utility of four regimens of 5-fluorouracil. A preliminary report. *Cancer,* 39:34–40.

11. Atkins, H., Falconer, M. A., Hayward, J. L., MacLean, K. S., and Schurr, P. H. (1966): The timing of adrenalectomy and of hypophysectomy in the treatment of advanced breast cancer. *Lancet,* 1:827–830.

12. Baker, L. H., Vaughn, C. B., Al-Sarraf, M., Reed, M. L., and Vaitkevicius, V. K. (1974): Evaluation of combination vs. sequential cytotoxic chemotherapy in the treatment of advanced breast cancer. *Cancer,* 33:513–518.

13. Band, P. R., Tormey, D. C., and Temkin, N., for the Eastern Cooperative Oncology Group (1976): Induction chemotherapy and maintenance chemo-hormonotherapy in metastatic breast cancer. *Proc. Am. Assoc. Cancer Res.,* 17:37.

14. Bates, T. D. (1975): A prospective clinical trial of post-operative radiotherapy delivered in three fractions per week versus two fractions per week in breast carcinoma. *Clin. Radiol.,* 26:297–304.

15. Bennett, M. B., Helman, P., and Palmer, P. (1975): Hormonal therapy of breast cancer with special reference to Masteril therapy. *S. Afr. Med. J.,* 49:2036–2040.

16. Bland, K. I., O'Leary, J. P., Woodward, E. R., and Dragstedt, L. R. (1975): Immediate oophorectomy and adrenalectomy in the treatment of stage III breast carcinoma. A ten year follow-up study. *Am. J. Surg.,* 129:277–285.

17. Blokhina, N. G., and Karev, N. I. (1974): Thio-tepa and endoxan in combined treatment of breast cancer (cooperative trial). *Radiobiol. Radiother.* (Berl.), 15:357–360.

18. Bonadonna, G., Rossi, A., Valagussa, P., Banfi, A., and Veronesi, U. (1977): The CMF program for operable breast cancer with positive axillary nodes: Updated analysis on the disease-free interval, site of relapse and drug tolerance. *Cancer,* 39:2904–2915.

19. Bonnet, J. D., Brownlee, R. W., Vaitkevicius, V. K., and Talley, R. W. (1973): Response of advanced breast cancer to two dosage regimens of 1,3-bis(2-chloroethyl)-1-nitrosourea (BCNU; NSC-409962). *Cancer Chemother. Rep.,* 57:231–234.

20. Boston, B., Mitchell, M., Farber, L., and Bertino, J. (1976): Combination vs. combination-sequential non-hormonal chemotherapy in advanced breast cancer. *Proc. Am. Soc. Clin. Oncol.,* 17:247.

21. Brambilla, C., De Lena, M., and Bonadonna, G. (1974): Combination chemotherapy with adriamycin (NSC-123127) in metastatic mammary carcinoma. *Cancer Chemother. Rep.,* 58:251–253.

22. Brambilla, C., De Lena, M., Rossi, A., Valagussa, P., and Bonadonna, G. (1976): Response and survival in advanced breast cancer after two non-cross-resistant combinations. *Br. Med. J.,* 1:801–804.

23. Brennan, M. J., and Talley, R. W. (1967): Implications of treatment sequence effects on responsiveness to 5-fluorouracil and cytoxan. In: *Current Concepts in Breast Cancer,* edited by A. Segaloff, K. K. Meyer, and S. Debakey, pp. 225–234. Williams & Wilkins, Baltimore.

24. Brinkley, D., and Haybittle, J. L. (1966): Treatment of stage-II carcinoma of the female breast. *Lancet,* 2:291–295.

25. Brinkley, D., and Haybittle, J. L. (1971): Treatment of stage-II carcinoma of the female breast. *Lancet,* 2:1086–1087.

26. Brown, I., and Ward, H. W. C. (1976): Doxorubicin in the treatment of advanced breast cancer; comparative studies of three combination chemotherapy regimes. *Clin. Oncol.,* 2:105–111.

27. Brunner, K. W., Sonntag, R. W., Martz, G., Senn, H. J., Obrecht, P., and Alberto, P. (1975): A controlled study in the use of combined drug therapy for metastatic breast cancer. *Cancer,* 36:1208–1219.

28. Bull, J., Tormey, D., Falkson, G., Blom, J., Perlin, E., and Carbone, P. (1975): A comparison of cyclophosphamide, adriamycin, and 5-fluorouracil versus cyclophosphamide, methotrexate, and 5-fluorouracil in metastatic breast cancer. *Proc. Am. Soc. Clin. Oncol.,* 16:246.

29. Burn, J. I. (1974): "Early" breast cancer: the Hammersmith trial. An interim report. *Br. J. Surg.,* 61:762–765.

30. Cancer Research Campaign (1976): Management of early cancer of the breast. Report on an international multicentre trial supported by the Cancer Research Campaign. *Br. Med. J.,* 1:1035–1038.

31. Canellos, G. P., Pocock, S. J., Taylor, S. G. III, Sears, M. E., Klaasen, D. J., and Band, P. R. (1976): Combination chemotherapy for metastatic breast carcinoma. Prospective comparison of multiple drug therapy with L-phenylalanine mustard. *Cancer,* 38:1882–1886.

32. Cantino, T. J., Eisenberg, E., and Gordan, G. S. (1966): Antitumor efficacy of 7α,17α-dimethyltestosterone in disseminated breast cancer. *Cancer,* 19:817–820.

33. Carey, R. W., Hall, T. C., and Finkel, H. E. (1963): A comparison of two dosage regimens for vincristine. *Cancer Chemother. Rep.,* 27:91–96.

34. Carter, S. K. (1976): Integration of chemotherapy into combined modality treatment of solid tumors. VII. Adenocarcinoma of the breast. *Cancer Treat. Rev.,* 3:141–174.

35. Charlson, M. E., and Feinstein, A. R. (1973): An analytic critique of existing systems of staging for breast cancer. *Surgery,* 73:579–598.

36. Chowdhury, M. S., Banks, A. J., Bond, W. H., Jones, W. G., and Ward, H. W. C. (1976): A comparison of drostanolone propionate (Masteril) and nandrolone decanoate (Decadurabolin) in the treatment of breast carcinoma. *Clin. Oncol.,* 2:203–206.

37. Clemmesen, J. (1965): *Statistical Studies in Malignant Neoplasms.* I. *Review and Results.* Munksgaard, København.

38. Coggins, P. R., Eisman, S. H., Elkins, W. L., and Ravdin, R. G. (1961): Cyclophosphamide therapy in carcinoma of the breast and ovary. A comparative study of intermittent massive vs continuous maintenance dosage regimens. *Cancer Chemother. Rep.,* 15:3–8.

39. Cole, M. P. (1975): A clinical trial of an artificial menopause in carcinoma of the breast. In: *Hormones and Breast Cancer,* edited by M. Namer and C. M. Lalanne, pp. 143–150. Inserm, Paris.

40. Cole, M. P., Todd, I. D. H., and Wilkinson, P. M. (1973): Cyclophosphamide and nandrolone decanoate in the treatment of advanced carcinoma of the breast—results of a comparative controlled trial of the agents used singly and in combination. *Br. J. Cancer,* 27:396–399.

41. Cooperative Breast Cancer Group (1961): Progress report: Results of studies by the Cooperative Breast Cancer Group—1956–60. *Cancer Chemother. Rep.,* 11:109–141.

42. Cooperative Breast Cancer Group (1964): Results of studies of the Cooperative Breast Cancer Group—1961–63. *Cancer Chemother. Rep.,* 41 (suppl 1):1–24.

43. Creech, R., Holroyde, C., Catalano, R., Koons, L., Miller, D., and Engstrom, P. (1976): Low dose CMF vs. CAMF treatment for metastatic breast cancer. *Proc. Am. Soc. Clin. Oncol.,* 17:259.

44. Cunningham, T. J., Nemoto, T., Rosner, D., Knight, E., Taylor, S., Rosenbaum, C., Horton, J., and Dao, T. (1974): Comparison of 5-azacytidine (NSC-102816) with CCNU (NSC-79037) in the treatment of patients with breast cancer and evaluation of the subsequent use of cyclophosphamide (NSC-26271). *Cancer Chemother. Rep.,* 58:677–681.

45. Dao, T. L. (1970): Early compared with late adrenalectomy. In: *The Clinical Management of Advanced Breast Cancer,* edited by C. A. F. Joslin and E. N. Gleave, pp. 68–72. Alpha Omega Alpha, Cardiff.

46. DeJager, R., Pinsky, C., Kaufman, R., Ochoa, M., Oettgen, H., and Krakoff, I. (1976): Chemotherapy of advanced breast cancer with a combination of cyclophosphamide, adriamycin, methotrexate, and 5-fluorouracil (CAMF) with and without *C. parvum. Proc. Am. Soc. Clin. Oncol.,* 17:296.

47. de Schryver, A. (1976): The Stockholm Breast Cancer Trial: Preliminary report of a randomized study concerning the value of pre-operative or post-operative radiotherapy in operable disease. *Int. J. Radiat. Oncol. Biol. Phys.,* 1:601–609.

48. Donegan, W. L. (1974): Extended surgical adjuvant thiotepa for mammary carcinoma. *Arch Surg.,* 109:187–192.

49. Duncan, W., Forrest, A. P. M., Gray, N., Hamilton, T., Langlands, A. O., Prescott, R. J., Shivas, A. A., and Stewart, H. J. (1975): New Edinburgh primary breast cancer trials. Report by Co-ordinating Committee. *Br. J. Cancer,* 32:628–630.

50. Eagan, R. T., Ahmann, D. L., Edmonson, J. H., Hahn, R. G., and Bisel, H. F. (1975): Controlled evaluation of the combination of adriamycin (NSC-123127), vincristine (NSC-67574), and methotrexate (NSC-740) in patients with disseminated breast cancer. *Cancer Chemother. Rep. Part 3,* 6:339–342.

51. Easson, E. C. (1968): Post-operative radiotherapy in breast cancer. In: *Prognostic Factors in Breast Cancer,* edited by A. P. M. Forrest and P. B. Kunkler, pp. 118–127. Williams & Wilkins, Baltimore.

52. Eastern Cooperative Group in Solid Tumor Chemotherapy (1967): Comparison of antimetabolites in the treatment of breast and colon cancer. *JAMA,* 200:770–778.

53. Edelstyn, G. A., Bates, T. D., Brinkley, D., MacRae, K. D., Spittle, M. F., and Wheeler, T. (1975): Comparison of 5-day, 1-day, and 2-day cyclical combination chemotherapy in advanced breast cancer. *Lancet,* 2:209–211.

54. Edland, R. W., Maldonado, L. G., Johnson, R. O., and Vermund, H. (1969): Postoperative irradiation in breast cancer. An evaluation of 291 cases treated at the University of Wisconsin Medical Center from 1955 through 1961. *Radiology,* 93:905–913.

55. Emery, E. W., and Trotter, W. R. (1963): Triiodothyronine in advanced breast cancer. *Lancet,* i:358–359.

56. Engelsman, E., Heuson, J. C. Blonk-Van Der Wijst, J., Drochmans, A. Maass, H., Cheix, F., Sobrinho, L. G., and Nowakowski, H. (1975): Controlled clinical trial of L-dopa and nafoxidine in advanced breast cancer: An E.O.R.T.C. study. *Br. Med. J.,* 2:714–715.

57. Falkson, G., van Dyk, J. J., van Eden, E. B., van der Merwe, A. M., and Falkson, H. C. (1974): Calusterone (NSC–88536): a poor substitute for fluoxymesterone (NSC–12165) in the treatment of advanced breast cancer. *Cancer Chemother. Rep.,* 58:939–941.

58. Feldman, E. B., and Carter, A. C. (1973): Diethylstilbestrol and circulating lipids in women with metastatic breast cancer: lack of dose response over three log units. *J. Clin. Endocrinol. Metab.,* 36:381–384.

59. Finney, R. (1971): Adjuvant chemotherapy in the radical treatment of carcinoma of the breast—a clinical trial. *Am. J. Roentgenol. Radium Ther. Nucl. Med.,* 111:137–141.

60. Firat, D., and Olshin, S. (1968): Treatment of metastatic carcinoma of the female breast with combination of hormones and other chemotherapy. *Cancer Chemother. Rep.,* 52:743–750.

61. Fisher, B., Glass, A., Redmond, C., Fisher, E. R., Barton, B., Such, E., Carbone, P., Economou, S., Foster, R., Frelick, R., Lerner, H., Levitt, M., Margolese, R., MacFarlane, J., Plotkin, D., Shibata, H., Volk, H. (and other cooperating investigators) (1977): L-phenylalanine mustard (L-PAM) in the management of primary breast cancer: An update of earlier findings and a comparison with those utilizing L-PAM plus 5-fluorouracil (5-FU). *Cancer,* 39:2883–2903.

62. Fisher, B., Ravdin, R. G., Ausman, R. K., Slack, N. H., Moore, G. E., and Noer, R. J. (1968): Surgical adjuvant chemotherapy in cancer of the breast: results of a decade of cooperative investigation. *Ann. Surg.,* 168:337–356.

63. Fisher, B., Slack, N. H., Cavanaugh, P. J., Gardner, B., and Ravdin, R. G. (1970): Postoperative radiotherapy in the treatment of breast cancer: Results of the NSABP Clinical Trial. *Ann. Surg.,* 172:711–732.

64. Fisher, B., Slack, N., Katrych, D., and Wolmark, N. (1975): Ten year follow-up results of patients with carcinoma of the breast in a co-operative clinical trial evaluating surgical adjuvant chemotherapy. *Surg. Gynecol. Obstet.,* 140:528–534.

65. Fisher, B., and Wolmark, N. (1975): New concepts in the management of primary breast cancer. *Cancer,* 36 (Suppl.):627–632.

66. Forrest, A. P. M., Roberts, M. M., Preece, P., Henk, J. M., Campbell, H., Hughes, L. E., Desai, S., and Hulbert, M. (1974): The Cardiff-St. Mary's trials. *Br. J. Surg.,* 61:766–769.

67. Gaertner, R. A., Lewison, E. F., Finney, G. G., Jr., and Montague, A. C. W. (1968): Combined hormone therapy in advanced breast cancer. Triple-blind study of 68 patients treated with dromostanolone and fluorometholone. *Johns Hopkins Med. J.,* 123:138–141.

68. Gold, G. L., Shnider, B. I., Salvin, L. G., Schneiderman, M. A., Colsky, J., Owens, A. H. Jr., Krant, M. J., Miller, S. P., Frei, E. III, Hall, T. C., Spurr, C. L., McIntyre, O. R., Hoogstraten, B., and Holland, J. F. (1970): The use of mechlorethamine, cyclophosphamide, and uracil mustard in neoplastic disease: A cooperative study. *J. Clin. Pharmacol.,* 10:110–120.

69. Goldenberg, I. S. (1969): Clinical trial of delta-1-testololactone (NSC 23759), medroxy progesterone acetate (NSC 26386) and oxylone acetate (NSC 47438) in advanced female mammary cancer. A report of the Cooperative Breast Cancer Group. *Cancer,* 23:109–112.

70. Goldenberg, I. S., Hayes, M. A., and Morin, J. E. (1965): Hormonal therapy of metastatic female breast carcinoma. V. Phenol, 4, 4'-(dl-1,2-diethyl-ethylene) di- and androst-4-en-3-one, 9-chloro-11 beta, 17 beta-dihydroxy-17-methyl-. *Cancer,* 18:447–449.

71. Goldenberg, I. S., McMahan, C. A., Escher, G. C., Volk, H., Ansfield, F. J., and Olson, K. B. (1973): Secondary chemotherapy of advanced breast cancer. *Cancer,* 31:660–663.

72. Goldenberg, I. S., Sedransk, N., Volk, H., Segaloff, A., Kelley, R. M., and Haines, C. R. (1975): Combined androgen and antimetabolite therapy of advanced female breast cancer. A report of the Cooperative Breast Cancer Group. *Cancer,* 36:308–310.

73. Goldenberg, I. S., Waters, M. N., Ravdin, R. S., Ansfield, F. J., and Segaloff, A. (1973): Androgenic therapy for advanced breast cancer in women. A report of the Cooperative Breast Cancer Group. *JAMA,* 223:1267–1268.

74. Gordan, G. S., Halden, A., Horn, Y., Fuery, J. J., Parsons, R. J., and Walter, R. M. (1973):

Calusterone (7β,17α-dimethyltestosterone) as primary and secondary therapy of advanced breast cancer. *Oncology*, 28:138–146.

75. Gottlieb, J. A., Rivkin, S. E., Spigel, S. C., Hoogstraten, B., O'Bryan, R. M., Delaney, F. C., and Singhakowinta, A. (1974): Superiority of adriamycin over oral nitrosoureas in patients with advanced breast carcinoma. A Southwest Cancer Chemotherapy Study Group study. *Cancer*, 33:519–526.

76. Guevara, E., Perlia, C. P., and Wolter, J. (1971): Estrogens in disseminated breast cancer: Comparative study of physiologic versus pharmacologic dose. *Rush-Presbyterian-St. Luke's Med. Bull*, 10:52–55.

77. Haines, C. R., Wallace, H. J. Jr., Nevinny, H. B., and Hall, T. C. (1969): Clinical evaluation of estrogen-androgen combination in advanced breast cancer. *Am. J. Surg.*, 117:589–594.

78. Hamilton, T., Langlands, A. O., and Prescott, R. J. (1974): The treatment of operable cancer of the breast: A clinical trial in the South-East region of Scotland. *Br. J. Surg.*, 61:758–761.

79. Hancock, B. M., Ribeiro, G. G., and Todd, I. D. H. (1976): Combination chemotherapy of advanced breast cancer. A random trial of two schedules. *Clin. Oncol.*, 2:101–104.

80. Harvey, H. A., Santen, R. J., Osterman, J., White, D., and Lipton, A. (1976): A comparative clinical trial of medical adrenalectomy vs. transsphenoidal hypophysectomy in advanced breast cancer. *Proc. Am. Assoc. Cancer Res.*, 17:219.

81. Haskell, C. M., Ossorio, R. C., Sarna, G. P., and Fahey, J. L. (1976): Chemoimmunotherapy of metastatic breast cancer with corynebacterium parvum (CP): A double blind randomized trial. *Proc. Am. Soc. Clin. Oncol.*, 17:265.

82. Haskell, C. M., Sparks, F. C., Graze, P. R., and Korenman, S. G. (1977): Systemic therapy for metastatic breast cancer. *Ann. Intern. Med.*, 86:68–80.

83. Hayward, J. (1974): Conservative surgery in the treatment of early breast cancer. *Br. J. Surg.*, 61:770–771.

84. Hayward, J. L., Atkins, H. J. B., Falconer, M. A., MacLean, K. S., Salmon, L. F. W., Schurr, P. H., and Shaheen, C. H. (1970): Clinical trials comparing transfrontal hypophysectomy with adrenalectomy and with transethmoidal hypophysectomy. In: *The Clinical Management of Advanced Breast Cancer,* edited by C. A. F. Joslin and E. N. Gleave, pp. 50–53. Alpha Omega Alpha, Cardiff.

85. Helman, P., Bennett, M. B., Louw, J. H., Wilkie, W., Madden, P., Silber, W., Sealy, R., and Heselson, J. (1972): Interim report on trial of treatment for operable breast cancer. *S. Afr. Med. J.,* 46:1374–1375.

86. Heuson, J. C., Engelsman, E., Blonk-Van der Wijst, J., Maass, H., Drochmans, A., Michel, J., Nowakowski, H., and Gorins, A. (1975): Comparative trial of nafoxidine and ethinyloestradiol in advanced breast cancer: An E.O.R.T.C. study. *Br. Med. J.*, 2:711–713.

87. Hoogstraten, B., George, S. L., Samal, B., Rivkin, S. E., Costanzi, J. J., Bonnet, J. D., Thigpen, T., and Braine, H. (1976): Combination chemotherapy and adriamycin in patients with advanced breast cancer. A Southwest Oncology Group study. *Cancer*, 38:13–20.

88. Horton, J., Dao, T., Cunningham, T., Nemoto, T., Sponzo, R., and Rosner, D. (1975): A comparison of 4 combination chemotherapies for metastatic breast cancer. *Proc. Am. Soc. Clin. Oncol.*, 16:240.

89. Horton, J., Olson, K. B., Cunningham, T., and Sullivan, J. (1968): Comparison of a combination of 5-fluorouracil (NSC-19893), mitomycin C (NSC-26980), triethylenethiophosphoramide (NSC-6396), and fluoxymesterone (NSC-12165) with 5-fluorouracil alone in patients with advanced cancer. *Cancer Chemother. Rep.*, 52:597–600.

90. Høst, H., and Brennhovd, I. O. (1975): Combined surgery and radiation therapy versus surgery alone in primary mammary carcinoma. I. The effect of orthovoltage radiation. *Acta Radiol., (Ther) (Stockh)* 14:25–32.

91. Irwin, L. E., Pugh, R., Sadoff, L., Hestorff, R., and Weiner, J., for the Western Cancer Study Group (1974): The influence on survival of combination chemotherapy vs. sequential single drug chemotherapy in patients with breast cancer. In: *Abstracts of the XI International Cancer Congress,* Florence, Italy, III, p. 597.

92. Israel, L. (1974): A randomized study of chemotherapy versus chemotherapy and immune therapy with *Corynebacterium parvum* in advanced breast cancer. *Proc. XI Int. Cancer Congr.*, Florence, 6:77–79.

93. Japanese Cooperative Group of Hormonal Treatment for Breast Cancer (1973): 2α,3α-epithio-5α-androstan-17β-ol in the treatment of advanced breast cancer. *Cancer*, 31:789–792.

94. Jones, V., Joslin, C. A. F., Jones, R. E., Davies, D. K. L., Roberts, M. M., Gleave, E. N., Campbell, H., and Forrest, A. P. M. (1971): Progestagens and advanced breast cancer. *Lancet*, 1:1049–1050.

95. Kaae, S., and Johansen, H. (1969): Simple mastectomy plus postoperative irradiation by the method of McWhirter for mammary carcinoma. *Ann. Surg.,* 170:895–899.
96. Kenis, Y. (1976): Roundtable discussion on curative treatment. In: *Breast Cancer, Trends in Research and Treatment,* edited by J. C. Heuson, W. H. Mattheiem, and M. Rozencweig, pp. 265–270. Raven Press, New York.
97. Kennedy, B. J. (1965): Diethylstilbestrol versus testosterone propionate therapy in advanced breast cancer. *Surg. Gynecol. Obstet.,* 120:1246–1250.
98. Kennedy, B. J., and Kiang, D. T. (1975): The effect of short-term cyclophosphamide on estrogen therapy in metastatic breast cancer. *Med. Pediatr. Oncol.,* 1:265–270.
99. Kennedy, B. J., and Yarbro, J. W. (1968): Effect of methenolone enenthate (NSC-64967) in advanced cancer of the breast. *Cancer,* 21:197–201.
100. Knight, E., Horton, J., Cunningham, T., Rhie, F., and Lagakos, S. (1975): Adriamycin-comparison of a five week schedule with a three week schedule in breast cancer and other tumors. *Proc. Am. Assoc. Cancer Res.,* 16:192.
101. Kuperminc, M., and Gelber, R., for the Eastern Cooperative Oncology Group. (1976): Tilorone: A phase II trial for advanced breast cancer. *Proc. Am. Soc. Clin. Oncol.,* 17:260.
102. Lacour, J., Bucalossi, P., Cacers, E., Jacobelli, G., Koszarowski, T., Le, M., Rumeau-Rouquette, C., and Veronesi, U. (1976): Radical mastectomy versus radical mastectomy plus internal mammary dissection. *Cancer,* 37:206–214.
103. Lemkin, S. R., and Dollinger, M. R. (1973): Combination vs single drug therapy in advanced breast cancer. *Proc. Am. Assoc. Cancer Res.,* 14:37.
104. Leone, L. A., and Rege, V. (1973): Treatment of metastatic, recurrent or inoperable carcinoma of breast with VCR/Pred/5-FU/MTX/Cyclo (reg I) vs. VCR/Pred/5-FU (reg II). *Proc. Am. Assoc. Cancer Res.,* 14:125.
105. Lloyd, R. E., Salmon, S. E., Jones, S. E., and Jackson, R. A. (1976): Randomized trial of low-dose adriamycin and cyclophosphamide ± calusterone for advanced breast cancer. *Proc. Am. Assoc. Cancer Res.,* 17:126.
106. Mansfield, C. M., Suntharalingam, N., Leeper, D. B., and Kramer, S. (1973): Effect of fractionation on skin reaction in tangential breast field $^{60}$Co treatment. Comparison of two regimes. *Radiology,* 109:723–724.
107. McDonald, A. M., Simpson, J. S., and MacIntyre, J. (1976): Treatment of early cancer of the breast: histological staging and role of radiotherapy. *Lancet,* 1:1098–1100.
108. Meakin, J. W., Allt, W. E. C., Beale, F. A., Brown, T. C., Clark, R. M., Fitzpatrick, P. J., Hawkins, N. V., Jenkin, R. D. T., Bulbrook, R. D., and Hayward, J. L. (1968): A preliminary report of two studies of adjuvant treatment of preliminary breast cancer. In: *Prognostic Factors in Breast Cancer,* edited by A. P. M. Forrest and P. B. Kunkler, pp. 157–163. Williams & Wilkins, Baltimore.
109. Montague, E. D. (1968): Experience with altered fractionation in radiation therapy of breast cancer. *Radiology,* 90:962–966.
110. Mrazek, R. (1970): Adjuvant chemotherapy with cancer of the breast at one institution. In: *Chemotherapy of Cancer,* edited by W. H. Cole, pp. 289–292. Lea & Febiger, Philadelphia.
111. Muss, H. B. (1975): A comparison of three drug and five drug combination chemotherapy in advanced breast cancer. *Proc. Am. Soc. Clin. Oncol.,* 16:255.
112. Muss, H. B., Cooper, M. R., Richards, F., Spurr, C. L. (1976): A randomized study of two five-drug regimens in advanced breast cancer. *Proc. Am. Soc. Clin. Oncol.,* 17:271.
113. Nemoto, T., Horton, J., Cunningham, T., Sponzo, R., Rosner, D., Diaz, R., and Dao, T. L. (1975): Up date report: Comparison of combination chemotherapy (FCP) vs adriamycin (ADM) vs adrenalectomy (ADX) in breast cancer. *Proc. Am. Assoc. Cancer Res.,* 16:46.
114. Nevinny, H. B., Hall, T. C., Haines, C., and Krant, M. J. (1968): Comparison of methotrexate (NSC-740) and testosterone propionate (NSC-9166) in the treatment of breast cancer. *J. Clin. Pharmacol.,* 8:126–129.
115. Nevinny, H. B., Nevinny, D., Rosoff, C. B., Hall, T. C., and Muench, H. (1969): Prophylactic oophorectomy in breast cancer therapy. A preliminary report. *Am. J. Surg.,* 117:531–536.
116. Nissen-Meyer, R. (1967): The role of prophylactic castration in the therapy of human mammary cancer. *Eur. J. Cancer,* 3:395–403.
117. Nissen-Meyer, R. (1973): Is prophylactic use of hormonal therapy or cytostatic chemotherapy beneficial in the outcome of breast cancer? *Recent Results Cancer Res.,* 42:122–129.
118. Oberfield, R. A., Nesto, R., Cady, B., Pazianos, A. G., and Salzman, F. A. (1975): A multidisciplined approach for the treatment of metastatic carcinoma of the breast. A review of five years' experience. *Med. Clin. North Am.,* 59:425–430.
119. O'Bryan, R. M., Gordon, G. S., Kelley, R. M., Ravdin, R. G., Segaloff, A., and Taylor,

S. G. III (1974): Does thyroid substance improve response of breast cancer to surgical castration? *Cancer,* 33:1082–1085.

120. Papac, R., Jacobs, E., Wong, F., Collom, A., Skoog, W., and Wood, D. A. (1962): Clinical evaluation of pyrimidine nucleosides 5-fluoro-2′-deoxyuridine and 5-iodo-2′-deoxyuridine. *Cancer Chemother. Rep.,* 20:143–146.

121. Priestman, T. J. (1975): Results of a prospective clinical trial comparing two cytotoxic regimes containing adriamycin in women with advanced breast cancer. *Clin. Oncol.,* 1:207–211.

122. Ramirez, G., Klotz, J., Strawitz, J. G., Wilson, W. L., Cornell, G. N., Madden, R. E., Minton, J. P., and the Central Oncology Group (1975): Combination chemotherapy in breast cancer. A randomized study of 4 versus 5 drugs. *Oncology,* 32:101–108.

123. Ravdin, R. G., Lewison, E. F., Slack, N. H., Dao, T. L., Gardner, B., State, D., and Fisher, B. (1970): Results of a clinical trial concerning the worth of prophylactic oophorectomy for breast carcinoma. *Surg. Gynecol. Obstet.,* 131:1055–1064.

124. Rieche, K., Berndt, H., and Prahl, B. (1972): Continuous postoperative treatment with cyclophosphamide in breast carcinoma—a randomized clinical study. *Arch Geschwulstforsch,* 40:349–354.

125. Robbins, G. G. (1962): Long-term survivals among primary operable breast cancer patients with metastatic axillary lymph nodes at level III. *Acta UICC,* 18:864–867.

126. Roberts, M. M. (1970): A comparison of transethmoidal hypophysectomy, yttrium 90 implant and adrenalectomy. In: *The Clinical Management of Advanced Breast Cancer,* edited by C. A. F. Joslin and E. N. Gleave, pp. 54–62. Alpha Omega Alpha, Cardiff.

127. Rojas, A. F., Mickiewicz, E., Feierstein, J. N., Glait, H., and Olivari, A. J. (1976): Levamisole in advanced human breast cancer. *Lancet,* 1:211–215.

128. Rossi, A., Brambilla, C., Bonadonna, G., and Veronesi, U. (1975): Controlled study with L-PAM and 5-FU (iv or po) plus or minus prednisone in advanced breast cancer. *Proc. Am. Assoc. Cancer Res.,* 16:189.

129. Rozencweig, M., and Heuson, J. C. (1975): Breast cancer: Prognostic factors and clinical evaluation. In: *Cancer Therapy: Prognostic Factors and Criteria of Response,* edited by M. J. Staquet, pp. 139–183. Raven Press, New York.

130. Rubens, R. D., Knight, R. K., and Hayward, J. L. (1975): Chemotherapy of advanced breast cancer: A controlled randomized trial of cyclophosphamide *versus* a four-drug combination. *Br. J. Cancer,* 32:730–736.

131. Segaloff, A., Cuningham, M., Rice, B. F., and Weeth, J. B. (1967): Hormonal therapy in cancer of the breast. XXIV. Effect of corticosterone or medroxyprogesterone acetate on clinical course and hormonal excretion. *Cancer,* 20:1673–1678.

132. Seidman, H. (1969): Cancer of the breast: statistical and epidemiological data. *Cancer,* 24:1355–1378.

133. Sellwood, R. A., Burn, I., and Fotherby, K. (1974): Clinical control of metastases in patients with advanced cancer of the breast. *Proc. R. Soc. Med.,* 67:854–857.

134. Smalley, R. V., Murphy, S., Huguley, C. M. Jr., and Bartolucci, A. A., for the Southeastern Cancer Study Group (1976): Combination *versus* sequential five-drug chemotherapy in metastatic carcinoma of the breast. *Cancer Res.,* 36:3911–3916.

135. Sponzo, R. W., Barkley, J. M., Longacre, D., Horton, J., and Cunningham, T. J. (1976): Treatment of recurrent postmenopausal breast cancer with estrogens or combination chemotherapy. *Proc. Am. Soc. Clin. Oncol.,* 17:254.

136. Stewart, H. J., Forrest, A. P. M., Roberts, M. M., Chinnock-Jones, R. E. A., Jones, V., and Campbell, H. (1969): Early pituitary implantation with yttrium-90 for advanced breast cancer. *Lancet,* 2:816–820.

137. Stott, P. B., Zelkowitz, L., and Tucker, W. G. (1973): Combination chemo-hormonal therapy for disseminated breast carcinoma. *Cancer Chemother. Rep.,* 57:106.

138. Talley, R. W., Haines, C. R., Waters, M. N., Goldenberg, I. S., Olson, K. B., and Bisel, H. F. (1973): A dose-response evaluation of androgens in the treatment of metastatic breast cancer. *Cancer,* 32:315–320.

139. Talley, R. W., O'Bryan, R. M., Burrows, J. H., and San Diego, E. L. (1970): Comparison of delta-1-testololactone (NSC-23759) and an estrogen-progestin combination (NSC-77622) in the treatment of metastatic breast cancer. *Cancer Chemother. Rep.,* 54:249–253.

140. Taylor, S. G., III, Pocock, S. J., Shnider, B. I., Colsky, J., and Hall, T. C. (1975): Clinical studies of 5-fluorouracil + premarin in the treatment of breast cancer. *Med. Pediatr. Oncol.,* 1:113–121.

141. Tejada, F., Moran, M., Zaharia, M., and Caceres, E. (1976): Combined therapy of stage III adenocarcinoma of the breast. *Proc. Am. Assoc. Cancer Res.,* 17:48.

142. Tormey, D. C. (1975): Combined chemotherapy and surgery in breast cancer: A review. *Cancer,* 36:881–892.
143. Tormey, D., Lippman, M., Bull, J., and Myers, C. (1976): Evaluation of tamoxifen dose in advanced breast cancer. *Proc. Am. Soc. Clin. Oncol.,* 17:276.
144. Urban, J. A., and Castro, E. B. (1971): Selecting variations in extent of surgical procedure for breast cancer. *Cancer,* 28:1615–1623.
145. Volk, H., Deupree, R. H., Goldenberg, I. S., Wilde, R. C., Carabasi, R. A., and Escher, G. C. (1974): A dose response evaluation of delta-1-testololactone in advanced breast cancer. *Cancer,* 33:9–13.
146. Ward, H. W. C. (1973): Anti-oestrogen therapy for breast cancer: A trial of tamoxifen at two dose levels. *Br. Med. J.,* 1:13–14.
147. von Wolff, G., and Prahl, B. (1973): Kontrollierter klinischer Versuch zur Hormon-und kombinierten Cyclophosphamid-Hormon-Behandlung des inkurablen Mammakarzinoms. *Arch Geschwulstforsch,* 41:363–372.
148. Yonemoto, R. H., Barton, D. R., Byron, R. L., and Riihimaki, D. U. (1973): Conservative mediastinal node dissection for the treatment of carcinoma of the breast. *Surg. Gynecol. Obstet.,* 136:417–420.
149. Yoshida, Y., Miura, S., Murai, H., and Takeuchi, S. (1973): Late results in combined chemotherapy for cure of breast cancer (axillary lymph node metastasis and therapeutic effect). In: *10th Annual Meeting of the Japanese Society for Cancer Therapy* (abstract 117).
150. Zubrod, C. G., Schneiderman, M., Frei, E. III, Brindley, C., Gold, G. L., Shnider, B. Oviedo, R., Gorman, J., Jones, R. Jr., Jonsson, U., Colsky, J., Chalmers, T., Ferguson, B., Dederick, M., Holland, J., Selawry, O., Regelson, W., Lasagna, L., and Owens, A. H. Jr. (1960): Appraisal of methods for the study of chemotherapy of cancer in man: Comparative therapeutic trial of nitrogen mustard and triethylene thiophosphoramide. *J. Chron. Dis.,* 11:7–33.

## Addendum to the References

Additional information can be found in the following papers that have been published since the submission of our manuscript:

151. Ahmann, D. L., O'Connell, M. J., Hahn, R. G., Bisel, H. F., Lee, R. A., and Edmonson, J. H. (1977): An evaluation of early or delayed adjuvant chemotherapy in premenopausal patients with advanced breast cancer undergoing oophorectomy. *N. Engl. J. Med.,* 297:356–360.
152. Brunner, K. W., Sonntag, R. W., Alberto, P., Senn, H. J., Martz, G., Obrecht, P., and Maurice, P. (1977): Combined chemo- and hormonal therapy in advanced breast cancer. *Cancer,* 39:2923–2933.
153. Carter, A. C., Sedransk, N., Kelley, R. M., Ansfield, F. J., Ravdin, R. G., Talley, R. W., and Potter, N. R. (1977): Diethylstilbestrol: Recommended dosages for different categories of breast cancer patients. Report of the Cooperative Breast Cancer Group. *J.A.M.A.,* 237:2079–2085.
154. Meakin, J. W., Allt, W. E. C., Beale, F. A., Brown, T. C., Bush, R. S., Clark, R. M., Fitzpatrick, P. J., Hawkins, N. V., Jenkin, R. D. T., Pringle, J. F., and Rider, W. D. (1977): Ovarian irradiation and prednisone following surgery for carcinoma of the breast. In: *Adjuvant Therapy of Cancer,* edited by S. S. Salmon and S. E. Jones, pp. 95–99. Elsevier/North-Holland Biomedical Press, Amsterdam.
155. Smalley, R. V., Carpenter, J., Bartolucci, A., Vogel, C., and Krauss, S. (1977): A comparison of cyclophosphamide, adriamycin, 5-fluorouracil (CAF) and cyclophosphamide, methotrexate, 5-fluorouracil, vincristine, prednisone (CMFVP) in patients with metastatic breast cancer: A Southeastern Cancer Study Group project. *Cancer,* 40:625–632.
156. Veronesi, U., Banfi, A., Saccozzi, R., Salvadori, B., Zucali, R., Uslenghi, C., Greco, M., Luini, A., Rilke, F., and Sultan, L. (1977): Conservative treatment of breast cancer: A trial in progress at the Cancer Institute of Milan. *Cancer,* 39:2822–2826.
157. Yonemoto, R. H., Tan, M. S. C., Byron, R. L., Riihimaki, D. U., Keating, J., and Jacobs, W. (1977): Randomized sequential hormonal therapy vs adrenalectomy for metastatic breast carcinoma. *Cancer,* 39:547–555.

*Randomized Trials in Cancer: A Critical Review by Sites,* edited by Maurice J. Staquet, Raven Press, New York © 1978.

# Ovarian Cancer

## William P. McGuire and Robert C. Young

*Combined Modality Branch and Medicine Branch, National Cancer Institute, Bethesda, Maryland 20014*

Ovarian carcinoma is the fifth most frequent cause of death from cancer among women and the most common cause of death from a gynecologic malignancy in the United States. With an annual incidence of 14,000 new cases and 10,000 deaths in the United States, the crude mortality rate of 70% bespeaks the lack of properly applied therapy for this common malignancy (27). Successful treatment of ovarian cancer has been compromised by the limited knowledge of the extent of activity of chemotherapy other than alkylating agents and by a general ignorance in selecting proper treatment for individual patients (2). Part of this ignorance stems from a paucity of prospective randomized clinical trials (14 published to date). Even within these trials there has been a failure to separate or stratify patients according to defined risk factors, for example, FIGO stage, histologic type, histologic grade, and extent of residual disease post-operatively, which makes comparisons among trials difficult or impossible (35). Furthermore, efforts to evaluate the efficacy of therapy in advanced disease are often hampered by lack of adequate response criteria. Response in ovarian cancer is difficult to access accurately because of the infrequency of palpable disease in many patients. Accurate clinical responses in patients without easily palpable disease must be documented by a "second-look" procedure such as peritoneoscopy and/or laparotomy (25,29).

A quick review of prognostic criteria is in order, since some prospective randomized trials take these factors into account in study design and all future trials should.

Staging should be in accordance with the classification adopted by the International Federation of Gynecology and Obstetrics (FIGO), and is outlined in Table 1. Stage at presentation is probably the single most important variable in determining eventual clinical course. Staging should be accomplished at the time of the initial surgical intervention, but may be supplemented by other procedures such as lymphangiogram, IVP, and barium enema. Most patients, however, have an exploratory laparotomy by a community physician and often a subumbilical incision is used that does not enable a careful search for disease

---

Received April 27, 1977.

TABLE 1. *Modified FIGO staging for primary carcinoma of the ovary*

|  |  |
|---|---|
| | Stage I: Growth limited to the ovaries |
| Stage Ia | Growth limited to one ovary; no ascites |
| | (i)   No tumor on the external surface; capsule intact |
| | (ii)  Tumor present on the external surface and/or capsule ruptured |
| Stage Ib | Growth limited to both ovaries; no ascites |
| | (i)   No tumor on the external surface; capsule intact |
| | (ii)  Tumor present on the external surface and/or capsule(s) ruptured |
| Stage Ic | Tumor either stage Ia or stage Ib, but ascites[a] present or positive peritoneal washings |
| | Stage II:  Growth involving one or both ovaries with pelvic extension |
| Stage IIa | Extension and/or metastases to the uterus and/or tubes |
| Stage IIb | Extension to other pelvic tissues |
| Stage IIc | Tumor either stage IIa or IIb, but with ascites[a] present or positive peritoneal washings |
| Stage III: | Growth involving one or both ovaries with intraperitoneal metastases outside the pelvis and/or positive retroperitoneal nodes (except pelvic node) |
| Stage IV: | Growth involving one or both ovaries with distant metastases (including vagina). If pleural effusion is present, there must be positive cytology to allot a case of stage IV. Parenchymal liver metastases equals stage IV. |

[a] Ascites is peritoneal effusion that in the opinion of the surgeon is pathologic and/or clearly exceeds normal amounts. Malignant cells must be present cytologically unless the volume is greater than 1,000 $cm^3$.

in the upper abdomen. If noninvasive procedures do not show advanced (stage III or IV) disease, then a second operative procedure may be necessary if the first gave a constricted view of the intraabdominal contents. Proper surgical staging should include not only the TAH–BSO but also a thorough search for disease in (a) lymph nodes in both pelvic and paraortic chains, (b) lateral pelvic walls, (c) omentum and mesentery, (d) both leaves of the diaphragm, and (e) Glisson's capsule. Furthermore, even if the disease is technically unresectable, as much tumor bulk as safely possible should be removed since patients with lesser amounts of postsurgical residual disease seem to respond better to therapy and have a prolonged survival.

Roentgenographic (including bipedal lymphangiography) and radionuclide imaging procedures allow FIGO upstaging in only a minority of patients. Since the most usual pattern of spread in ovarian cancer is via multiple intraperitoneal implants, which may not be visualized or palpable through the common Pfannenstiehl incision made to evaluate most adnexal masses, some form of extended surgical incision is indicated to assure that a patient does not have disease outside the confines of the pelvis. This is particularly important since therapy of stage I and II disease has often consisted of local modalities only, for example, surgery and/or lower abdominal radiotherapy (24). Utilization of peritoneoscopy in patients referred to the National Cancer Institute detected unsuspected involvement of the diaphragm or Glisson's capsule in two-thirds of the patients (3), so adequate surgical staging is of utmost importance.

Histologic pattern of the tumor may have a significant bearing on course of the disease, although this has not been conclusively demonstrated to be independent of stage. Of the 90% of primary ovarian tumors of epithelial origin, patients with mucinous, endometrioid, or mesonephroid histology have a better prognosis than those with serous or undifferentiated histology (1,21). Unfortunately, in the former three histologic types, presentation was with stage III and IV disease in only 20% of the cases; in the latter two cell types advanced presentation was seen in approximately 50% of the cases. These differences in initial stage would be expected to influence survival greatly, independent of histologic type. At least until this question is resolved, future clinical trials should stratify patients according to cell type.

Histologic grade of ovarian carcinoma also shows correlation with survival according to some authors (10,20). Newer information suggests that it may be of greatest value in earlier stages of disease (4). Certainly for trials studying all stages of disease, protocols should stratify patients according to both stage and histologic grade.

Finally, several studies have shown in patients with disease not totally resectable that the amount of residual disease after the completion of surgery bears directly on prognosis. Patients with residual lesions < 2 cm in diameter appear to do much better than those with residual lesions >2 cm in diameter (17,32).

## LOCALIZED DISEASE TRIALS: FIGO STAGE I AND II

Only four published studies have investigated the adjuvant use of radiotherapy and/or chemotherapy in patients with localized disease in a randomized manner. Several other studies are currently under way, but results are as yet preliminary.

The earliest study (12), although not randomized, was designed to establish if the intraperitoneal instillation of radiogold in patients with stage I disease with rupture of a cyst at surgery was beneficial in preventing recurrences. Twenty-five patients received 140 mCi of radiogold and 22 stage I patients, well matched to the treated group, had only surgery. Five-year survival for the treated group was 80% and 43% for the untreated controls. These statistically significant differences in survival between the two groups supports the need for additional therapy in such patients. Whether or not radiogold is the optimal therapy in such patients is unknown. Several other stages were treated in the same manner in this study with and without external radiation therapy with no apparent benefit.

A study from M. D. Anderson Hospital was designed to look at the efficacy of additional radiotherapy or single-agent chemotherapy postoperatively in patients with stages I–III who had complete surgical resection or debulking such that no patient had residual disease >2 cm (31). Staging was adequate and patients were stratified according to age and histologic type but not histologic grade or stage. One hundred forty-nine patients were randomized to one of the following treatment regimens:

1. L-PAM, 0.2 mg/kg daily × 5 every 4 weeks × 12 cycles.
2. Abdominal strip irradiation (2,600 to 2,800 rads midplane) and pelvic irradiation (2,000 rads midpelvis) (13).

Follow-up is now 3 to 6 years with the following percentages of disease-free patients by stage and treatment:

| | | |
|---|---|---|
| Stage I | L-PAM (*n* = 28) | 90% |
| | RT (*n* = 14) | 85% |
| Stage II | L-PAM (*n* = 29) | 58% |
| | RT (*n* = 37) | 55% |
| Stage III | L-PAM (*n* = 21) | 35% |
| | RT (*n* = 19) | 53% |

There were no statistically significant differences in these data. Berkson-Gage projections of 5-year survivals show a trend in favor of radiotherapy in stage I and chemotherapy in stage III. Numbers of patients, however, are small, and Berkson-Gage projections are often meaningless with small numbers of patients and short follow-up. Simply stated, this study shows no demonstrated preference for either chemotherapy or radiotherapy as a surgical adjuvant in ovarian carcinoma.

The Gynecologic Oncology Group has recently completed a three-arm trial in stage I disease (18). One hundred eleven patients with stage Ia and Ib disease (no stratifications) were randomly assigned to one of the following arms postoperatively:

1. Observation
2. Pelvic irradiation (5,000 rads midpelvis)
3. L-PAM, 0.2 mg/kg daily × 5 every 4 weeks × 18 cycles

Not all patients had visualization of the upper abdominal contents, so the population may include some stage III patients. A recent update in recurrence rates shows a trend in favor of chemotherapy:

1. 5/29 (17%) recurrence
2. 8/22 (36%) recurrence
3. 3/30 (10%) recurrence

The smaller numbers of patients in the radiotherapy arm is due to the high numbers of protocol deviations requiring exclusion from the study. These results are in contrast to those of Smith et al. Patient numbers and median follow-up are both greater in this trial, but staging and stratification factors are less stringent. Therefore, the question of efficacy of either postoperative radiotherapy or chemotherapy in stage I remains unanswered. The Ovarian Cancer Study Group (Mayo Foundation; M. D. Anderson Hospital; Roswell Park Memorial Institute; and the Medicine Branch, National Cancer Institute) has recently initiated a study in stage I patients with favorable histology to attempt to resolve this issue. Extensive and uniform staging and complete stratification for prognostic factors have been included in this trial, which randomizes patients to observation or L-PAM.

A recently completed trial from the Princess Margaret Hospital in Toronto, Canada, looks at the relative benefits of postoperative radiotherapy and/or chemotherapy (9). Patients with stage Ia were randomly assigned to observation or pelvic irradiation following surgery. Only 30 patients have been entered, and it is too early for analysis. Because of a prior retrospective study that showed that patients with stage Ib and II disease had similar survivals, these patients were pooled for purposes of the prospective study. Stratification was by age, stage, histologic type, and histologic grade. Staging of patients, however, was not done by laparoscopy or repeat laparotomy in the larger percentage of referred patients. One hundred twenty-five stage Ib and II patients were randomly allocated to one of the three following treatment strategies:

1. Pelvic irradiation (4,500 rads midpelvis)
2. Pelvic irradiation (4,500 rads midpelvis) and abdominal strip irradiation (2,250 rads midplane)
3. Pelvic irradiation (4,500 rads midpelvis) and chlorambucil (6 mg/day $\times$ 24 months) starting immediately after radiation

No statistical difference was seen among any of the three arms when all patients were analyzed together. If, however, patients who had a complete TAH–BSO (most of these patients would have $< 2$ cm residual mass) were analyzed separately, an interesting trend was seen. In patients with incomplete TAH–BSO, there were no significant differences. In patients with complete TAH–BSO, there were fewer recurrences and progressions in patients who received extrapelvic therapy (i.e., chemotherapy or abdominal irradiation). Median follow-up is 30 months with the following percentages of disease-free patients:

1. Pelvic RT ($n = 29$): 45%
2. Pelvic + abdominal RT ($n = 29$): 77%
3. Pelvic RT + CT ($n = 36$): 77%

Although these data are not statistically significant to date, there is certainly a trend suggesting benefit in "localized" disease (FIGO Ib and II) after maximal surgical resection of application of additional extrapelvic (i.e., abdominal RT or chemotherapy) modalities for control of unsuspected abdominal micrometastases.

In summary, the relatively few prospective randomized trials in FIGO stage I and II disease suggest the need for application of therapies directed outside the pelvis. Clearly surgery is necessary for adequate staging and tumor debulking. Pelvic radiotherapy may assist in prevention of local recurrence, although no study has been designed to test this hypothesis. A second major problem in early ovarian cancer is prevention of intraabdominal progression. This will require use of regional therapies (i.e., radioactive colloids, abdominal strip irradiation, and chemotherapy), but the proper combination and/or sequence of application of these additional therapies is as yet not known.

## ADVANCED DISEASE TRIALS: FIGO STAGES III AND IV

In contrast to early disease where physicians have only recently recognized the need to study various adjuvant therapies following surgical resection, there are several randomized trials utilizing single modalities or combinations in stage III and IV disease. This willingness to utilize additional therapy for patients who present with advanced disease or for those who develop recurrence is due to lack of surgical resectability and to the availability of other therapies that produce responses and prolong survival.

### Radiotherapy

Only a single published trial studied the effect of radiotherapy alone given postsurgery in patients with FIGO stages III and IV (16). Fifty patients were assigned to radiotherapy following surgery using either the open-field technique (4,000 rads midplane) or the moving-strip technique (3,000 rads midplane). All stages of disease were included and, because of lack of stratification, the open-field technique had an abundance of stage III/IV patients, patients with residual disease, and patients with serous histology. Neither treatment produced significantly different results. Of note, however, is the disease-free survival of 7/24 (28%) at 2 years with either treatment, which is the range seen with other therapies in more advanced disease.

### Chemotherapy

Several trials have studied the efficacy of single-agent or combination chemotherapy in advanced ovarian cancer.

Two different alkylating agents were compared for efficacy in advanced disease (34). Twenty-four stage III and IV patients were randomly allocated to:

1. L-PAM, 0.2 mg/kg daily × 5 every 4 weeks
2. Ctx, 40 mg/kg, i.v., q. 12 hours × 2 every 4 weeks

Response rate, remission duration, and median survivals were as follows:

1. 64%; 6 months; 14 months
2. 60%; 5 months; 15 months

Therefore, high-dose intravenous alkylating agent (Ctx) had no increased benefit over standard oral therapy (L-PAM), and the toxicity of the former was much greater.

In a similar fashion, two standard dose alkylating agents were compared in a trial completed by the Southwest Oncology Group (26). Patients with stage III or IV ovarian cancer were randomized to receive:

1. L-PAM, 6 mg/m², days 1–6 q. 6 weeks
2. Chlorambucil, 6 mg/m² daily for 6 weeks followed by 4 mg/m² daily thereafter

Responses were judged clinically and were as follows:

1. 3/24 (12.5%) response: 2 CR and 1 PR
2. 5/23 (21.7%) response: 2 CR and 3 PR

No patient who failed one therapy responded to the other, showing the expected cross-resistance between alkylating agents. Median survivals were as follows:

1. 68 weeks
2. 38 weeks

A comparison between two different classes of chemotherapeutic agents was also made (14). Thirty-nine patients were randomly assigned to either:

1. L-PAM, 6 mg/m² daily × 5 every 4 weeks
2. ADR, 75 mg/m² q. 3 weeks (maximum dose 600 mg/m²)

There was no stratification by histologic grade or amount of residual disease, and responses were based on clinical assessment alone. Response rates and median duration of responses were as follows:

1. 4/20 (25%): 6.5 months
2. 8/19 (42%): 5.0 months

The differences between response rates and response duration are not statistically significant; however, the lack of cross-resistance between these two agents was seen when patients were crossed over to the other therapy. Four of six (66%) patients responded to ADR after L-PAM failure, and 4/12 (33%) responded to L-PAM after ADR failure.

Other active single agents have been identified in studies conducted at the M. D. Anderson Hospital (30). Ninety-six patients with advanced ovarian cancer were randomized to one of three drugs:

1. L-PAM, 0.2 mg/kg, days 1–5 q. 4 weeks
2. Hexamethylmelamine, 8 mg/kg, p.o., q.d.
3. 5-FU, 15 mg/kg, weekly

Responses to these agents were as follows:

1. 15/50 (30%) response
   11/15 (73%) complete response

2. 10/22 (45%) response
   7/10 (70%) complete response
3. 4/24 (16%) response
   4/4 (100%) complete response

Crossover therapy was effective only with L-PAM, although other more recent studies (unpublished) have shown hexamethylmelamine to be active in 15 to 20% of patients who are no longer responsive to alkylating agents.

## COMBINATION CHEMOTHERAPY

Unfortunately, the dramatic results seen in such diseases as lymphoma, Wilm's tumor, and testicular tumors when active single agents were combined have not as yet been established for ovarian cancer.

The first study utilizing combination chemotherapy (32) compared a standard alkylating agent therapy, L-PAM, to a three-drug combination (ActFuCy). Ninety-seven patients were randomized (there were no stratifications by histology type or histology grade and all patients had residual masses >2 cm) to one of the following regimens:

1. L-PAM, 0.2 mg/kg, daily × 5 every 4 weeks
2. Act-D, 0.5 mg, i.v., daily × 5
   5-FU, 8 mg/kg, i.v., daily × 5 every 4 weeks
   Ctx, 7 mg/kg, i.v., daily × 5

Response rates and 2-year survivals were

1. 42%; 17%
2. 45%; 17%

Thus response rate, response duration, and survival were not improved using that drug combination in place of a single alkylating agent.

The Eastern Cooperative Oncology Group compared L-PAM to a three-drug combination (6). Two hundred sixty-eight patients were randomized (no stratification for residual disease or extent of previous therapy) to receive either:

1. L-PAM, 7 mg/m², days 1–5 q. 5 weeks
2. 5-FU, 400 mg/m², days 1 and 8
   Mtx, 15 mg/m², days 1 and 8
   Ctx, 400 mg/m², days 1 and 8

Response rates and duration of responses were similar in both groups, and the combination was more toxic. Approximately 12% of patients in both groups attained CR, and these were somewhat more durable in the group treated with L-PAM. Unfortunately, the failure to stratify for previous therapy and residual disease makes interpretation of this data difficult. Including significant numbers of patients with previous radiotherapy or chemotherapy will always result in lowered overall response rates as well as fewer complete remissions.

Studies performed at the Mayo Clinic (15) comparing cytoxan alone or in combination with adriamycin showed similar discouraging results. Sixty previously untreated patients with advanced ovarian cancer were randomized to receive:

1. Ctx, 1,000 mg/m$^2$, q. 3 weeks
2. Ctx, 500 mg/m$^2$, q. 3 weeks
   Adr, 40 mg/m$^2$, q. 3 weeks

Patients were stratified according to whether or not they had measurable disease and performance status. Response rates were determined clinically and were

1. 10/31 (32%) response
2. 12/29 (45%) response

The higher response with the combination was not statistically better, and the duration of response and survival, although slightly better, was not significantly so and was at the expense of more toxicity.

More recent studies, however, utilizing other drug combinations appear to have more impact on survival. A recent study at the National Cancer Institute (36) shows significant superiority of a four-drug combination. Fifty-six previously untreated patients with advanced ovarian cancer were randomly assigned to:

1. L-PAM, 0.2 mg/kg, days 1–5 q. 4 weeks
2. Hexamethylmelamine, 150 mg/m$^2$, days 1–14
   Ctx, 150 mg/m$^2$, days 1–14
   5-FU, 600 mg/m$^2$, days 1 and 8
   M + x, 40 mg/m$^2$, days 1 and 8
   Cycles repeated every 4 weeks

Patients were stratified according to stage, age, histologic type, and amount of residual disease. Response rates are as follows (responses documented by second-look laparoscopy and/or laparotomy):

1. 16/26 (61%) with 5/26 (19%) CR
2. 19/24 (79%) with 8/24 (33%) CR

Median survivals are

1. 17 months with 11/28 (39%) alive
2. Not yet reached with 17/28 (61%) alive

This is the first combination regimen in which a higher response rate from a combination eventuated in prolonged remission duration and survival. Unfortunately, the combination is significantly more toxic than the single agent.

A group of investigators at M. D. Anderson Hospital have, however, found that the additoin of hexamethylmelamine to an alkylating agent (a less toxic combination) appears to have a good overall response and complete remission rate (28). In this study, patients previously untreated with advanced disease who were clinically free of disease after chemotherapy usually had some second-look procedure for documentation of CR. Consequently, although overall response rates to L-PAM are similar to older studies, the percentage attaining CR is significantly lower. Patients were randomized to one of four chemotherapeutic regimens as follows:

1. L-PAM, 0.2 mg/kg daily × 5 every 4 weeks
2. Hexamethylmelamine, 8 mg/kg daily
3. Adr, 60 mg/m² every 3 weeks
4. Hexamethylmelamine, 4 mg/kg daily × 14 each month with Ctx, 250 mg/m² daily × 5 every 4 weeks

Responses are as follows:

1. 10/33 (30%) with 4/33 (12%) CR
2. 7/33 (22%) with 1/33 (3%) CR
3. 10/34 (29%) with 4/24 (12%) CR
4. 17/32 (53%) with 10/32 (31%) CR

At the present time it is too early to comment on response duration or survival in this study, but if the high response rate with the combination translates into prolonged survival, this will make a significant impact on treatment of advanced ovarian cancer.

Another active agent for ovarian cancer has recently been identified (33) and confirmed by prospective studies at Mt. Sinai Hospital (7). *cis*-Platinum was used alone and in combination with adriamycin and compared to a combination regimen of thiotepa and methotrexate. Patients in this study were not stratified, resulting in a greater percentage of older patients in the thiotepa arm, but a higher percentage of poorly differentiated histologies in the adriamycin plus platinum arm. Responses were determined clinically. Patients received one of the following:

1. Adr, 50 mg/m² every 3 weeks
   *cis*-Platinum, 50 mg/m² every 3 weeks
2. *cis*-Platinum, 50 mg/m² every 3 weeks
3. Thiotepa, 15 mg daily × 5 (loading)
   Mtx, 2.5–12.5 mg daily at various intervals

Responses were as follows:

1. 12/18 (66%) with 6/18 (33%) CR
2. 7/17 (41%) with 3/17 (18%) CR
3. 6/17 (35%) with 2/17 (12%) CR

Again, results are preliminary and the completeness of remission only assessed clinically, but the drug combination of platinum plus adriamycin appears to give better responses when compared to single-agent platinum or thiotepa plus methotrexate (8).

## NEW DRUGS FOR OVARIAN CANCER

Drug combinations are usually more toxic than single agents, and to date have not been shown conclusively to be significantly more advantageous in the therapy of advanced ovarian cancer. Therefore, there are continued efforts to identify new agents that are active and can be combined with existing regimens or utilized after initial therapy has failed.

Both cytembena and epipodophyllotoxin were compared at Mayo Clinic (15), and there were no responses to either drug.

Investigators at Roswell Park (5) compared high-dose methotrexate alone or combined with cyclophosphamide in patients who had failed prior single alkylating agent or combination chemotherapy. Patients were stratified according to whether or not they had failed single-agent or combination therapy. Patients received either:

1. Mtx-CF, 450–500 mg/m² with CF every 6 hr X 12 starting 6 hr after Mtx
2. Mtx-CF, as above
   Ctx, 250 mg/m² daily X 5

Responses (all partial) were as follows:

1. 2/11 (18%)
2. 6/13 (46%)

Previous therapy with L-PAM did not preclude response to either second-line therapy. Thus high doses of an antimetabolite with standard doses of alkylating agent appear to be beneficial as second-line therapy, and this is yet another combination that needs to be tested as initial therapy.

In summary, numerous agents have been identified that are active in advanced ovarian cancer. At the present time, use of single-agent alkylating therapy (e.g., L-PAM, cytoxan, chlorambucil, and thiotepa) produces responses in approximately 40% of patients and improves their overall survival. A minority (5 to 10%), however, will have long-term survival with this approach. Combinations of active single agents have not yet been tremendously successful, and toxicity has been substantial. Only recently have combinations employing newer classes of agents (e.g., hexamethylmelamine, adriamycin, and *cis*-platinum) been successful in producing higher response rates, and one study has demonstrated more durable responses and longer survival. What role combination chemotherapy has and specifically which agents in combination offer the best therapeutic index still remains to be answered. Even so, there is still a need for defining new active agents to be used alone or in combination in patients failing standard methods of therapy.

## Combination Modalities

There have been five trials that compared radiation therapy and chemotherapy alone or in combination.

The first published study (11) used various schedules of radiotherapy as a surgical adjuvant in previously untreated patients with advanced disease with or without the addition of cytoxan. Actually there were five groups, but the first two are the only comparable groups as they received the same schedule of radiotherapy, that is, 3,500 rads midplane via opposed anterior and posterior portals. Cytoxan was given to group II at 400 mg i.v. ×4 days followed by radiation and then cytoxan was again administered at 50 to 150 mg p.o. daily for as long as response was noted. Thirty-five patients were followed for time to recurrence and survival. Time to recurrence was the more valid figure, since various treatments were utilized after relapse. The results were:

RT alone: median time to recurrence, 3.0 months; median survival, 7.0 months
RT + Ctx: median time to recurrence, 8.0 months; median survival, 13.0 months

The results were not analyzed statistically, but the addition of cytoxan to surgical debulking and abdominal irradiation was clearly beneficial.

A study from Sweden (22) compared radiation therapy alone and in combination with thiotepa in stage III disease. Two hundred nineteen patients received either:

1. Abdominal RT: 2,000 rads midplane
2. Radiation therapy: as above
   Thiotepa: 10 mg every 2nd day (dose varied from 50 to 200 mg)

Responses were defined clinically and there was no stratification. Response rate and median survival were as follows:

1. 41/88 (47%), 6.5 months
2. 114/131 (87%), 12.5 months

The high response rates are most likely due to less stringent criteria for response than is required today. Of possible significance, however, is the apparent survival benefit when the two modalities are combined as was seen in the previous study.

Because of apparent benefit of the addition of cytoxan to radiation at the Mayo Clinic (see above) a random trial was conducted comparing cytoxan alone and in combination with radiation (19). Fifty patients were randomly assigned to receive either:

1. Cytoxan, 500 mg daily × 3, then 50 mg daily
2. Cytoxan, as above
   Abdominal RT, 2,250 rads midplane

There were no statistically significant differences in survival in either group (≃10% at 5 years), although there was a slight benefit up to 2 years in the group treated with the combination. This study demonstrates in a prospective randomized trial that chemotherapy alone produces results equivalent to that achieved with whole abdominal radiotherapy.

The Eastern Cooperative Oncology Group (23) conducted a trial comparing abdominal radiation and chlorambucil alone or in combination. Fifty-one patients were assigned to receive either:

1. Abdominal RT, 3,500 rads midplane
2. Chlorambucil, 0.2 mg/kg daily × 8 weeks
3. Combination of RT + CT, as above

All patients were untreated and had stage III disease; there was no stratification and responses were clinical. Response rates and median survivals were as follows:

1. 9/17 (52%), 33.5 weeks
2. 9/18 (50%), 94.9 weeks
3. 11/16 (69%), 42.2 weeks

Major problems in interpretation of these data arise because of the small numbers of patients and the variations in doses among the participating institutions. Furthermore, the chemotherapy was administered for only 8 weeks, which is not an adequate duration for optimal response.

Finally, a recently completed trial from the Princess Margaret Hospital in Toronto (9) compared the efficacy of either no further therapy, pelvic radiation and abdominal radiation, or pelvic radiation and chlorambucil in stage III asymptomatic patients. Patients were stratified by histologic grade only and responses were clinically defined. Patients were randomized after maximal surgical debulking to receive:

1. No therapy until symptoms appear
2. Pelvic RT, 4,500 rads midpelvis
   Abdominal strip RT, 2,250 rads midplane
3. Pelvic RT, as above
   Chlorambucil, 6 mg/day × 2 years

If all asymptomatic patients are grouped, there is no significant difference in survival among any of the three arms. Of those patients with complete TAH–BSO ($n = 23$), there have been 7 recurrences and 1 progression or 35% failure rate, whereas in those without complete surgery ($n = 35$), there have been 18 recurrences and 9 progressions, or 77% failure rate. The numbers are too small for statistical significance among the different treatment groups.

In summary, the relatively small number of trials with small numbers of patients in each trial make assessment of the efficacy of various combinations of chemotherapy and radiotherapy impossible. Often therapeutic doses of either regimen are altered in combination because of added toxicity, so one is not really comparing a single modality against the combination. Both modalities have additive effects on the bone marrow reserve, and radiation alters the vascularity within the radiation field, perhaps partially preventing adequate distribution of the chemotherapeutic agent. Newer combined modality trials will probably involve a "sandwich technique," that is, chemotherapy followed by radiotherapy followed by additional chemotherapy. The use of a third modality, immunotherapy, has just begun to be explored in ovarian cancer. Future trials must be carefully designed to ensure well-balanced, accurately staged patient groups for comparison. The treatment regimens proposed must be utilized in such a way that the benefits and toxicities of each modality utilized may be assessed.

## CONCLUSION

Ovarian cancer is a common malignancy and usually a lethal one. Surgery, chemotherapy, and radiotherapy are each capable of destroying malignant cells, and some patients may even be rendered free of macroscopic disease. Nevertheless, a majority of these "responders" will eventually succumb to recurrent or progressive ovarian cancer.

Surgery has an important role both from a diagnostic and a staging point of view, and also as a tumor debulking procedure. Several studies cited above have suggested that patients with small amounts of residual disease enjoy improved survival. Whether this survival is related to the surgical debulking itself or related to an intrinsically less aggressive tumor is unknown.

Radiotherapy is effective although it is not entirely clear in which stages it should be applied. Bulky postoperative residual pelvic disease is one area where radiotherapy has had the greatest impact. Newer radiotherapeutic techniques are being developed that allow delivery of larger doses with less normal tissue toxicity. In addition, newer approaches utilizing radiation ports designed to include the paraaortic nodes and the diaphragmatic reflections may improve the effectiveness of radiotherapy in advanced disease.

Chemotherapy remains the only modality capable of destroying diffuse intraperitoneal disease. Whether one should use single alkylating agents or one of the more aggressive combinations remains to be answered, although very early data would suggest that some combinations are superior.

Immunotherapy in this disease is still in its infancy. Suffice it to say that immune reconstitution or stimulation offers benefit only in the presence of minimal residual disease. Due to the high propensity for patients rendered macroscopically disease free by surgery, radiotherapy, and/or chemotherapy to develop recurrence, immune therapy will likely have its greatest impact in patients who are first treated with some combination of these three modalities.

Gynecologists are increasingly aware of the necessity of adequate staging, definition of other risk factors, and usefulness and need of other modalities of therapy in addition to surgery. Properly designed clinical trials in the future should be able to answer the questions of how much, how many, and when the three nonsurgical modalities of therapy should be applied to increase the survival rate in the large number of women who have highly responsive yet very deadly ovarian cancer.

## REFERENCES

1. Aure, J. C., Hoeg, K., and Kolstad, P. (1971): Clinical and histologic studies of ovarian carcinoma: Long term followup of 990 cases. *Obstet. Gynecol.,* 37:1–9.
2. Bagley, C. M., Young, R. C., Canellos, G. P., and DeVita, V. T. (1972): Treatment of ovarian carcinoma: Possibilities for progress. *N. Engl. J. Med.,* 287:856–862.
3. Bagley, C. M., Young, R. C., Schein, P. S., Chabner, B. A., and DeVita, V. T. (1973): Ovarian carcinoma metastatic to diaphragm—frequently undiagnosed at laparotomy. *Am. J. Obstet. Gynecol.,* 116:397–400.
4. Barber, H. R. K., Sommers, S. C., Snyder, R., and Kwon, T. H. (1975): Histologic and nuclear grading and stromal reactions as indices for prognosis in ovarian cancer. *Am. J. Obstet. Gynecol.,* 121:795–807.
5. Barlow, J. J., and Piver, M. S. (1976): Methotrexate with citrovorum factor rescue, alone and in combination with cyclophosphamide, in ovarian cancer. *Cancer Treatment Rep.,* 60:527–533.
6. Brodovsky, H. S., Pocock, S. J., and Sears, M. (1977): A comparison of melphalan with 5-fluorouracil, cytoxan and methotrexate in patients with ovarian cancer. *Proc. Am. Soc. Clin. Oncol. (in press).*
7. Bruckner, H. W., Cohen, C. J., Gusberg, S. B., Wallach, R. C., Kabakow, B., Greenspan, E. M., and Holland, J. F. (1976): Chemotherapy of ovarian cancer with adriamycin (ADM) and cis-platinum (DDP). *Proc. Am. Soc. Clin. Oncol.,* 17:287.
8. Bruckner, H. W., Cohen, C. J., Kabakow, B., Wallach, R. C., Greenspan, E. M., Gusberg, S. B., and Holland, J. F. (1977): Combination chemotherapy of ovarian carcinoma with platinum: Improved therapeutic index. *Proc. Am. Soc. Clin. Oncol.* 18:339.
9. Bush, R. S., Allt, W. E. C., Beale, F. A., Bean, H., Pringle, J. F., and Sturgeon, J. (1977): *Am. J. Obstet. Gynecol.* 127:692–704.
10. Decker, D. G., Malkasian, G. D., and Taylor, W. F. (1975): Prognostic importance of histologic grading in ovarian cancer. *Natl. Cancer Inst. Monogr.,* 42:9–11.
11. Decker, D. G., Mussey, E., Malkasian, G. D., and Johnson, C. E. (1967): Adjuvant treatment for advanced ovarian malignancy. *Am. J. Obstet. Gynecol.,* 97:171–180.
12. Decker, D. G., Webb, W. J., and Holbrook, M. A. (1973): Radiogold treatment of epithelial cancer of the ovary: Late results. *Am. J. Obstet. Gynecol.,* 115:751–758.
13. Delclos, L., and Smith, J. P. (1973): Tumors of the ovary. In: *Textbook of Radiotherapy,* pp. 690–702. Lea & Febiger, Philadelphia.
14. dePalo, G. M., DeLena, M., DiRe, F., Luciani, L., Volagussa, P., and Bonadonna, G. (1975): Melphalan versus adriamycin in the treatment of advanced carcinoma of the ovary. *Surg. Gynecol., Obstet.,* 141:899–902.
15. Edmonson, J. H. (1975): Status report of Mayo Clinic studies. *Natl. Cancer Inst. Monogr.,* 42:167–168.
16. Fazekas, J. T., and Maier, J. G. (1974): Irradiation of ovarian carcinomas. A prospective comparison of the open-field and moving-strip techniques. *Am. J. Roentgenol. Radium Ther. Nucl. Med.,* 120:118–123.
17. Griffiths, C. T., Grogan, R. H., and Hall, T. C. (1972): Advanced ovarian cancer: Primary treatment with surgery, radiotherapy and chemotherapy. *Cancer,* 29:1–7.

18. Hreschchyshyn, M. M. (1975): Results of the gynecologic oncology group trials on ovarian cancer: Preliminary report. *Natl. Cancer Inst. Monogr.,* 42:155–165.
19. Johnson, C. E., Decker, D. G., Van Henrik, M., Mussey, E., Malkasian, G. D., and Jorgensen, E. O. (1972): Advanced ovarian cancer: Therapy with radiation and cyclophosphamide in a random series. *Am. J. Roentgenol. Radium Ther. Nucl. Med.,* 114:136–141.
20. Kottmeier, H. L. (1962): Modern trends in the treatment of patients with semimalignant and malignant ovarian tumors. In: *Carcinoma of the Uterine Cervix, Endometrium and Ovary,* pp. 285–298. Year Book Medical Publishers, Chicago.
21. Kottmeier, H. L. (1968): Clinical staging in ovarian cancer. In: *Ovarian Cancer* (IUCC Monograph Series, Vol. 11), pp. 146–156. Springer-Verlag, New York.
22. Kottmeier, H. L. (1968): Treatment of ovarian cancer with thiotepa. *Clin. Obstet. Gynecol.,* 11:428–438.
23. Miller, S. P., Brenner, S., Horton, J., Stolbach, L., Shnider, B. I., and Pocock, S. (1975): Comparative evaluation of combined radiation-chlorambucil treatment of ovarian carcinomatosis. *Cancer,* 36:1625–1630.
24. Piver, M. S., Lele, S., and Barlow, J. J. (1976): Preoperative and intraoperative evaluation in ovarian malignancy. *Obstet. Gynecol.,* 43:312–315.
25. Rosenoff, S. H., DeVita, V. T., Hubbard, S., and Young, R. C. (1975): Peritoneoscopy in the staging and follow-up of ovarian cancer. *Seminars in Oncology,* 2:223–228.
26. Rossof, A. H., Drukker, B. H., Talley, R. W., Torres, J., Bonnet, J., and Brownlee, R. W. (1976): Randomized evaluation of chlorambucil and melphalan in advanced ovarian cancer. *Proc. Am. Soc. Clin. Oncol.,* 18:300.
27. Silverberg, E., and Holleb, A. I. (1972): Cancer Statistics 1972. *Cancer,* 22:2–20.
28. Smith, J. P. (1977): *Personal communication.*
29. Smith, J. P., Delgado, G., and Rutledge, F. (1976): Second look operation in ovarian carcinoma. *Cancer,* 38:1438–1442.
30. Smith, J. P., and Rutledge, F. N. (1975): Random study of hexamethylmelamine, 5-fluorouracil and melphalan in treatment of advanced carcinoma of the ovary. *Natl. Cancer Inst. Monogr.,* 42:169–172.
31. Smith, J. P., Rutledge, F. N., and Delclos, L. (1975): Postoperative treatment of early cancer of the ovary: A random trial between postoperative irradiation and chemotherapy. *Natl. Cancer Inst. Monogr.,* 42:149–153.
32. Smith, J. P., Rutledge, F., and Wharton, J. T. (1972): Chemotherapy of ovarian cancer. *Cancer,* 30:1565–1571.
33. Wiltshaw, E., and Kroner, T. (1976): Phase II study of cis-dichlorodiammine-platinum (II) (NSC-119875) in advanced adenocarcinoma of the ovary. *Cancer Treatment Rep.,* 60:55–60.
34. Young, R. C., Canellos, G. P., Chabner, B. A., Schein, P. S., Hubbard, S. P., and DeVita, V. T. (1974): Chemotherapy of advanced ovarian carcinoma: A prospective randomized comparison of phenylalanine mustard and high dose cyclophosphamide. *Gynecol. Oncol.,* 2:489–497.
35. Young, R. C., and DeVita, V. T. (1975): Ovarian carcinoma: Cinical trials, prognostic factors and criteria for response. In: *Cancer Therapy: Prognostic Factors and Criteria of Response,* edited by M. Staquet, pp. 319–335. Raven Press, New York.
36. Young, R. C., DeVita, V. T., and Chabner, B. A. (1976): A prospective trial of melphalan (PAM) and combination chemotherapy in advanced ovarian cancer. *Proc. Am. Soc. Clin. Oncol.,* 17:279.

*Randomized Trials in Cancer: A Critical Review by Sites,* edited by Maurice J. Staquet, Raven Press, New York © 1978.

# Endometrial, Cervical, and Vulva Cancer

Mark W. Pasmantier, Morton Coleman, Richard T. Silver, and Stanley J. Birnbaum

*Division of Hematology–Oncology, Department of Medicine and the Department of Obstetrics and Gynecology, The New York Hospital–Cornell Medical Center, New York, New York 10021*

Although the value of prospective randomized controlled clinical trials in oncology is beyond dispute, only a few such studies have been conducted in patients with carcinoma of the endometrium, cervix, and vulva. Nevertheless, in the past few years a greater interest has developed in the randomized trial as an appropriate vehicle for research in gynecologic oncology. Most such trials are currently in progress, thus precluding detailed comment on them now. As an alternative we shall sketch the current treatment programs in these three disease entities and emphasize where randomized trials might have impact.

## ENDOMETRIAL CANCER

Adenocarcinoma of the endometrium remains the most common gynecologic malignancy. In the United States 27,000 new cases and approximately 3,500 deaths occurred in 1975 (23). The major conceptual advances, including the determination of extent of disease, the prognostic implications of stage and histology, and the implementation of multiple modality therapy, have been employed by gynecological oncologists in their approach to endometrial adenocarcinoma. In endometrial cancer the staging workup currently suggested by the International Federation of Gynecologists and Obstetricians (FIGO) (16) is outlined in Table 1. The FIGO staging system is shown in Table 2 (16). The stage of the patient clearly has prognostic and therefore therapeutic implications. The relation of stage to survival, as demonstrated by the 15th Annual Report from Stockholm (15) on corpus cancer, is shown in Table 3.

The literature contains a marked variation in survival of stage I patients from various groups (22,25), with 5-year survivals reported as high as 87%. This in part is related to other accessible parameters in the mix of these stage I patients. Stage I, for instance, can be subdivided on the basis of histology of the tumor and the length of the uterus (see Table 2). If just these two parameters

---

Received May 17, 1977.

TABLE 1. *Staging procedures for carcinoma of the uterus by FIGO (16)*

A. Required
   1. Palpation
   2. Inspection
   3. Coloposcopy
   4. Endocervical curettage
   5. Hysterography
   6. Hysteroscopy
   7. Cystoscopy
   8. Proctoscopy
   9. IVP
   10. Chest and skeletal X-ray

B. Optional
   1. Lymphangiogram
   2. Arteriography
   3. Venography
   4. Laparoscopy

are utilized, the 5-year survival of $IaG_1$ approximates 95%, whereas that of $IbG_3$ is close to 50% (11). Nodal status also has prognostic and therapeutic importance. In a literature review and utilizing the FIGO classification, Morrow, Di Saia, and Townsend (18) found that 10.6% of stage I patients had positive nodes, whereas 36.5% stage II had positive nodes. Nodal involvement probably should be incorporated into the staging system.

The evolution of the current therapeutic approaches is well outlined by Gusberg (8) and can be traced back to a time before the meaning of adequate

TABLE 2. *Staging of carcinoma of the endometrium by FIGO (16)*

| | |
|---|---|
| Stage 0 | Carcinoma in situ. Histological findings suspicious of malignancy. |
| | Cases of Stage 0 should not be included in any therapeutic statistics. |
| Stage I | The carcinoma is confined to the corpus including the isthmus |
| Stage Ia | The length of the uterine cavity is 8 cm or less |
| Stage Ib | The length of the uterine cavity is more than 8 cm |

The stage I cases should be subgrouped with regard to the histological type of the adenocarcinoma as follows:

G1 Highly differentiated adenomatous carcinoma
G2 Differentiated adenomatous carcinoma with partly solid areas
G3 Predominantly solid or entirely undifferentiated carcinoma

| | |
|---|---|
| Stage II | The carcinoma has involved the corpus and the cervix, but has not extended outside the uterus |
| Stage III | The carcinoma has extended outside the uterus, but not outside the true pelvis |
| Stage IV | The carcinoma has extended outside the true pelvis or has obviously involved the mucosa of the bladder or rectum; bullous edema as such does not permit a case to be allotted to stage IV |
| Stage IVa | Spread of the growth to adjacent organs |
| Stage IVb | Spread to distant organs |

TABLE 3. *15th Annual Report Stockholm on corpus cancer (15)*

| Stage | Number of patients treated | Percent of cases | Survival |
|---|---|---|---|
| I | 3025 | 72.0 | 70.0% |
| II | 595 | 14.2 | 47.4 |
| III | 428 | 10.2 | 28.0 |
| IV | 149 | 3.6 | 4.7 |
| Total | 4197 | 100.0 | 60.2 |

staging was understood. Important therapeutic advances include the development of the hysterectomy in 1870, the use of radium in 1920 (12), the use of external radiation, and the importance of postoperative vaginal vault radiation (14).

Standardization of staging procedures and therapeutic advances made possible the individualization of treatment pioneered by Gusberg (9,10). Several acceptable and relatively successful contemporary treatment plans have been outlined by Boronow (2) (Table 4), but these have been developed without controlled clinical trials. To distinguish the relative merits of the programs outlined for stage I, II, and III diseases, randomized trials are needed and several are under way. The Gynecological Oncology Group (GOG; Protocol 16) is testing preoperative versus postoperative irradiation in the treatment of stage I, and grade 2 and 3 adenocarcinoma of the endometrium. These include patients both in stage

TABLE 4. *Currently acceptable treatment plans (2)*

Stage I
  1. Uterus normal size for age and parity; and well-differentiated cancer (FIGO stage IaGl
     and some IbGl)
     a. Surgery alone or
     b. Preoperative vaginal and uterine radium or
     c. Preoperative whole pelvis irradiation
  2. Uterus enlarged or tumor histology less than well differentiated (FIGO stage IaG2, IaG3,
     IbGl, IbG2, IbG3)
     a. Preoperative vaginal and uterine radium or
     b. Preoperative whole pelvis irradiation

Stage II
  1. Subclinical cervical involvement
     a. Uterine and vaginal radium as for stage I, then hysterectomy or
     b. Preoperative whole pelvis irradiation as for stage I, then hysterectomy or
     c. Primary radical hysterectomy and pelvic lymphadenectomy
  2. Clinical cervical involvement
     a. Treat with radium and external beam therapy as cervix cancer, then add conservative
        hysterectomy or
     b. Radium and external beam therapy without hysterectomy or
     c. Primary radical hysterectomy and pelvic lymphadenectomy

Stage III
  Treat as cervical cancer of comparable clinical findings; add hysterectomy rarely only,
  selectively

Ia and Ib FIGO classification considered medically suitable for hysterectomy. These patients are assigned to either preoperative radiation or postoperative whole pelvic radiation, or selective postoperative treatment based on the surgical pathologic findings. This protocol was activated in December 1974 and is still accruing patients.

The GOG (Protocol 18) is also involved in testing three treatment regimens for stage II endometrial adenocarcinoma or adenoacanthoma. The treatment regimens include the following: regimen I: radical hysterectomy (TAH), bilateral salpingo-oöphorectomy (BSO), and pelvic lymphadenectomy; regimen II: external radiation plus tandem and ovoids, plus TAH BSO; regimen III: external radiation plus tandem ovoids (if persistence of disease after 3 months, TAH plus BSO). This protocol was activated August 8, 1974, and is still accruing patients.

The treatment of extrapelvic metastatic endometrial cancer has met with only limited success. The progestational agents have been said to produce objective response rates in the range of 30% (21). Younger women (under 50) and women with well-differentiated tumors seem to respond better. Pulmonary metastases are said to respond better than bulky pelvic recurrences.

The role of nonhormonal chemotherapy in endometrial cancer is not well defined. In the review by De Vita et al. (5) the effect of single-agent chemotherapy was not clear. Of 30 relatively widely used chemotherapeutic drugs, only three were considered adequately evaluated. The data that is available has been obtained from phase II studies and not from randomized controlled clinical trials, although several prospective randomized controlled clinical trials are under way.

The development of additional therapy for disseminated disease will also be important for developing successful adjuvant therapy. Adjuvant therapy has already been tried in endometrial carcinoma. One large-scale trial compared depo provera and a placebo as adjuvant to surgery or surgery plus radiotherapy (17).

The treatment of uterine sarcoma is also now being subjected to rigors of randomized controlled clinical trials. The GOG (Protocol 20) has an adjuvant protocol for stage I and II uterine sarcoma. In this study Adriamycin® as an adjuvant is compared to no treatment. The study was activated in later 1973 and accrual continues. The GOG (Protocol 21) is also testing Adriamycin versus Adriamycin and dimethyl triazeno imadizole carboxamide in advanced uterine sarcoma. This study was activated in November 1973 and is still accruing cases.

## CERVICAL CARCINOMA

The American Cancer Society 1975 figures show there were 19,000 new cases of cervical cancer in 1975 and 7,800 deaths in the United States. As in endometrial carcinoma, progress has been made without conspicuous utilization of the prospective randomized controlled clinical trial. Clearly the most significant advance in cervical cancer has not been in treatment but in detection. Here

TABLE 5. *Cancer of the uterus incidence rates (3) for Connecticut 1935–1972, Cervix*

| Year | Total | Invasive | In situ |
|------|-------|----------|---------|
| 1935–1939 | 21.2 | 21.2 | |
| 1940–1944 | 18.9 | 18.9 | 0.0 |
| 1945–1949 | 21.1 | 20.0 | 1.1 |
| 1950–1954 | 22.3 | 18.7 | 3.6 |
| 1955–1959 | 28.7 | 19.5 | 9.2 |
| 1960–1964 | 31.9 | 17.7 | 14.2 |
| 1965–1968 | 37.2 | 11.7 | 25.5 |
| 1969–1972 | 41.9 | 10.9 | 31.0 |

the increased utilization of the Pap smear, which contributes to early diagnosis (Table 5) (3), has resulted in a major impact on the disease. Other improvements, that is, in management, stem from the application of the extent of disease workup and the value of the multimodality therapy.

The staging system proposed by FIGO is outlined in Table 6 (16). As might have been predicted, the stage of disease has some correlation with involvement of both pelvic and para-aortic nodes (1,6,13,20).

Therapy is based in part on the stage. Both radiation and surgery are recognized modalities for carcinoma of the cervix, and each has its vocal proponents. No single therapeutic recommendation can be made now for, unfortunately,

TABLE 6. *FIGO staging classification for cervical cancer (16)*

| | |
|---|---|
| | Preinvasive carcinoma |
| Stage 0 | Carcinoma *in situ,* intraepithelial carcinoma |
| Cases of stage 0 should not be included in any therapeutic statistics for invasive carcinoma. | |
| | Invasive carcinoma |
| Stage I | Carcinoma strictly confined to the cervix (extension to the corpus should be disregarded) |
| Stage Ia | Microinvasive carcinoma (early stromal invasion) |
| Stage Ib | All other cases of stage I; occult cancer should be marked "occ" |
| Stage II | The carcinoma extends beyond the cervix, but has not extended on to the pelvic wall. The carcinoma involves the vagina, but not the lower third. |
| Stage IIa | No obvious parametrial involvement |
| Stage IIb | Obvious parametrial involvement |
| Stage III | The carcinoma has extended on to the pelvic wall. On rectal examination there is no cancer-free space between the tumor and the pelvic wall. The tumor involves the lower third of the vagina. All cases with a hydronephrosis or nonfunctioning kidney |
| Stage IIIa | No extension on to the pelvic wall |
| Stage IIIb | Extension on to the pelvic wall and/or hydronephrosis or nonfunctioning kidney |
| Stage IV | The carcinoma has extended beyond the true pelvis or has clinically involved the mucosa of the bladder or rectum. A bullous oedema as such does not permit a case to be allotted to stage IV. |
| Stage IVa | Spread of the growth to adjacent organs |
| Stage IVb | Spread to distant organs |

no prospective, randomized controlled clinical trial has been performed to settle the issues involved. Gusberg (7) has reviewed an extensive number of patients and has shown little difference in 5-year survival in stage I and II with either modality. Although the numbers were large, the groups were not totally comparable; thus the results must be viewed with some skepticism.

The treatment of stage III disease is no clearer an issue. There are still advocates of radical surgery and those who recommend extensive radiation. Still others have proposed and tested a variety of combinations of surgery and radiation (4,24). Again there are no randomized, controlled studies, and the issues remain unsettled.

There has been some systematic activity in the evaluation of chemotherapeutic agents in cervical cancer, although the number of randomized controlled clinical trials is small. Several agents including cyclophosphamide, 5-fluorouracil, methotrexate, and perhaps bleomycin, hydroxyurea, vincristine, adriamycin, and hexamethylmelamine have been demonstrated to have some activity in stage IV cervical cancer.

The existence of single agents with some activity in cervical cancer has led to interest in testing drug combinations. The Southwest Oncology Group (Protocol 7412) is comparing vincristine, mitomycin C, and bleomycin to vincristine, mitomycin C, and bleomycin infusion.

The demonstration that drugs have activity in advanced disease leads to their use in adjuvant programs. One such adjuvant study reported by Piver et al. (19) was a double-blind, randomized study comparing radiation plus hydroxyurea to radiation alone in IIB or IIIB previously untreated patients. At 2 years postevaluation, there were fewer patients with evidence of recurrence in the group treated with hydroxyurea. A study by the Gynecologic Oncology Group (Protocol 4) includes patients with untreated squamous cell carcinoma of the cervix in stages IIIB and IV, stratified by stage and randomly assigned to radiotherapy plus hydroxyurea or radiotherapy alone. This study was activated in June 1971. It has been completed and it is now being evaluated.

The management of cervical cancer has been determined for the most part without the benefit of randomized controlled clinical trials. Many important issues remain and may best be settled only by the use of the randomized controlled trial which, fortunately, is being increasingly employed.


## VULVA CANCER

In 1975 (GOG Protocol 4) the incidence of carcinoma of the vulva in the United States was 18 per 100,000. It caused approximately 500 deaths. There is a growing awareness of the value of staging, and there is some recent interest in the possibilities of a combined modality approach.

At this point little interest has been shown to mount a randomized controlled clinical trial.

## SUMMARY

The success of the gynecological oncologist in dealing with early carcinoma of the endometrium, cervix, and vulva is impressive when compared to that in other solid tumors. This in part is related to the possibility of early diagnosis, the relative ease of examination, and the surgical and radiotherapeutic techniques available. The success in these cancers has been achieved for the most part without the use of the randomized controlled clinical trial. From a review of the studies currently being planned and in progress it would appear that the randomized trial will play an increasingly important role in the generation of the data necessary for further advancement in the successful treatment of these diseases.

## ACKNOWLEDGMENTS

This investigation was supported by grants CA 07968 and C01–CN–35025 from the National Cancer Institute, Bethesda, Maryland.

## REFERENCES

1. Averette, H. E., Dudan, R. C., and Ford, J. R. (1972): Exploratory celiotomy for surgical staging of cervical cancer. *Am. J. Obstet. Gynecol.,* 113:1095–1096.
2. Bonorow, R. C. (1969): Therapeutic considerations in endometrial cancer. *J. Miss. State Med. Assoc.,* 10:451.
3. *Cancer Facts and Figures, 1975,* American Cancer Society.
4. Decker, D. G., Aaro, L. A., Hunt, A. B., Johnson, L. E., and Smith, R. A. (1965): Sequential radiation and operation in carcinoma of the uterine cervix. *Am. J. Obstet. Gynecol.,* 92:35–43.
5. De Vita, V. T., Wasserman, T. H., Young, R. C., and Carter, S. K. (1976): Perspectives on research in gynecologic oncology. *Cancer,* 38(1 Suppl.):509–525.
6. Fletcher, G. H., and Rutledge, F. N. (1972): Extended field technique in the management of cancer of the uterine cervix. *Am. J. Roentgenol. Radium Ther. Nucl. Med.,* 114:116–122.
7. Gusberg, S. B. (1970): Surgical treatment for cervical cancer. In: *Oncology, Vol. IV, Diagnosis and Management of Cancer,* edited by R. L. Clark, R. W. Cumley, T. McCory, et al., pp. 250–263. Year Book Medical Publishers, Chicago.
8. Gusberg, S. B. (1976): The evolution of modern treatment of corpus cancer. *Cancer,* 38 (1 Suppl.):603–609.
9. Gusberg, S. B., Jones, H. C., Jr., and Tovell, H. M. M. (1960): Selection of treatment for corpus cancer. *Am. J. Obstet. Gynecol.,* 80:374–380.
10. Gusberg, S. B., and Yannopoulos, D. (1964): Therapeutic decisions in corpus cancer. *Am. J. Obstet. Gynecol.,* 88:157–162.
11. Hemesley, H. O., Borman, R. C., and Lewis, J. L., Jr. (1976): Treatment of adenocarcinoma of the endometrium at the Memorial-James Ewing Hospital 1949–1965. *Obstet. Gynecol.* 47:100–105.
12. Heyman, J. (1927): Radiological or operative treatment of cancer of the uterus. *Acta Radiol.,* 8:363–409.
13. Javert, C. T. (1954): The lymph nodes and lymph channels of the pelvis. In: *Surgical Treatment of the Cancer of the Cervix,* edited by J. V. Meigs. Grune & Stratton, New York.
14. Kottmeier, H. L. (1955): Place of radiation therapy and of surgery in the treatment of uterine cancer. *J. Obstet. Gynaecol. Br. Commonw.,* 62:737–773.
15. Kottmeier, H. L. (ed.) (1973): *Annual Report on the Results of Treatment in Carcinoma of the Uterus, Vagina and Ovary,* Vol. 15. International Federation of Gynecology and Obstetrics, Stockholm.

16. Kottmeier, H. L. (ed.), and Kolstad, P. (asst. ed.) (1976): *Annual Report on the Results of Treatment in Carcinoma of the Uterus, Vagina and Ovary.* International Federation of Gynecology and Obstetrics, Stockholm.

17. Lewis, G. C., Jr., Slack, N. H., Moertel, R., and Bross, I. D. J. (1974): Adjuvant progestogen therapy in the primary definitive treatment of endometrial cancer. *Gynecol. Oncol.,* 2(2–3):368–376.

18. Morrow, C. P., Di Saia, P. J., and Townsend, D. T. (1973): Current management of endometrial cancer. *Obstet. Gynecol.,* 42:399–406.

19. Piver, M. S., Barlow, J. J., Vongtoma, V., and Webster, J. (1974): Hydroxyurea and radiation therapy in advanced cervical cancer. *Am. J. Obstet. Gynecol.,* 120(7):969–972.

20. Piver, M. S., Wallace, S., and Castro, J. R. (1971): The accuracy of lymphangiography in carcinoma of the uterine cervix. *Am. J. Roentgenol. Radium Ther. Nucl. Med.,* 111:278–283.

21. Reifenstein, E. C., Jr. (1971): Hydroprogesterone caproate therapy in advanced endometrial cancer. *Cancer,* 27:485–502.

22. Sall, S., Sonnenblick, B., and Stone, M. L. (1970): Factors affecting survival of patients with endometrial adenocarcinoma. *Am. J. Obstet. Gynecol.,* 107:116–123.

23. Silverberg, E. (1975): *Gynecologic Cancer: Statistical and Epidemiological Information.* American Cancer Society Professional Education Publication.

24. Stallworthy, J. (1964): Radical surgery following radiation treatment for cervical carcinoma. *Ann. R. Coll. Surg. Engl.,* 34:161–178.

25. Welander, C., Griem, M. L., and Newton, N. (1972): Staging and treatment of endometrial carcinoma. *J. Reprod. Med.,* 8:41–46.

*Randomized Trials in Cancer: A Critical Review by Sites,* edited by Maurice J. Staquet, Raven Press, New York © 1978.

# Bronchogenic Carcinoma

## Martin H. Cohen

*NCI-VA Medical Oncology Section, Veterans Administration Hospital, Washington, D.C. 20422*

In lung cancer, as in other malignancies, superiority of a treatment regimen can be demonstrated only when comparable patient groups are evaluated. Prospective randomized trials are the first step in assuring comparability since differences in diagnostic and staging procedures and in supportive care techniques for the various treatment groups should be minimal. Prerandomization stratification by important prognostic variables is a second essential for assuring patient comparability. Finally, adequate numbers of patients must be entered into the trial to assure that more than one patient falls into each prognostic stratum (97).

The following discussion divides lung cancer treatment into surgical adjuvant trials, radiation therapy studies, combined radiation therapy-chemotherapy trials, treatment programs for small cell bronchogenic carcinoma, chemotherapy trials in non-small cell (epidermoid, adenocarcinoma, and large cell anaplastic) lung cancer, and immunotherapy studies. For each of these treatment areas study design, in terms of appropriate stratification, and therapeutic results are considered.

## SURGICAL ADJUVANT THERAPY

The principal prognostic factor for surgical adjuvant studies is stage of disease. In surgical studies stage can best be defined in the TNM system (15,70). Patients in a numerically or alphabetically lower-stage category have a better prognosis than individuals in a higher category. Precision of staging increases as one goes from clinical staging, which generally underestimates the extent of tumor dissemination (70), to surgical staging with evaluation of gross disease within the thorax to pathologic staging based on histologic evaluation of resected lymph nodes. Patients staged pathologically would have a better prognosis than those staged clinically.

For surgical adjuvant studies tumor histology, possibly excluding small cell carcinoma (69), is a less important prognostic factor. Several studies indicate

Received February 14, 1977.

TABLE 1. Surgical adjuvant studies

| Group | Treatment | No. of pts. studied | Stratification | | | Results by | | | Conclusion | Ref. |
| | | | Histology | Stage of disease | Histology | Stage of disease | Histology | TNM stage | | |
|---|---|---|---|---|---|---|---|---|---|---|
| VA Surgical Adjuvant Lung Cancer Group | CTX, 6 mg/kg for 5 doses starting at surgery; repeat 5-day course at 8 mg/kg week 5 vs. control | 1,008 | No | No | Yes | | No | | Benefit in small cell; no benefit for other histologies | Higgins et al., 1969–1972 (45,46) |
| Swiss Group for Clinical Cancer Research | CTX, 12 mg/kg weekly for 8 or 9 doses every 4 months vs. control | 189 | No | No | Partial—small cell + large cell anaplastic are one group | | No | | CTX worse for each histology | Brunner et al., 1973 (13) |
| Moscow Herzen Oncologic Institute (partially randomized last 4 years of 13-year trial) | CTX, 1 g i.v. every 5 days to dose of 8–12 g, or thiotepa, 20 mg every other day to 280–380 mg; 50% of dose preop 50% post-op, or control | 301 | No | No | Partial—small cell and large cell together | | No | | Benefit for all cell types except adeno | Pavlov et al., 1973 (72) |
| Austrian Study Group | Partially randomized CTX, 12 mg/kg; 5-FU, 12 mg/kg; MTX, 0.5 mg/kg; Vlb, 0.1 mg/kg weekly X3; then 10 more doses over 3 years | 82 | Partial | Partial | No | | Only stage I | | Possible benefit for stage I | Karrer et al., 1973 (54) |
| VA Surgical Adjuvant Group | CTX, 8 mg/kg/ day X 5 alternate at 5-week intervals with MTX 10 mg/day X 5 for 18 months vs. control | 260 | No | No | No | | No | | No benefit | Shields et al., 1974 (84) |

| Group | Regimen | No. of patients | | | | | Results | Reference |
|---|---|---|---|---|---|---|---|---|
| Working Party-Lung (WP-L) stage I and II resected epidermoid, adeno, and large cell carcinoma | CCNU, 130 mg/m² every 6 weeks for 2 years vs. control | Ongoing | Yes | Yes | Too soon for results | Yes | Ongoing | — |
| (WP-L) stage III adeno or large cell carcinoma no residual disease | CCNU, 130 mg/m² every 6 weeks for 2 years vs. control | Ongoing | Yes | Yes | Too soon for results | No | Ongoing | — |
| VA Surgical Adjuvant Lung Group | CTX, 8 mg/kg/day × 5 i.v. every 5 weeks vs. control | 248 | No | No | Incomplete | No | No benefit; no harm | Shields et al., 1974 (84) |
| Br. Med. Res. Council | CTX, 200 mg/day p.o. × 10 then 75–150 mg/day × 2 years vs. control | 483 | Yes | No | Yes | No | No benefit at 24 months | Miller et al., 1971 (66) |
| Poulsen | CTX, 50–200 mg daily orally for 21 months | 106 | Yes | No | Only evaluated differentiated epidermoid carcinoma | No | Benefit. Follow-up about 1 year | Poulsen, 1962 (75) |
| Crosbie | Vinblastine, 0.1 mg/kg/week or more based on hematologic toxicity for 3 months vs. control | 167 | Yes | No | Yes | No | Possible benefit for pts. with positive lymph nodes and for small cell pts. at 1 year | Crosbie et al., 1966 (24) |
| Br. Med. Res. Council | Busulfan, 4 mg/day then 1.5–3 mg/day × 2 years vs. control | 492 | Yes | No | Yes | No | No benefit at 24 months | Miller et al., 1971 (66) |
| University Surgical Adjuvant Lung Project | HN2, 0.3–0.4 mg/kg divided dose for 3–4 days starting on day of surgery vs. control | 1,192 | No | Partial | Partial; anaplastic tumors considered together | Evaluated tumor size and neg. vs. positive nodes | No benefit of HN2 | Slack, 1970 (85) |
| VA Surgical Adjuvant Lung Cancer Group | HN2, same as above | 1,142 | No | No | No | No | No benefit of HN2 | Shields, 1973 (81) |

that 5-year survival after an apparently curative resection is similar for all histologies (6,47,91). Other less important prognostic factors are the age and sex of the patient and the presence or absence of underlying lung disease.

The Veterans Administration Surgical Adjuvant Group demonstrated that patients less than 60 years old did better than individuals above this age (82). Similar results were obtained by Bergh and Schersten (8). Females had a better prognosis than males, probably because of the higher frequency of peripheral adenocarcinoma and especially bronchioloalveolar carcinoma in the female population (6,21). The presence of preexisting lung disease may preclude adequate resectional surgery.

In designing surgical adjuvant chemotherapy programs current concepts indicate that drugs should be given intermittently to avoid prolonged immunosuppression and that treatment should be continued for at least 1 year to ensure tumor eradication (16); Table 1 lists randomized surgical adjuvant chemotherapy trials. As is evident, the only drug used in more than a single trial is cyclophosphamide. Even with this drug, however, studies are generally inadequate. Of six trials using cyclophosphamide, two gave the drug on a daily schedule (66,75), two treated for only a short period of time (45,72), and in one study the drug was given weekly for 8 or 9 doses every 4 months (13). Only one trial gave the drug optimally, by present standards (84). Results of this study showed no benefit from cyclophosphamide treatment.

Another major difficulty in evaluating the above studies is the lack of stratification by clinical or pathologic stage of disease. Patients entered into these studies could range from individuals with small asymptomatic pulmonary nodules treated by lobectomy to patients with mediastinal lymph node involvement treated by radical pneumonectomy. Thus firm conclusions as to the efficacy of cyclophosphamide as a surgical adjuvant cannot be made. The drug appears useful in small cell carcinoma, but few of these patients come to surgery (45). The studies of Pavlov et al. (72) and Poulsen (75) suggest benefit for adjuvant cyclophosphamide, but patient follow-up in these trials is either brief or incompletely documented.

Similar conclusions as those made above for cyclophosphamide could be made for studies of vinblastine, nitrogen mustard, and busulfan. Treatment was either for a short period of time (24,81,85) or it involved daily drug administration (66). Only one of these studies partially stratified patients by stage of disease (85).

A well-designed surgical adjuvant study was recently initiated by the Working Party for Lung Cancer (WP–L). In this study patients are staged in the TNM system according to criteria established by the American Joint Commission for Cancer Staging and End Results Reporting (70). Resected patients with stage I or II non-small cell carcinoma were stratified by stage and histology to receive cyclohexyl-chloroethyl nitrosourea (CCNU) or placebo every 6 weeks for 2 years. This study is actively accruing patients in the United States and in the Soviet Union.

Only two published studies have used two or more drugs either sequentially or in combination. The Veterans Administration Surgical Adjuvant Group treated with cyclophosphamide alternating with methotrexate (84), whereas the Austrian Study Group used a combination of cyclophosphamide, 5-fluorouracil, methotrexate, and vinblastine (54). Neither study was optimally stratified. Although results of the latter study appear promising, there are insufficient numbers of patients for firm conclusions.

From the above discussion it appears that chemotherapy has not had an adequate trial as a surgical adjuvant. Since single-agent chemotherapy of non-small cell cancer patients with advanced disease is relatively ineffective, future chemotherapy adjuvant studies will probably employ active drug combinations or will await discovery of new active single agents.

## SURGERY PLUS RADIATION THERAPY

Radiation therapy has been given either preoperatively or postoperatively. Potential advantages of the former mode of treatment are that a percentage of patients with regional tumor extension might be converted from nonresectable to resectable by radiation therapy and secondly by decreasing tumor cell viability preoperative radiation might lessen the possibility of tumor dissemination at surgery. The purpose of postoperative irradiation is to sterilize residual tumor left in the chest after surgery. In addition, by giving radiation postoperatively, one avoids the potential for radiation side effects seen with preoperative radiation therapy including delayed wound healing and increased incidence of intrathoracic infection (10). Further, one does not have to delay surgery for postoperative radiation.

Assessment of both preoperative and postoperative radiation trials is difficult because of lack of proper stratification in three of the four trials listed in Table 2. Despite demonstrable tumor sterilization in patients receiving preoperative radiation, there was no benefit or even a slight disadvantage to this form of treatment. Postoperative radiation therapy should be most useful in patients with epidermoid carcinoma who have residual tumor in mediastinal lymph nodes (38). The study by Bangma (7) was particularly disappointing in that it failed to show benefit in this group of patients. However, patient numbers were very small, with only 5 of 36 radiated patients having positive mediastinal nodes.

Somewhat disturbing in Paterson and Russell's (71) postoperative radiation study was the finding of an increased incidence of systemic metastasis, especially to the liver and brain, in irradiated patients. Other authors, however, have not confirmed this finding (1).

As with chemotherapy adjuvant studies, it is difficult to draw firm conclusions on the efficacy of adjuvant radiation therapy. In future trials it would appear that postoperative radiation therapy studies would be more useful than preoperative studies. Using the former approach, patients whose tumor was completely

TABLE 2. *Surgery-radiation therapy*

| R.T. given | Dose/ treatment duration | No. of pts. studied | Stratification by | | Results by | | Conclusion | Ref. |
|---|---|---|---|---|---|---|---|---|
| | | | Histology | Stage | Histology | Stage | | |
| Preop | 4,000–5,000 rads/ 4–6 weeks | 331 | Partially | No, but included only central lesions | No | No | No benefit even in pts. with tumor sterilization after radiation | Shields, 1970; 1972 (80,83) |
| Preop | 4,000–5,200 rads/ 4–6 weeks | 568 | Yes | No | Yes | No | No benefit | Collaborative Study, 1969–1975 (19,20) |
| Postop patients with curative resection | 4,500 rads/5 weeks | 73 | Yes | Yes | Yes | Yes | No benefit even in localized epidermoid carcinoma | Bangma, 1971 (7) |
| Postop | 4,500 rads/4 weeks | 202 | Yes | No | Partially | No | No benefit | Paterson and Russell, 1962 (71) |

resected and who had negative lymph nodes would be spared from further, presumably unnecessary, local treatment. Also, as mentioned previously, surgery would not be delayed.

In designing either chemotherapy or radiation therapy, surgical adjuvant studies must assure that adequate numbers of patients will be entered in the trial. Thus for patients who have stage I disease (70), after pathologic examination of resected tissues one might expect a 50% 5-year survival from surgery alone. Of patients who die, approximately 14% will die of causes unrelated to their cancer (82). Consequently, surgical adjuvant treatment would be expected to benefit only a third of all entered patients. For stage II disease $(T_2N_1M_0)$, with a 5-year survival of about 25% and with 14% deaths unrelated to cancer, about 60% of entered patients might benefit from treatment.

## RADIATION THERAPY

With the exception of two randomized trials comparing radiation therapy to surgery, the majority of studies have attempted to control local disease and improve survival of nonresectable patients who clinically have disease confined to one hemithorax with or without ipsilateral supraclavicular nodes (limited disease) (Table 3).

In the radiation therapy versus surgery studies, Morrison, Deeley, and Cleland (68) included 28 radiation therapy patients and 30 surgically resected patients evenly matched as to histology, age, and suspected mediastinal node involvement. Radiation therapy (4500 rads/4 weeks) was given by an 8-MeV accelerator. Overall 4-year survival for surgically treated patients was 23% versus 7% for radiation therapy patients. For patients with epidermoid carcinoma 4-year survivals were 30% versus 6% for surgery and radiation therapy, respectively. For anaplastic tumors, as one might expect, because of the high metastatic potential of these tumors, there was no difference in 4-year survival by type of local treatment.

A second radiation therapy versus surgery study was conducted in patients with "operable" small cell lung cancer by the British Medical Research Council (67). No patient treated with surgery survived 5 years, whereas 6% of radiation therapy patients survived that interval.

The majority of randomized radiation therapy trials have attempted to define optimal time-dose relationships for treatment. The end point of most of these studies is patient survival. Results of autopsy evaluation of the frequency of tumor sterilization within the irradiated field are rarely reported. The difficulty with survival as the principal determinant of radiotherapy efficacy is that for many patients treatment failure, with resultant early death, is due to unrecognized disease outside of the radiation port.

Prognostic parameters to be used in stratifying radiation therapy trials include histologic cell type, stage of disease, performance status, and immune status. Histology is important because of differences in radiation sensitivity of the various

TABLE 3. *Radiation therapy*

| Purpose of study | No. of patients | Radiation dose(s) Treatment duration | Stratified by | | Conclusions | Ref. |
| | | | Histology | Stage | | |
| --- | --- | --- | --- | --- | --- | --- |
| RT vs. placebo | 554 | 4,000–5,000 rads 4–5 weeks 90% orthovoltage | Yes | Limited disease only | No significant difference in survival | Wolf et al., 1966 (95) |
| RT vs. surgery | 58 | 4,500 rads/4 weeks supervoltage | Yes | Operable patients; 33% with mediastinal nodes | Surgery significantly better for epidermoid carcinoma (30% vs. 6% 4-year survival) | Roswit et al., 1968 (77) Morrison et al., 1963 (68) |
| 3,000 rads vs. 4,000 rads | 102 | 3,000 or 4,000 rads 4 weeks supervoltage | Anaplastic carcinoma only | Limited disease | Median survival 9.3 months in 3,000-rad group, 6.0 months in 4,000-rad group, significant at 0.05 level | Deeley, 1966 (25) |
| RT vs. surgery: small cell carcinoma | 144 | Variable radiation doses and schedules vs. surgery | Small cell only | Operable | Median survival significantly better for radiotherapy; 6% 5-year survival with RT 0% for surgery | Miller et al., 1969 (67) |
| Continuous vs. split course | 25 | 6,000 rads/6 weeks vs. 1,800 rads/3 days; 28 day rest; 1,800 rads/3 days | Epidermoid carcinoma only | Limited disease | No difference in survival, but not enough patients | Levitt et al., 1966 (62) |
| Continuous vs. split course | 349 | 5,000–6,000 rads/5–6 weeks continuous and 8–9 weeks split | Yes | Inoperable | No difference in survival; less toxicity with split | Holsti, 1973 (48) |
| Continuous vs. split course | 84 | 6,000 rads/6 weeks vs. 2,000 rads/1 week; 3 week rest; 2,000 rads/1 week | Yes | Limited disease | Significant increase in 1-year survival with split-course treatment | Abramson and Cavanaugh, 1970 (2) |
| Time-dose relationship for split course | 250 | 3,000 rads/3 weeks; 2 week rest 2,000 rads/2 weeks vs. 2,000 rads/1 week; 3 week rest; 2,000 rads/1 week | Yes | Limited disease | Ongoing | Working Party for Lung Cancer (WP-L), protocol 7312 |

| Objective | No. | Dose schedule | Histology | Stage/disease | Results | Reference |
|---|---|---|---|---|---|---|
| Time-dose relationship for split course | 91 | 3,000 rads/2 weeks; 1 month rest; 3,000 rads/2 weeks vs. 2,000 rads/1 week; 1 month rest; 2,000 rads 1 week | No | Limited disease | 1-year survival significantly better for 3,000 rads schedule; survival difference not significant at 18 months | Guthrie et al., 1973 (40) |
| Continuous vs. split course | 188 | 5,000 rads/4–5 weeks vs. 5,000 rads/7–9 weeks (3–4 week rest in the middle of treatment) | Yes | Yes | No significant difference; large cell carcinoma responded better to split-course therapy | Lee et al., 1976 (60) |
| Time-dose relationships for radiation therapy | — | 2,000 rads/1 week; 2 week rest; 2,000 rads/1 week vs. 4,000 rads/4 weeks vs. 5,000 rads/5 weeks vs. 6,000 rads/6 weeks | Yes; epidermoid, adeno, and large cell | Yes T3 any N or N2 with any T | Ongoing | Radiation Therapy Oncology Group, protocol 5173 |
| Time-dose relationships | — | 5,000 rads/5 weeks vs. Brain RT 2,000 rads/2 weeks given to 50% of patients on both arms | No | Limited disease | Ongoing | Veterans Administration Lung Cancer Group, protocol VALG 15 |
| Adjuvant radiotherapy known residual disease | — | 2,000 rads/1 week; 3 week rest; 2,000 rads/1 week vs. 3,000 rads/3 weeks; 2 week rest 2,000 rads/2 weeks | Epidermoid | III | Ongoing | Working Party for Lung Cancer (WP–L), protocol 75–11 |
| Adjuvant radiotherapy no known residual disease | — | Surgery alone vs. surgery + RT 4,800 rads/4 weeks | Epidermoid | III | Ongoing | WP–L 75–12 |
| Time-dose relationships | — | 2,000 rads/1 week; 3 week rest; 2,000 rads/1 week vs. 800 rads/d1, 8, 22 then 500 rads/d36, 43, 49, 56, 63, 70 | Epidermoid | Limited | Ongoing | WP–L 75–13 |
| Time-dose relationships | 100 | 4,800 rads/4 weeks vs. 2,800 rads/4 fractions of 700 rads in 10 days conventional or 35 MeV electrons | No | Limited | Similar survival and disease control in all arms | Johnson et al., 1973 (53) |

types of lung cancer (78). Most studies do stratify by histology. Stage of disease is most often expressed as limited (disease confined to one hemithorax with or without ipsilateral supraclavicular node involvement) or extensive disease. Unfortunately, most authors do not indicate their routine staging workup, so that it is difficult to determine the precision with which the classification of limited versus extensive disease is made. Although staging in the TNM system is more precise and would allow a firmer estimate of treatment benefit, it is unlikely that most institutions could stage patients in this fashion. Performance status is a very important prognostic factor. Ambulatory asymptomatic individuals survive considerably longer than their counterparts who are bedridden secondary to disease symptoms (96). Delayed hypersensitivity skin testing also correlates with survival. Patients who react to one or more recall skin tests live longer than anergic individuals (52). Most studies have not been stratified by these latter two variables.

As indicated above, there is little information on optimal dose–time relationships for local tumor control of the various lung cancer histologies. The two principal treatment techniques are either continuous treatment to a planned dose or split-course treatment. The latter implies that treatment is interrupted one or more times before completion. Split-course radiation may utilize standard 200-rad doses, 5 days a week, with a break in the middle of treatment, or it may be given as large fractions of radiation over a short time period. The theoretical basis for the latter is that small fractional doses might only injure tumor cells sublethally. The cells might then be able to repair sublethal damage before the next scheduled treatment. Practically, the advantage of this approach is that a patient has to come less frequently for radiation therapy.

When split-course radiation therapy is compared with continuous radiation therapy with patient survival as the end point of study, little difference between the two methods of radiation therapy are noted (2,48,60,62). Despite the lack of survival benefit in randomized studies, split-course radiation therapy has two advantages over continuous treatment: It is accompanied by less toxicity, and because it is interrupted therapy it allows time for detection of newly appearing systemic metastases, thus saving the patient possible toxicity from further futile X-irradiation.

## RADIATION THERAPY AND CHEMOTHERAPY

The addition of chemotherapy to radiation therapy is, in part, to control disease outside of the radiation field. However, since several of the tested drugs are considered to be radiosensitizers, tumor kill within the radiation field might also increase. Stratification for these studies should include those listed for radiation therapy alone (see above). In studies summarized in Table 4 it is evident that although radiation therapy doses and schedules are adequate, chemotherapy is given for only a short period of time, generally for the duration of radiation therapy. This is too short a drug exposure. Also, although most studies stratify by histology, few are stratified by patient performance status.

TABLE 4. Radiation therapy plus chemotherapy (single agents)

| Study plan | No. of patients | Radiation dose/ duration of treatment | Chemotherapy dose and schedule | Stratified by Histology | Stratified by Stage | Conclusions | Ref. |
|---|---|---|---|---|---|---|---|
| RT ± CTX | 115 | 4,000 rads/4 weeks | 1 g/m² q. 3 weeks for 4 or 8 courses | Small cell vs. epidermoid and large cell | Limited | Greatest benefit for small cell, less for other histologies | Bergsagel et al., 1972 (9) |
| RT ± CTX | 94 | 6,000 rads/6 weeks | 200 mg/day preceding irradiation | Yes | Limited | No survival benefit | Brouet, 1968 (11) |
| RT ± CTX | 14 | 5,000 rads split course: 1,500 rads/1.5–2 weeks; 4–5 week rest; 1,500 rads/1.5–2 weeks; 4–5 week rest etc. | 400 mg daily for 3–4 days then 200 mg 3 times weekly until toxicity or RT completion | No | Limited | No benefit but small numbers | Gollin et al., 1964 (36) |
| RT ± CTX | 149 | 4,000–5,000 rads/4–6 weeks | 400 mg daily to total dose of 40 mg/kg. Then 100 mg daily | Small cell epidermoid | Limited | Slight benefit for CTX In small cell ca., median survival 8.5 vs. 5.5 months | Host, 1973 (51) |
| RT vs. CTX | 22 | 1,500 rads/12 days; 1–2 week rest; 2,250 rads/12 days | 50 mg/kg d1 and 35 | Small cell | Limited | Better survival with CTX than with RT | Tucker et al., 1973 (88) |
| RT ± CTX vs. CTX vs. BCNU | 239 | 4,000–5,000 rads/4–6 weeks | CTX alone—300 mg/m²/ day × 5, then 200 mg/ day; CTX + RT—200 mg/day BCNU—185 mg/m² q. 6 weeks | Yes | Limited | RT alone best for epidermoid, although results highly variable in consecutive studies; otherwise median survival similar for all treatment groups | Kaung et al., 1974 (55) |
| RT ± 5-FU | 62 | 2,000 rads/2 weeks 2,000 rads/2 weeks + 5-FU 4,000 rads/4 weeks | 5 mg/kg/day throughout radiation course | Yes | Limited | Median survival similar in all arms | Cohen et al., 1971 (17) |
| RT ± 5-FU | 188 | 4,500–5,000 rads in 4–9 weeks continuous or split course | 10 mg/kg daily × 5; only 1 course with continuous RT, 2 courses with split | Yes | Limited | Possible benefit for 5-FU in adenocarcinoma; 2-yr survival 27% vs. 5% | Carr et al., 1972 (14) |
| RT ± 5-FU | 44 | 5,000–6,000 rads/8–9 weeks split | Uncertain | Yes | Limited | No benefit | Holsti, 1973, (48) |

TABLE 4—Cont.

| Study plan | No. of patients | Radiation dose/ duration of treatment | Chemotherapy dose and schedule | Stratified by | | Conclusions | Ref. |
|---|---|---|---|---|---|---|---|
| | | | | Histology | Stage | | |
| RT ±5-FU or ACT-D | 342 | 5,000 rads/5–8 weeks ortho- or supervoltage | 5-FU, 5 mg/kg/day ACT-D, 4 μg/kg/day both started 4 days before RT and continued throughout RT | No | Mostly limited | No benefit from addition of chemotherapy | Hall et al., 1967 (41) |
| RT ±5-FU or ACT-D or MTX | 27 | 4,000 rads/4 weeks | 5-FU, 5 mg/kg/day ACT-D, 4 μg/kg/day MTX, 5 mg/day all started 2 days before RT | No | Limited | Pilot study; no conclusions | Hosley et al., 1962 (50) |
| RT + 5-FU RT + IUDR RT + CTX | 100 | 4,000–5,000 rads/4–5 weeks | 5-FU, 10–12 mg/kg/day X3, then t.i.w. IUDR, 15 mg/kg/day CTX, 400 mg/day X 3, then 200 mg t.i.w. | Yes | Limited | Survival similar for all groups and similar to historical radiation alone controls | Gollin et al., 1967 (37) |
| RT ± mechlorethamine during or before RT | 219 | 4,000–6,000 rads/4–6 weeks | Simultaneous HN2, 0.1 mg/kg/day X 4; 2 week rest; then 0.1 mg/kg/ w X 4 Prior HN2, 0.2 mg/ kg, d1 & 3; 2 week rest; then 0.1 mg/kg/w X 4 | No | Limited | Similar survival for all arms | Krant et al., 1963 (56) |
| Observation vs. RT ± HN2 or HN2 | 249 | 4,000 rads/4 weeks | HN2 alone, 0.2–0.3 mg/kg d1, 3, 11 RT + HN2, 0.1–0.2 mg/kg d1, 3, 11 | Partially; large cell and small cell together | Limited | Similar survival for all arms | Durrant et al., 1971 (28) |
| RT ± chlorambucil | 30 | 5,000 rads/4–5 weeks | Chlorambucil, 2–8 mg/day after completing RT | Partially; large cell and small cell together | Limited | Median survival 5 months vs. 7.5 months in favor of RT + chlor | Horwitz et al., 1965 (49) |
| RT ± hydroxyurea vs. hydroxyurea vs. observation | 111 | 4,000–6,000 rads/6–8 weeks | HU, 80 mg/kg q.3d. | No | Limited | Similar surival for all arms | Scheer et al., 1974 (79) |

| Treatment | N | Dose | Drug/dose | Randomized | Result | Reference |
|---|---|---|---|---|---|---|
| RT ± procarbazine or hydroxyurea | 98 | 5,000 rads/5–8 weeks | Procarbazine, 100 mg/day HU, 1,000 mg/day throughout RT | Yes | Similar response and survival for all arms | Hall et al., 1976 (42) |
| RT ± hydroxyurea | 53 | 3,000 rads/2 weeks; 4 week rest; 3,000 rads/2 weeks | 30 mg/kg/day | No | Similar survivals | Landgren et al., 1974 (58) |
| RT ± hydroxyurea | 26 | 6,000 rads/6 weeks | 10 mg/kg/day | No | Similar survivals | LePar et al., 1967 (61) |
| RT ± vinblastine | 194 | 4,000 rads/twice weekly in 4 weeks | 5 mg, 7.5 mg, 10 mg, and 10 mg prior to RT treatments 1, 3, 5, 7 | No | Similar survivals | Coy, 1970 (23) |
| RT ± procarbazine | 67 | 5,000–6,000 rads/5 weeks | 100–125 mg/m²/day, duration unspecified | | RT alone better | Landgren et al., 1973 (59) |
| RT ± methotrexate | 20 | 3,000 rads/12 days | 5 mg i.v. daily during RT | Only epidermoid | Better survival in MTX group | Tucker et al., 1973 (89) |

The best results for radiation therapy plus single-agent chemotherapy have been in patients with small cell cancer. In the trial of Bergsagel et al. (9), the median survival of patients treated with radiation plus cytoxan was 291 days versus 149 days for radiation alone. For other histologies corresponding median survivals were 327 days and 273 days, respectively. Similar results were obtained by Host (51).

Randomized studies of combination chemotherapy and radiation therapy are few, and data are generally unavailable at present (Table 5). The planned duration of chemotherapy in these studies is longer than 1 year, an improvement over most single-agent trials. As in other radiation therapy studies, patient stratification is often not completely satisfactory.

## SMALL CELL CARCINOMA RADIATION THERAPY PLUS CHEMOTHERAPY

Small cell carcinoma is highly sensitive to both chemotherapy and radiation therapy. Since disease is often disseminated at the time of presentation, chemotherapy is the principal therapeutic modality. Radiation therapy is used primarily to control "bulky" disease and to eradicate tumor cells in chemotherapy sanctuaries such as the brain.

In conducting clinical trials small cell patients should be stratified by stage of disease (limited versus extensive), by performance status, and by whether or not they had previous chemotherapy or radiation therapy. If sufficient numbers of patients are included in the trial stratification by immune status, sex and age should also be included. At present we do not know if particular sites of metastatic involvement by small cell cancer, such as bone marrow, liver, or brain, confer a worse prognosis than other metastatic sites. Future studies should look at this question, since new treatment strategies may have to be developed for resistant sites.

Table 6 lists randomized radiation therapy plus chemotherapy trials specifically in small cell carcinoma. Many of the trials listed in Table 3 also include small cell patients. As in other lung cancer studies, a deficiency in these trials is the lack of a uniform staging workup and a lack of stratification by patient performance status.

An important question in current and future small cell treatment programs is whether or not the addition of radiation therapy to chemotherapy results in prolongation of survival. It is evident that one obtains higher response rates of chest lesions when radiation therapy is added and possibly there is delayed recurrence of thoracic disease. The price paid for these benefits includes a decreased tolerance to chemotherapy (proportional to radiation dose, fractionation, and field size), an increased incidence of chemotherapy side effects, and a decreased ability, because of radiation pneumonitis and fibrosis, to use the chest roentgenogram for following tumor changes.

A question of lesser importance, at present, is the value of prophylactic brain

TABLE 5. *Radiation therapy and chemotherapy (drug combinations)*

| Study plan | No. of patients | Radiation dose Duration of treatment | Stratification Histology | Stratification Stage | Results | Ref. |
|---|---|---|---|---|---|---|
| RT + 5-FU + DTIC + VCR + BCNU vs. RT + CCNU + hyproxyurea | 57 | 2,000 rads/2 weeks; 5 week rest; 1,200 rads/1 week; 5 week rest; 1,200 rads/1 week; etc. | Partially | No information | Neither regimen gave better results than historical controls receiving RT alone or RT + 5-FU | Van Der Merwe et al., 1973 (90) |
| RT alone vs. RT + CCNU + hydroxyurea | Ongoing | 5,000–5,500 rads/ 4–6 weeks | Yes | Limited | Ongoing | Veterans Administration Lung Group, protocol 13 |
| RT alone vs. RT + CCNU + CTX + MTX | Ongoing | 3,000 rads/3 weeks; 2 week rest 2,000 rads/2 weeks | Adeno and large cell only | Limited | Ongoing | Working Party for Lung Cancer (WP-L), protocol 73–31 |
| Surgery + RT vs. Surgery + RT + CCNU + CTX + MTX | Ongoing | As in WP–L 73–31 above | Adeno and large cell | III either N2 lesions or T3 lesions, residual disease | Ongoing | WP–L 75–52 |
| Radiotherapy vs. CCNU + CTX + MTX ± BCG vs. BCG | Ongoing | Unknown | Unknown | Limited | Ongoing | E.O.R.T.C. |

TABLE 6. *Radiation therapy and chemotherapy: small cell carcinoma*

| Study plan | No. of patients | Radiation dose duration of treatment | Stratification by stage | Results | Ref. |
|---|---|---|---|---|---|
| RT + CTX + VCR + MTX + citrovorum vs. RT + CTX ± MTX 50% of patients receive brain RT | Ongoing | Thoracic disease, 3,200 rads/ 12 days; brain, 3,000 rads/ 12 days | No | Ongoing | Cancer and Leukemia Group B, CALGB 7283 |
| RT + CCNU + CTX ± brain RT 50% start chemotherapy at start of RT. Remainder start chemotherapy at disease progression | Ongoing | Thoracic, 4,500 rads/5–6 weeks; brain, 3,000 rads/2 weeks | Limited disease | Ongoing | Radiation Therapy Oncology Group and Eastern Cooperative Oncology Group, RTOG 7503/ ECOG 1575 |
| RT + CCNU + CTX + MTX ± brain RT | Ongoing | Thoracic, 3,000 rads/ 3 weeks; 2 week rest; 2,000 rads/2 weeks; brain, 3,000 rads/10 days | Limited disease | Ongoing | Working Party for Lung Cancer, 72–21 |
| CCNU + CTX + MTX ± RT to chest, brain, and upper abdomen | Ongoing | Brain, 3,000 rads/10 days, then chest, 2,000 rads/2 weeks, then abdomen, 2,000 rads/2 weeks | Extensive disease | Ongoing | Working Party for Lung Cancer, 72–22 |
| CTX + VCR + MeCCNU ± | 35, 19 randomized | Thoracic, 4,000 rads/4 weeks | Limited and extensive | Less thoracic recurrences with RT survivals similar | Donovan et al., 1976 (27) |
| PROC + VCR + CTX + CCNU + RT vs. CTX + VCR + MTX + RT or PROC + VCR + CTX + CCNU + RT vs. PROC + VCR + CTX + | 39 | Not specified | Not specified | POCC ± RT longer survival then COM + RT; no difference yet in results of POCC ± RT | Glatstein, 1976 (35) |

radiotherapy. This question should be addressed after regimens are developed that yield a high percentage of long-duration complete responders. At present, many patients receiving prophylactic brain radiation never achieve a complete response and relapse systemically within a few months of the onset of treatment. Death of these patients impairs the determination of efficacy of brain radiation therapy.

Considering the studies listed in Table 6, the Cancer and Leukemia Group B (CALGB) study is designed to determine if three active drugs plus radiation therapy are better than one or two active drugs with the same radiation therapy. Prophylactic brain radiotherapy is also tested. Generally these are not important questions, as most literature results indicate that combinations of three or four active drugs give better responses and longer survivals than single drugs alone or two-drug combinations (32,43,44).

The Radiation Therapy Oncology Group/Eastern Cooperative Oncology Group (RTOG 7503/ECOG 1575) protocol for limited small cell cancer principally concerns the timing of chemotherapy administration relative to radiation therapy and also tests prophylactic brain irradiation. From knowledge of the natural history of disease one would predict that patients starting effective chemotherapy at the same time as radiation therapy would do better than patients whose treatment is delayed until disease progression.

The Working Party for Lung Cancer (WP–L) protocol 72–21 for limited disease patients only questions the value of prophylactic brain irradiation. As indicated previously, this is not an important question at present.

WP–L protocol 72–22 asks an interesting and pertinent question as to whether or not addition of chest, brain, and upper abdominal radiation therapy to three-drug combination chemotherapy will improve response rate and survival. Results of this study will be important with regard to future combined chemotherapy–radiation therapy trials.

Trials conducted by Donovan et al. (27) and Glatstein (35), although hampered by small patient numbers, also ask appropriate questions as to whether or not combined modality treatment is better than chemotherapy alone.

Chemotherapy alone trials in small cell cancer (Table 7) have attempted to define active single agents (31,38,55,92), to determine if combinations of active agents were better than single-drug treatment (31,32), to investigate if simultaneous use of active drugs was better than sequential administration of the same drugs (4), and to determine if intensive chemotherapy, yielding significant leukopenia and thrombocytopenia, was better than using the same drugs in more standard fashion (18). Generally speaking, results show that two-drug combinations give better results than single agents, that three-drug combinations are often better than two-drug combinations, and that certain four-drug combinations may be better than three drugs. Going beyond four-drug combinations does not seem to be beneficial. Simultaneous administration of active drugs is better than sequential administration, and intensive induction chemotherapy yields a higher response rate and longer survivals than does standard dose treat-

TABLE 7. *Chemotherapy: small cell carcinoma*

| Study plan | No. of patients | Drug dose (mg/m²)/Schedule | Stratified by Stage | Stratified by Performance status | Results | Ref. |
|---|---|---|---|---|---|---|
| CCNU + CTX + MTX vs. CTX + MTX | 62 | CCNU 50 q.6w. CTX 500 or 1,100 q.3w. MTX 10 or 20 b.i.w. | Extensive only | No | Nonsignificant increase in response rate and survival for 3-drug combination | Hansen et al., 1976 (44) |
| Simultaneous or sequential MTX + CTX + PROC +VCR | 39 | Simultaneous: MTX 20 q.w. VCR 1.2 q.w., CTX 60 q.d. p.o. PROC 80 q.d. p.o. Sequent: MTX 25 q.w. × 2, CTX 150 q.d. p.o. × 14 days, PROC 150 q.d.p.o. × 14 days, VCR 1.2 q.w. × 2 | No | No | Higher response rate for simultaneous admin. 65% vs. 36%, no survival data | Alberto et al., 1976 (4) |
| Intensive vs. standard induction treatment with CCNU, CTX, MTX | 32 | CTX 1,000 or 500 q.3w. CCNU 100 or 50 q.6w. MTX 15 or 10 b.i.w. | Yes | Yes | 96% PR + CR, 25% CR with high dose vs. 45% PR + CR, 0% CR standard dose | Cohen et al., 1976 (18) |
| CCNU + CTX + MTX ± VCR | 96 | CCNU 70 q.4w. CTX 700 q.4w. MTX 20 d18 + 21 q.4w. VCR 1.5 q.w. × 4 then q.4w. | Extensive only | Not specified | Response rate 3 drugs 75%, 4 drugs 83%; median survival; 3 drugs 6.5 months, 4 drugs 9 months | Hansen and Hansen, 1976 (43) |
| CCNU + CTX vs. CTX | 258 | CCNU 70 q.6w. CTX 700 or 1,000 q.3w. | No | Yes | Response rate CCNU + CTX 43% CTX 22% No difference in median survival | Edmonson et al., 1976 (32) |
| VP-16 vs. CTX, VCR, MTXvs. VCR, BLEO, ADR | 35 | VP 16 125–140 mg d1, 3, 5, q.4–5 w. or CTX 1,500 d1, VCR 1.4 d1, MTX 25 d22 q.4–5w. or VCR 1.2 d1 + 5, Bleo 12.5 d1 + 5 (6 hr after VCR), ADR 50 d2 q.4–5 w. | Extensive only | Yes | Similar response & survival to all regimens; many patients also received thoracic RT | Eagan et al., 1976 (31) |
| Survival prolongation with various single agents | 142 | L-ASP 150 IU/kg/week × 6 L-ASP 1,500 IU/kg/week × 6 DBD (dibromodulcitol) 400 q.w. p.o. × 6 | Extensive only | No | High-dose L-ASP and dibromodulcitol inferior to CTX; other drugs had comparable survival to cytoxan | Kaung et al., 1974 (55) |

| Regimen comparison | No. | Doses/Schedule | Extent | Randomized | Results | Group/Reference |
|---|---|---|---|---|---|---|
| | | CCNU 130 q.6-8w. PROC 150 q.d. Hexamethylmelamine 8 mg/kg/day Streptozotocin 1,000 q.w. × 10 DTIC 325 q.d. × 5 q.4w. | | | | |
| BCNU vs. CTX (2 doses) | Unknown | CTX 1,100 q.3w. CTX 300 q.d. × 5 q.5w. CTX 1.1 q.d. q.3w. BCNU 185 q.6w. | Extensive only | No | Shorter survival when CTX was given q.5w. BCNU and CTX q.3w. similar survival | Whittington et al., 1972 (92) |
| HN₂ vs. CTX vs. placebo | 341 | HN₂ 0.4 mg/kg q.6w. × 2 CTX 8 mg/kg/day × 5; repeat at 30 days and 60 days | Extensive only | No | CTX significantly better than placebo; nitrogen mustard had a slight effect on survival | Green et al., 1969 (38) |
| CCNU + CTX ± procarbazine induction; fixed crossover to ADR or ADR + VCR at 6 weeks if no response or progression | Ongoing | CCNU 70 q.6w. CTX 700 q.3w. PROC 70 q.d. × 7 q.3w. ADR 60 q.3w. VCR 1.2 q.3w. | Limited + extensive | Yes | Ongoing | Eastern Cooperative Oncology Group, No. 1574 |
| CTX vs. CTX, ADR, DTIC for induction; maintenance CTX vs. CTX, ADR, DTIC vs. CTX + VCR, HU, MTX vs. CTX, ADR, DTIC, VCR, HU, MTX | Ongoing | CTX 1,100 q.3w. × 2 vs. CTX 500 q.3w. × 2 + ADR 50 q.3w. × 2+ DTIC 250 q.3w. × 2 Maint: Above regimens q.28d. +: VCR 2 mg d8, 15 HU 2,000 d22, 24 MTX 20 d22, 24 | Limited + extensive | Yes | Ongoing | Southeast Group, No. 357 |
| CTX vs. CCNU vs. MeCCNU vs. CCNU + CTX + HU (sequential) | Ongoing | CTX 1,100 q.3w. CCNU 130 q.6w. MeCCNU 220 q.6w. | Extensive | Yes | Ongoing | VALG #13 |
| CTX vs. CTX + CCNU vs. CTX + ADR vs. CCNU + ADR | Ongoing | CTX 70 q.6w. × 3 + CTX 700 q.3w. × 2, then Hu 1,000 b.i.w. × 12w; repeat cycle q.18w. CTX 1,100 q.3w. vs. CTX 700 q.3w., ADR 40 q.3w. vs. CTX + ADR 40 q.3w. vs. CCNU 70 q.6w., ADR 40 q.3w. vs. CCNU 70 q.6w., CTX 700 q.3w., CCNU 70 q.6w. | Extensive | Yes | Ongoing | VALG #14 |

ment. A problem with developing drug combinations for small cell cancer is that nearly all active drugs except vincristine have myelosuppression as their principal toxicity.

Since several active drug combinations are now available, the next question to answer is how best to use them. All authors indicate that small cell cancer responds rapidly to treatment. Maximal therapeutic response is usually manifest within 6 to 12 weeks of treatment. Since a complete response to treatment appears necessary for prolonged survival, it appears reasonable to change to a new regimen in all patients who do not achieve a complete response within a reasonable time period. The Eastern Cooperative Oncology Group (ECOG 1574) and the Southeast Oncology Group (SEG 357) are partially testing this hypothesis.

Future studies should continue to explore cyclic alternating chemotherapy with active drug combinations. The role of radiation therapy for remission induction and/or maintenance will also have to be defined further. Future studies should also pay closer attention to stratification by important prognostic variables as listed earlier.

## NON-SMALL CELL CANCER CHEMOTHERAPY

Table 8 lists single agent trials in non-small cell lung cancer and Table 9 considers the efficacy of drug combinations. A common study design is to randomize a test drug or drug combination against "standard" treatment. The standard treatment most often chosen is cyclophosphamide, 1,000 to 1,100 mg/$m^2$, every 3 weeks. Prognostic variables for such trials should include histology, disease stage, performance status, prior therapy, and possibly immune status. Patients with metastatic disease have a worse prognosis than those with regional extension only, patients bedridden because of tumor have a worse prognosis than ambulatory asymptomatic individuals, patients who received prior chemotherapy or radiation therapy have lower response rates than previously untreated cases, and anergic individuals have a worse prognosis than patients with intact delayed hypersensitivity.

Because most chemotherapy regimens tested in non-small cell carcinoma yield response rates of 20% or less, serious consideration should be given to including only good-prognosis patients on treatment protocols. Activity of a new drug or combination might be missed if most patients are in the poor-prognosis categories listed above. Reporting of results in terms of median survival also poses a problem. Since none of the regimens in Tables 8 and 9 have a response rate of 50%, median survival should not be influenced. Many authors compare survival of responders versus nonresponders. Reporting results in this way has certain advantages. Thus if a regimen is highly toxic, the response rate might be high but survival of responders would not greatly exceed survival of nonresponders. Secondly, since response rates are generally low, one can look at the survival of nonresponders, weighted by the various prognostic factors listed

TABLE 8. Chemotherapy (single agents only): non-small cell carcinoma

| Study plan | No. of patients | Chemotherapy doses (mg/m²) and schedules | Stratified by | | Results | Ref. |
| | | | Stages | Performance status | | |
|---|---|---|---|---|---|---|
| Survival studies by Veterans Administration Lung Group | over 600 | CTX, 1100 q.3w. DTIC, 325 q.d. × 5 q.4w. L-ASP, 1,500 IU/kg/ wk × 6 L-ASP, 150 IU/kg/ wk × 6 DBD, 400 q.w. × 6 CCNU, 130 q.6w. PROC, 150 q.d. HMM, 8 mg/kg/day Streptozotocin, 1,000 q.w. × 10 | Extensive | No | High-dose L-ASP associated with shortest survival; median survival time similar for other treatments | Kaung et al., 1974 (55) |
| DBD vs. HMM | 250 | Not specified | Limited and extensive | No | Patients dying in 6 weeks nonevaluable; HMM better for epidermoid MS 31w. vs 22W; DBD better for adeno MS 35 vs. 22W | Wilson et al., 1975 (94) |
| HN₂ vs. CTX vs. placebo | over 300 | HN₂, 0.4 mg/kg/d1 and 42 CTX, 8 mg/kg/day × 5 d1, 30, 60 | Extensive | No | HN₂ superior to CTX and placebo in epidermoid; neither better than placebo in adeno | Green et al., 1969 (39) |
| 5-FU vs. CTX | 61 ⅓ prior therapy | 5-FU, 600 q.d. × 5 q.2w. CTX, 1,100 q.3w. | No | No | Less than 10% responses; only cell type with sufficient patients was epidermoid | Brugarolas et al., 1975 (12) |
| CCNU vs. MeCCNU | 124 12% prior therapy | CCNU, 130 q.7w. MeCCNU, 200, then 150 q.7w. | Yes | Yes | Less than 10% responses | Eagan et al., 1974 (29) |
| BCNU vs. CTX | 48 | BCNU, 75–100 q.d. × 3 q.8w. CTX, 370 q.d. × 3 q.4w. | Limited vs. extensive disease | No | 10% or less responses | Ahmann et al., 1972 (3) |

TABLE 8—Cont.

| Study plan | No. of patients | Chemotherapy doses (mg/m²) and schedules | Stratified by | | | Results | Ref. |
| --- | --- | --- | --- | --- | --- | --- | --- |
| | | | Stages | Performance status | | | |
| BCNU vs. CTX q.3.w. vs. CTX q.5w. | Over 300 | BCNU, 185 q.6w. CTX, 1,100 q.3w. CTX, 300 q.d. × 5 q.5w. | Extensive only | No | | 1-year survival-BCNU 13%, CTX q.3w. 8% CTX q.5w. 4% (includes small cell patients) | Whittington et al., 1972 (92) |
| MTX (2 doses) vs. placebo | 227 | MTX, 0.6 mg/kg b.i.w. MTX, 0.2 mg/kg/b.i.w. Placebo | Limited vs. extensive disease | Retrospectively | | Best response rate (21%) with MTX 0.6 mg/kg MS responders 34 weeks vs. 11 weeks for nonresponders | Selawry, et al. (1977) |
| ADR (2 doses) vs. CTX | 714 | ADR, 50 or 75 q.3w. CTX, 1,000 q.3w. | Limited vs. extensive disease | No | | CTX better for large cell; otherwise no differences in response rates or survival | Perlia and Stolbach, 1976 (73) |

TABLE 9. *Chemotherapy non-small cell carcinoma: combinations and/or single agents*

| Study plan | No. of patients | Chemotherapy doses (mg/m²) and schedules | Stage | Histology | Performance | Results | Ref. |
|---|---|---|---|---|---|---|---|
| HN₂ + CCNU vs. HN₂; prior therapy allowed | 237 | HN₂ 10 q.3w. + CCNU 70 q.6w. vs. HN₂ 15 q.3w. | No | Epidermoid and large cell only | No | Response rate 11% or less; no difference in survival; MS approximately 11 weeks | Edmonson et al., 1976 (33) |
| CTX + CCNU vs. CTX; prior therapy allowed | 185 | CTX 700 q.3w. + CCNU 70 q.6w. vs. CTX 1,000 q.3w. | No | Adeno only | No | Response rate 12% both arms; survival better with combination; $p = 0.07$ | Edmonson et al., 1976 (32) |
| VCR + Bleo + ADR vs. ICRF-159; prior therapy allowed | 63 | VCR 1.2 d1, 5, Bleo 12.5 d1, 5 (6 hr after VCR) ADR 50 d2 vs. ICRF 330 t.i.d. × 3d; all treatment repeated q.4–5w. | No But only 4 pts had limited disease | Yes | Yes | Response rate 20% combination 8% to ICRF; thus ICRF of little benefit alone in advanced disease | Eagan et al., 1976 (30) |
| Simultaneous vs. sequential MTX + CTX + PROC + VCR; prior therapy allowed | 61 | Simultaneous, MTX 20 q.w. VCR 1.2 q.w., CTX 60 q.d. p.o. PROC 80 q.d. p.o. Sequent: MTX 25 q.w. × 2w., then CTX 150 q.d. p.o. × 2w., then PROC 150 q.d. p.o. × 2w., then VCR 1.2 q.w. × 2 | No | No | No | Response rates EPID 33% vs. 13% simultaneous better; too few adeno and large cell patients; survival of patients with response or no change superior to nonresponders | Alberto et al., 1976 (4) |
| CTX or HN₂ + MTX vs. CTX or HN₂ + MTX + CCNU CTX for adeno, HN₂ for epid. and large cell, no prior therapy | 125 | CTX 1,100 q.3w. or HN₂ 15 q.3w. + MTX 20 b.i.w. vs. CTX 500 q.3w. or HN₂ 10 q.3w. + MTX 10 b.i.w. + CCNU 50 q.6w. | Extensive only | Yes | No | Epidermoid and large cell less than 10%; responses for adeno 3 drugs better than 2: 38% vs. 6% with corresponding improved survival | Hansen et al., 1976 (44) |
| CTX + CCNU vs. CTX + ADR vs. CCNU + ADR vs. CTX; prior RT, no prior chemo | 220 | CTX 700 q.3w. CCNU 70 q.6w. CTX 700 q.3w. ADR 40 q.3w. CCNU 70 q.6w. ADR 40 q.3w. only | Extensive | Yes | Yes | Early results suggest that all combinations better than CTX alone for well-differentiated epidermoid | Lowe et al., 1976 (64) |
| MeCCNU vs. MeCCNU + VCR vs. MeCCNU + VCR + MTX; 40–50% no prior therapy | 77 | MeCCNU 150 q.6w. vs. MeCCNU 150 q.6w. + VCR 0.025 mg/kg d1, 8, 15 q.6w. MeCCNU 100 q.6w. + VCR as above + MTX 0.15 mg/kg b.i.w. × 3 q.6w. | Limited vs. extensive | Yes | Yes | MeCCNU alone inferior; MeCCNU + VCR + MTX was best arm at time of report | Richards et al., 1975 (76) |
| BACON vs. NAC; no prior chemotherapy | 110 | HN₂ 8 + ADR 40 d1 and q.4w. CCNU 65 q.8w. VCR 0.75–1 mg q.w. × 6 Bleo 30 U q.w. × 6 vs. HN₂ + ADR + CCNU in doses and schedules listed above | Extensive only | Epidermoid only | Yes | No difference in response rate; survival of responders and stable disease patients on BACON 36 + weeks vs. 24 weeks for NAC $p < .05$ | Livingston et al., 1976 (63) |

TABLE 9—Cont.

| Study plan | No. of patients | Chemotherapy doses (mg/m²) and schedules | Stratified by | | | Results | Ref. |
|---|---|---|---|---|---|---|---|
| | | | Stage | Histology | Performance | | |
| COMB vs. CTX | 64 | MeCCNU 100 and CTX 800 q.4w. VCR 0.5 followed by Bleo 8 mg b.i.w. X 12 weeks vs. CTX 1,100 q.3w. | Extensive | Epidermoid only | Yes | Response rates of 5% on both arms; MS 14.4 weeks for CTX 10.9w for COMB | Wilson et al., 1976 (93) |
| Combination or single-agent chemotherapy vs. observation; symptomatic patients all entered treatment arms; only asymptomatic patients considered here | 118 | HN₂ 0.15 mg/kg + VLB 0.25 mg/kg d1, 7, PROC 2.5 mg/kg + PRED 40 mg d1, 14, repeat treatment q.28d. vs. PROC 2.5–5.0 mg/kg/day vs. observation | No | No | No | In asymptomatic individuals observation yielded best survival; for symptomatic individuals no difference in treatment arms | Laing et al., 1975 (57) |
| CTX + CCNU vs. MeCCNU vs. CCNU + CTX + HU (sequential) | Ongoing | CTX 1,100 q.3w. CCNU 130 q.6w. MeCCNU 220 q.6w. CCNU 70 q.6w. X 3 + CTX 700 q.3w. X 2 then HU 1,000 b.i.w. X 12w Repeat cycle q.18w. | Yes | Yes | Yes | Ongoing | VALG #13 |
| HMM + ADR vs. CTX + CCNU + VCR + Bleo | Ongoing | HMM 60 q.i.d. X 21d; rest d22–42 ADR 40 q.3w. CCNU 50 q.28d., CTX 400 q.28d. VCR 0.75 + Bleo 15 mg b.i.w. X 6w | No | Partially | No | Ongoing | Western Cancer Group Group No. 159 |
| ADR + PROC vs. CCNU + CTX + MTX | Ongoing | ADR 60 q.3w. + PROC 100 q.d. X 21 q.6w. vs. CCNU 50 q.6w. + CTX 500 q.3w. + MTX 10 b.i.w. | Extensive only | Adeno + large cell only | Yes | Ongoing | WP-L 74–52 |
| CCNU + ADR + HMM vs. CCNU + Bleo + HMM | Ongoing | CCNU 100 q.6w. + ADR 15 q.w. + HMM 50 q.i.d. vs. CCNU 100 q.6w. + Bleo 15 U q.w. + HMM 50 q.i.d. | No | Epidermoid only | No | Ongoing | Central Oncology Group No. 7532 |
| CTX + CCNU vs. VCR + Bleo + MTX vs. CTX + MTX vs. Baker's antifol vs. Melphalan vs. Act-D vs. Galactitol vs. Mitomycin C vs. MTX + ADR + CTX + CCNU vs. CTX + Cis-plat + Bleo No prior therapy | Ongoing | CTX 700 q.3w. CCNU 70 q.6w. VCR 1 2–6 hr before Bleo 20 MTX 40; all drugs q.w. CTX 1,100 q.3w. MTX 20 b.i.w. starting 9 days after CTX Baker's (Triazinate) 500 q.w. Melphalan 3.5 mg b.i.d. X 5 days q.5w. Act-D 2.5 q.3w. Galactitol 30 q.d. X 5 q.5w. MITO. C 20 q.3w. MTX 40 + ADR 40 + CTX 400 + CCNU 30 q.3w. CTX 500 Pt 30 Bleo 20 d1, 8 q.4w. | Limited vs. extensive | Epidermoid only | Yes | Ongoing | ECOG 2575 |

| | N | Treatment | Stage | Histology | Randomized | Results | Reference |
|---|---|---|---|---|---|---|---|
| CTX + CCNU vs. HMM + ADR + MTX vs. 5FU + PROC vs. CTX + MTX vs. BAKER'S ANTIFOL vs. DBD + ADR vs. Ftorafur vs. MTX + ADR + CTX + CCNU vs. Piperazinedione vs. ADR + 5-FU + cis-platinum No prior therapy | Ongoing | CTX 700 q.3w. + CCNU 70 q.6w. ADR 40 + MTX 40 q.3w. HMM 100 mg q.d. 5-FU 500 q.d. × 5 q.4w. PROC 200 mg q.d. × 14 q.4w. CTX 1,100 q.3w. MTX 20 b.i.w. starting d9 q.3w. BAKERS 500 q.w. DBD 140 q.d.×10 + ADR 40 q.4w. Ftorafur 4,000 q.2w. MTX 40 + ADR 40 + CTX 400 + CCNU 30 q.3w. Piperazinedione 15 q.3w. ADR 25 + 5-FU 400 + Pt 30 d1, 8 q.4w. | Limited vs. extensive | Adeno and large cell only | Yes | Ongoing | EST 2575 |
| VM-26 vs. ascorbic acid Failures on above protocols | | VM 26 67. q.w. Ascorbic acid 3,000–5,000 q.d. | Limited vs. extensive | Epid vs. adeno vs. large cell | Yes | Ongoing | EST 2575 |
| CTX ± heparin + coumadin | 53 | CTX 1,000 q.3w. | Not specified | Not specified | Not specified | No difference in the 2 groups | Conroy et al., 1976 (22) |

above, to ensure that a given treatment does not shorten the expected survival of nonresponders. If survival was decreased it would be unreasonable to recommend that treatment for general use.

One must question the need for randomized trials in advanced non-small cell carcinoma. At present only marginal benefit has been achieved by chemotherapy, with only occasional patients obtaining a complete response. The principal effort in the immediate future will be to discover new active single agents and drug combinations. If regimens show activity it is almost certain, given the large number of lung cancer patients available for study, that other groups will test these treatments further. At that time randomized trials might be initiated in an attempt to improve an active regimen either by addition of new drug(s) or by removal of drug(s) not thought to contribute to the activity of the combination.

## IMMUNOTHERAPY

Immunotherapy has been used in a surgical adjuvant setting and has been combined with radiation therapy or chemotherapy for nonresectable patients. In surgical adjuvant trials the principal prognostic variable for stratification is stage of disease, hopefully defined pathologically, in the TNM classification. Age and the presence or absence of preexisting lung disease may also be important variables in that they might prevent optimal surgery from being performed. If a "curative" resection has been performed, histology is a less important prognostic factor (6,47,91), and the large majority of patients having tumor resections should have good performance status.

Results of surgical adjuvant immunotherapy trials appear promising. Table 10 lists these studies. Reports by McKneally, Maver, and Kausel (65), Amery (5), and Stewart, Hollinshead, and Harris (86) all indicate that specific subgroups of patients benefit from immunotherapy with delayed tumor recurrence and prolonged survival over that seen in patients treated with surgery alone. A difficulty in evaluating Amery's data is that patients are not staged by currently accepted criteria, and the problem with Stewart et al.'s study is that too few patients are entered so that for analysis patients with several disease stages were lumped together. Also there is not a randomized control group receiving surgery only.

In nonresectable lung cancer patients immunotherapy may also be beneficial. Prognostic factors for stratifying these trials are those already mentioned for advanced disease radiation therapy and chemotherapy trials and include disease stage, performance status, histology, prior therapy, and immune status. Only abstracts are available for the studies of Dimitrov et al. (26) and Takita and Moayeri (87), and stratification of patients was not mentioned. In the published report of Pines no stratification was used (74).

In conclusion, several points need to be stressed: (a) The need for stratification of patients by important prognostic variables is evident. (b) Uniform criteria

TABLE 10. *Immunotherapy*

| Study plan | No. of patients | Drug doses (mg/m²) and schedules | Stratified by | | | Results | Ref. |
|---|---|---|---|---|---|---|---|
| | | | Stage | Histology | Performance status | | |
| Surgery ± intrapleural BCG | 60 | BCG (TICE) 10⁷ viable units via chest tube 3–5 days postpneumonectomy; INH 300 mg/day × 3 mo. started 14 days after BCG | Yes | No | No | Stage I BCG pts have fewer disease recurrences; no difference in stage II or III | McKneally et al., 1976 (65) |
| Surgery + levamisole | 111 | Levamisole 50 mg t.i.d. × 3d q.2w. | No | No | No | More advanced surgical patients have delayed tumor recurrence with levamisole treatment | Amery, 1975 (5) |
| Surgery + BCG | Ongoing; 500 thus far | BCG (Glaxo) 500,000 units subdermally postop | Not specified | | | Ongoing | Edwards and Whitwell 1974 (34) |
| MTX + citrovorum + soluble lung cancer antigens in Freund's adjuvant vs. antigen alone after surgical resection; coincident controls | Ongoing; 38 thus far | MTX 1,000 mg (300 push 700 over 6 hr) then CF 10 mg q.6h. ×10 doses | Yes | No | No | Patients receiving antigens with or without MTX appear to be doing better | Stewart et al., 1976 (86) |
| Surgery + aerosol BCG | Ongoing | BCG (Tice) 2 × 10⁷ viable organisms by nebulization | Not specified | | | Ongoing | C. L. Cusumano |
| Surgery + oral BCG | Recently closed | BCG (Connaught) 120 mg p.o. | Not specified | | | Undergoing analysis | A. B. Miller |
| ADR + C. parv. | 57 | ADR 60 q.3w. C. parv. 4.2 mg s.c. (multiple sites) q.w. | Not specified | Epidermoid or adenocarcinoma | Not specified | Decreased leukopenia and increased survival in C. parv. group | Dimitrov et al., 1976 (26) |
| MeCCNU + VLB + C. parv. | 32 | MeCCNU 220 + VLB 0.25 mg/kg q.6–8w. C. parv. intravenous Dose not specified | Not specified | | | Increased median survival in C. parv. group | Takita and Moayeri, 1976 (87) |
| Surgery, radiotherapy or chemotherapy as appropriate alone or with BCG or with BCG + allogenic tumor cells (irradiated) | Ongoing | BCG (Pasteur) 150 mg scarification cells 5 × 10⁷ i.d. and s.c. | Not specified | Yes | Not specified | Ongoing | W. J. Heim E. Perlin J. W. Reid |

TABLE 10—Cont.

| Study plan | No. of patients | Drug doses (mg/m²) and schedules | Stratified by | | | Results | Ref. |
|---|---|---|---|---|---|---|---|
| | | | Stage | Histology | Performance status | | |
| Surgery alone or with BCG or with BCG + allogenic cells (irradiated + neuraminidase treated) | Ongoing | BCG (Chicago Research) Multiple puncture | Not specified | | | Ongoing | W. V. Young |
| Radiation therapy + BCG | 48 | RT 4,000–6,000 rads/4–5w BCG (Glaxo) 2.5–12.5 × 10⁷ organisms multiple puncture q.w. after RT | No | Epidermoid | No | Some prolongation of survival and decreased systemic metastases with BCG | Pines 1976 (74) |
| Radiation + BCG | Ongoing | Not specified | Limited | Not specified | | Ongoing | S. S. Stefani |
| No treatment or BCG | Ongoing | Not specified | Not specified | | | Ongoing | S. E. Warren |
| CTX + MTX + ADR + VCR alone or with BCG or with C. parv. | Ongoing | BCG 4 × 10⁸ viable units i.d. C. parv. (Burroughs Wellcome) 2.5 mg/m² i.v. | Not specified | | | Ongoing | J. L. Fahey |
| MER before or after radiation | Ongoing | MER 2 mg i.d. | Stage III (Mo) completely resected | Epidermoid only | No | Ongoing | R. T. Eagan |
| Surgery + C. parv. | Ongoing | C. parv. 5 mg/m² s.c. | Not specified | | | Ongoing | A. Lipton |

of response should be adopted. If patients with stable disease are included as responders, this should be emphasized in the report. (c) There should be a uniform reference time to determine patient survival; whereas most authors determine survival from the first day of treatment, other reports use date of presentation, date of diagnosis, or date of first symptoms for survival calculations. (d) Criteria of patient evaluability for study reporting are variable; some authors exclude patients because of early death, whereas other authors include all eligible patients in their reports. Exclusion of early deaths serves to increase both response rate and survival duration.

## REFERENCES

1. Abadir, R., and Muggia, F. M. (1975): Irradiated lung cancer. An autopsy analysis of spread pattern. *Radiology,* 114:427–430.
2. Abramson, N., and Cavanaugh, P. J. (1970): Short-course radiation therapy in carcinoma of the lung. *Radiology,* 96:627–630.
3. Ahmann, D. L., Carr, D. T., Coles, D. T., and Hahn, R. G. (1972): Evaluation of cyclophosphamide (NSC 26271) and BCNU (NSC 409962) in the treatment of patients with inoperable or disseminated lung cancer. *Cancer Chemother. Rep.,* 56:401–403.
4. Alberto, P., Brunner, K. W., Martz, G., Obrecht, J. P., and Sonntag, R. W. (1976): Treatment of bronchogenic carcinoma with simultaneous or sequential combination chemotherapy, including methotrexate, cyclophosphamide, procarbazine and vincristine. *Cancer,* 38:2208–2216.
5. Amery, W. (1975): Immunopotentiation with levamisole in resectable bronchogenic carcinoma: A double-blind controlled trial. *Br. Med. J.,* 3:461–464.
6. Ashor, G. L., Kern, W. H., Meyer, B. W., Lindesmith, G. G., Stiles, Q. R., Tucker, B. L., and Jones, J. C. (1975): Long term survival in bronchogenic carcinoma. *J. Thorac Cardiovasc. Surg.,* 70:581–589.
7. Bangma, P. J. (1971): Post operative radiotherapy. In: *Modern Radiotherapy. Carcinoma of the Bronchus,* edited by T. H. Deeley. Appleton-Century-Crofts, New York.
8. Bergh, N. P., and Schersten, T. (1965): Bronchogenic carcinoma. A follow-up study of a surgically treated series with special reference to the prognostic significance of lymph node metastases. *Acta Chir. Scand.,* Suppl. 347:1–42.
9. Bergsagel, D. E., Jenkin, R. D. T., Pringle, J. F., White, D. M., Fetterly, J. C. M., Klaasen, D. J., and McDermot, R. S. R. (1972): Lung cancer: Clinical trial of radiotherapy alone vs. radiotherapy plus cyclophosphamide. *Cancer,* 30:621–627.
10. Bloedorn, F. G., Cowley, C. A., Cuccia, R., Mercado, R., Jr., Wizenberg, M. J., and Linberg, E. J. (1964): Preoperative irradiation in bronchogenic carcinoma. *Am. J. Roentgenol.,* 92:77–87.
11. Brouet, D. (1968): Results of a trial using radiotherapy and chemotherapy in bronchial cancer. *Eur. J. Cancer,* 4:437–445.
12. Brugarolas, A., Rivas, A., Lacave, A. J., Gonzalez-Palacios, F., and Froufe, A. (1975): 5-Fluorouracil (NSC 19893) compared to cyclophosphamide (NSC 26271 in bronchogenic carcinoma). Results of a clinical study. *Cancer Chemother. Rep.,* 59:1025–1026.
13. Brunner, K. W., Marthaler, T., and Muller, W. (1973): Effects of long term adjuvant chemotherapy with cyclophosphamide (NSC 26271) for radically resected bronchogenic carcinoma. *Cancer Chemother. Rep.,* 4:125–132.
14. Carr, D. T., Childs, D. S., Jr., and Lee, R. E. (1972): Radiotherapy plus 5FU compared to radiotherapy alone for inoperable and unresectable bronchogenic carcinoma. *Cancer,* 29:375–380.
15. Carr, D. T., and Mountain, C. F. (1974): The staging of lung cancer. *Semin. Oncol.,* 1:229–234.
16. Carter, S. K. (1973): Some thoughts on surgical adjuvant studies in lung cancer. *Cancer Chemother. Rep.,* 4:109–117.
17. Cohen, J. L., Krant, M. J., Shnider, B. I., Matias, P. I., Horton, J., and Baxter, D. (1971):

Radiation plus 5-fluorouracil (NSC 19893). Clinical demonstration of an additive effect in bronchogenic carcinoma. *Cancer Chemother. Rep.,* 4:253–258.

18. Cohen, M. H., Fossieck, B. E., Creaven, P. J., and Minna, J. D. (1976): Intensive chemotherapy of small cell bronchogenic carcinoma. *Proc. Am. Assoc. Cancer Res. and ASCO,* 17:273.

19. Collaborative Study (1969): Preoperative irradiation of cancer of the lung. *Cancer,* 23:419–430.

20. Collaborative Study (1975): Preoperative irradiation of cancer of the lung: Final report of a therapeutic trial. *Cancer,* 36:914–925.

21. Connelly, R. R., Cutler, S. J., and Baylis, P. (1966): End results in cancer of the lung: Comparison of male and female patients. *J. Natl. Cancer Inst.,* 36:277–287.

22. Conroy, J., Brodsky, I., Kahn, S. B., and Elias, E. (1976): Anticoagulation in the treatment of inoperable lung cancer. *Proc. Am. Assoc. Cancer Res. and ASCO,* 17:277.

23. Coy, P. (1970): A randomized study of irradiation and vinblastine in lung cancer. *Cancer,* 26:803–807.

24. Crosbie, W. A., Kamdar, H. H., and Belcher, J. R. (1966): A controlled trial of vinblastine sulphate in the treatment of cancer of the lung. *Br. J. Dis. Chest,* 60:28–35.

25. Deeley, T. J. (1966): A clinical trial to compare two different tumor dose levels in the treatment of advanced carcinoma of the bronchus. *Clin. Radiol.,* 17:299–301.

26. Dimitrov, N. V., Singh, T., Conroy, J., and Suhrland, G. L. (1976): Combination therapy with *C. parvum* and adriamycin in patients with lung cancer. *Proc. Am. Assoc. Cancer Res. and ASCO,* 17:292.

27. Donovan, M., Baxter, D., Sponzo, R., Cunningham, T., and Horton, J. (1976): The rationale for combined modality management in small cell cancer of the lung. *Proc. Am. Assoc. Cancer Res., and ASCO,* 17:100.

28. Durrant, K. R., Ellis, F., Black, J. M., Berry, R. J., Ridehalgh, F. R., and Hamilton, W. S. (1971): Comparison of treatment policies in inoperable bronchial carcinoma. *Lancet,* 1:715–719.

29. Eagan, R. T., Carr, D. T., Coles, D. T., Dines, D. E., and Ritts, R. E., Jr. (1974): Randomized study comparing CCNU (NSC 79037) and methyl-CCNU (NSC 95441) in advanced bronchogenic carcinoma. *Cancer Chemother. Rep.,* 58:913–918.

30. Eagan, R. T., Carr, D. T., Coles, D. T., Rubin, J., and Frytak, S. (1976): ICRF-159 versus polychemotherapy in non-small cell lung cancer. *Cancer Treatment Rep.,* 60:947–948.

31. Eagan, R. T., Carr, D. T., Frytak, S., Rubin, J., and Lee, R. E. (1976): VP-16–213 versus polychemotherapy in patients with advanced small cell lung cancer. *Cancer Treatment Rep.,* 60:949–951.

32. Edmonson, J. H., Lagakos, S. W., Selawry, O. S., Perlia, C. P., Bennett, J. M., Muggia, F. M., Wampler, G., Brodovsky, H. S., Horton, J., Colsky, J., Mansour, E. G., Creech, R., Stolbach, L., Greenspan, E. M., Levitt, M., Israel, L., Ezdinli, E. Z., and Carbone, P. P. (1976): Cyclophosphamide and CCNU in the treatment of inoperable small cell carcinoma and adenocarcinoma of the lung. *Cancer Treatment Rep.,* 60:925–932.

33. Edmonson, J. H., Lagakos, S., Stolbach, L., Perlia, C. P., Bennett, J. M., Mansour, E. G., Horton, J., Regelson, W., Cummings, F. J., Israel, L., Brodsky, I., Shnider, B. I., Creech, R., and Carbone, P. P. (1976): Mechlorethamine (NSC 762) plus CCNU (NSC 79037) in the treatment of inoperable squamous and large cell carcinoma of the lung. *Cancer Treatment Rep.,* 60:625–627.

34. Edwards, F. R., and Whitwell, F. (1974): Use of BCG as an immunostimulant in the surgical treatment of carcinoma of the lung. *Thorax,* 29:654–658.

35. Glatstein, E. (1976): Combined chemotherapy-radiotherapy of oat cell cancer of the lung. *Proc. Am. Assoc. Cancer Res. and ASCO,* 17:262.

36. Gollin, F. F., Ansfield, F. J., and Vermund, H. (1964): Clinical studies of combined chemotherapy and irradiation in inoperable bronchogenic carcinoma. *Am. J. Roentgenol.,* 92:88–95.

37. Gollin, F. F., Ansfield, F. J., and Vermund, H. (1967): Continued studies of combined chemotherapy and irradiation in inoperable bronchogenic carcinoma. *Cancer Chemother. Rep.,* 51:189–192.

38. Green, N., Kurohara, S. S., George, F. W., and Crews, Q. E., Jr. (1975): Postresection irradiation for primary lung cancer. *Radiology,* 116:405–407.

39. Green, R. A., Humphrey, E., Close, H., and Patno, M. E. (1969): Alkylating agents in bronchogenic carcinoma. *Am. J. Med.,* 46:516–525.

40. Guthrie, R. T., Ptacek, J. R., and Hass, C. A. (1973): Comparative analysis of two regimens of split course radiation in carcinoma of the lung. *Am. J. Roentgenol.,* 117:605–608.
41. Hall, T. C., Dederick, M. M., Chalmers, T. C., Krant, M. J., Shnider, B. I., Lynch, J. J., Holland, J. F., Ross, C., Koons, C. R., Owens, A. H., Jr., Frei, T., III, Brindley, C., Miller, S. P., Brenner, S., Hosley, H. F., and Olson, K. B. (1967): A clinical pharmacologic study of chemotherapy and X-ray therapy in lung cancer. *Am. J. Med.,* 43:186–193.
42. Hall, T. C., Pocock, S., and Horton, J. (1976): Procarbazine and hydroxyurea as radiosensitizers in lung cancer. *Med. Pediatr. Oncol. (in press).*
43. Hansen, H. H., and Hansen, M. (1976): A comparison of 3 and 4 drug combination chemotherapy for advanced small cell anaplastic carcinoma of the lung. *Proc. Am. Assoc. Cancer Res. and ASCO,* 17:129.
44. Hansen, H. H., Selawry, O. S., Simon, R., Carr, D. T., Van Wyk, C. E., Tucker, R. D., and Sealy, R. (1976): Combination chemotherapy of advanced lung cancer. A randomized trial. *Cancer,* 38:2201–2207.
45. Higgins, G. A., Jr. (1972): Use of chemotherapy as an adjunct to surgery for bronchogenic carcinoma. *Cancer,* 30:1383–1387.
46. Higgins, G. A., Humphrey, E. W., Hughes, F. A., and Keehn, R. J. (1969): Cytoxan as an adjuvant to surgery for lung cancer. *J. Surg. Oncol.,* 1:221–228.
47. Higgins, G. A., Shields, T. W., and Keehn, R. J. (1975): The solitary pulmonary nodule. 10 year follow-up of Veterans Administration Armed Forces cooperative study. *Arch. Surg.,* 110:570–575.
48. Holsti, L. R. (1973): Alternative approaches to radiotherapy alone and radiotherapy as part of a combined therapeutic approach for lung cancer. *Cancer Chemother. Rep.,* 4:165–169.
49. Horwitz, H., Wright, T. L., Perry, H., and Barrett, C. M. (1965): Suppressive chemotherapy in bronchogenic carcinoma. A randomized prospective clinical trial. *Am. J. Roentgenol.,* 93:615–638.
50. Hosley, H. F., Marangoudakis, S., Ross, C. A., Murphy, W. T., and Holland, J. F. (1962): Combined radiation-chemotherapy for bronchogenic carcinoma—Pilot study. *Cancer Chemother. Rep.,* 16:467–471.
51. Host, H. (1973): Cyclophosphamide (NSC 26271) as an adjuvant to radiotherapy in the treatment of unresectable bronchogenic carcinoma. *Cancer Chemother. Rep.,* 4:161–164.
52. Israel, L., Muggica, J., and Chahinian, P. H. (1973): Prognoses of early bronchogenic carcinoma. Survival curves of 451 patients after resection of lung cancer in relation to the results of preoperative tuberculin skin test. *Biomedicine,* 19:68–72.
53. Johnson, R. J. R., Walton, R. J., Lim, L. M., Zylak, C. J., and Painchaud, L. A. (1973): A randomized study on survival of bronchogenic carcinoma treated with conventional or short fractionation radiation. *Clin. Radiol.,* 24:494–497.
54. Karrer, K., Pridun, N., and Zwintz, E. (1973): Chemotherapeutic studies in bronchogenic carcinoma by the Austrian Study Group. *Cancer Chemother. Rep.,* 4:207–213.
55. Kaung, D. T., Wolf, J., Hyde, L., and Zelen, M. (1974): Preliminary report on the treatment of nonresectable cancer of the lung. *Cancer Chemother. Rep.,* 58:359–364.
56. Krant, M. J., Chalmers, T. C., Dederick, M. M., Hall, T. C., Levene, M. B., Muench, H., Shnider, B. I., Gold, G. L., Hunter, C., Bersack, S. R., Owens, A. H., Jr., DeLeon, N., Nickson, R. J., Brindley, C., Brace, K. C., Frei, E., III, Gehan, E., and Salvin, L. (1963): Comparative trial of chemotherapy and radiotherapy in patients with nonresectable cancer of the lung. *Am. J. Med.,* 35:363–373.
57. Laing, A. H., Berry, R. J., Newman, C. R., and Smith, P. (1975): Treatment of small cell carcinoma of bronchus. *Lancet,* 1:129–132.
58. Landgren, R. C., Hussey, D. H., Barkley, H. T., Jr., and Samuels, M. L. (1974): Split-course irradiation compared to split course irradiation plus hydroxyurea in inoperable bronchogenic carcinoma. *Cancer,* 34:1598–1601.
59. Landgren, R. C., Hussey, D. H., Samuels, M. L., and Leary, W. V. (1973): A randomized study comparing irradiation alone to irradiation plus procarbazine in inoperable bronchogenic carcinoma. *Radiology,* 108:403–406.
60. Lee, R. L., Carr, D. T., and Childs, D. S., Jr. (1976): Comparison of split-course radiation therapy and continuous radiation therapy for unresectable bronchogenic carcinoma: 5 year results. *Am. J. Roentgenol.,* 126:116–122.
61. LePar, E., Faust, D. S., Brady, L. W., and Beckloff, G. L. (1967): Clinical evaluation of the

adjunctive use of hydroxyurea (NSC 32065) in radiation therapy of carcinoma of the lung. *Radiol. Clin. Biol.*, 36:32–40.

62. Levitt, S. H., Condit, P. T., and Bogardus, C. R., Jr. (1966): Split-dose intensive radiation therapy in the treatment of patients with advanced carcinoma of the lung. *Radiology*, 85:738–739.

63. Livingston, R., Thigpen, T., and Hart, J. (1976): Comparison of 3 drug and 5 drug combination chemotherapy in extensive squamous lung cancer. *Proc. Am. Assoc. Cancer Res. and ASCO*, 17:273.

64. Lowe, W. C., Mietlowski, W., and Phillips, R. (1976): Combination chemotherapy aids lung cancer. *JAMA*, 236:2480–2482.

65. McKneally, M. F., Maver, C., and Kausel, H. W. (1976): Regional immunotherapy of lung cancer with intrapleural BCG. *Lancet*, 1:377–379.

66. Miller, A. B., Fox, W., Somasundaram, P. R., and Tall, R. (1971): Study of cytotoxic chemotherapy as an adjuvant to surgery in carcinoma of the bronchus. Report by a Medical Research Council Working Party. *Br. Med. J.*, 1:421–428.

67. Miller, A. B., Fox, W., and Tall, R. (1969): Five year follow-up of the Medical Research Council trial of surgery and radiotherapy for the primary treatment of small-celled or oat-celled carcinoma of the bronchus. *Lancet*, 2:501–505.

68. Morrison, R., Deeley, T. J., and Cleland, W. P. (1963): The treatment of carcinoma of the bronchus. A clinical trial to compare surgery and supervoltage radiotherapy. *Lancet*, 1:683–684.

69. Mountain, C. F. (1973): Keynote address on surgery in the therapy of lung cancer: Surgical prospects and priorities for clinical research. *Cancer Chemother. Rep.*, 4:19–24.

70. Mountain, C. F., Carr, D. T., and Anderson, W. A. (1974): A system for the clinical staging of lung cancer. *Am. J. Roentgenol.*, 120:130–138.

71. Patterson, R., and Russell, M. H. (1962): Clinical trials in malignant disease. IV. Lung cancer. Value of postoperative radiotherapy. *Clin. Radiol.*, 13:141–144.

72. Pavlov, A., Pirigov, A., Trachtenberg, A., Volkova, M., Maximov, T., and Mateeva, T. (1973): Results of combination treatment of lung cancer patients: Surgery plus radiotherapy and surgery plus chemotherapy. *Cancer Chemother. Rep.*, 4:133–135.

73. Perlia, C. P., and Stolbach, L. (1976): Adriamycin and cytoxan in the treatment of inoperable lung cancer. *Proc. Am. Assoc. Cancer Res. and ASCO*, 17:27.

74. Pines, A. (1976): A five year controlled study of BCG and radiotherapy for inoperable lung cancer. *Lancet*, 1:380–381.

75. Poulsen, O. (1962): Cyclophosphamide. An evaluation of its cytostatic effects on surgically treated carcinoma of the lung. *J. Int. Coll. Surg.*, 37:177–187.

76. Richards, F., II, Cooper, M. R., Hayes, D. M., and Spurr, C. L. (1975): Combination chemotherapy vs. single agent chemotherapy in advanced bronchogenic carcinoma. *Proc. Am. Assoc. Cancer Res. and ASCO*, 16:268.

77. Roswit, B., Patno, M. E., Rapp, R., Veinbergs, A., Feder, B., Stuhlbarg, J., and Reid, C. B. (1968): The survival of patients with inoperable lung cancer. A large scale randomized trial of radiation therapy versus placebo. *Radiology*, 90:688–697.

78. Salazar, O. M., Rubin, P., Brown, J. C., Feldstein, M. L., and Keller, B. E. (1976): Predictors of radiation response in lung cancer. A clinico-pathobiological analysis. *Cancer*, 37:2636–2650.

79. Scheer, A. C., Wilson, R. F., and Kalisher, L. (1974): Combined radiotherapy and hydroxyurea in the management of lung cancer. *Clin. Radiol.*, 25:415–418.

80. Shields, T. W. (1972): Preoperative radiation therapy in the treatment of bronchial carcinoma. *Cancer*, 30:1388–1394.

81. Shields, T. W. (1973): Status report on adjuvant cancer chemotherapy trials in the treatment of bronchial carcinoma. *Cancer Chemother. Rep.*, 4:119–124.

82. Shields, T. W., Higgins, G. A., and Keehn, R. J. (1972): Factors influencing survival after resection of bronchogenic carcinoma. *J. Thorac Cardiovasc. Surg.*, 64:391–399.

83. Shields, T. W., Higgins, G. A., Jr., Lawton, R., Heilbrunn, H., and Keehn, R. J. (1970): Preoperative X-ray therapy as an adjuvant in the treatment of bronchogenic carcinoma. *J. Thorac Cardiovasc. Surg.*, 59:49–61.

84. Shields, T. W., Robinette, D., and Keehn, R. J. (1974): Bronchial carcinoma treated by adjuvant cancer chemotherapy. *Arch. Surg.*, 109:329–333.

85. Slack, N. H. (1970): Bronchogenic carcinoma: Nitrogen mustard as a surgical adjuvant and factors influencing survival. University Surgical Adjuvant Lung Project. *Cancer*, 25:987–1002.

86. Stewart, T. H. M., Hollinshead, A. C., and Harris, J. (1976): Immunochemotherapy of lung cancer. *Proc. Am. Assoc. Cancer Res. and ASCO*, 17:305.
87. Takita, H., and Moayeri, H. (1976): Effects of *Corynebacterium parvum* and chemotherapy in lung cancer. *Proc. Am. Assoc. Cancer Res. and ASCO*, 17:292.
88. Tucker, R. D., Sealy, R., Van Wyk, C., LeRoux, P. L. M., and Soskolne, C. L. (1973): A clinical trial of cyclophosphamide (NSC 26271) and radiation therapy for oat cell carcinoma of the lung. *Cancer Chemother. Rep.*, 4:159–160.
89. Tucker, R. D., Sealy, R., Van Wyk, C., Soskolne, C. L., and LeRoux, P. L. M. (1973): A clinical trial of methotrexate (NSC 740) and radiation therapy for squamous cell carcinoma of the lung. *Cancer Chemother. Rep.*, 4:157–158.
90. Van Der Merwe, A. M., Falkson, G., Sandison, A. G., Van Dyk, J. J., and Falkson, H. C. (1973): Advanced lung cancer. A clinical trial of radiotherapy plus two drug combination regimens. *S. Afr. Med. J.*, 47:2219–2222.
91. Vincent, R. G., Takita, H., Lane, W. W., Gutierrez, A. C., and Pickren, J. W. (1976): Surgical therapy of lung cancer. *J. Thorac Cardiovasc. Surg.*, 71:581–591.
92. Whittington, R. M., Fairly, J. L., Majima, H., Patno, M. E., and Prentice, R. (1972): BCNU (NSC 409962) in the treatment of bronchogenic carcinoma. *Cancer Chemother. Rep.*, 56:739–743.
93. Wilson, H., Lagakos, S., Bodey, G., Gutierrez, A., Selawry, O., Sealy, R., and Ryall, R. D. (1976): Therapy of advanced epidermoid carcinoma. *Proc. Am. Assoc. Cancer Res. and ASCO*, 17:294.
94. Wilson, W. L., Van Ryzin, J., Weiss, A. J., Frelick, R. W., and Moss, S. E. (1975): A phase III study in lung cancer comparing hexamethylmelamine to dibromodulcitol. *Oncology*, 31:293–309.
95. Wolf, J., Patno, M. E., Roswit, B., and D'Esopo, N. (1966): Controlled study of survival of patients with clinically inoperable lung cancer treated with radiation therapy. *Am. J. Med.*, 40:360–367.
96. Zelen, M. (1973): Keynote address on biostatistics and data retrieval. *Cancer Chemother. Rep.*, 4:31–42.
97. Zelen, M. (1975): Importance of prognostic factors in planning therapeutic trials. In: *Cancer Therapy: Prognostic Factors and Criteria of Response*, edited by M. J. Staquet, pp. 1–6. Raven Press, New York.

Randomized Trials in Cancer: A Critical
Review by Sites, edited by Maurice J.
Staquet, Raven Press, New York © 1978.

# Cancer of the Head and Neck

## Yves Cachin

*Institut Gustave-Roussy, 94800 Villejuif, France*

This chapter analyzes 23 studies, whose results have been published, involving randomized clinical trials in patients with head and neck cancers. Some of the results presented are definitive, but more often they are of a preliminary nature.

It is certain that this review is incomplete. Out of 39 therapeutic trials registered with the Information Office of the UICC at the end of 1976, only eight have so far let to publication. Four studies were abandoned before completion, and the results of the other 27 have not yet been published. Furthermore, a number of clinical trials were sought by a careful review of the world's literature, thereby increasing the chances of omission.

The 21 randomized studies whose results are available can be grouped into the following categories: Ten deal with chemotherapy; one with immunotherapy; one with combined immunotherapy and chemotherapy; four with radiotherapy; and five with combined surgery and radiotherapy.

### THERAPEUTIC TRIALS INVOLVING CHEMOTHERAPY

The majority of the published reports deal with chemotherapy used in association with radiotherapy; however, two concern the various treatment modalities involved in chemotherapy, and one deals with its combined use with immunotherapy. The drugs were given systematically in 10 of the studies and intraarterially in three. Methotrexate and 5-fluorouracil were the drugs most often used, but bleomycin, hydroxyurea, IUdR, and 6-mercaptopurine were also tested.

Five studies were designed to test the value of chemotherapy administered concurrently with radiotherapy. The object of these studies was to see if chemotherapy, given during the course of radiotherapy, or even during the actual treatment sessions, could potentiate the effects of the radiation. The earliest of these studies is that of Fletcher et al. from 1963 (6), in which radiotherapy was used in combination with 5-fluorouracil (5-FU). In a randomized study of 19 patients with cancer of the pharingeal wall, treated with radiotherapy (6,000 rads by telecobalt), alone or in combination with intravenously administered

---

Received May 1977.

5-FU, Fletcher observed no difference in the regression rates of lesions of the tonsillar region, soft palate, or epiglottis, but the number of patients was small.

In 1976 Lo et al. (13) published the results of a large therapeutic trial that was begun in 1961 to evaluate combined therapy with radiation and 5-FU. The study group consisted of 136 patients with advanced cancers of the oral cavity and oropharynx, for whom there was a minimum of 2 years follow-up. All patients received radiation to a dose of 6,000 to 7,000 rads. The combined treatment group received, in addition, intravenously 5-FU in a dose of 10 mg/kg/day for the first 3 days of radiotherapy. This was followed by a dose of 5 mg/kg three times a week for the duration of the radiotherapy treatment period. The 5-FU was given intraarterially during the first years of the study. Local tumor control and survival were both better in the combined treatment group (5-year survival, 31%) than in the control group (5-year survival, 14%), but the difference was statistically significant only in the case of the oral cavity lesions (5-year survival 40% versus 13%). Acute treatment and late complications were both more frequent in the combined treatment group. Both groups showed the same incidence of second primary lesions and of metastases developing in the face of local control.

Doggett, Bagshaw, and Kaplan (4) compared three groups of patients. The first group was treated by radiotherapy alone. The second group was treated by radiotherapy, combined with a prolonged intraarterial infusion of methotrexate, according to the technique of Sullivan (total dose between 700 mg in 18 days and 2,160 mg in 44 days). A third group was treated with radiotherapy and 6-mercaptopurine. The results are difficult to interpret because the number of patients was small and the length of follow-up short.

Stefani, Eells, and Abbate (18), in a study of 126 patients, compared a group treated by radiotherapy alone (6,000 to 10,000 rads) with a group treated simultaneously with radiotherapy and hydroxyurea, given orally in twice-weekly doses of 80 mg/kg. No statistically significant differences were found when primary tumor regression, cervical nodal response, and early survival were compared. Distant metastases subsequently developed in 22.8% of the combined treatment group, but in only 7.5% of the group receiving radiotherapy alone.

A randomized E.O.R.T.C. (Head and Neck Cooperative Group) study (2) was designed to compare radiotherapy and concurrently administered bleomycin with radiotherapy alone in the treatment of epidermoid carcinomas of the oropharynx. The radiotherapy was delivered in a maximum dose of 7,000 rads in 7 to 8 weeks by telecobalt. Bleomycin was given in a dose of 15 mg, either i.v. or i.m., twice a week, from the start of radiotherapy for a period of 5 weeks (total dose 150 mg). Each injection of bleomycin was given 2 hr before a session of radiotherapy. In the 186 patients evaluated in this study, no significant difference was found in the degree of response of the two groups. A complete regression of the primary tumor was found in approximately 67% of the patients in both groups. The same was true with respect to the response rate of clinically involved lymph nodes and with respect to the length of survival. There was a higher early death rate in the bleomycin-treated group, because of a higher rate of major complications.

In summary, all therapeutic trials except one (13), conclude that the effectiveness of radiotherapy in the treatment of advanced head and neck cancers is not improved by the addition of simultaneously administered chemotherapy. Local and systemic complications are more frequent when the two treatment modalities are combined. One cannot ignore, however, the finding by Lo et al. (13) that there is a statistically significant improvement in local tumor control and in survival in oral cavity lesions when 5-FU is given concurrently with radiotherapy.

Three therapeutic trials were designed to test the value of chemotherapy administered before the start of radiotherapy, to see if the effectiveness of radiotherapy could be improved when the volume of the tumor and the proportion of viable tumor cells had been reduced by previously administered chemotherapy. Kligerman et al. (10) compared two groups of advanced cancers treated by radiotherapy, one of which was treated with chemotherapy (methotrexate, 0.2 mg/kg/day i.v. for 5 days) 15 days before the start of radiotherapy. The average survival was not significantly different in the two groups, but the number of patients was small.

Von Essen et al. (22) compared four groups of patients from Southern India (total of 100 patients) with advanced cancers of the oral cavity. The first group was treated by radiotherapy alone (6,500 rads in 6 weeks). The three other groups received prior chemotherapy, one dose per day i.v. for 5 days, using methotrexate (7 mg/m$^2$), IUdR (2.84 mg/m$^2$), or 5-FU (520 mg/m$^2$). They noted complete regression of the primary tumor in 53% of the group treated with radiotherapy alone, and in 82%, 62%, and 67% of the chemotherapy groups, respectively, but in the majority of cases the lesions recurred. Although prior chemotherapy improved the quality of the tumor regression observed after radiotherapy, the fraction showing tumor "control" was unchanged.

Richard et al. (16) compared two groups of patients with advanced cancers of the oral cavity and oropharynx, treated with a combination of intraarterial chemotherapy followed by radiotherapy, or with radiotherapy alone. The drug used for the local infusion was methotrexate (50 mg/day, to a total dose of 300 to 600 mg). Telecobalt was begun 14 days after the completion of chemotherapy. Tumor regression was far greater after combined treatment (40%) than after radiotherapy alone (10%). Median survival was 6 months in the group receiving only radiotherapy and 9 months in the group receiving combined treatment. However, when survival rates were examined after all patients had been followed for 5 years, the difference between the two groups disappeared toward the eighteenth month of follow-up. The results of the three trials were in agreement, therefore, in reporting an improvement in initial tumor regression and average survival, with no change in long-term survival.

There were two trials whose object was to assess different schedules of administration of methotrexate (MTX). Richard et al. (15) demonstrated by sequential trial that, in terms of tumor regression, treatment with high-dose methotrexate (50 mg/day by infusion over 10 hr) was superior to treatment with low-dose methotrexate (5 mg/day without leucovorin) in advanced cancers of the oral cavity and oropharynx. No difference in response rate was noted by Vogler and Jacobs (21) among the three methotrexate treatment schedules that they tested: A: (large and repeated doses of MTX), 125 mg/m² p.o., q.6h. for 4 doses, every week for 12 weeks, combined with leucovorin (LCV) q.6h. for 6 doses beginning 36 hr after the first dose of MTX; B: (small and repeated doses of MTX), 15 mg/m² p.o., q.6h. for 4 doses, every week for 12 weeks; C: (single weekly i.v. dose of MTX), 60 mg/m² i.v. every week.

A therapeutic trial of Richman et al. (17) compared the results obtained using chemotherapy with those obtained using chemotherapy and immunotherapy combined, in the treatment of 34 patients with recurrent head and neck cancers. Chemotherapy consisted of the multiple drug regimen, BACON (bleomycin, adriamycin, CCNU, vincristine, and mechlorethamine), and immunotherapy was accomplished by scarification with BCG. Patients treated with BACON and BCG had significantly longer survival (mean of 30.5 weeks) than those treated with BACON alone (13.5 weeks). Five deaths due to drug toxicity, four of which occurred in the group receiving BACON alone, were observed during the first 8 weeks of treatment.

It is regrettable that there are no published results available concerning the value of chemotherapy administered routinely after standard treatment for head and neck cancers.

## THERAPEUTIC TRIALS INVOLVING IMMUNOTHERAPY

Amiel, Sancho, and Vandenbrouck (1) have published preliminary results, after 2 years of observation, of an immunotherapy trial in 55 patients treated for laryngeal and hypopharyngeal cancers by surgery and postoperative radiotherapy. During the month following the completion of radiotherapy, the patients were randomized into two groups, one to receive weekly BCG by scarification for 1 year, and the other to be observed only. As judged by the number of local recurrences, by the number of metastases, and by the number of second primary tumors, the BCG-treated group would appear to be the favorable one, but the period of observation is as yet too short to allow any conclusions to be drawn. The preliminary results of this study, in conjunction with the interesting findings of Richman et al. (17), should encourage further interest in this area of study, namely, the immunotherapy of head and neck cancers, which until now has received little attention.

## THERAPEUTIC TRIALS INVOLVING RADIOTHERAPY
## TREATMENT MODALITIES

Two randomized therapeutic trials were designed to examine the effect of varying radiation delivery schedules. Percarpio and Fischer (14) looked at the effect of two dosage schedules in a randomized study of 35 patients with advanced head and neck cancers. The first group received 200 rads/day to a dose of 6,000 to 7,000 rads (30 to 35 treatment sessions). The second group received 400 rads/day to a dose of 4,000 to 4,800 rads (10 to 12 treatment sessions). There was better local control and better survival (1-year actuarial survival 44.5%, no recurrence in 35%) in the group receiving 400 rads/day than in the group receiving 200 rads/day (1-year survival 15.5%, all with recurrences). However, these differences are not significant, nor was the period of observation very long.

Dutreix et al. (5) looked at the effects of two dosage schedules in a study of 88 patients with carcinomas of the tonsillar region. The first group received three treatments per week of 330 rads each for a total dose of 4,600 rads (14 treatment sessions). The second group received a split course of treatment, beginning with two sessions of 850 rads given 48 hr apart, followed in 3 weeks by five sessions of 330 rads, given at a rate of three sessions per week (dose equivalent of 4,600 rads). In both groups treatment was complemented by a neck dissection and by $^{192}$Ir implants. Tumor regression and mucosal reaction occurred significantly earlier in the second group (modified fractionation), but no significant difference in 5-year survival was documented.

Catterall, Sutherland, and Bewley (3) studied the comparative effects of neutron and photon radiotherapy (cobalt or linear accelerator) in the treatment of 102 advanced cancers of the head and neck. After randomization, one group was treated with photons (X-rays or gamma rays) in the standard manner at doses of 4,500 to 6,800 rads. Another group was treated with neutrons in three treatment sessions per week for 4 weeks, for a dose of 1,440 rads. In 37 of 52 patients treated with neutrons, and in 16 of 50 treated with photons, there was complete regression of the primary tumor. Tumor later recurred in 9 of the 16 photon-treated patients with complete regression, but there was no local recurrence in any of the 37 neutron-treated patients. Although this represents a highly significant difference in the degree of local control, there was no difference in survival noted.

Henk (8) compared the results obtained by radiotherapy, performed either in room air or in hyperbaric oxygen, in 83 patients with laryngeal cancers. All patients were treated by the same technique, receiving 4,000 to 4,500 rads in 10 sessions spread over 20 days, but one group of patients was in room air during the treatment sessions, and the other was in hyperbaric oxygen. No difference in survival rates was observed, but the group treated under hyperbaric oxygen showed better local control of tumor, as well as a much higher rate of complications. It is important to point out that the period of observation in this study was quite short (6 to 20 months).

## THERAPEUTIC TRIALS INVOLVING COMBINED
## SURGERY AND RADIOTHERAPY

The goal of these trials was to test the value of preoperative radiotherapy, to clarify treatment modalities, and to compare the results obtained with pre-

and postoperative radiotherapy. Three trials were designed to compare the results of treatment by surgery alone with those of treatment by surgery preceded by radiotherapy.

Strong et al. (19) reported on the first randomized clinical trial conducted on the value of preoperative radiotherapy on the cervical lymph nodes. This clinical trial, carried out from 1960 to 1967, compared several groups of patients suffering from head and neck cancers (the great majority being cancers of the oral cavity and oropharynx). A group of 164 patients received 2,000 rads in five fractions over 5 days preoperatively, which was immediately followed by surgery. Two other groups of patients (111 and 58) were treated by surgery alone.

The results were assessed on the percentage of lymph node recurrences. When preoperative radiotherapy was administered, 22.5% recurred. Recurrence rate in the two "surgery only" groups was 33.1% and 32.8%. The difference is hardly significant, but becomes very significant in patients with lymph node involvement, which histologically showed grade N+ involvement: 30.9% against 50%.

This work is of some interest, but does not show any significant difference as far as the 3-year survival rate is concerned.

Ketcham et al. (9), in a technically valid prospective study, compared two groups of patients suffering from malignant tumors of the head and neck region (especially of the oral cavity and pharynx). All underwent resection of the primary tumor and radical neck dissection. The first group (60 cases) received 1,000 rads preoperative during 1 session 24 hr before surgery, the second group (19 cases) underwent surgery alone. No significant difference was observed as far as local recurrences or metastases were concerned.

Lawrence et al. (12), in a random clinical trial, studied another way of giving preoperative radiotherapy. In this study, two-thirds of the patients had cancer of the oral cavity and of the oropharynx and one-third cancer of the hypopharynx. They were treated by resection of the primary tumor and radical neck dissection. The first group (69 cases) received preoperative radiation (1,400 rads in 2 sessions; 24 and 48 hr before surgery); the second group (74 cases) underwent surgery alone. The results show that there was no significant difference between the two groups as far as the survival rate, the percentage of local or regional lymph node recurrences, or metastases were concerned. The method used in this trial was valid, but the follow-up period was somewhat short for some of the patients.

Based on these three trials, it is not possible to draw any definite conclusions about the overall value of preoperative radiotherapy. It is possible to say that the benefits are rather modest in the treatment of head and neck cancers, for the techniques utilized (total doses, fractionation, delay between radiotherapy and surgery). Preoperative radiotherapy may sometimes improve local control (reduced local and nodal recurrences), but it does not improve survival.

Hendrickson (7), in a randomized clinical trial of the larynx, compared two ways of administering preoperative radiotherapy, either at low doses (2,000 rads in 2 weeks) or at high doses (5,000 rads in 4 weeks). The survival rates do not show any marked difference between the two groups. The 4-year survival rate was 58% in the first group (29 cases) and 50% in the second group (42 cases).

In a prospective, randomized clinical trial, Vandenbrouck et al. (20) evaluated preoperative versus postoperative radiotherapy in the treatment of patients with tumors of the hypopharynx. A statistically significant difference ($p = 0.01$), in favor of postoperative radiotherapy, was found, relative to survival rates, complication rates, and quality of life. The 5-year survival was 56% for the postoperative radiotherapy group and 20% for the preoperative group. The most noteworthy aspect of this study is that it gives a positive value to postoperative radiotherapy, at least in the case of hypopharyngeal carcinomas.

## CONCLUSIONS

In spite of the incomplete nature and the small number of the randomized therapeutic trials concerning head and neck cancers, it is still possible to come to some conclusions. The studies involving chemotherapy have been concerned mostly with its use before and during radiotherapy. It is interesting to note that initial tumor regression, and even local control, have been improved by the use of chemotherapy. However, survival has not been prolonged, except in the case of oral cavity lesions in the study of Lo et al. (13). In many cases, local and systemic toxicity have caused severe complications or have prompted undesirable modifications in the course of the associated radiotherapy.

In the studies involving radiotherapy, no great differences have seemed to follow the application of different fractionations or the use of hyperbaric oxygen. Neutron radiotherapy appears to improve local tumor control, but it does not prolong survival. The studies dealing with radiotherapy combined with surgery cast doubt on the usefulness of preoperative radiotherapy, at least in the manner in which it was used in these trials.

In the future it will be important to extend and standardize the use of randomized therapeutic trials. Results can be obtained more quickly when several medical centers partake in a study. It will be of particular interest to look at the effectiveness of chemotherapy employed in a systematic manner *after* radiotherapy or surgery, over extended periods of time. The same is true for immunotherapy.

## REFERENCES

1. Amiel, J. L., Sancho, H., and Vandenbrouck, C. (1976): Note préliminaire sur un essai d'immunothérapie par le BCG pour des tumeurs ORL. *Bull. Cancer Paris,* 2:287–288.
2. Cachin, Y., Jortay, A., Sancho, H., Eschwege, F., Madelain, M., Desaulty, A., and Gerard, P. (1977): Preliminary results of a randomized E.O.R.T.C. study comparing radiotherapy and concomitant bleomycin to radiotherapy alone in epidermoïd carcinomas of the oro-pharynx. *Eur. J. Cancer,* 13:1389–1395.

3. Catterall, M., Sutherland, I., and Bewley, D. K. (1975): First results of a randomized clinical trial of fast neutrons compared with X or gamma rays in treatment of advanced tumours of the head and neck. *Br. Med. J.,* 2:653–656.

4. Doggett, R. L. S., Bagshaw, M. A., and Kaplan, H. S. (1967): Combined therapy using chemotherapeutic agents and radiotherapy. In: *Modern Trends in Radiotherapy,* edited by Deeley and Wood, pp. 107–131. London.

5. Dutreix, J., Hayem, M., Pierquin, B., Zummer, K., Hesse, C., and Wambersie, A. (1974): Epitheliomas de la région amygdalienne. Comparaison entre fractionnement classique et irradiation en deux séries (split-course). *Acta Radiol.,* 13:167–184.

6. Fletcher, G. H., Suit, H. D., Howe, C. D., Samuels, M., Jesse, R. H., and Villareal, R. V. (1963): Clinical method of testing radiation-sensitizing agents in squamous cell carcinoma. *Cancer,* 16:355–363.

7. Hendrickson, F. R. (1970): The results of low dose preoperative radiotherapy for advanced carcinoma of the langue. *Front Radiat. Ther. Oncol.,* 5:123.

8. Henk, J. M. (1975): The influence of oxygen and hypoxia on laryngeal cancer management. *Laryngoscope,* 85:1134–1144.

9. Ketcham, A. S., Hoye, R. C., Chretien, P. B., and Brace, K. L. (1969): Irradiation twenty four hours preoperatively. *Ann. J. Surg.,* 118:691.

10. Kligerman, M. M., Hellman, S., Vonessen, C. F., and Bertino, J. R. (1966): Sequential chemotherapy and radiotherapy. Preliminary results of clinical trial with methotrexate in Head and Neck cancer. *Radiology,* 86:250.

11. Kramer, S. (1975): Methotrexate and radiotherapy in the treatment of advanced squamous cell carcinoma of the oral cavity, oropharynx, supraglottic larynx and hypopharynx. Preliminary report of a controlled clinical trial of the radiotherapy oncology group. *Can. J. Otolar.,* 4:213–218.

12. Lawrence, W., Terz, J. J., Rogers, C., King, R. E., Wolf, J. S., and King, E. R. (1974): Preoperative irradiation for head and neck cancer = a prospective study. *Cancer,* 33:318.

13. Lo, T., Wiley, A. L., Ansfield, F. J., Brandenburg, J. H., Davis, H. L., Gollin, F. F., Johnson, R. O., Famirez, G., and Vermund, H. (1976): Combined radiation therapy and 5-Fluorouracil for advanced squamous cell carcinoma of the oral cavity and oropharynx: A randomized study. *Cancer,* 126:229–235.

14. Percarpio, B. and Fischer, J. J. (1976): Irradiation of advanced head and neck cancer with large daily fractions. *Radiology,* 2:489–490.

15. Richard, J., Sancho, H., Brugere, J., and Vandenbrouck, C. (1973): Intraarterial methotrexate in head and neck tumors. *Eur. J. Cancer,* 9:847–851.

16. Richard, J. M., Sancho, H., Lepintre, Y., Rodary, J., and Pierquin, B. (1974): Intraarterial methotrexate chemotherapy and telecobaltherapy in cancer of the oral cavity and oro-pharynx. *Cancer,* 34:491–496.

17. Richman, S. P., Livingston, R. B., Gutterman, J. V., Suen, J. Y., and Hersh, E. M. (1976): Chemotherapy versus chemo-immunotherapy of head and neck cancer: Report of a randomized study. *Cancer Treatment Rep.,* 5:535–539.

18. Stefani, S., Eells, R. W., and Abbate, J. (1971): Hydroxyurea and radiotherapy in head and neck cancer. Results of a prospective controlled study in 126 patients. *Radiology,* 101:391–396.

19. Strong, E. W., Henschke, U. K., Nickson, J. J., Frazell, E. L., Tolefson, H. K., and Hilaris, B. S. (1966): Preoperative X-ray therapy as an adjunct to radical neck dissection. *Cancer,* 19:1509–1516.

20. Vandenbrouck, C., Sancho, H., Lefur, R., Richard, J. M., and Cachin, Y. (1977): Results of a randomized clinical trial of preoperative irradiation versus post-operative in treatment of tumours of the hypopharynx. *Cancer,* 39:1445–1449.

21. Vogler, W. R., and Jacobs, J. (1975): Methotrexate with leucovorin rescue low oral divided methotrexate vs single dose i.v. methotrexate in advanced cancers of head, neck, breast, and colon. *Proc. AACR-ASCO,* 16:266.

22. Von Essen, C. F., Joseph, L. B. M., Simon, G. T., Singh, A. D., and Singh, S. P. (1968): Sequential chemotherapy and radiation therapy of buccal mucosa carcinoma in South India. Methods and preliminary results. *Ann. J. Roentgenol.* 102:530–540.

*Randomized Trials in Cancer: A Critical Review by Sites,* edited by Maurice J. Staquet, Raven Press, New York © 1978.

# Malignant Melanoma

*Ferdy J. Lejeune and **Gilbert De Wasch

* Department of Surgery and ** Department of Internal Medicine, Institut Jules Bordet, 1000 Bruxelles, Belgium

This chapter analyzes and compares the results of properly controlled and randomized trials. For convenience, the treatment of the three clinical stages of malignant melanoma is reviewed separately, according to the international staging: stage I, primary melanoma; stage II, loco-regional metastasis: (a) in transit metastasis, (b) lymph node metastasis; stage III, distant metastasis (21).

Some of the data are preliminary but are shown because there are statistical analyses.

## STAGE I MALIGNANT MELANOMA

### Treatment of Primary Tumor

It is generally accepted that the surgical excision of skin malignant melanoma should be wide. Most current protocols require a clearance of 3 to 5 cm from the borders of the tumor.

Although some authors claim that 80% of not widely excised melanoma will recur (33), no randomized trial has ever been designed to study the optimal diameter of excision.

In addition, the question of leaving or not leaving the muscular fascia was discussed by Olsen (28), who assumed that it constitutes a barrier to tumor cell dissemination through the muscle vessels. For this point, no controlled trial seems to have been carried out, so the question still remains open.

### Prophylactic Lymph Node Dissection

In contrast, the problem of whether or not to perform prophylactic dissection of clinically uninvolved regional lymph nodes has been the subject of many uncontrolled studies. It is not surprising that the conclusions have been contradictory (23). This prompted the W.H.O. Melanoma Group to perform a randomized prospective trial (36). From 1967 to 1974, 553 cases of melanoma of the limbs

Received July 4, 1977.

TABLE 1. *Malignant melanoma: randomized trials in stages I and II—surgery and immunotherapy*

| Ref. | Author and year | Stage | No. of patients | Criteria | Treatments | | |
|---|---|---|---|---|---|---|---|
| 36 | Veronesi et al., WHO MG, 1977 | I | 553 | Survival 5 yr | Excision + node dissection 73% | | Excision only 71% |
| 35 | Spitler et al., MCCG, 1976 | I and II | 132 | Recurrence 15 mo | Levamisole 30% | | Placebo 30% |
| 20 | Cunningham et al., ECOG, 1976 | I and II | 127 | Disease Free | Excision + BCG 65% | | Excision only 86% |
| 26 | Morton, UCLA, 1976 | I and II | 89 | Recurrence<br>Survival | BCG 41%<br>81% | BCG + cells 34%<br>76% | Surgery only 50%<br>57% |
| 30 | Pinsky et al., MSKCC, 1976 | II | 47 | Recurrence<br>Survival | BCG 58%<br>110.5 wk | | 57%<br>107 wk |
| 24 | McIllmurray et al., 1977 | IIb | 15 | Recurrence 6 mo<br>Death 6 mo<br>Death 12 mo | BCG —<br>4/8<br>3/8<br>4/7 | | 2/7<br>0/7<br>0/5 |

entered the study. The patients were randomized to receive either wide excision of the primary only or excision and elective lymph node dissection; inguino–iliac dissection or axillary dissection.

The main results were the following:

1. The 8-year actuarial survival curves of the 286 cases submitted to excision only and of the 267 cases operated in the lymph nodes were identical.

2. Microscopical metastasis were found in 18.3% of the 267 cases subjected to elective node dissection ($N_{0+}$).

3. The 5-year survival of patients with microscopical metastasis ($N_{0+}$) was 39.4%, and it was 32.5% for patients who developed clinical lymph node metastasis (biopsy proven) during the 5-year follow-up period. This difference was not significant.

The main conclusion of this study was that there is no indication for elective node dissection in melanoma of the limbs. This conclusion should be interpreted only in a therapeutic sense. However, this study clearly showed (36) that elective lymph node dissection can select from the beginning those patients having a worse prognosis: the 5-year survival of lymph node-operated patients with no microscopical involvement was 69%, whereas it was only 30% where there were micrometastases.

Long after the start of the W.H.O. study, Clark, From, and Bernardino (14) and Breslow (10) demonstrated that melanoma invasion and its correlate, melanoma thickness, are the most important criteria for assessing the prognosis of primary melanoma. In addition, it was shown by several authors (21,37) that the rate of regional lymph node microscopical involvement increases according to the degree of invasion.

For this reason ongoing trials on stage I melanoma are based on the histological status of the regional lymph nodes, in addition to the histological grading of the primary tumor (6,13,32). For example, grade III of more that 1.5 mm thickness, and grade IV and V melanoma with no histological lymph node metastasis can be eligible in trials as cases of high risk for hematogenous micrometastasis (13).

## IMMUNOADJUVANT TREATMENT IN STAGE I HIGH-RISK MELANOMA AND STAGE II

BCG[1] and levamisole were used as immunoadjuvant after surgical removal of primary melanoma of high-risk and stage II patients (Table 1).

Cunningham et al. (20) reported on a BCG trial with 127 all localizations stage I and extremity stage II melanoma. Although this procedure mixed two different stages of the disease, the distribution of the patient characteristics was equal. After 1 year, the disease-free rate was 86% after surgery only and

---

[1] All abbreviations are explained at the end of the chapter.

65% after BCG with the prong technique. This difference was not signifiant ($p = 0.18$).

Levamisole versus placebo was studied by Spitler et al. (35) in patients with high-risk melanoma. The 15-month follow-up of 132 patients showed the same 30% recurrence rate, but stage I and II were mixed together.

In contrast, Morton (26) recently confirmed the previous unrandomized studies showing an improvement with BCG. After wide local excision and lymph node dissection, 89 stage I and II patients were randomized to receive either no further treatment or BCG by scarification or BCG plus allogeneic cultured melanoma cells. The results show a delay of the recurrences and a reduction of the death rate. The recurrence rate was 50% in control against 41% and 34% in the immunotherapy groups. The death rate was 36% in control against 19% and 24% in the immunotherapy group.

It seems to be much too early to draw any definite conclusion: The results of these trials are either preliminary or presented with no distinction between prognosis criteria.

## STAGE II MALIGNANT MELANOMA

### Immunotherapy Only as Adjuvant Treatment After Surgery

Pinsky et al. (29) reported on the effect of BCG administration on the recurrence and survival of operated stage II melanoma. They introduced an immunological selection criterion: The patients had to be either tuberculine or DNCB positive on the skin test. BCG, 4 to $6 \times 10^7$ viable units, was applied by means of a multiple tine technique once a week. When the reaction was too strong, the dose of BCG was diminished. Forty-seven patients entered the trial. The prognosis factor distribution was not homogenous, but the balance was acceptable. The analysis was made 160 days after lymph node dissection. There was no difference between the two groups in the actual curves for recurrence rate and survival rate. These results of 1975 were confirmed 1 year later (30): The recurrence rate was 57% and 58%, the median survival 107 weeks and 110.5 weeks for surgery only and surgery plus BCG, respectively (Table 2).

McIllmurray et al. (24) recently reported on adverse effect of immunotherapy given after surgery in stage IIb patients. The immunotherapy regimen was i.d. injections on day 14 only after operation, of a mixture of $3 \times 10^7$ live units of BCG and $5 \times 10^7$ autologous irradiated cells. In vaccinated patients, early widespread recurrences were seen and 4 of 7 patients died within 12 months, whereas none out of the 5 evaluable controls did so. This small trial, 15 cases, nevertheless demonstrated a striking unfavorable effect of immunotherapy. The authors decided to stop this trial.

These five trials seem to be in conflict with each other. However, the BCG treatment conditions differed the origin of the vaccine, and the method of administration was not the same. Therefore, no definite conclusion can be proposed.

## Chemotherapy Versus Chemotherapy Plus Immunotherapy as Adjuvant Treatment After Surgery in Stage II Melanoma

In all the three studies reported here, DTIC and BCG were the only treatment chosen.

Cunningham et al. (20) compared the effects of BCG with DTIC plus BCG in 78 stage II cases of trunk melanoma. No control with surgery only was made. After 1 year 66% BCG cases were free of disease, compared to 47% in the DTIC plus BCG group. This difference was not significant ($p = 0.11$).

Simmons (34) made a study comparing the effect on recurrence of immunotherapy and chemotherapy alone or a combination of both treatments. Fifty patients entered. After surgery, they were randomized to receive BCG plus neuraminidase-treated autologous tumor cells, DTIC, or a combination of the two treatments. The median disease-free interval was almost identical: 72 weeks.

The W.H.O. Melanoma Group (9) started a clinical trial for comparing DTIC, BCG, DTIC plus BCG, and no adjuvant treatment after lymph node dissection for stage II melanoma of all localization and stage II of the trunk (Clark III to V). DTIC was given intravenously at 200 mg/m² from day 1 to 5 every 28 days. Lyophilized BCG from the Institut Pasteur, 2 ampules of 37.5 mg containing 5 to $9 \times 10^8$ viable units, was applied with the Heaf gun technique, once a week or monthly when the reaction became ++.

A preliminary analysis (9) of the first 196 patients showed, on the actuarial curves, a nonstatistically significant longer disease-free interval in patients receiving BCG and DTIC. A more recent analysis (38) of the first 293 evaluable patients consisted of 146 previously untreated and 147 previously treated cases. In the first group, all three adjuvant treatments provided a doubled median disease-free interval. In the second group, DTIC + BCG was the only treatment to produce this effect. However, these figures are not statistically significant and should still be considered as preliminary data.

## STAGE III MALIGNANT MELANOMA

### Chemotherapy Alone

A great variety of chemotherapeutic trials have been conducted in the treatment of melanoma. Only a minority were properly controlled. For reasons of convenience, the different studies cited below are discussed according to the same criteria. In the presentation of the results we would like to draw the attention to the importance of the classical response criteria, which should be defined as follows:

1. CR (complete remission): disappearance of all manifestation of disease.
2. PR (partial response or remission): should be defined as a regression of 50% or more of the initial size of measurable lesions (defined as a reduction by 50% of the sum of the products of the two longest perpendicular diameters

TABLE 2. *Malignant melanoma: randomized trials in stages I and II—chemotherapy + immunotherapy*

| Ref. | Author and year | Stage | No. of points | Criteria | Treatments | | | |
|------|-----------------|-------|---------------|----------|------|-----|-----------|--------|
| | | | | | DTIC | BCG | DTIC + BCG | Surgery only |
| 20 | Cunningham et al., ECOG, 1976 | II | 78 | Disease-free 1 yr | — | 66% | 47% | — |
| 34 | Simmons, 1976 | II | 50 | Median disease free | 72 wk | — | 72 wk (+ cells) | — |
| 38 | W.H.O., MG, 1977 | IIb | 146 | Median disease free: previously untreated | 24 mo | 22 mo | 24 mo | 11.84 mo |
| 38 | W.H.O., MG, 1977 | IIb | 147 | Previously treated | 11.6 | 14.1 | 17.1 | 9.1 |

of all tumors for at least 1 month) without progression or appearance of any new lesions at any site. The order of the reported studies is based on the number of drugs used for treatment and time of publication (Table 3).

Ahman, Hahn, and Bisch (2) made in 1972 a clinical evaluation with DTIC, 275 to 400 mg/m$^2$/day $\times$ 5 days i.v./4 weeks; hydroxyurea (HU), 70 to 100 mg/kg/day $\times$ 5 days; or MPH, 0.25 mg/kg/day p.o. $\times$ 5 days. The study included a total of 35 patients (19 men and 16 women), and all were evaluable. Randomization was well balanced for primary and secondary treatment. Therapeutical results were not impressive, with only 2 clinical responses out of 12 trials with primary DTIC treatment. No response was noted on the other treatment arms. It should be pointed out that, with the limited number of included patients, divided over three treatment arms (including 12 patients for each primary treatment), one cannot claim with 95% certainty that a 20% active treatment has not been missed. Further, secondary treatment is not an equivalent of primary treatment in cancer therapy, and the authors pool this together. Response criteria are not the generally accepted ones.

If a classical response analysis was used, no response could be claimed from the whole study. Two deaths can be retained for DTIC on a hematological basis, but the dose regimen of this drug was varying in the study and we do not know at which level it occurred, or whether it was for primary or secondary treatment. The overall impression is negative, and no valuable conclusion can be drawn from this study.

Costanza et al. (16) initiated in 1971 an ECOG prospective randomized trial with two treatment arms: DTIC, 150 mg/m$^2$/day i.v. $\times$ 5 days; and triazeno imidazole carboxamide mustard (TIC), 800 mg/m$^2$/day i.v. $\times$ 5 days, a structure equivalent. Dose modifications in function of hematologic toxicity were included. Response criteria were correctly defined. A total of 178 patients were included in the study, of which 150 were evaluable: 80 in the DTIC group and 70 in the TIC group. The two groups were quite comparable for performance status, free interval, prior chemotherapy, radiotherapy, disease distribution, age, and sex.

The response rate for DTIC (15/79 or 19%) was significantly better than TIC, with 4/66 (6.1%) even in the different categories where performance status, prior chemotherapy, surgery, and prior radiotherapy were taken into account. Toxicity in the two treatment arms was comparable and within acceptable limits. The authors conclude correctly that DTIC was significantly better ($p \leqslant 0.03$) than TIC mustard and confirmed the therapeutic usefulness of DTIC in stage III melanoma. Their experience with crossover treatment showed clearly lesser results with DTIC (3/39 or 8%) and TIC (1/23 or 4%).

In view of the very poor results in treatment of stage III melanoma with single agents, several authors have tried a great variety of combinations. Only a minority of the trials were conducted as controlled and prospectively randomized trials.

TABLE 3. Malignant melanoma: randomized trials in stage III—chemotherapy

| Ref. | Author and year | No. of patients | Criteria | Treatments | | | |
|---|---|---|---|---|---|---|---|
| 2 | Ahman et al., 1972 | | PR + CR | DTIC 2/12 | MPH 0/12 | HU 0/11 | |
| 16 | Costanza et al., ECOG, 1976 | 178 (150) | PR + CR | DTIC 18.2% 15/79 | TIC mustard 5.8% 4/66 | | |
| 17 | Costanza et al., ECOG, 1972 | 140 (112) | PR + CR | DTIC 17.9% 9/51 | DTIC + BCNU 19.5% 12/61 | | |
| 25 | Moon et al., 1975 | 120 (98) | PR + CR | DTIC/day 24% 6/25 | DTIC q.8h. 29% 6/21 | BCNU-VCR 16% 8/51 | |
| 7 | Bellet et al., MCCG, 1976 | 50 (46) | PR + CR | DTIC 29% 7/24 | BCNU + VCR 23% 5/22 | | |
| 15 | Costanza and Nathanson, ECOG, 1974 | 84 (73) | PR + CR | DTIC 12.5% 3/24 | MeCCNU 8.7% 2/23 | DTIC + MeCCNU 23.1% 6/26 | |
| 3 | Ahman et al., 1972 | 37 | PR | DTIC + VCR 4/18 | CCNU 1/19 | | |
| 4 | Ahman et al., 1974 | 38 | PR | DTIC + VCR 4/19 | MeCCNU 5/19 | | |
| 1 | Ahman et al., 1976 | 44 | PR | DTIC + MeCCNU 28% 6/21 | ADM | | |
| 19 | Costanzi et al., SWOG, 1975 | 228 (178) | CR + PR | BCNU-HU-DTIC 27% 24/89 | BCNU-HU 0/23 | DTIC + VCR 30% 27/89 | |
| 5 | Ahman et al., 1975 | 40 | PR | DTIC-VCR 2/20 | MeCCNU-CPA 1/20 | | |
| 11 | Byrne, 1976 | 19 (16) | PR | CPA-VCR 3/10 | CPA-VCR-PCZ 2/6 | | |
| 8 | Beretta et al., WHO-MG, 1976 | 463 (274) | CR + PR | DTIC-VCR-BCNU 20.9% 27/129 | DTIC-VCR-HU 20.2% 17/84 | DTIC-ACD-BCNU 31.1% 19/61 | |
| 12 | Carter et al., COG, 1976 | 270 | CR + PR | DTIC-BCNU-VCR 23% 15/65 | DTIC 16% 8/48 | DTIC-CCNU-VCR 16% 11/67 | DTIC-BCNU-HU 13% 8/63 |

TABLE 4. *Malignant melanoma: randomized trials in stage III—chemotherapy versus chemoimmunotherapy*

| Ref. | Author and year | No. of patients | Criteria | | Treatments | |
|---|---|---|---|---|---|---|
| 18 | Costanzi, SWOG, 1976 | 232 | PR + CR | BCNU–DTIC–HU<br>28%<br>21/75 | id. + BCG<br>29%<br>25/87 | DTIC + BCG<br>20%<br>14/70 |
| 22 | Mastrangelo et al., 1976 | 50 | PR + CR | MeCCNU + VCR<br>23%<br>6/26 | id. + BCG +<br>16.6%<br>4/24 | |
| 31 | Presant et al., 1976 | 69<br>(56) | | CPA + DTIC<br>28% | id. + *C. parvum*<br>33% | |

Costanza et al. (17) reported in 1972 an ECOG study comparing DTIC, 150 mg/m² day i.v. × 5 days to DTIC, 100 mg/m²/day i.v. × 5 days + BCNU, 75 mg/m² d2 and 3 i.v. One-hundred-forty patients were entered into the study: 65 were allocated to the DTIC treatment and 77 to the combination; 28 were not evaluable. The two treatment groups were nearly identical in terms of organ involvement, sex, age, prior chemotherapy or radiotherapy, and surgery. The 9/51 or 17.9% response yield for DTIC according to correct criteria for CR and PR was completely within the expected range, and so was the toxicity. The combination treatment yielded no better results (12/61 or 19.5%) with regard to the ratio of complete or partial responders, duration of the response, or survival. The expected reduction of the incidence of CNS lesions by BCNU was not observed. The authors concluded on a correct basis that the combination of BCNU to DTIC failed to demonstrate a superiority of DTIC alone. They confirmed the value of DTIC in therapy and the benefit obtained on survival time by obtention of remission.

Moon et al. (25) reported in 1975 a study conducted by ALGB comparing the combination BCNU, 150 mg/m²/i.v., + VCR, 2 mg/m² i.v., and two dose schedules of DTIC (regimen A: 300 mg/m²/day × 6 days i.v.; regimen B: 100 mg/m²/8 hr × 6 days i.v.). A total of 120 patients were entered within a 2-year interval (1969–1970) and randomly attributed to one of the three treatment arms. Half of the patients were treated with BCNU + VCR. Response criteria used are correct. The three treatment groups were reported comparable for sex, age, free interval, and tumor distribution. Response rates were, respectively, 16% for BCNU + VCR, 24% for the daily DTIC, and 29% for DTIC q.8h. Special attention can be drawn to CNS recurrence after remission, which is the same for BCNU or DTIC regimens.

The number of patients included in the study did not show any significant difference between BCNU–VCR versus DTIC-treated patients. No schedule dependency for DTIC was demonstrated, but the limited number (25 and 21) should not have raised any hope of this. It is important to note that the authors found a complete absence of response in crossovers, although no conclusion can yet be drawn about cross-resistance: The number of patients treated in that way does not exclude a 20% response rate after treatment crossing.

Bellet et al. (7) reported in 1976 a quite similar study as above comparing in a randomized trial DTIC, 2 mg/kg/day × 10 days i.v., versus BCNU + VCR. A total of 50 consecutive patients were randomized, allocating 50 to each treatment arm. Response criteria used for CR and PR were correct. No data are available about the similarity of the two treatment groups, but analysis of the responders revealed no difference between the two treatment arms with regard to sex, age, tumor distribution, or tumor burden. This phase III study showed no difference in the overall response rate comparing primary DTIC treatment (29%) or BCNU + VCR (23%) treated patients.

Nor was any difference found in the response rate to secondary treatment. The authors made an interesting analysis of response rate according to tumor burden (defined as the 24-hr melanin elimination), showing a significantly better response for both treatments in low burden as compared to high burden. Unfortunately, such subdivision is always subjective. No difference in median survival time was found between the two arms for responders and nonresponders, respectively.

DTIC, used as reference therapy in the studies above, has been extensively combined with other agents, but these combinations have seldom been compared to DTIC alone.

Costanza and Nathanson (15) presented for the ASCO a study, although incomplete, comparing DTIC, 200 mg/m$^2$/day i.v. X 5 days + MeCCNU, 200 mg/m$^2$ p.o., and DTIC, 150 mg/m$^2$/day i.v. X 5 days + MeCCNU, 130 mg/m$^2$/p.o. d2. With 84 patients randomized, of which 73 were evaluable, divided over the three arms, no significant difference in response rate have been found noting, respectively, 12.5% for DTIC (24p), 8.7% for MeCCNU (23p) and 23.1% for MeCCNU + DTIC (26p).

Ahman, Hahn, and Bisch (3) compared DTIC + VCR versus CCNU in a study published in 1972. Only 37 patients were randomized in the two treatment arms. Visceral disease was predominant (34/37), and patients were randomized after stratification for this parameter. An analysis of comparability between the two randomization arms is not available. Response criteria used are correct for partial remission. All patients were evaluable, although again the low patient number does not allow one to find a significant difference between the two treatments, showing 1 response/19p for CCNU (5.5%) for 4/18 for DTIC + VCR (22%). No difference was observed for toxicity with an exception for neurologic toxicity by VCR and a slightly more frequent alopecia in the DTIC–VCR group. The authors consider CCNU as a not very useful treatment in melanoma, but this conclusion was not based on a statistically significant difference.

Ahman, Hahn, and Bisch (4) again conducted a nearly identical study, reported in 1974, comparing MeCCNU to their combination DTIC + VCR. Thirty-eight patients were randomized. After stratification for visceral and nonvisceral disease, 19 were allocated to the MeCCNU (225 mg/m$^2$/6 weeks) arm and 19 to the DTIC (325 mg/m$^2$/day X 5 days i.v./4 weeks) plus VCR (1.4 mg/m$^2$/day 1 and 5 i.v.) branch. All were evaluable. No further analysis of the similarity of the treatment arms was done. Response criteria defined only PR. They observed responses in respectively 5/19 or 26.3% (MeCCNU) and 4/19 or 21.5% of the primary treated cases. There was no unexpected toxicity from the therapeutic schedule. The authors conclude correctly that MeCCNU has a definite activity, which is on a statistical range of 20%, in the treatment of melanoma. No further conclusions can be drawn, the number being too small to show any difference between the two treatment schedules.

Ahman et al. (1) also compared in a controlled study adriamycin and a combination of DTIC + MeCCNU. A total of 44 patients were admitted to the study. Thirty-six of these had visceral involvement. Patients were stratified by this discriminant before randomization either to ADM treatment (60 mg/m² i.v./4 weeks) or the combination treatment with DTIC (150 mg/m²/day i.v. X 5 days) plus MeCCNU (125 mg/m² p.o. day 1). No further analysis of the treatment arms is described. Response criteria defined only PR. Objective responses were observed in 28% of the combination treatment (primary treatment); none was seen in the ADM group. They observed one toxic death by blood loss in a patient who received the combination treatment and developed a profound thrombocytopenia. All responses concerned patients with long and/or node involvement. They conclude correctly that, in their hands, ADM failed to show any evidence of activity in the treatment of melanoma. Statistically we can be more than 95% sure that ADM (60) does not have a 20% activity range in melanoma. However, attention should be drawn to the fact that ADM was used at 60 mg/m²/4 weeks and not at the classic 75 mg/m²/3 weeks dosage level. They claimed a definite activity for the association of DTIC + MeCCNU, but with the occurrence of one toxic death we would need proof of the advantage of this combination over DTIC or MeCCNU alone. For this the ECOG study, started in 1974, should be followed with great interest.

Several authors started comparing immediately drug combinations that showed hopeful results on screening. Chronologically we found the following publications of this kind:

Costanzi (19) published in 1975 the study of the SOG that started in 1971. A total of 228 patients were registered in the study. At the time of publication 40 were too early to evaluate. Two treatment arms were included. The patients were treated with either BCNU, 150 mg/m² i.v. d1 every other course, plus hydroxyurea, 1,480 mg/m²/day p.o. X 5 days, and DTIC, 150 mg/m²/day i.v. X 5 days, or the same regimen plus VCR, 1.4 mg/m² i.v. d1 and 5. These schedules were repeated every 28 days. One-hundred-eleven patients were randomized to the BHD arm and 117 to the BHD–V arm. After removing the 40 patients who were too early to evaluate, 5 protocol violations, 4 inadequate trials by reason of toxicity, and 1 lost patient, 178 remained evaluable, 89 in each treatment arm. No (detailed) analysis of patient characteristics between the two treatment arms is available. Early deaths (before 28 days) were equally distributed (25 for BHD, 21 for BHD–V). The analysis of the total response rates (27% for BHD and 30% for BHD–V) or analysis of CR and PR, respectively, do not show any advantage in adding VCR to the BCNU–HU–DTIC combination. The overall results do compare well to other treatment schedules, but the authors state that the majority of the responders had metastases confined to skin, lungs, and/or lymph nodes and we do not know definitively which percentage these patients represented, nor the way they were distributed over the two treatment arms. It appears that the combination of BCNU, hydroxyurea, and DTIC is an effective regimen in patients with disseminated melanoma, particularly if they have skin, lung, and/or lymph node involvement. This deserves further investigation and, for instance, a comparative study to DTIC alone.

Ahman et al. (5) reported in 1975 a comparative study of DTIC–VCR versus MeCCNU–CPA. A homogenous group of 40 patients (36 with visceral involvement) was randomized into the two treatment arms. The first arm received DTIC, 300 to 340 mg/m²/day i.v. X 5 days, and VCR, 1.4 mg/m² i.v. d1 and 5 (max. 2 mg) every 4 weeks; the second arm received MeCCNU, 150 mg/m² p.o. d1, and CPA, 500 to 800 mg/m² i.v. d1, to be repeated every 6 weeks. Patients were stratified with regard to visceral disease. The two arms of 20 patients each are comparable. Toxicity showed constant nausea and vomiting and neurologic toxicity for the DTIC–VCR group. The 10% (DTIC–VCR) and 5% (MeCCNU–CPA) remission rate (only PR defined) are within the same statistical range and do not differ from the results of this author reported earlier. Here again the low number should not have raised hope of finding a difference. They do show that both regimens have some activity in treatment of melanoma, but the results do not even suggest a better therapeutic range than DTIC or MeCCNU alone. A comparative trial of this kind has not been published yet, but ECOG is comparing under Protocol 1672 a MeCCNU versus DTIC versus DTIC + MeCCNU program, and up to now they obtain a 20% response rate in each arm.

A minor study was published by Byrne (11) in 1976 comparing CPA, 1,000 mg/m² i.v., and VCR, 1.4 mg/m² i.v. d1, versus the same regimen plus procarbazine (PCZ), 100 mg/m²/day X 7 days. Cycles were repeated every 3 weeks. The low total number of patients (19), allowing only 10 evaluable cases for the CV arm and 6 for the CVP arm, does not allow any meaningful analysis. It should be noted that the overall response was about 30% of evaluable cases. Only PR was defined.

W.H.O. (8) reported in 1976 a cooperative study comparing three combination regimens. In fact, the study, including 463 patients, was initially designed with four treatment arms, all including DTIC: regimen A: DTIC, 100 mg/m²/day X 5 days, VCR, 1.4 mg/m² i.v. d1 and 15, and BCNU, 100 mg/m² i.v. d1; regimen B: DTIC, VCR, and HU, 10 mg/kg d7, 10, 13, 17, 21, and 25; regimen C: DTIC, BCNU, and ACD, 0.05 mg/kg d1 and 15; regimen D: DTIC–ACD–HU. Cycles were repeated every 4 weeks. Dose-reduction schedules were included. Treatment was considered adequate for evaluation if a minimum of two courses were administered or if remission occured before. For this reason or for protocol violations 166 patients (35.8%) became inevaluable. Further, the nonclassical way of randomization, assigning only two regimens to each center, resulted in an even greater numerical imbalance of the four arms. For this reason regimen D (23 evaluable patients) was discarded for analysis, leaving 274 patients divided over three treatment arms: regimen A, 129 evaluable for 207 entered; regimen B, 84 (122); regimen C, 61 (98). The analysis of the respective response rates of 20.9%, 20.2%, and 31% failed to show a superiority of one of the three treatment arms. The 20.9% response for regimen A was within the expected range. Survival analysis confirmed that responders live longer than nonresponders but, unfortunately, the study also shows that CR was limited to a small fraction of patients with skin, node, and/or lung involvement. Further and most important is that BCNU failed to delay the development of CNS metastases.

Carter et al. (12) reported in 1976 a study from the Central Oncology Group comparing three combination treatments to DTIC, 4.5 mg/kg $\times$ 10, alone: regimen A: 2.7 mg/kg i.v. d1–5, CCNU, 1.5 mg/kg d2, VCR, 0.027 mg/kg d1 and 5; regimen B: DTIC, BCNU, 2 mg/kg i.v. d2, and VCR; regimen C: DTIC, BCNU, and HU, 30 mg/kg d2, 5, 9, 12, 16, 19. All treatment cycles were repeated every 6 weeks. Two-hundred and seventy patients were entered in the study, of whom 243 were evaluable. Patients were stratified according to prior treatment and presence of brain or liver metastases. Thirty-one patients already treated with DTIC were randomized to one of the combination treatments. Treatment arms were numerically well balanced and comparable. Definition for CR and PR were correct. The response rates were, respectively, 16% for DTIC (48 patients), 16% for DCV (67 patients), 23% for DBV (64 patients), and 13% for DBH (63 patients). These differences were not significant. Nor was there any difference found in median response duration, age group, sex, or survival. When survival was examined by patient response, however, a highly significant difference was found comparing response versus nonresponse versus ($p = <0.001$) progression. Examining response rate by toxicity, a significantly better response rate was found for patients having some degree of toxicity (except for the DBH arm).

The overall conclusion is that the combination treatments are not better than DTIC alone. Crossover, however showed that prior DTIC treatment did not preclude a subsequent response to one of the combinations.

The enumeration and brief discussion of comparative chemotherapeutic trials in stage III melanoma did not show, at any moment, a definitely superior treatment. According to the studies of Ahman and Costanza, we can positively discard ADM, 60 mg/m² i.v./4 weeks, and TIC mustard in the treatment of melanoma.

## Chemotherapy Versus Chemoimmunotherapy

Several authors have recently published very encouraging results of addition of immunotherapy to single- or multiple-agent chemotherapy. However, only one comparative study has been published. Others presented their results at the National Cancer Institute Conference on Immunotherapy in Man in October 1976 (Table 4).

Newlands et al. (27) published in 1976 a comparative study of the Westminster Hospital, London. Two regimens were compared: DTIC, 100 mg/m²/day i.v. $\times$ 5 days, and ICRF 159 (1,2-di-(3,5-dioxopiperazin–1–y1 propane), 125 mg twice daily for 5 days versus the same treatment plus interdermal autologous irradiated tumor cells (2 $\times$ 10⁷) and BCG (Glaxo) (50 mg). BCG only was administered for two cycles. Of 56 patients included in the study, 17 were not evaluable.

Unfortunately, they entered in their study stage III and stage IIb patients (17). The chemotherapy group received 20 stage III and 9 stage IIb patients (with 1 IIb and 9 III p. NE), the chemoimmunotherapy group, respectively, $19 + 8$ cases (with 2 IIb and 5 III patients NE).

The definition of CR was correct, but their definition of PR included patients with mixed response or possible progressive disease elsewhere, and this is incorrect. Therefore we take into account only the survival analysis of the study showing no difference between the two treatment arms. Important is the significant ($p < 0.05$) difference in 1-year survival between the stage IIb (75%) and stage III patients (20%).

Costanzi (18) reported in 1976 a randomized study from SWOG comparing their earlier described association of BCNU, HU, and DTIC versus the same regimen plus BCG scarifications versus DTIC + BCG. Until now, a total of 286 patients have been included in the study. A stratification was done for brain metastases that received 3,000 rads on brain + steroids and for patients with liver metastasis who received hepatic artery perfusion with DTIC. A total of 286 patients were entered and were numerically well distributed over the three treatment arms. No analysis in terms of prognostic factors is yet available. The response rates of the three groups were 29% for BHD (91 p.), 28% for BHD + BCG (99 p.), and 18% for DTIC + BCG (96 p.). These differences were not significant. It is therefore felt that the addition of BCG by scarification does not increase the response rate. Neither was there any difference on careful analysis of the survival.

Mastrangelo, Bellet, and Berd (22) conducted a controlled study including 50 patients using a more specific kind of immunotherapy. Patients were randomized to receive either (A) MeCCNU, 200 mg/m$^2$ p.o. q.8w., and VCR, 2 mg i.v. q.4w. $\times$ 2, or (B) the same chemotherapy with BCG + irradiated (6,000 rads) allogeneic melanoma cells ($10^8$) intradermally. No analysis of treatment groups in terms of prognostic factors is yet available. No difference was noted for response rates, respectively 23 and 16.6%, median duration of remission, and median survival duration.

Presant et al. (31) reported a study of the Southeast Cancer Study Group comparing DTIC, 200 mg/m$^2$ i.v./day $\times$ 5 days, plus CPA, 600 mg/m$^2$ i.v. d1, or the same chemotherapy plus *C. parvum,* 5 mg/m$^2$ i.v. d1, 8, and 15. Treatment cycles were repeated every 3 weeks. Sixty-nine patients were randomized, of whom 56 are evaluable. Analysis of results showed no difference in response rate (respectively, 28 and 33%), median remission duration, and median survival. The authors concluded that the addition of CP does not improve therapeutic results but only produces additional toxicity.

## DISCUSSION AND CONCLUSIONS

Most randomized clinical trials showed no beneficial effect of adjuvant treatment with chemotherapy, immunotherapy, or chemoimmunotherapy, in the so-called minimum residual disease, high-risk cases of stage I and II malignant melanoma. That is in contrast with the consistency of low objective response rates obtained with chemotherapy in stage III advanced malignant melanoma. In the latter, only two types of drugs were found to be active: DTIC and nitrosourea derivatives. However, the response rates using single drugs averaged 20%. There was no improvement when these drugs were combined, nor when other agents were associated.

These poor results in advanced disease raise the question of the adequacy of adjuvant treatment in stage II and I melanoma. The main point is that only 20% of stage III patients responding to therapy will experience a prolonged survival, so it is not surprising that such an effect will be barely detectable in groups composed of long-surviving stage II patients.

Therefore, we feel that the limiting factor for the assessment of adjuvant treatment in melanoma is the methodology itself.

There is an overwhelming amount of reports claiming the effectiveness of immunotherapy. Most of them were based on uncontrolled studies. Among the very few randomized trials that we found, the results were either difficult to interpret or, in one instance, there was a tumor enhancement. The disappointing results of immunotherapy might well be due to the fact that the experimental bases of immunotherapy are still incomplete and that clinical immunotherapy developed too quickly. More work will be needed to select new immunotherapy agents, with a defined chemical structure and nontoxicity when administered systemically.

In conclusion, the analysis of recent randomized trials in the treatment of malignant melanoma clearly indicates that the therapeutical possibilities consist of only two types of chemotherapy. There is an important need for improving the methodology in many respects: the clinical workup of malignant melanoma, the selection of cases to avoid the meaningless study of too small or nonhomogeneous groups; and knowledge of the *in vivo* and *in vitro* mechanisms of action of chemotherapeutical and so-called immunotherapeutical agents.

## SUMMARY

The authors reviewed 26 controlled randomized studies on the treatment of human malignant melanoma. Of these, 10 trials dealt with stage I and II disease: No adjuvant treatment (chemotherapy, immunotherapy, chemoimmunotherapy) was definitively proven to be useful. Sixteen studies concerned stage III advanced malignant melanoma: only two types of drugs, DTIC and nitrosourea derivatives (BCNU, MeCCNU, CCNU) were found to be effective with an overall 20% response rate, that is, percentage of objective remissions. Combinations of drugs did not improve the results. Conflicting results were found after adding immunotherapy to the chemotherapy.

## ABBREVIATIONS

### Drugs

| | |
|---|---|
| ACD | Actinomycin-D |
| ADM | Adriamycin |
| BCG | Bacille Calmette-Guérin |
| BCNU | *bis*-Chloroethyl nitrosourea |
| C. parvum | *Corynebacterium parvum* |
| DTIC | Dimethyl triazeno imidazole carboxamide |
| HU | Hydroxyurea |
| MPH | Melphalan (phenyl alanin mustard) |
| MeCCNU | Chloroethyl-methylcyclohexyl nitrosourea |
| PCZ | Procarbazine |
| VCR | Vincristine |

### Groups

| | |
|---|---|
| COG | Central Oncology Group |
| ECOG | Eastern Cooperative Oncology Group |
| MCCG | Melanoma Clinical Cooperative Group |
| MSKCG | Memorial-Sloan-Kettering Cancer Center |
| SWOG | Southwest Oncology Group |
| UCLA | University of California Los Angeles |
| WHO-MG | World Health Organization Melanoma Group |
| EORTC MG | European Organization for Research on Treatment of Cancer, Melanoma Cooperative Group |

## REFERENCES

1. Ahman, D. L., Bisch, H. F., Edmonson, J. H., Hahn, R. G., Eagan, R. T., O'Conord, M. J., and Frytak, S. (1976): Clinical comparison of ADM and a combination of MeCCNU and DTIC in disseminated malignant melanoma. *Clin. Pharmacol. Ther.*, 19:821–824.
2. Ahman, D. L., Hahn, G. R., and Bisch, H. F. (1972): Clinical evaluation of DTIC, melphalan and hydroxyurea in the treatment of malignant melanoma. *Cancer Chemother. Rep.*, Part 1, 56:369–372.
3. Ahman, D. L., Hahn, K. G., and Bisch, H. F. (1972): A comparative study of CCNU and DTIC and VCR in the palliation of disseminated malignant melanoma. *Cancer Res.*, 32:2432–2434.
4. Ahman, D. L., Hahn, R. G., and Bisel, H. F. (1974): Evaluation of MeCCNU versus combined DTIC and VCR in the palliation of disseminated malignant melanoma. *Cancer*, 33:615–618.
5. Ahman, D. L., Hahn, R. G., Bisch, H. F., Eagan, R. T., and Edmonson, J. H. (1975): Comparative study of MeCCNU with CPA and DTIC with VCR in patients with disseminated malignant melanoma. *Cancer Chemother. Rep.*, Part 1, 59:451–453.
6. Balch, C. (1977): In: *Minutes of Melanoma Meeting NIH Bethesda, January 1977*, edited by H. Davis, A. Louie, and E. Jacobs.
7. Bellet, R. E., Mastrangelo, M. J., Laucius, J. F., and Bodurtha, A. J. (1976): Randomized

prospectove trial of DTIC alone versus BCNU plus VCR in the treatment of metastatic malignant melanoma. *Cancer Treatment Rep.,* 60:595–600.

8. Beretta, G., Bonadonna, G., Cascinelli, N., Moralito, A., and Veronesi, U. (1976): Comparative evaluation of three regimens for advanced malignant melanoma; Results of an international cooperative study. *Cancer Treatment,* 60:33–40.

9. Beretta, G., et al. (1978): Controlled study for prolonged chemotherapy, immunotherapy and chemotherapy plus immunotherapy as an adjuvant to surgery in stage I-II malignant melanoma: Preliminary report. In: *Immunotherapy of Cancer: Present Status of Trials in Man,* edited by W. D. Terry and D. Windhorst, pp. 65–72. Raven Press, New York.

10. Breslow, A. (1970): Thickness, cross-sectional areas and depth of invasion in the prognosis of cutaneous melanoma. *Ann. Surg.,* 172:902–908.

11. Byrne, M. J. (1976): Cyclophosphamide, vincristine and procarbazine in the treatment of malignant melanoma. *Cancer,* 38:1922–1924.

12. Carter, K. D., Krementz, E. T., Hill, G. J., Metter, G. E., Fletcher, W. S., Golomb, F. M., Grange, T. B., Minton, J. P., and Sparks, F. C. (1976): DTIC and combination therapy for melanoma. I studies with DTIC, BCNU, CCNU, VCR and Hydroxyurea. *Cancer Treatment Rep.,* 60:601–609.

13. Cesarini, J. P., Lejeune, F. J., and Silvester, R. (1976): An assessment of chemotherapy versus immunotherapy in the treatment of high risk patients after surgical removal of a primary malignant melanoma of the skin. (1) Limbs: with histologically negative lymph nodes ($N_0$-); (2) Head and neck and trunk: with no palpable lymph nodes ($N_0$), Protocol 18761, E.O.R.T.C. Malignant Melanoma Cooperative Group.

14. Clark, W. H., Jr., From, L., and Bernardino, E. A. (1969): The histogenesis and biologic behavior of primary human malignant melanomas of the skin. *Cancer Res.,* 29:705–727.

15. Costanza, M. E., and Nathanson, L. (1974): Combination of DTIC and MeCCNU versus single agents in disseminated melanoma. *Am. Soc. Clin. Oncol.,* Abstracts 1974, p. 758.

16. Costanza, M. E., Nathanson, L., Costello, W. G., Wolter, J., Brunk, F., Colsky, J., Hall, T., Oberfield, R. A., and Regelson, W. (1976): Results of a randomized study comparing DTIC with TIC mustard in malignant melanoma. *Cancer,* 37:1654–1659.

17. Costanza, M. E., Nathanson, L., Lenhard, R., Wolter, J., Colsky, J., Oberfield, R. A., and Schilling, A. (1972): Therapy of malignant melanoma with an imidazole carboxamide and BCNU. *Cancer,* 30:1457–1461.

18. Costanzi, J. J. (1978): Chemotherapy and BCG in the treatment of disseminated malignant melanoma. In: *Immunotherapy of Cancer: Present Status of Trials in Man,* edited by W. D. Terry and D. Windhorst, pp. 87–93. Raven Press, New York.

19. Costanzi, J. J., Vaitkevicius, V. K., Quagliana, J. M., Hoogstraten, B., Coltman, C. A., and Delaney, F. C. (1975): Combination chemotherapy for disseminated malignant melanoma. *Cancer,* 35:342–346.

20. Cunningham, T. J., Schoenfeld, D., Wolters, J., Nathanson, L., Cohen, M., and Patterson, B. (1978): A controlled study of adjuvant therapy (BCG,BCG-DTIC) with stage I and II melanoma. In: *Immunotherapy of Cancer: Present Status of Trials in Man,* edited by W. D. Terry and D. Windhorst, pp. 19–26. Raven Press, New York.

21. Goldsmith, H., Sham, J. P., and Kim, D. H. (1970): Prognostic significance of lymph node dissection in the treatment of malignant melanoma. *Cancer,* 26:606–609.

22. Mastrangelo, M. J., Bellet, K. E., and Berd, D. (1978): A randomized prospective trial comparing MeCCNU + VCR to MeCCNU + VCR + BCG + allogeneic tumor cells in patients with metastatic malignant melanoma. In: *Immunotherapy of Cancer: Present Status of Trials in Man,* edited by W. D. Terry and D. Windhorst, pp. 95–102. Raven Press, New York.

23. Matton, G., and Van Calster, E. (1974): Surgical treatment of melanoma. In: *Melanoma of the Skin,* edited by A. Castermans, F. Lejeune, and G. Matton. *Acta Chir. Belg.,* 73:189–236.

24. McIllmurray, M. B., Embleton, M. J., Reeves, W. G., Langman, M. J. S., and Deane, M. (1977): Controlled trial of active immunotherapy in management of stage IIb malignant melanoma. *Br. Med. J.,* 1:540–542.

25. Moon, J. H., Gailani, S., Cooper, M. R., Hayes, D. M., Reye, V. B., Blom, J., Falkson, G., Maurice, P., Brunner, K., Glidenell, O., and Holland, J. F. (1975): Comparison of the combination of BCNU and VCR with two dose schedules of DTIC in the treatment of disseminated malignant melanoma. *Cancer,* 35:368–371.

26. Morton, D. L. et al., (1978): Adjuvant immunotherapy of malignant melanoma: preliminary results of a randomized trial in patients with lymph node metastases. In: *Immunotherapy of*

*Cancer: Present Status of Trials in Man,* edited by W. D. Terry and D. Windhorst, pp. 57–64. Raven Press, New York.

27. Newlands, E. S., Oon, C. J., Roberts, J. T., and Elliott, P. (1976): Clinical trial of combination chemotherapy and specific active immunotherapy in disseminated melanoma. *Br. J. Cancer,* 34:174–179.

28. Olsen, G. (1966): The malignant melanoma of the skin. New theories based on a study of 500 cases. *Acta Chir. Scand.* (Suppl.), 365:128–136.

29. Pinsky, C. M., Hirshaut, Y., Wanebo, M. J., Fortner, J. G., Mike, V., Schottenfeld, D., and Oettgen, H. F. (1975): Randomized trial of Bacillus Calmette-Guérin (percutaneous administration) as surgical adjuvant immunotherapy for patients with stage II melanoma. *Ann. N.Y. Acad. Sci.,* 277:187–194.

30. Pinsky, C. M., Hirshaut, Y., Wanebo, M. J., Fortner, J. G., Mike, V., Schottenfeld, D., and Oettgen, H. F. (1978): Surgical adjuvant immunotherapy with BCG in patients with malignant melanoma. Results of a prospective, randomized trial. In: *Immunotherapy of Cancer: Present Status of Trials in Man,* edited by W. D. Terry and D. Windhorst, pp. 27–34. Raven Press, New York.

31. Presant, C. A., Bartolucci, A., Swalley, R., Vogler, W. R., and the Southwest Oncology Group (1978): Effect of *C. Parvum* on the combination chemotherapy of metastatic malignant melanoma. In: *Immunotherapy of Cancer: Present Status of Trials in Man,* edited by W. D. Terry and D. Windhorst, pp. 113–121. Raven Press, New York.

32. Raker, J. 1977: In: *Minutes of the Melanoma Meeting NIH Bethesda, January 1977,* edited by H. Davis, A. Louie, and E. Jacobs.

33. Rosenberg, S. A. (1976): Surgical treatment of malignant melanoma. *Cancer Treatment Rep.,* 60:159–163.

34. Simmons, R. L. (1978): Active specific immunotherapy for advanced melanoma utilizing neuroaminidase-treated autochthonous tumor cells. In: *Immunotherapy of Cancer: Present Status of Trials in Man,* edited by W. D. Terry and D. Windhorst, pp. 123–134. Raven Press, New York.

35. Spitler, L., Sagebiel, R., Wong, P., Malm, T., Chase, R., and Gonzales, R. (1976): A randomized double blind trial of adjuvant therapy with levamisole in patients with malignant melanoma. In: *Immunotherapy of Cancer.* Raven Press, New York *(in press).*

36. Veronesi, U., Adamus, J., Bandiera, D., Brennhovd, I., Caceres, E., Cascinelli, N., Claudio, F., Ikonopisov, R., Javorskj, J., Kirov, S., Kulakowski, A., Lacour, J., Lejeune, F., Mechel, Z., Morabito, A., Rode, I., Sergeev, S., Van Slooten, E., Szczygiel, K., Trapeznikov, N., and Wagner, R. (1977): Inefficiency of immediate node dissection in stage I melanoma of the limbs. *N. Engl. J. Med.,* 297:627–630.

37. Wanebo, H. J., Woodruff, J., and Fortner, J. G. (1975): Malignant melanoma of the extremities: a clinicopathologic study using levels of invasion (microstage). *Cancer,* 35:666–676.

38. W.H.O. Collaborating Centres for evaluation of method of diagnosis and treatment of melanoma, U. Veronesi, Chairman: Minutes of the meeting held in Milano, March 1977.

*Randomized Trials in Cancer: A Critical Review by Sites,* edited by Maurice J. Staquet, Raven Press, New York © 1978.

# Soft Tissue Sarcoma in Adults

*Herbert M. Pinedo, **Bruce A. Chabner, †Maria G. Nieuwenhuis, and ‡Steven A. Rosenberg

*Oncology Unit, Department of Internal Medicine, University Hospital, Utrecht, The Netherlands; ** Clinical Pharmacology Branch, National Cancer Institute, Bethesda, Maryland 20014; †Department of Internal Medicine, University Hospital, Utrecht, The Netherlands; ‡Surgery Branch, National Cancer Institute, Bethesda, Maryland 20014*

Soft tissue sarcomas include all primary mesenchymal tumors of anatomic sites other than the bones. These include fibrosarcoma, leiomyosarcoma, rhabdomyosarcoma, synovial cell sarcoma, liposarcoma, hemangiosarcoma, hemangiopericytoma, neurofibrosarcoma, and undifferentiated sarcoma; mesothelioma is often included with soft tissue sarcomas, because it shares some of the characteristics of these tumors. Also, Kaposi's sarcoma may be included, although the sensitivity of this tumor to chemotherapeutic drugs is quite different as compared to that of the other soft tissue sarcomas. The relative incidence of the different histological types in several series is shown in Table 1, and survival following surgical treatment of the primary tumor is shown in Table 2. The survival from the time of discovery of the first metastases has not been well documented for untreated patients or for patients treated with single agents. However, Gottlieb mentioned a survival of 6 months after establishing metastatic disease in patients with soft tissue sarcoma who received no treatment, versus a median survival of 8 months for patients on adriamycin. These latter data were gathered from nonrandomized trials.

In order to provide an overview of current therapeutic efforts, we have compiled information on the treatment protocols and the therapeutic results of the major randomized trials in the area of soft tissue sarcomas. Unless otherwise indicated, a partial response was defined as a 50% or greater decrease in the product of perpendicular diameters of measurable lesions for a minimum of 4 weeks with no increase in any other indicator lesions, and without appearance of new lesions. In complete response there was disappearance of all evidence of disease.

Received December 29, 1976.

TABLE 1. Relative incidence of histologic types of soft tissue sarcomas

| | Pack and Ariel (8) | Martin et al. (7) | Hare and Cerny (6) | Shieber and Graham (12) | Ferrell and Frable (4) | Stout and Lattes (13) | Average |
|---|---|---|---|---|---|---|---|
| Unclassified | 36.4 | 14.8 | 28.5 | — | — | — | 13.3 |
| Liposarcoma | 14.6 | 26.9 | 11.5 | 16.0 | 17.0 | 24.6 | 18.4 |
| Rhabdomyosarcoma | 13.9 | 20.6 | 5.0 | 16.0 | 30.0 | 10.3 | 16.0 |
| Synoviosarcoma | 8.4 | 3.0 | 2.5 | 0.8 | 2.5 | 4.3 | 3.6 |
| Kaposi's sarcoma | 6.7 | 1.0 | — | — | 6.0 | 3.1 | 2.8 |
| Neurilemmal sarcoma | 6.4 | — | — | 3.2 | — | 4.3 | 2.3 |
| Fibrosarcoma | 5.4 | 24.1 | 43.0 | 44.0 | 33.0 | 24.8 | 29.1 |
| Dermatofibrosarcoma protuberans | 5.4 | — | 3.0 | — | — | — | 1.4 |
| Angiosarcoma | 2.6 | 0.3 | — | 4.8 | — | 3.2 | 1.3 |
| Leiomyosarcoma | — | 6.3 | 6.5 | 6.4 | 4.0 | 5.9 | 3.9 |
| Mesenchymoma | — | — | — | — | — | 8.1 | 1.4 |
| Other | — | 3.0 | — | 8.8 | 7.5 | 11.4 | 3.2 |
| Total cases | 717 | 398 | 200 | 125 | 117 | 1,771 | 3,328 |

TABLE 2. Survival following surgical treatment of soft tissue sarcomas

| | Pack and Ariel (8) 5-yr NED | Martin et al. (7) 5-yr survival | Hare and Cerny (6) | | Shieber and Graham (12) 5-yr survival | Ferrell and Frable (4) | |
|---|---|---|---|---|---|---|---|
| | | | 5-yr survival | 10-yr survival | | 5-yr survival | 10-yr survival |
| Unclassified | 39.2 | 43 | 39 | 30 | — | — | |
| Liposarcoma | 40.8 | 47 | 78 | 53 | 27 | 77 | 64 |
| Rhabdomyosarcoma | 35.9 | 26 | 10 | 0 | 8 | 29 | 25 |
| Synoviosarcoma | 21.6 | 40 | — | — | | — | — |
| Malignant neurilemmoma | 59.4 | 20 | — | — | | — | — |
| Fibrosarcoma | 55.6 | 44 | 60 | 43 | 39 | 82 | 73 |
| Dermatofibrosarcoma protuberans | 69.1 | | 100 | 100 | | — | |
| Kaposi's sarcoma | 28.6 | | | | | — | — |
| Hemangiosarcoma | 27.3 | | | | — | — | — |
| Overall | 39.2 (of 418) | 39.8 (of 183) | 39% (of 200) | | | | |

## ADRIAMYCIN VERSUS CYCLOLEUCINE (EASTERN COOPERATIVE ONCOLOGY GROUP, EST 1372)

*Objective:* The objective of this study was to compare the effectiveness of adriamycin to that of cycloleucine (NSC 1026) (9).

*Pretreatment:* Unknown.

*Extent of disease:* Unknown.

*Stratification:* The patients were stratified according to the following tumor groups: (a) fibrous tissue origin; (b) fatty tissue origin; (c) muscle origin; (d) vascular origin; and (e) unclassified origins.

*Randomization:* After stratification the patients were randomized to either adriamycin, 20 mg/m² i.v. daily X 3 every 3 weeks, or cycloleucine, 300 mg/kg/day i.v. for 8 days (repeated every 28 days) (Table 3).

Later the dose of cycloleucine was reduced to 200 mg/kg because of central nervous system toxicity. The patients were crossed over to the other arm after failure on the first arm. Most of the tumors were of fibrous or muscle tissue origin.

*Number of patients entered on study:* Although at the time of the original abstract a total number of 160 patients have been treated, the number entered on the study had increased to 232 patients at the time the study was terminated.

*Conditions for evaluability:* Not specified.

*Number of evaluable patients:* 172.

*Treatment results:* The response rates to adriamycin and to cycloleucine were 17.6% and 12.3%, respectively. The difference between these numbers was not statistically significant.

*Toxicity:* There was serious central nervous system toxicity in the group of patients treated with cycloleucine.

*Discussion:* The results of this study have not been published.

## ADRIAMYCIN PLUS DTIC VERSUS CYCLOPHOSPHAMIDE, VINCRISTINE PLUS METHOTREXATE (MILAN, WHO)

This study was part of a larger WHO study in which combination regimens including DTIC were studied in malignant melanomas, soft tissue sarcomas, and Hodgkin's disease (2).

*Objective:* Because of the favorable results obtained by Gottlieb with adriamycin plus DTIC in soft tissue sarcomas and sarcomas originating in the bones, Beretta et al. started a controlled study at the National Cancer Institute of

TABLE 3. *Outline of treatments: adriamycin versus cycloleucine (9)*

| Drug | Dose and schedule | Rest period |
|------|-------------------|-------------|
| Adriamycin | 20 mg/m², d1–3 | d4–21 |
| Cycloleucine | 300 mg/kg, d1–8 | d9–28 |

TABLE 4. *Outline of treatments: ADIC versus CPA–VCR–MTX (2)*

| Intravenous treatment | Dose and schedule | Rest period |
|---|---|---|
| Regimen I | | |
| Adriamycin | 60 mg/m², d1 | d6–21 |
| DTIC | 250 mg/m², d1–5 | |
| Regimen II | | |
| Cyclophosphamide | 1 g/m², d1 | |
| Vincristine | 1.4 mg/m², d1, 8 | d6–21 |
| Methotrexate | 20 mg/m², d1, 8 | |

Milan to test the therapeutic effects and cross-resistance of two independent combinations in patients with advanced soft tissue sarcomas.

*Previous treatment:* Not specified.

*Extent of disease:* The extent of disease was not indicated precisely, but the performance status was greater than 40 in all patients and the life expectancy was greater than 4 weeks.

*Stratification:* There was no stratification prior to randomization of the patients.

*Randomization:* Table 4 outlines the treatment schemes. After random allocation, treatment was continued in both groups until either progression or relapse after an initial response was evident. In the absence of severe myelosuppression, each cycle was repeated on day 22. In the presence of moderate myelosuppression (decrease in leukocyte count to levels between 2,000 and 3,999 cells/mm³), the dose of each drug was decreased by 50%. In 3 patients crossover was carried out automatically because the total dose of adriamycin was approaching 550 to 600 mg/m². On further progression after secondary treatment, actinomycin D was administered (1.5 to 2 mg/m²/week).

*Number of patients entered on study:* The total number of patients entered on study was 63.

TABLE 5. *Response to primary treatment*

| | ADIC | CPA–VCR–MTX |
|---|---|---|
| No. of patients entered | 31 | 32 |
| No. of patients evaluable | 21 | 28 |
| CR | 19% | 11% |
| PR | 38% | 4% |
| Objective improvements | 29% | 28% |
| CR + PR | 57% | 15% |
| Total responses | 86% | 43% |
| Median duration in mo. (range) of | | |
| CR | 7.5 (3 − 10+) | 10 (2+ − 13+) |
| PR | 3 (1+ − 9+) | 2 |
| CR + PR | 5 (1+ − 10+) | 6 (2 − 13+) |

*Conditions for patient evaluability:* Patients were considered evaluable if they received a minimum of two cycles of either of the two regimens.

*Number of evaluable patients:* 49.

*Treatment results:* Data on the response rate of the two regimens are given in Table 5. The total response rate of ADIC was 57%, which is significantly higher than the 15% response rate obtained with CPA–VCR–MTX. The number of complete remissions on ADIC was 4, whereas that on CPA–VCR–MTX was 3. The numbers of total or partial remissions were 8 and 1, respectively. The median duration of survival for complete and partial responders was 10+ months for the ADIC regimen and 9+ for the CPA–VCR–MTX regimen. In nonresponders these medians were 6 and 5.5 months, respectively. Response as related to the histologic subgroups is shown in Table 6. In the DIC group, 5 of 5 patients with undifferentiated histologic type responded, whereas only 1 of 6 patients with fibrosarcoma responded.

After crossing over, ADIC was given to 17 patients. A short-term remission was induced in only 2 of these patients (during 1 and 5 months, respectively). Secondary therapy with the triple combination induced a remission in 1 of 7 patients who relapsed on ADIC.

*Toxicity:* Besides the toxic effects related to vincristine (paresthesias) and cyclophosphamide (cystitis), thrombocytopenia, mucositis, and alopecia were more often encountered during ADIC than during CPA–VCR–MTX. No patient showed cardiomyopathy, and there were no drug-related deaths. The percentage of optimal dose administered was adriamycin, 92%; DTIC, 91%; cyclophosphamide, 85%; methotrexate, 81%; and vincristine, 82%.

*Conclusion of the authors:* The combination of adriamycin plus DTIC is superior to the triple combination of the three conventional agents, and this is probably due to the fact that adriamycin combined with DTIC is synergistic in man as well as in experimental systems.

*Discussion:* The weak point of the study is the limited number of patients in both arms. It is doubtful if the results on the remission duration are of any

TABLE 6. *CR + PR related to histologic subgroups*

| Histologic type | No. of responses/total no. of evaluable patients receiving | |
|---|---|---|
| | ADIC | CPA–VCR–MTX |
| Undifferentiated | 5/5 | 0/3 |
| Fibrosarcoma | 1/6 | 1/7 |
| Leiomyosarcoma | 1/1 | 0/3 |
| Liposarcoma | 2/2 | 0/5 |
| Rhabdomyosarcoma | 1/2 | 1/5 |
| Synovial cell sarcoma | 0/2 | — |
| Angiosarcoma | — | 1/2 |
| Neurofibrosarcoma | 2/3 | 0/2 |

significance as there are only 4 responding patients in the CPA–VCR–MTX arm.

## VINCRISTINE, ADRIAMYCIN PLUS DTIC (VADIC) VERSUS VINCRISTINE, ACTINOMYCIN D PLUS CYCLOPHOSPHAMIDE (VAC) VERSUS METHYL CCNU (MAYO CLINICS)

*Objective:* Comparison of three regimens (Table 7) in patients with advanced sarcomas (3).

*Previous chemotherapy:* Very few patients (only 5) had received prior chemotherapy.

*Extent of disease:* 73 of the 80 patients had visceral-dominant disease and 6 had only bone or soft tissue sarcomas.

*Stratification:* There was no stratification.

*Randomization:* The patients were randomized to one of the three treatment groups. With progression the patients were randomized to one of the alternative two other arms. Treatment was repeated every 5 weeks for regimens I and II and every 7 weeks for regimen III. Because of objective progression, 50 patients were randomized to the alternative regimens. Methyl CCNU was excluded from the study after 11 consecutive patients failed to respond.

*Patients entered on study:* 80. There were 42 males and 38 females.

*Conditions for evaluability:* The patients were considered evaluable for response after they received a minimum of one treatment cycle. Other conditions for evaluability are unknown. All 80 patients entered on study were evaluable.

*Treatment results:* The VADIC regimen gave a response rate of 11% in 31 patients, whereas 8% of 38 patients responded to primary treatment with VAC. After crossing over to VADIC, 3 of 23 (13%) patients responded; the corresponding number for those crossing over to VAC was 2 of 23 (9%) patients. No patient responded on methyl CCNU.

*Conclusion of the authors:* The authors conclude that their findings in both

TABLE 7. *Outline of treatments: VCR-ADM-DTIC versus VCR-ACD-CPR versus methyl CCNU*

| Treatment | Dose and schedule | Rest period |
|---|---|---|
| Regimen I | | |
| Vincristine | 1.2 mg/m², i.v., d1, + 5 | d5–35 |
| Adriamycin | 50 mg/m², i.v., d3 | |
| DTIC | 250 mg/m², i.v., d1–5 | |
| Regimen II | | |
| Vincristine | 1.2 mg/m², i.v., d1, 5 | d5–35 |
| Actinomycin D | 325 µg/m², i.v., d1–5 | |
| Cyclophosphamide | 250 mg/m², i.v., d1, 3, 5 | |
| Regimen III | | |
| Methyl-CCNU | 200 mg/m², d1, orally | d2–49 |

regimens are disappointing as compared to previous data published in the literature.

*Discussion:* The response rate to the VADIC regimen is indeed very low as compared to that of the ADIC regimen of the previous study. Although the response rates for ADIC are higher in the previous studies than one would expect from data from nonrandomized studies, the results of the Mayo Clinics have probably been influenced by (a) the long intervals between each cycle, (b) the administration of adriamycin on day 3 of each cycle, and (c) the fact that the patients have been evaluated after only 1 cycle of treatment. In nonrandomized studies it has been shown that remissions may be seen after 2 or even 3 cycles of ADIC. Because of the low number of responders, no meaningful data could be obtained for remission duration or duration of survival. It should also be mentioned that 16 of the 80 patients had osteosarcoma.

This is one of the few studies in which all patients have been evaluated by a single center.

## CYCLOPHOSPHAMIDE, VINCRISTINE, ADRIAMYCIN PLUS DTIC (CYVADIC) VERSUS CYCLOPHOSPHAMIDE, VINCRISTINE, ADRIAMYCIN PLUS ACTINOMYCIN D (CYVADACT) (SOUTH WESTERN ONCOLOGY GROUP, SWOG 7402)

*Objective:* Comparison of two four-drug regimens (Table 8). The South Western Oncology Group has previously shown in a nonrandomized trial (SWOG 7302) that CYVADIC gives a 59% response rate in soft tissue sarcomas (5). However, in the SWOG 7402 trials cyclophosphamide and adriamycin have been administered on day 2 instead of on day 1, because it has been shown that vincristine and cyclophosphamide are synergistic in an experimental system when vincristine is administered 1 day prior to the cyclophosphamide. In addition, vincristine was given weekly in this SWOG 7402 trial, starting on day 1. The purpose of the study was to evaluate if DTIC could be replaced by actinomycin D (1).

*Previous chemotherapy:* Eight patients were considered ineligible because they had received prior chemotherapy with agents used in the protocol.

*Extent of disease:* Not specified.

*Stratification:* Prior to randomization the patients had been stratified on histological types and bone marrow reserve.

*Randomization:* The patients were randomized to one of the two arms as indicated in Table 8. The doses were reduced to 80% of the initial dose in the case of an inadequate marrow reserve.

*Number of patients entered:* The number of patients entered on CYVADIC was 282 and on CYVADACT 271.

*Conditions of patient evaluability:* The patients were evaluated for responses after two courses of treatment had been given. There were 221 fully evaluable patients on CYVADIC and 225 patients on CYVADACT.

TABLE 8. *CYVADIC versus CYVADACT (SWOG-7402)*[a]

| Drugs | Regimen used with | |
|---|---|---|
| | Adequate marrow reserve | Inadequate marrow reserve |
| Regimen I | | |
| Cyclophosphamide | 500 mg/m², d2 (i.v.) | 400 mg/m², d2 (i.v.) |
| Vincristine | 1.5 mg/m² (top dose 2 mg), d1 and weekly X 7 wks | 1.5 mg/m² (top dose 2 mg), d1 and weekly X 7 wks |
| Adriamycin | 50 mg/m², d2 | 40 mg/m², d2 |
| DTIC | 250 mg/m²/day, d1–5 | 200 mg/m²/day, 1–5 |
| Regimen II | | |
| Cyclophosphamide | 500 mg/m², d2 (i.v.) | 400 mg/m², d2 (i.v.) |
| Vincristine | 1.5 mg/m² (top dose 2 mg), d1 and weekly X 7 wks | 1.5 mg/m² (top dose 2 mg), d1 and weekly X 7 wks |
| Adriamycin | 50 mg/m², d2 | 40 mg/m², d2 |
| Actinomycin D | 0.3 mg/m²/day (top daily dose 0.5 mg), d3–5 | 0.2 mg/m²/day (top daily dose 0.3 mg), d3–5 |

[a] All patients stratified by histologic cell type and marrow reserve status prior to randomization. Regimen repeated at 3-week intervals if blood counts have recovered.

*Treatment results:* In Table 9 the response rates are shown in both eligible and evaluable patients. The total response rate on CYVADIC was 50% and on CYVADACT 39%, with 14 and 12% complete responders, respectively. The difference in response rate was statistically significant ( $p = 0.02$ ). In both studies 72% of the patients responded with either a remission or remained stable.

Duration of remission on CYVADIC was significantly longer than on CYVADACT ( $p = 0.03$ ). The median duration of complete remission on CYVADIC had not been reached when the data on this study were presented at the Meetings of the American Society of Clinical Oncology in May 1976 but could not be less than 7 months and was projected to be 14 months. The median duration of complete remission on CYVADACT was 5.5 months. The median duration of partial remissions was 5 months for CYVADIC and 4 months for CYVADACT. The median duration of survival of patients responding to CYVADIC was 19 months, which was superior to the corresponding 12 months for patients on CYVADACT ( $p = 0.005$ ). The median duration of survival for complete responders on both regimens had not been reached at the time the data were presented. Response rates of different histologic types did not differ significantly, either in the CYVADIC arm or in the CYVADACT arm.

*Toxicity:* The toxicity of patients on CYVADIC did not differ significantly from that of patients on CYVADACT.

*Conclusion of the authors:* The conclusion of the authors was that the addition

TABLE 9. *Outline of treatments. Induction: ADM versus ADM-VCR-DEX; mainte-nance CBL-ARAC versus CBL-ARAC-ADM-VCR-DEX*

| Treatment | Dose and schedule |
|---|---|
| *Induction treatment* | |
| Regimen I | |
|   Adriamycin | 40 mg/m² i.v., d1, 14, and 28 |
| Regimen II | |
|   Adriamycin | 40 mg/m² i.v., d1, 14, and 28 |
|   Vincristine | 1 mg/m², i.v., d1, 7, 14, and 21 |
|   Dexamethasone | 10 mg/m² orally/day |
| *Maintenance treatment* | |
| Regimen III | |
|   Chlorambucil | 4 mg/m² orally/day |
|   Cytosine arabinoside | 40 mg/m² s.c., weekly |
| Regimen IV | |
|   Chlorambucil | 4 mg/m² orally/day |
|   Cytosine arabinoside | 40 mg/m² s.c., weekly |
|   Adriamycin | 30 mg/m² i.v., q.4w. |
|   Vincristine | 1 mg/m² i.v., q.4w. |
|   Dexamethasone | 10 mg/m² orally/day |

of DTIC to the three-drug combination of adriamycin, cyclophosphamide, and vincristine is superior to the addition of actinomycin D in terms of remission rate, remission duration, and survival. Adriamycin and DTIC form the backbone of the most active combination regimens available at present.

*Discussion:* There are various interesting points to be discussed in this study. As with most studies in soft tissue sarcomas in which large numbers of patients are evaluated, many centers participated. It is well known that this will have some influence, especially on evaluation of the responses. Apparently the protocol did not exclude patients without measurable disease from entering the study. Also, the number of patients that were ineligible was unacceptably high in both treatment arms. Of the eligible patients 19% were nonevaluable.

Second, the 50% response rate is lower than the 59% response rate that had been achieved with soft tissue sarcomas in the previous nonrandomized CYVADIC protocol (SWOG 7302). One might explain this difference in response rates on the basis of differences in the schedules of the two CYVADIC regimens. The lower response rate for CYVADACT again could be attributed to the same phenomenon, whereas in addition there are indications of an existing antagonism between adriamycin and actinomycin D. We think the response rates of the eligible patients, which were 42 and 34%, respectively, should also be emphasized and should raise the question as to whether the CYVADIC regimen is better than the ADIC regimen, which gave a response rate of 46% in a nonrandomized study performed in the South Western Oncology Group, and a 57% response rate in the study performed by Beretta et al.

## ADRIAMYCIN VERSUS ADRIAMYCIN PLUS VINCRISTINE AND CORTICOSTEROIDS IN INDUCTION TREATMENT; CHLORAMBUCIL, CYTOSINE ARABINOSIDE VERSUS CHLORAMBUCIL, CYTOSINE ARABINOSIDE PLUS ADRIAMYCIN, VINCRISTINE, AND CORTICOSTEROIDS IN MAINTENANCE TREATMENT (SCHWEIZERISCHE ARBEITSGRUPPE FUR KLINISCHE KREBSFORSCHUNG, SAKK 23/72)

*Objective:* The primary objective of this study was to compare the response rates to adriamycin and to a combination regimen of adriamycin, vincristine, and corticosteroids for remission induction in inoperable and/or disseminated soft tissue sarcoma (10,11). In addition, the results of maintenance treatment as described below were evaluated.

*Previous treatment:* Four patients had received prior chemotherapy.

*Extent of disease:* Not specified.

*Stratification:* There was no stratification prior to randomization.

*Randomization:* Patients were randomized to receive either adriamycin, 40 mg/m$^2$ i.v. on days 1, 14, and 28 of the treatment schedule (regimen I) or, in addition, vincristine, 1 mg/m$^2$ i.v. on days 1, 7, 14, and 21, and dexamethasone, 10 mg/m$^2$ p.o. daily (regimen II).

After induction treatment, patients without tumor progression were again randomized for maintenance treatment, consisting of either chlorambucil plus cytosine arabinoside (regimen III) or, in addition, monthly pulse doses of adriamycin, vincristine, and corticosteroids (regimen IV) (Table 10). Maintenance treatment was terminated when tumor progression occurred.

*Number of patients entered on study:* There were 50 patients, 23 men and 27 women, with a mean age of 49 and 50.4 years on regimens I and II, respectively.

*Conditions for evaluation:* Patients were considered evaluable if treatment had been continued up to day 35.

TABLE 10. *Outline of treatments: ADM versus VCR–CPA–ADM and VCR–CPA–ACD*

| Intravenous treatment | Dose and schedule |
|---|---|
| Regimen I | |
| Adriamycin | 70 mg/m$^2$ q.3w. |
| Regimen II | |
| Vincristine | 1.4 mg/m$^2$ q.3w. |
| Cyclophosphamide | 750 mg/m$^2$ q.3w. |
| Adriamycin | 50 mg/m$^2$ q.3w. |
| Regimen III | |
| Vincristine | 1.4 mg/m$^2$ q.3w. |
| Cyclophosphamide | 750 mg/m$^2$ q.3w. |
| Actinomycin D | 0.4 mg/m$^2$ q.3w. |

*Number of evaluable patients:* 44.

*Toxicity:* There were 2 cardiac deaths possibly related to adriamycin after total doses of 230 and 410 mg, respectively, had been administered.

*Treatment results:* Induction treatment: there were no complete remissions. The partial response rates showed a statistically significant ($p < 0.01$) difference for patients on regimen I and II: 13% (3/25) and 47% (9/19), respectively.

Maintenance treatment: median duration of remission was only 2 ½ months after both induction regimens. Median survival was 6+ months. A significant difference in survival was found between patients showing primary tumor progression with a median survival of only 3 months, and patients attaining either partial remission or objectively stable disease, with a median survival of 10+ months.

The percentage of patients with partial remission or stable disease that will survive for 2 years or more is expected to be about 25%.

*Conclusion of the authors:* On account of the unfavorable results in terms of complete remission rate and duration of remission, possibly partly due to suboptimal dosage of adriamycin, a second study (SAKK 23/75) is ongoing with other drug combinations.

*Discussion:* Comparison with other studies is difficult because in the Swiss study partial remission was defined as a 25% or greater decrease in cross-sectional areas of measurable lesions. When more stringent criteria are applied, as in most studies, the partial remission rate would have been even less. The fact that six centers participated in this study with less than 50 patients may have made uniform evaluation difficult.

One wonders if there were more complications of treatment in regimen IV than in regimen III, as a result of the long-term dexamethasone administration.


# ADRIAMYCIN; VINCRISTINE, CYCLOPHOSPHAMIDE, AND ADRIAMYCIN VERSUS VINCRISTINE, CYCLOPHOSPHAMIDE, AND ACTINOMYCIN D (EASTERN COOPERATIVE ONCOLOGY GROUP, EST 2374)


*Objective:* The objective of this study was to compare the response rate of (a) adriamycin as a single agent, (b) vincristine, cyclophosphamide, and adriamycin, and (c) vincristine, cyclophosphamide, and actinomycin D. When progression was observed on regimen I, treatment was switched to regimen III. In the case of progression on regimen II the treatment was continued with actinomy-cin D as a single agent (0.4 mg/m$^2$, days 1 to 5, q. 28 days). Progression during treatment with regimen III led to a change to adriamycin as a single agent (70 mg/m$^2$, q. 3 weeks). The study included osteogenic sarcoma and Ewing's sarcoma.

*Stratification:* Patients were stratified to: (1) the initial performance status; (2) tissue type, and (3) extent of disease. The tissue type included four groups: (a) chondrosarcoma, (b) Ewing's sarcoma and mesothelioma, (c) osteogenic sarcoma and liposarcoma, and (d) fibrosarcoma, leiomyosarcoma, angiosarcoma, and undifferentiated sarcoma.

*Randomization:* The patients were randomized to one of the three treatment groups (Table 10).

*Number of patients entered on study:* A total of 206 patients had been entered in the study, which has been closed to accrual, by September 15, 1976. Conditions for patients to enter the study were (a) progression of primary disease after the definite surgery and/or radiation, or recurrence at the primary site with no possible surgical treatment, or distant metastases; (b) measurable disease had to be present and might include both pulmonary and osteolytic lesions; and (c) all patients should have recovered from surgery and an interval of at least 4 weeks since prior radiation or chemotherapy should have passed.

*Conditions for patient evaluability:* Patients with stable disease should receive three full courses in order to be evaluable; with progressive disease, two full courses are considered sufficient.

*Number of evaluable patients:* 115. There were no evaluable patients with osteogenic sarcoma or Ewing's sarcoma.

*Treatment results:* Of the 39 patients on adriamycin alone, 11 (28%) showed a response, 3 of whom had a complete remission. The response rate for patients on vincristine, adriamycin, and cyclophosphamide was 13% (5/38) and for those on vincristine, actinomycin D, and cyclophosphamide 5% (2/38), with 1 patient showing a complete remission in both groups.

The median duration of response for all responders was 5 months. Median survival for responders was 15 months as compared to 8 months for nonresponders.

The number of patients in each histopathological group was too small to evaluate response in a given tissue type.

*Toxicity:* There was no difference in toxicity among the three groups. Three episodes of life-threatening toxicity were encountered with adriamycin, whereas one such episode occurred with each of the combination regimens.

*Conclusion of the authors:* From the data available thus far, the study chairman concludes that treatment with vincristine, actinomycin D, and cyclophosphamide is inferior to the other two regimens. Adriamycin alone is expected to give better statistically significant results than the combination treatment with adriamycin, vincristine, and cyclophosphamide; the difference in adriamycin dose may account for the difference in response rate.

*Discussion:* Although a final analysis of the data is not yet possible, results seem inferior to the ADIC and CYVADIC regimens.

The authors are planning a new study, with high-dose methotrexate with leucovorin rescue in one of the treatment arms.

## ACTINOMYCIN D VERSUS CYCLOPHOSPHAMIDE IN KAPOSI'S SARCOMA (UGANDA CANCER INSTITUTE)

*Objective:* Actinomycin D and cyclophosphamide were compared as single agents in patients with florid and infiltrative types of Kaposi's sarcoma (15). Thus, patients with nodular and lymphadenopathic disease were excluded from the study.

*Previous treatment:* None.

*Extent of disease:* There were only 2 patients with regional lymphnode metastases; the others had localized disease. However, several patients had local infiltration of bone.

*Stratification:* None.

*Randomization:* The patients were selected at random to receive one of the following three treatment regimens: (a) actinomycin D, 370 $\mu g/m^2$/day i.v. until toxicity occurred; (b) cyclophosphamide, 370 mg/m$^2$/day i.v. for 5 days; and (c) cyclophosphamide, 370 mg/m$^2$/day orally for 5 days. Patients with evidence of tumor regression after the first course of therapy were given additional courses of the same regimen until complete regression or relapse. If there was a reduction of less than 50% in tumor size after the second course, the patients were considered treatment failures and crossed over to an alternative regimen. Cyclophosphamide failures subsequently received actinomycin D, whereas actinomycin D failures received one of the cyclophosphamide regimens.

*Number of patients entered:* 14.

*Conditions for evaluability:* All patients were evaluated after one course of treatment.

*Number of evaluable patients:* 14.

*Treatment results:* Of the 14 patients treated, 6 initially received actinomycin D and 8 received cyclophosphamide. Of the 6 patients initially treated with actinomycin D, there were 1 complete and 2 partial remissions. The other 3 patients failed to respond. Of the 8 patients receiving cyclophosphamide (either intravenously or orally), one had tumor regression. Six of 7 patients failing to respond to cyclophosphamide were treated with actinomycin D, and of these 1 had a complete remission and 5 a partial remission. Two patients who initially failed to respond to actinomycin D therapy also failed to respond to cyclophosphamide.

*Conclusion of the authors:* When combining the results a total of 10 patients received cyclophosphamide, of whom only one responded to treatment. However, of 12 patients treated with actinomycin D, 9 showed a partial or complete tumor regression. The 2 patients with complete remission remained free of tumor 44+ and 54+ weeks from the start of therapy. Three patients with partial remission remained in remission. Their duration of remission was 24+, 20+, and 28+ weeks. The remaining 4 patients with partial remission relapsed during therapy.

In general, patients with florid tumors showing the mixed or monocellular histological pattern responded well to therapy. Of 3 patients with florid tumors showing the anaplastic variant pattern, only one showed a transient response. Four patients with infiltrative lesions (associated with underlying bone lesions) responded slowly or not at all.

*Discussion:* This study demonstrated that actinomycin D was more effective than cyclophosphamide in the treatment of florid and infiltrative types of Kaposi's sarcoma. The authors do not mention clearly the interval between each cycle of treatment. Neither is it clear if treatment was discontinued at the moment complete remission had been reached or whether a few additional cycles were given.

## ACTINOMYCIN D VERSUS VINCRISTINE PLUS ACTINOMYCIN D IN KAPOSI'S SARCOMA (UGANDA CANCER INSTITUTE)

This study has been published as an abstract (14). The conclusion of the study was that in the 25 patients randomized, a combination of actinomycin

D and vincristine was superior to actinomycin D used alone. No further discussion is possible on this study.

## REFERENCES

1. Benjamin, R. S., Gottlieb, J. A., Baker, L. O., and Sinkovics, J. G. (1976): CYVADIC vs CYVADACT—A randomized trial of cyclophosphamide (CY), and adriamycin (A), plus dacarbazine (DIC), or actinomycin D (DACT) in metastatic sarcomas. *Proc. Am. Assoc. Cancer Res.,* 17:256.
2. Beretta, G., Bonadonna, G., Bajetta, E., Tancini, G., De Lena, M., Azzarelli, A., and Veronesi, U. (1976): Combination chemotherapy with DTIC (NSC-45388) in advanced malignant melanoma, soft tissue sarcomas, and Hodgkin's disease. *Cancer Treatment Rep.,* 60:205–211.
3. Cregan, E. T., Hahn, R. G., Ahmann, D. L., Edmonson, J. H., Bisel, H. F., and Eagan, R. T. (1977): A comparative clinical trial evaluating the combination adriamycin (NSC-123127), imidazole carboxamide (NSC-45388), vincristine (NSC-67574); the combination actinomycin (NSC-3053), cyclophosphamide (NSC-26271), vincristine, and a single agent, methyl-CCNU (NSC-95441), in advanced sarcomas. *Cancer Treatment Rep. (in press).*
4. Ferrell, H. W., and Frable, W. J. (1972): Soft part sarcomas revisited. Review and comparison of a second series. *Cancer,* 30:475–480.
5. Gottlieb, J. A., Baker, L. H., O'Bryan, R. M., Sinkovics, J. G., Hoogstraten, B., Quagliana, J. M., Rivkin, S. E., Bodey, G. P., Sr., Rodriguez, V. T., Blumenschein, G. R., Saiki, J. H., Coltman, C., Jr., Burgess, M. A., Sullivan, P., Thigpen, T., Bottomley, R., Bakerzak, S., and Moon, T. E. (1975): Adriamycin (NSC-123127) used alone and in combination for soft tissue and bony sarcomas. *Cancer Treatment Rep.,* Part 3, 6:271–282.
6. Hare, H. F., and Cerny, M. F. (1963): Soft tissue sarcoma: A review of 200 cases. *Cancer,* 16:1332–1337.
7. Martin, R. G., Butler, J. J., and Albores-Saavedra, J. (1965): Soft tissue tumors: Surgical treatment and results. In: *Tumors of Bone and Soft Tissue.* At the 8th Annual Clinical Conference on Cancer, 1963, at the University of Texas, Anderson Hospital and Tumor Institute, Houston Texas.
8. Pack, G. T., and Ariel, I. M. (1965): *Treatment of Cancer and Allied Diseases, Vol. VIII, Tumors of the Soft Somatic Tissues and Bone,* edited by G. T. Pack and I. M. Ariel. Harper & Row, New York.
9. Savlov, E. D., Knight, E., and Costello, W. (1974): Study of adriamycin versus cycloleucine in the treatment of sarcomas. *Proc. Am. Assoc. Cancer Res.,* 15:168.
10. Senn, H. J. (1974): Adriamycin versus adriamycin + vincristine + corticosteroids in the treatment of inoperable and/or disseminated soft tissue sarcomas (SAKK-study 23/72) 1974. *XIII Int. Cancer Congress, Florence, Italy.*
11. Senn, H. J., and Jungi, W. F. (1975): Adriamycin versus adriamycin + vincristine + corticosteroids bei disseminierten und/oder inoperablen Weichteilsarkomen. In: *Ergebnisse der Adriamycin-Therapie (Adriamycin Symposium Frankfurt am Main,* edited by M. Gione, J. Fetzer, and H. Maier. Springer-Verlag, Berlin/Heidelberg/New York.
12. Shieber, W., and Graham, P. (1962): An experience with sarcomas of the soft tissues in adults. *Surgery,* 52:295–398.
13. Stout, A. P., and Lattes, R. (1967): *Atlas of Tumor Pathology, Fascicle I,* Armed Forces Institute of Pathology Publishers, Washington, D.C.
14. Vogel, C. L., Dhru, D., Primack, A., and Kyalwazi, S. K. (1972): Chemotherapy of Kaposi's sarcoma. *Proc. Am. Assoc. Cancer Res.,* 13:49.

15. Vogel, C. L., Templeton, C. J., Templeton, A. C., Taylor, J. F., and Kyalwazi, S. K. (1972): Treatment of Kaposi's sarcoma with actinomycin D and cyclophosphamide: Results of a randomized clinical trial. *Int. J. Cancer,* 8:136–143.

*Randomized Trials in Cancer: A Critical Review by Sites,* edited by Maurice J. Staquet, Raven Press, New York © 1978.

# Malignant Gliomas

Jerzy Hildebrand and Claire Nouwynck

*Service de Médecine et Laboratoire d'Investigation Clinique Henri Tagnon, Institut Jules Bordet, 1000 Bruxelles, Belgium*

Today, surgery followed by radiation therapy may be considered as the standard treatment of malignant brain gliomas, despite the fact that this association almost invariably fails to cure the patient. Malignant brain gliomas are highly infiltrating, sometimes multifocal tumors involving a vital organ; their resection is therefore always incomplete. The benefit of neurosurgery has never been tested in prospective and randomized studies; and such a clinical approach even appears unrealistic for several reasons: (a) biopsy, which is *per se* a neurosurgical procedure, is a prerequisite for any randomized trial; (b) the extent of tumor resection, which is related to its nature (kystic, necrotic, vascular, etc.) and its location, is difficult to standardize; and (c) it would be difficult for many neurosurgeons to limit voluntarily the resection of the tumor in cases where the bulk of the neoplastic tissue can be easily removed. Retrospective analyses indicate that the survival time is longer and of better quality when the resection is exhaustive (10), and this is particularly true when patients who underwent a simple biopsy are compared with other types of resection.

Of course the difference may be due, at least partially, to the fact that limited resections are performed more frequently in elderly patients, or in most infiltrating, deeply located tumors, which have a poor prognosis.

This review is thus limited to randomized trials testing radiotherapy, chemotherapy, or immunotherapy in patients with histologically proven malignant gliomas.

## RADIATION THERAPY

The evidence that postoperative radiation therapy is able to prolong the survival time of patients with malignant brain glioma has been based for a long time on studies using historical controls (3,16). The favorable conclusions of these authors have been recently confirmed in randomized trials designed primarily to test chemotherapeutic agents or immunotherapy. Table 1 summarizes the main characteristics of these studies.

---

Received August 18, 1977.

TABLE 1. *Randomized trials testing radiation therapy in malignant brain gliomas*

| Dosage and schedule of radiation therapy | Number of patients | | Age mean (range) | Sex ratio M/F | Evaluation criteria | Therapeutic effect of radiation therapy | Reference |
|---|---|---|---|---|---|---|---|
| | Randomized (no. of arms) | Evaluated | | | | | |
| 6,000 rads whole head in 6–8 wks | — (4 arms) | 180 Controls BCNU (see Table 2) RT BCNU + RT | | — | Median survival | Increased from 17 to 28 mo ($p < 0.01$) (as compared to best supportive care) | Walker and Gehan, 1972, (21) |
| 5,000 rads in 25–28 fractions over 30 to 39 days, by parallel opposed fields | 75 (3 arms) | 63 22 p. CCNU alone 22 p. RT alone 19 p. RT + CCNU | 52.3 yr (31–70) 53 yr (22–70) 58 yr (47–77) | — | Median survival | Increased from 6.6 to 12 mo ($p < 0.02$) As compared to CCNU 130 mg/m² every 8 wks | Reagan et al., 1976, (12) |
| 5,000 rads | — (4 arms) | 65 10 received IMT 18 received IMT + RT 20 received RT 17 received supportive care | | — | Median survival | Increased from 5.4 to 7.5 mo ($p = 0.005$) | Trouillas, 1973 (17) |
| Average dose of 4,398 rads in 33 days whole-brain irradiation vs. average dose of 5,272 rads in 28 days limited-volume irradiation | — (2 arms) | 34 13 whole-brain RT 21 delineated RT | | — | Median survival | No difference: 11.6 mo vs. 11.5 mo (in randomized patients) | Ramsey and Brand, 1973 (11) |
| 3,000 rads in 9 fractions in 18 days vs. same RT + metronidazole 6 g/m² 4 hr before each radiation | 36 (2 arms) | 31 15 p. received RT 16 p. received RT + metronidazole | 54.5 yr ± 13.8 51.1 yr ± 10.7 | — | Median survival | Increased by 4½ mo ($p = 0.02$) | Urtasun, et al., 1976 (19) |

| | | | | | Median survival | Increase in the survival time not statistically significant | Shapiro and Young, 1976 (15) |
|---|---|---|---|---|---|---|---|
| 4,500 rads to the whole brain + 1,500 rads to the tumor | 33 (2 arms) | 33 | BCNU 80 mg/m$^2$ × 3 every 5–8 wks + VCR + RT | 58 yr | 11/6 | | |
| | | 17 | | | | | |
| | | 16 | BCNU: 80 mg/m$^2$ × 3 every 3–8 wks + VCR | 60 yr | 11/5 | | |

Abbreviations: RT, radiation therapy; IMT, immunotherapy.

The first randomized trial, showing a 65% increase in survival time after 6,000 rads postoperative radiotherapy, was reported by the NCI Brain Tumors Study Group (21).

Trouillas (17) also showed that postoperative 5,000 rads produced a 35% increase in the survival time.

In these two studies, patients treated by radiation therapy were compared to controls receiving best supportive care but no specific antineoplastic treatment other than surgery.

In a third study, performed at the Mayo Clinic (12), an 83% increase in survival time after radiations was demonstrated by comparing patients receiving CCNU alone to those treated with CCNU plus 5,000 rads.

The prolongation of survival time by radiation therapy was also observed by retrospective analysis of a randomized study aiming to test the effect of mithramycin (20).

In a recent study of Shapiro and Young (15), the addition of radiotherapy to BCNU and vincristine increased survival time by nearly 50%. The observed difference was not statistically significant, but the total number of patients included was relatively low (33 patients).

The dosage of radiotherapy usually varies from 4,500 to 6,000 rads. The best dosage remains to be established. It has not been demonstrated that 6,000 rads are superior to lower doses. On the other hand, 6,000 rads may be more toxic for brain tumors than 4,500 to 5,000 rads.

The choice of limited versus whole brain irradiation is another parameter that has been insufficiently investigated. In the study of Ramsey and Brand (11), the two types of radiation gave the same survival time in 34 randomized patients, whereas in 26 selected cases limited radiation was followed by a longer survival. However, the patients selected for small-field treatments were usually the most favorable cases. Perhaps a more precise localization of the tumoral tissue with the C.A.T. scan will allow a better selection of patients for limited versus whole brain irradiation.

Although radiosensitizers have been used previously in brain gliomas (13), the efficiency of one of them, metronidazole, has been demonstrated only recently in a prospective and randomized study (19). In this investigation, patients were stratified according to functional level, and radiotherapy was limited to 3,000 rads.

In summary, at least three randomized trials have confirmed that postoperative irradiation of 5,000 to 6,000 rads is able to produce a 35 to 82% increase in survival time of patients with malignant glioma. However, the choice of the best total dosage and delimitation of irradiation fields still remains to be established. Further, a recent randomized trial has indicated that the use of radiosensitizers (metronidazole) may be beneficial.

## CHEMOTHERAPY

Three parameters have been measured in chemotherapeutic trials performed in patients with brain glioma: (a) prolongation of survival time, (b) rate and importance of objective remission, and (c) prolongation of the free interval.

Randomized studies, summarized in Table 2, evaluating one of these parameters are few as compared to uncontrolled reports, which have been reviewed by Shapiro and Ausman (14).

### Studies Evaluating Survival Time

Starting from the operation day, the duration of survival time is remarkably constant in patients with malignant gliomas receiving only supportive care. In the randomized studies summarized in this chapter, the duration of the survival time was, respectively: 17 weeks (21), 24 weeks (17), 15 weeks (20), and 17 weeks (5). This parameter has been measured in at least five controlled trials (Table 2).

Two drugs, 5-fluorouracil (4) and mithramycin (20), have been found ineffective in prolonging survival time. Radiotherapy was given to all patients in the study with 5-fluorouracil and to some patients in the mithramycin investigation. The negative results found for mithramycin contrast with favorable data reported by Kennedy, Brown, and Yorbo (8).

Nitrosourea derivatives were tested in the three remaining trials. In the NCI Brain Tumors Study Group, BCNU has been found to prolong survival time when combined with radiation therapy but not when used alone (21). This group has recently confirmed the increase in survival time by BCNU-irradiation association over radiotherapy (6,000 rads) used alone, methyl-CCNU, or the combination of methyl-CCNU and radiation therapy (23). CCNU, the third currently used nitrosourea, has been found to prolong survival in a small group of selected patients by the E.O.R.T.C. Brain Tumor Group (5). However, this result was not confirmed by Reagan et al. (12). The discrepancy may be due to differences in patient selection, the scheduled doses of CCNU, and the dose of the drug actually given.

### Studies Evaluating the Rate and Length of Objective Remissions

This parameter is usually evaluated in patients with signs of brain tumor recurrence, in phase II-type studies where controls may be omitted if only one drug is tested. In such *nonrandomized* trials the three commonly used nitrosoureas, BCNU, CCNU, and methyl-CCNU, and procarbazine have been shown to produce objective remissions. The rate and length of these remissions are summarized in Table 3.

Randomized trials are necessary when the effects of two or more drugs are compared. An example of such a controlled investigation is provided by the study of Fewer et al. (6), demonstrating that the addition of vincristine to BCNU does not increase the rate of objective remissions in patients with recurring malignant brain gliomas.

TABLE 2. *Randomized trials testing chemotherapeutic drugs in malignant gliomas*

| Drug tested | Dosage Scheduled | Dosage Given | Number of patients Randomized (number of arms) | Number of patients Evaluated | Age mean (range) | Sex ratio M/F | Evaluation criteria | Therapeutic effect of chemotherapy | Reference |
|---|---|---|---|---|---|---|---|---|---|
| Mithramycin | 1st course: 25µg/kg/day for 21 days 2nd & 3rd course: 21 µg/kg/day | Median number of doses received: 21 | 116 (2 arms) | 96 52 treated by ChT 44 controls | 53 yr | 4/1 | Median survival (certain patients received RT) | None | Walker et al., 1976 (20) |
| 5-Fluorouracil | Single course 1st day 2nd day }10 mg/kg 3rd day 4th day 5 mg/kg | — | 32 (2 arms) | 32 15 treated by ChT 17 controls | Treated by ChT 50 yr (19–66) Controls 49 yr (30–63) | 2/1 | Median survival (all patients received RT) | None | Edland et al., 1971 (4) |
| CCNU | 130 mg/m² p.o. every 8 weeks | — | 75 (3 arms) | 63 22 received RT 22 received CCNU 19 received RT + CCNU | Treated by RT 52.3 yr (31–70) 53 yr (22–70) 58 yr (47–77) | | Median survival | None | Reagan et al., 1976 (12) |
| CCNU | 130 mg/m² p.o. every 3 weeks | — | 35 (3 arms) | 35 CCNU RT (4,500 rads) CCNU + RT | — | | Median time to progression (MPG or free interval) | Improved by RT + CCNU as compared to the two other groups where RT or CCNU were given before recurrence | Band et al., 1974 (1) |
| CCNU (trial 26741) | | 80% during free interval period | 100 (2 arms) | 81 45 received CCNU after surgery 36 controls received CCNU after relapse | 50 yr (21–71) | 1.6/1 | 1. Free interval 2. Rate of objective remissions | None 25% (4/16) | E.O.R.T.C. Brain Tumor Group, 1976 (5) |

| | Dose | Cures | No. (arms) | Arms/Patients | Age | | Endpoint | Results | Reference |
|---|---|---|---|---|---|---|---|---|---|
| (trial 26742) | 130 mg/m² p.o. every 6 weeks | — | 23 (2 arms) | 17 9 treated with CCNU 8 controls | 56 yr (20–72) | 1/2 | Median survival | Prolonged 33 weeks vs. 17 weeks in controls ($p < 0.05$) | Walker and Gehan, 1972 (21) |
| BCNU | 80 mg/m² for 3 days every 6 weeks | 2 cures or more | 180 (4 arms) | Controls BCNU RT BCNU + RT | | | Median survival | Not increased by BCNU alone Increased when BCNU combined with RT ($p < 0.1$) | |
| BCNU | 80 mg/m² for 3 days every 6–8 weeks | 2 cures or more | 332 (4 arms) | MeCCNU RT MeCCNU + RT BCNU + RT | | | Median survival | Increased by BCNU but not by MeCCNU as compared to RT alone | Walker and Strike, 1976 (23) |
| MeCCNU | 220 mg/m² one every 6–8 weeks | | | | | | | | |

TABLE 3. *Rate and length of remissions in malignant gliomas treated with single-agent chemotherapy*

| Treatment | Number of patients | Responses Rate (%) | Responses Duration (months) | Reference |
|---|---|---|---|---|
| BCNU: 80–90 mg/m² × 3 q. 6–8 wks | 57 | 47 | 9 | Wilson et al., 1976 (24) |
| BCNU: 100–125 mg/m²/day × 3 q. 6–8 wks | 16 | 60 | — | Walker and Hurwitz, 1970 (22) |
| CCNU: 120–130 mg/m² q. 6–8 wks | 36 | 44 | 6 | Wilson et al., 1976 (24) |
| CCNU: 150 mg/m² q. 6 wks | 24 | 29 | 7 (+) | E.O.R.T.C. Brain Tumor Group, 1976 (5) |
| CCNU: 130 mg/m² q. 6 wks | 16 malignant glioma 6 other glioma | 25 66 | 8 9 | Hildebrand et al., 1975 (7) |
| CCNU: 130 mg/m² q.8 wks | 17 | 24 | — | Reagan et al., 1976 (12) |
| Methyl–CCNU: 130–170 mg/m² q. 6–8 wks | 28 | 18 improved 32 stabilized | 8 (+) 8 (+) | Levine et al., 1974 (9) |
| Procarbazine: 150 mg/m²/day × 30 | 27 | 52 | 6 | Wilson et al., 1976 (24) |

## Studies Evaluating the Duration of the Free Interval

Free interval is the period that separates surgical removal from the relapse of neurological deterioration. It is not present in all individuals operated for brain glioma, but it can be measured with reasonable accuracy in a selected group of patients. The effect of CCNU on the duration of the free interval was investigated in two studies. The reported results are contradictory: in the E.O.R.T.C. Brain Tumor Group study (5) CCNU was found ineffective in prolonging the free interval, whereas in the study of Band et al. (1), the free interval (median time to progression) was increased. The scheduled doses of CCNU were the same in both studies and the discrepancy is difficult to explain. In the E.O.R.T.C. trial, the use of corticosteroids was not allowed before relapse, and the number of patients evaluated was larger as compared to the study of Band et al. (1).

In summary, in controlled and randomized studies, only nitrosourea derivatives have been found to have some activity against malignant brain glioma. Three parameters—(a) survival time after operation, (b) objective remission, and (c) free interval—have been measured in assays using nitrosoureas. The apparent discrepancy of the reported results may be due in part to the fact that the three parameters do not measure the same phenomenon but also to the fact that the activity of single drugs and associations tested so far is weak. The available data indicate that: (a) BCNU, CCNU, and methyl-CCNU used alone are able to produce objective remissions in patients with recurring signs of malignant glioma; (b) BCNU added to radiation therapy prolongs the postoperative survival time. The results of studies reporting the effects of CCNU on the survival time are conflicting, and this point requires additional investigation. (c) CCNU is probably ineffective in prolonging the free interval, at least when given at the actual dose of 106 mg/m$^2$ once every 6 weeks.

## IMMUNOTHERAPY

Two randomized and controlled studies testing active immunotherapy were performed so far and reported conflicting results (Table 4). Technical differences may account for this discrepancy. In the study of Trouillas (17), where 4 to 10 injections of saline tumor extract were given postoperatively, survival was prolonged by 35%. The use of corticosteroids was avoided in Trouillas' study, but Freund adjuvant was used. In the trial of Bloom et al. (2), one to three injections of irradiated tumor cells did not increase the survival time.

Interesting results were recently reported by Young, Kaplan, and Regelson (25) after intratumoral injections of autologous lymphocytes. The efficacy of this passive immunotherapy, however, requires further confirmation in controlled studies.

In summary, because of the limited number of studies and the conflicting results they report, the role of immunotherapy in the treatment of malignant gliomas cannot be assessed at the present time.

TABLE 4. *Randomized trials testing immunotherapy in malignant gliomas*

| Form and schedule of immunotherapy | Number of patients | | Evaluation criteria | Therapeutic effect of immunotherapy | Reference |
| | Randomized (arms) | Evaluated | | | |
| --- | --- | --- | --- | --- | --- |
| 4 to 10 injections of autologous tumors homogenate in saline + Freund's adjuvant | — (4 arms) | 65 {10 IMT<br>28 {18 IMT + RT<br>37 {20 RT<br>{17 controls | Median survival | Increased by 35% ($p < 0.005$) | Trouillas, 1973 (17) |
| Irradiated autologous tumor cells (15,000 rads)<br>17 p. had 1 inject.<br>1 p. had 2 inject.<br>9 p. had 3 inject. | 75 (2 arms) | 62<br>27 IMT<br>35 controls | Median survival | None | Bloom et al., 1973 (2) |

Abbreviations as in Table 1.

# REFERENCES

1. Band, P. R., Weir, B. K. A., Urtasun, R. C., Blain, G., McLean, D., Wilson, F., Mielke, B., and Grace, M. (1974): Radiotherapy and CCNU in grade III and IV astrocytoma. *ASCO Abstract,* 15:161.
2. Bloom, H. J. G., Peckham, M. J., Richardson, A. E., Alexander, P. A., and Payne, P. H. (1973): Glioblastoma multiforme: A controlled trial to assess the value of specific active immunotherapy in patients treated by radical surgery and radiotherapy. *Br. J. Cancer,* 27:253–267.
3. Bloor, R. J., Templeton, A. W., and Quick, R. S. (1962): Radiation therapy in treatment of intracranial tumors. *Am. J. Roentgenol. Radium Ther. Nucl. Med.,* 87:463–472.
4. Edland, R. W., Javid, M., and Ansfield, F. J. (1971): Glioblastoma multiforme. An analysis of the results of post operative radiotherapy alone versus radiotherapy and concomitant 5-fluorouracil. *Am. J. Roentgenol.,* III:337–342.
5. E.O.R.T.C. Brain Tumor Group (1976): Effect of CCNU on survival, rate of objective remission and duration of free interval in patients with malignant brain glioma. First evaluation. *Eur. J. Cancer,* 12:41–45.
6. Fewer, D., Wilson, C. B., Boldrey, E. B., Enot, K. J., and Powell, M. R. (1972): The chemotherapy of brain tumors: Clinical experience in the carmustine (BCNU) and vincristine. *JAMA,* 222:549–552.
7. Hildebrand, J., Brihaye, J., Wagenknecht, L., Michel, J., and Kenis, Y. (1973): Combination chemotherapy with CCNU, vincristine and methotrexate in primary and metastatic brain tumors. *Eur. J. Cancer,* 11:585–587.
8. Kennedy, B. J., Brown, J. H., and Yarbo, J. W. (1965): Mithramycin (NSC-24559) therapy for primary glioblastomas. *Cancer Chemother. Rep.,* 48:59–63.
9. Levine, M. A., Walker, M. D., and Weiss, H. D. (1974): Intravenous methyl-CCNU in the treatment of malignant glioma (phase II). *ASCO Abstracts,* p. 167.
10. Penman, J., and Smith, M. C. (1954): Intracranial gliomata. *Med. Res. Counc. (Lond.),* 384:1–70.
11. Ramsey, R. G., and Brand, W. N. (1973): Radiotherapy of glioblastoma multiforme. *J. Neurosurg.,* 39:197–202.
12. Reagan, T. J., Bisel, H. F., Childs, D. S., Jr., Layton, D. D., Jr., Rhoton, A. L., Jr., and Taylor, W. F. (1976): Controlled study of CCNU and radiation therapy in malignant astrocytoma. *J. Neurosurg.,* 44:186–190.
13. Sano, K., Sato, F., Hoshino, T., and Nagai, M. (1968): Radio sensitization of brain tumor cells with a thymidine analogue (bromouridine). *J. Neurosurg.,* 28:530–538.
14. Shapiro, W. R., and Ausman, J. I. (1969): The chemotherapy of brain tumors. A clinical and experimental review. In: *Recent Advances in Neurology,* edited by F. Plum, pp. 149–235. Davis, Philadelphia.
15. Shapiro, W. R., and Young, D. F. (1976): Treatment of malignant glioma. *Arch. Neurol.,* 33:494–500.
16. Taveras, J. M., Thompson, H. G., and Pool, J. L. (1962): Should we treat glioblastoma multiforme? *Am. J. Roentgenol. Radium Ther. Nucl. Med.,* 87:473–479.
17. Trouillas, P. (1973): Immunologie et immunothérapie des tumeurs cérébrales. Etat actuel. *Rev. Neurol.,* 128:23–38.
18. Urtasun, R. C., Band, P. R., Chapman, J. D., and Feldstein, M. L. (1977): Radiation plus metronidazole for gliomas. *N. Engl. J. Med.,* 296:757.
19. Urtasun, R., Band, P., Chapman, J. D., Feldstein, M. L., Mielke, B., and Fryer, C. (1976): Radiation and high-dose metronidazole in supratentorial glioblastomas. *N. Engl. J. Med.,* 294:1374–1367.
20. Walker, M. D., Alexander, E., Jr., Hunt, W. E., Leventhal, C. M., Mahaley, M. S., Jr., Norrell, H. A., Owens, G., Ransonoff, J., Wilson, C. B., and Gehan, E. A. (1976): Evaluation of mithramycin in the treatment of anaplastic gliomas. *J. Neurosurg.,* 44:655–667.
21. Walker, M. D., and Gehan, E. A. (1972): An evaluation of 1-3-bis (2-chloroethyl)-1-nitrosourea (BCNU) and irradiation done and in combination for the treatment of malignant glioma. In: *Proceedings of the 63rd Meeting of the AACR (Proc. Am. Assoc. Cancer Res.,* 13).
22. Walker, M. D., and Hurwitz, B. S. (1970): BCNU (1,3,-bis(2-chloroethyl)-1-nitrosourea (NSC-409962) in the treatment of malignant brain tumors. A preliminary report. *Cancer Chemother. Rep.,* 54:263–271.

23. Walker, M. D., and Strike, T. A. (1976): An evaluation of methyl-CCNU, BCNU and radiotherapy in treatment of malignant glioma. *Proc. AACR Meeting,* Toronto, p. 163.
24. Wilson, C. B., Gutin, P., Boldrey, E. B., Crafts, D., Levin, V. A., and Enot, J. (1976): Single agent chemotherapy of brain tumors. *Arch. Neurol.,* 33:739–744.
25. Young, H., Kaplan, A., and Regelson, W. (1976): Clinical regression of recurrent glioblastoma due to autologous lymphocyte infusion. *ASCO Abstracts,* p. 259.

*Randomized Trials in Cancer: A Critical Review by Sites,* edited by Maurice J. Staquet, Raven Press, New York © 1978.

# Carcinoma of the Prostate

André Coune

*Service de Médecine et Laboratoire d'Investigation Clinique Henri Tagnon, Institut Jules Bordet, 1000 Bruxelles, Belgium*

Although prostatic adenocarcinoma is the second most frequent cancer in the human male, only a few prospective randomized therapeutic trials have been performed. Most of the available data concern clinical studies carried out in selected patients or in patients treated without an adequate control group. This accounts for the lack of precise knowledge about the value of radical prostatectomy and radiation therapy for localized prostatic cancer, as well as about the remission rate induced by the endocrine treatments in the disseminated stages of the disease. The randomized clinical trials for which results have been published are collected in Table 1.

A new era started in this field in 1960, when the Veterans Administration Cooperative Urological Research Group (VACURG) launched its first prospective randomized clinical trial for the treatment of prostatic adenocarcinoma at its several stages (25). This cooperative group consisted of 14 Veterans Administration hospitals with a full-time urologist on their staff. Patients were admitted to the first study until 1967. A second clinical trial was begun at that time, patients being admitted until 1969 (1,6,7). A third study has been started thereafter. This latter trial will not be reviewed here because of the lack of significant results at the present time.

More recently, chemotherapeutic trials were performed in spite of the lack of information on potentially useful antimitotic drugs for prostatic cancer (27). The results of two randomized clinical trials using chemotherapeutic regimens are discussed (16,20,23,24).

## VACURG CLINICAL TRIALS

The first VACURG study was undertaken in order to evaluate the most widely used treatments for prostatic cancer. The second trial was performed to answer some of the questions raised by some unexpected results of the former study. An ancillary randomized trial, called the Focal Carcinoma Study, including only patients not eligible to the first VACURG study, was performed at the same time (11). The results of all three studies have been published.

Received August 22, 1977.

TABLE 1. *Prospective randomized clinical trials in human prostatic adenocarcinoma*

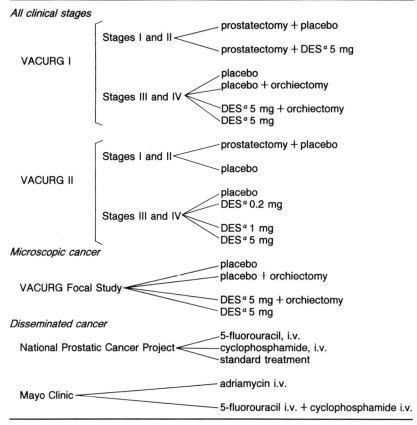

All clinical stages

VACURG I

Stages I and II
- prostatectomy + placebo
- prostatectomy + DES[a] 5 mg

Stages III and IV
- placebo
- placebo + orchiectomy
- DES[a] 5 mg + orchiectomy
- DES[a] 5 mg

VACURG II

Stages I and II
- prostatectomy + placebo
- placebo

Stages III and IV
- placebo
- DES[a] 0.2 mg
- DES[a] 1 mg
- DES[a] 5 mg

Microscopic cancer

VACURG Focal Study
- placebo
- placebo + orchiectomy
- DES[a] 5 mg + orchiectomy
- DES[a] 5 mg

Disseminated cancer

National Prostatic Cancer Project
- 5-fluorouracil, i.v.
- cyclophosphamide, i.v.
- standard treatment

Mayo Clinic
- adriamycin i.v.
- 5-fluorouracil i.v. + cyclophosphamide i.v.

[a] DES = diethylstilbestrol oral, daily dose indicated in the table.

The same criteria of eligibility and of evaluation of the therapeutic response were used for the two main studies (7).

Patients were admitted provided that they had a histological proof of prostatic cancer, had received no previous treatment, had no second malignancy, no psychosis, were in good physical condition, and were cooperative.

A staging system based on information collected by physical examination of the patient and by some unsophisticated laboratory tests was used (25):

Stage I patients had no evidence of prostatic cancer at rectal examination as well as no evidence of metastasis. The serum prostatic acid phosphatase level was normal. The microscopic examination of some prostatic tissue removed for a nonmalignant disease of the gland had shown incidentally a carcinoma.

Stage II patients presented at rectal examination a nodule with no signs of extension of the disease beyond the capsule, no evidence of metastasis, and no elevation of the serum prostatic acid phosphatase level.

Stage III patients had no evidence of distant metastasis and no elevation of the serum prostatic acid phosphatase; rectal examination disclosed extension of the tumor into the periprostatic tissues.

Stage IV patients had evidence of distant metastasis of the tumor, or an increased serum prostatic acid phosphatase level, or both, regardless of the findings of the rectal examination. Radiologic evidence of bone metastasis or biopsy proof of a tissue taken from a distant site was considered as indicative of stage IV.

The response to the treatment was mainly evaluated by the duration of survival from the start of the therapy, although supplementary criteria of evaluation were used for some groups of patients, as indicated further on.

Although the patients were randomized at their entry to the study, every clinician had the possibility to modify the allocated treatment of any patient whose condition was deteriorating.

### First VACURG Study

Of the previously untreated patients with prostatic adenocarcinoma consulting at the participating Veterans Administration hospitals, 74% were eligible to the clinical trial. The total number of patients amounted to 2,314. The maximum follow-up period from the time of admission was 15 years. Table 2 gives the distribution of the patients' deaths according to their causes, the clinical stage of the tumor, and the treatment received (7).

Stage I and II patients were randomly allocated to either radical prostatectomy plus placebo (Px + P) or radical prostatectomy plus diethylstilbestrol (DES) per o.s., at a daily dosage of 5 mg (Px + E). Although there was no significant difference between the mortality rate of stage II patients in both therapeutic groups, stage I patients receiving DES had a higher mortality rate (61%) than patients taking the placebo (50%); the excess of mortality was clearly related to deaths due to a cardiovascular accident: 42% for the (Px + E) group versus 33% for the (Px + P) group. Even after an 11-year follow-up, stage I patients treated with a placebo after the prostatectomy have a much higher survival rate than those treated with DES (8).

Stage III and IV patients were randomly assigned to one of the following four therapeutic regimens: placebo (P), DES per o.s. 5 mg daily (E), orchiectomy plus placebo (O + P), orchiectomy plus DES, per o.s., 5 mg daily (O + E). As shown in Table 2, there was for stage III patients an excess of mortality due to cardiovascular causes and a lower rate of death due to cancer in groups (E) and (O + E), whereas the reverse was observed in the two groups receiving no estrogen. Such differences were not found among the stage IV patients. Using actuarial survival curves, it could be statistically demonstrated that stage III patients allocated to the (P) and (O + P) groups had a better survival than patients receiving the estrogen compound.

TABLE 2. *First VACURG study: deaths by stage, treatment, and cause (7)*

| Stage | I | | II | | III | | | | IV | | | |
|---|---|---|---|---|---|---|---|---|---|---|---|---|
| Treatment[a] | Px+P | Px+E | Px+P | Px+E | P | E | O+P | O+E | P | E | O+P | O+E |
| Number of patients | 60 | 60 | 85 | 94 | 262 | 265 | 266 | 257 | 223 | 211 | 203 | 216 |
| Cancer of prostate | 3 | 2 | 8 | 2 | 46 | 18 | 35 | 25 | 105 | 82 | 97 | 82 |
| Cardiovascular | 20 | 25 | 25 | 32 | 88 | 112 | 95 | 108 | 55 | 76 | 56 | 59 |
| Other causes | 7 | 10 | 9 | 12 | 43 | 50 | 54 | 48 | 29 | 23 | 29 | 40 |
| Total deaths | 30 | 37 | 42 | 46 | 177 | 180 | 184 | 181 | 189 | 181 | 182 | 181 |

[a]Px = radical prostatectomy; P = placebo; E = DES, 5.0 mg daily, per o.s.; O = orchiectomy.

Survival curves for stage III and IV patients constructed for cancer deaths only showed that the placebo was the worst treatment and that the estrogen alone appeared to be the best overall treatment, although it was superior to orchiectomy and DES only during the first 2 years of the therapy. Moreover, no significant difference between (O + P) and (O + E) could be demonstrated, both therapeutic regimens having nearly identical curves for the first 5 years.

On the other hand, survival curves of the same patients, constructed for cardiovascular deaths only, showed a small but distinct difference between the treatments without DES and the treatments with DES, the latter being associated with a higher mortality rate. Separate analysis of stages III and IV showed that this association was much stronger for stage III patients (6,7).

The cardiovascular causes of death associated with DES included myocardial infarction, congestive heart failure, arteriosclerotic heart disease, cerebrovascular accident, and pulmonary embolism. The risk of such a death was the highest during the first year of administration of the estrogen.

Although the stage III patients initially treated with a placebo had a better survival rate than the patients treated with DES and orchiectomy, the probability of going from a stage III to a stage IV prostatic carcinoma was significantly higher in the placebo group. The orchiectomy and placebo treatment was also associated with a higher probability of transition to stage IV than DES alone.

Analysis of the survival of stage III patients developing complications due to their disease showed that the shortest median survival time (8 months) was associated with the appearance of upper urinary tract obstruction; the median survival time of the patients developing a marked increase in the serum prostatic acid phosphatase level (equal or superior to 10 King-Armstrong units) was 10 months, whereas the median survival time of the patients developing bone metastases was 11 months (26). It must be stressed that these latter patients died at a faster rate than stage IV patients who already had osseous involvement at the time they were admitted to the study.

Objective and subjective criteria were used for the evaluation of the response to treatment of stage III and IV patients admitted to this study and treated at the Minneapolis Veterans Administration hospital (3). The DES and placebo groups were studied according to a double-blind method. Remission was considered to occur in stage III patients if the size of the prostatic tumor was reduced by 50% or more compared to its pretreatment size. In stage IV patients, the following criteria were evaluated in addition: diminution or disappearance of bone pain, increase in strength or in appetite, decrease in the density of the bone metastases, and a 50% or greater decrease in the serum prostatic acid phosphatase level. Using these criteria, the investigators were unable to demonstrate that DES at a daily dose of 5 mg improved the status of the patient or halted the progression of the disease in a significantly higher percentage than did the placebo. In spite of this lack of difference, it must be remembered as indicated previously that the initial placebo treatment was associated in all stage III patients admitted to the VACURG study with a higher transition rate to clinical stage IV. These discrepancies stressed the big difficulties encountered in the objective evaluation of the response to therapy in prostatic cancer (13).

Analysis of the cardiovascular deaths of all stage I and II patients entered to the first VACURG study revealed that these deaths occured more frequently in people already suffering from a cardiovascular disease at the time of admission (6). The review of the cases from the Minneapolis Veterans Administration hospital also showed the association of cardiovascular deaths with previous cardiovascular diseases.

## VACURG Focal Carcinoma Study

This clinical trial was started to accommodate some stage I patients not eligible for the first VACURG study (11). These patients were either in too poor health to undergo a radical prostatectomy or too old to expect a significant lengthening of their survival time, or so concerned about the complications of the radical prostatectomy that they refused the operation. As a matter of fact, these patients had a median age 5 years higher than that of the patients admitted to the first VACURG study, the proportion of patients older than 75 years being 34% in the Focal Carcinoma Study and only 5% among the stage I patients in the first VACURG study. The three different groups of patients were randomly assigned to one of the same four therapeutic regimens studied in stage III and IV patients entered to the first VACURG study, that is, placebo, placebo + orchiectomy, DES 5 mg daily + orchiectomy, or DES 5 mg daily. From 1964 to 1969, 148 patients were admitted to the study. An appraisal of the situation on April 1, 1972, revealed that 72 patients had died, all from another cause than prostatic cancer. In 22 of these 72 patients, a postmortem examination was performed; residual carcinoma was found in only one case. Evidence of advancing disease, provided by the examination of the follow-up records, was found in only 6.8% of the patients.

No significant differences in the death rate according to the four different therapeutic regimens were detected, even after a 7-year follow-up period (8). Patients who had refused the prostatectomy had a better survival rate than the patients entered to the study, because of another reason.

## Second VACURG Study

As several important points were raised by the first VACURG study, a second clinical trial was started in 1967 in order to gain more information. Methods identical to those used in the first study were utilized (6,7).

The number of patients eligible to the study was 561. Stage I and II patients were randomly assigned to prostatectomy plus placebo or placebo alone. Although the follow-up period of these patients is too short to draw any valid conclusion, it should be noted that 5 years after the beginning of the trial no difference was yet observed between these two groups of patients with regard to survival time and the rate of progression of their disease, as measured by the appearance of an increased serum acid phosphatase or by the appearance of metastases.

Stage III and IV patients were randomized to one of the following four therapeutic conditions: placebo; DES, 0.2 mg daily dose; DES, 1 mg daily dose; DES, 5 mg daily dose, the estrogen being taken by mouth. After 2 years, new patients were no longer admitted to the study, because clear-cut differences in the survival of the patients were obvious. Stage III and IV patients treated with the two highest DES doses had fewer cancer deaths than those receiving placebo or 0.2 mg of DES. However, in stage III patients, the 5-mg DES dosage was associated with an excess of cardiovascular deaths as compared with the placebo and two lowest DES dosages. More recent data suggest that in patients older than 75 years, even 1.0 mg of DES may lead to an increased number of cardiovascular deaths (8).

Here again, constructed survival curves showed that for stage III patients, placebo was significantly better than 5-mg DES. On the other hand, curves for stage IV patients indicated that daily doses of 1 mg and 5 mg of DES were significantly better than placebo without any significant difference from each other. Curves constructed for cardiovascular deaths of stage III patients showed that the cardiovascular toxicity associated with the 5-mg dose occurred during the first year of the treatment. Curves for cancer deaths in stage IV patients revealed no difference between the patients treated with 1 mg or 5 mg of DES; both groups had a significant longer survival than the groups treated with 0.2 mg of DES or with placebo.

The better efficacy of the two highest DES doses was also shown by the low transition rates from clinical stage III to stage IV in patients treated with 1 or 5 mg of DES; much higher transition rates were observed in the two other therapeutic groups. Both higher doses of DES were also more efficient in decreasing the prostatic tumor size and the serum prostatic acid phosphatase level (7).

## Discussion of the VACURG Clinical Trials

It should be stressed that these clinical trials were very carefully designed and that proper statistical methods were used for the evaluation of the data. However, as soon as the unexpected results of the first study were known, several criticisms arose, a lot of people considering the association of cardiovascular deaths with estrogen treatment as due to a bias in the study.

It occurs to me that the following points concerning the VACURG studies deserve some discussion. As a matter of fact, adequate information about most of them was provided by the VACURG investigators themselves.

1. The first trial was planned to determine the best treatment to be offered

to the patients suffering from prostatic cancer at the different stages of their disease. The duration of the survival from the start of the initial therapy was the only criterion used for evaluating the response. As prostatic adenocarcinoma has in a high percentage of cases a rather slow development, a long follow-up period, of a maximal duration of 15 years, had to be considered. This was not an ideal criterion for evaluation, as 45% of patients with prostatic cancer, older than 70 years, died of an intercurrent disease and not of their neoplasm (26). Nevertheless, this choice turned out to be a fortunate one, because of its ability to reveal the higher death rate associated with the estrogenic treatment.

2. All participating hospitals belonged to the Veterans Administration. This was an important factor in the planning of such a clinical trial necessitating for the most favorable cases, a long follow-up period. As the patients treated at these hospitals were probably rather sedentary and were seen regularly at the same hospital, a major pitfall of long follow-ups was avoided.

Some bias could be introduced by the high number of participating centers located throughout the United States. For instance, the staging system used considered as disseminated a patient with prostatic cancer having an increased serum prostatic acid phosphatase; as this determination might be influenced by several factors, including the sensitivity of the utilized substrate to the several acid phosphatase isoenzymes, one might wonder if the clinical stage of some patients would not be different in hospitals using different methods for the determination of the serum acid phosphatase. To obviate such difficulties several measures were taken by the cooperative group. All serum acid phosphatase determinations were performed in a central laboratory, which had investigated the best means of taking and shipping the blood specimens in order to avoid all possible *in vitro* loss of enzymatic activity (15). Several other blood components were analyzed in the same laboratory, which investigated the effect of the estrogens on several blood proteins and lipids. The biopsies of all patients were reviewed by a referee pathologist, and all questionable X-rays had to be sent to a referee radiologist who gave a final decision.

3. The criteria of admission to the trials were precisely defined and seemed quite valid. Entering patients with a very low performance status as well as patients suffering from a psychosis or a second malignancy, and patients already receiving another treatment would have introduced marked bias in the results. Therefore it was no wonder that 27% of all untreated patients with prostatic adenocarcinoma seen at the several participating hospitals were not entered into the first VACURG study (5). The rejection rate was of the same order of magnitude in the second study.

4. The clinical stage for each patient was determined according to the data of the physical examination and of some unsophisticated laboratory tests. As some patients reported as clinical stage II were discovered at the operation as having a periprostatic involvement, the possibility of a frequent confusion between these two stages at the rectal examination had to be raised. In fact, 208 prostatectomy specimens of stage I and II patients from the first VACURG

study were analyzed and compared with the rectal examination findings (10). Although 80% of the prostates considered as having a single nodule in fact contained several, very good agreement was found as far as the periprostatic involvement was concerned, 79% of the cases of capsular involvement having been correctly diagnosed and 78% of the cases of seminal involvement having been detected by the clinical examination. On the other hand, as stated previously, several measures were taken to avoid a wrong assignment to stage III or stage IV because of erroneous interpretation of the bone X-rays or because of *in vitro* degradation of the serum prostatic acid phosphatase activity. Clinical staging could have been ameliorated by exploratory laparotomies and histological examination of the pelvic lymph nodes, but such a procedure probably would have resulted in a higher number of rejected patients, some of them being unable to undergo the operation or refusing the procedure (14).

5. A very disturbing point concerning this study was the choice of the survival period as the single criterion of response when all the patients were not treated with the same sequential therapeutic regimens. It would have been, of course, unethical to refuse a patient initially treated by a prostatectomy or a placebo another treatment when his clinical status started deteriorating. Such a modification of the treatment occurred in 20% of the patients entered to the first study (5). Although one might consider that analysis of the results would have been done after exclusion of the patients whose treatment had been changed, such a procedure might introduce another bias. In fact, as worsening of the patients was probably occurring in the groups receiving the less active treatments, exclusion of these patients would result in an apparent lengthening of the survival period of these groups, the statistical evaluation taking into account only the patients with the less aggressive tumors. This point of view seemed to be corroborated by the observation that 80% of the patients whose primary treatment had to be changed had been assigned initially to a group receiving a placebo (5).

6. The unexpected conclusions of the first study, as well as the results of the second study, were based on the analysis of the causes of death. How reliable was this criterion? It is well known that determination of the cause of death may be very difficult in these old patients, who frequently suffer from several intercurrent diseases (6).

A committee of five members was set up by the VACURG in order to investigate the cause of all deaths. The analysis was based on the review and if necessary on the discussion of the death certificate, of the autopsy report if available, of the patient's records, of the final hospital summary or of a report of the last illness from the attending physician if the patient had died outside the hospital (5). The members of this committee were not aware of the treatment to which the patients had been assigned at their entry into the study.

A major drawback to this analysis was the absence of a postmortem examination in a rather high percentage of cases. This happened because most of the patients died at home. In the first study, an autopsy was carried out in 36%

of all deaths, the range being from 16 to 47%, according to the several participating hospitals. In the second VACURG study, the mean rate dropped to 26%, with a very wide range, from 7 to 80% (8). Nevertheless, it must be stressed that the complications due to a 5-mg daily dose of DES frequently resulted in a medical emergency requiring the immediate help of a physician who usually ordered several laboratory investigations. These data could be used later by the VACURG Review Committee for the determination of the cause of death.

7. Another drawback to these clinical trials was linked to the oral route of administration of the DES. It was highly probable that some of the patients assigned to the estrogen did not take the drug. The higher the percentage of these patients, the more likely a bias could be present in the study. Fortunately, there is a dose-related increase of the plasma transcortin level induced by DES (4). The determination of the plasma concentration of this protein was used to detect the patients who were not taking the drug. This amounted to about 10% of all patients allocated to the estrogen treatment. Admission of these patients to the hospital resulted in a major lowering of the percentage of the cheaters; thereafter only 2 of 100 patients persisted in refusing to take the prescribed drug (5).

8. There was a lot of discussion about the selected dosage of DES in the first VACURG study. It has to be remembered that from the start of the endocrine therapy for prostatic cancer until the publication by the VACURG of the results of its first study, the dosage of DES varied considerably, the daily doses ranging from less than 1 mg to 1,000 mg. The dosage selected by the group was considered to be an average value of the usual dosages prescribed by the urologists at that time (6).

9. Although the patients admitted to the first VACURG study had been randomly allocated to the several therapeutic regimens, nothing was known about their pretreatment cardiovascular status or the presence of disorders predisposing to cardiovascular diseases. It could be considered that the unexpected results of the clinical trial resulted from a higher number of these latter patients in the estrogen-treated groups. As a matter of fact, at the time the study was launched, nobody knew about the possible cardiovascular side effects of the estrogens. The initial results of the Coronary Drug Research Project were not yet known (12). The salt-retaining capacity of estrogenic compounds, used at pharmacological doses in some female patients for disseminated breast cancer, should have been a warning to the investigators. In spite of the absence of data concerning the pretreatment cardiovascular status of all patients included in the first study, analysis of the data for the stage III and IV patients treated at the Veterans Administration Hospital at Minneapolis showed no significant difference between the placebo-treated and the DES-treated groups, when clinical conditions known to predispose to cardiovascular diseases (obesity, diabetes, moderate to severe hypertension) were taken into account (5).

At the time of entry to the study, 26% of the patients assigned to the placebo and 37% of those randomized to DES had an excellent cardiovascular status.

Analysis of the patients with no previous history of cardiovascular diseases showed a much higher percentage of cardiovascular complications in the DES-treated groups (36%) than in the placebo-treated groups (13%); such a difference was statistically significant ($p < 0.01$). An analysis of the clinical data of all stage I and II patients admitted to the first study showed, in the patients treated with DES, an association between a previous cardiovascular disease and the occurrence of lethal cardiovascular complications (6).

Other studies comparing estrogen-treated patients and age-matched controls failed to disclose any possible connection between the stage of atherosclerosis of the coronary arteries and of the aorta and the estrogen administration (18). It is highly probable that the cardiovascular side effects associated with the estrogen treatments were not due to a dramatic progression of preexisting atherosclerotic lesions, but were induced by other mechanisms, such as the activation of some circulating blood clotting factors. If the complications were due to the worsening of a preexisting atherosclerotic disease, one would expect an increase of the lethal side effects proportional to the duration of the treatment, whereas most cardiovascular deaths occurred during the first year of the administration of DES.

Another surprising observation concerning the first VACURG study has been made: The excess of mortality due to cardiovascular complications quite evident in stage I patients was not found in stage II patients. No clear-cut explanation is available. However, stage I cases were in fact patients suffering from a symptomatic benign prostatic hypertrophy, whereas stage II patients had no clinical symptoms of a prostatic disease. In the stage I patients, the hypertrophy might be associated with modifications of some other physiological functions, favoring the cardiovascular side effects of DES. Likewise, the lethal estrogen side effects detected in stage III were not conspicuous in stage IV patients; however, actuarial curves constructed only for cardiovascular deaths showed the phenomenon to be true for the whole set of stage III and IV patients. The apparent absence of lethal side effects of DES in stage IV patients could be ascribed to the modification of the treatment in a nonnegligible percentage of the patients assigned to the placebo therapy at the time their status was worsening and to the much shorter life expectancy of stage IV patients due to the advanced state of their disease.

Moreover, during this first VACURG study, a similar observation was made as far as another complication of the estrogen treatment was concerned: The moderate lowering of the hemoglobin level resulting from the administration of DES, although well apparent in stage III patients was not seen in stage IV patients who had in most cases osseous metastases associated with a slight or moderate anemia (25).

Contrary to the former clinical trials, the Focal Carcinoma trial was performed on a selected population; these patients did not undergo a radical prostatectomy, either because they were in a poor state of health or because they refused the operation. After a 7-year follow-up, no significant difference between the four therapeutic regimens had been observed, although there was a trend suggesting a higher death rate from cardiovascular diseases in the patients treated with DES. The lack of significance of these differences was probably due in part to the smaller number of patients in these therapeutic groups as compared to the groups of the first VACURG study. In fact, the population of patients admitted to the Focal Carcinoma study was a mixed one, as shown by the much longer survival time of the patients who had refused the prostatectomy than that of the patients considered too old to undergo such an operation (11). These latter patients amounted to 41% of all the patients entered to this study. Their high mortality rate during the first year of the follow-up period might have prevented the detection of the cardiovascular side effects of the estrogen in a group of patients much smaller than the groups of the first VACURG study.

The second VACURG study was designed to determine if a radical prostatectomy had to be performed in stage I and II patients and to evaluate the therapeutic value and the frequency of the cardiovascular side effects of DES, given at doses smaller than 5 mg.

Two years after the beginning of this clinical trial, a significant difference between the therapeutic groups emerged in stage III and IV patients (1). This observation precluded the study to be continued. The admission of new patients was stopped, although rather small numbers of stage I and II patients had been entered. As many of these tumors are growing slowly, no valid conclusion can be drawn today, the follow-up period being too short. Nevertheless, it should be stressed that appearance of an increased acid phosphatase or of metastases is as common in the patients treated with the radical prostatectomy as in those treated with the placebo (8).

The annual mortality rates of stage III patients treated with a placebo or with 5 mg of DES were similar to the rates of the same therapeutic groups in the first VACURG study. These findings corroborated that most DES-associated cardiovascular deaths occurred during the first year of treatment. Analysis of the survival curves of stage III patients showed that the placebo treatment was associated with a lower overall mortality than the 5-mg DES dosage, although the placebo patients as well as those receiving the lowest DES dosage had the highest progression rate from clinical stage III to stage IV. The fact that this transition was not associated with a high mortality rate pointed out how needless it was to start an estrogen treatment in asymptomatic stage III patients, the benefits of the therapy being offset by the mortality due to the side effects of the drug.

Comparison of the overall mortality rates of stage IV patients in the first and second VACURG studies disclosed a striking difference: Within the former trial, the survival rates were similar whatever the therapeutic group, whereas in the latter trial, the placebo group had a much lower survival rate, due mainly to the progression of the cancer (6).

Two different factors at least played a role in this situation: More patients with a lower performance status were admitted into the second study—candidates to the first study had to be eligible to an orchiectomy—and, placebo administration was continued for a longer period in this second study, before a treatment of known efficacy was started in cases showing progression of their disease.

10. Some criticism was raised because DES was used in the studies instead of a steroidal estrogen. As DES was, and still is, widely used in several countries, the choice of this compound as the standard additive endocrine therapy for prostatic cancer was quite appropriate. This selection was not an unfortunate one, as shown later, when the Coronary Drug Project Research Group published its results indicating in male patients an association of nonlethal cardiovascular diseases with the use of equine conjugated estrogens, given in order to reduce the frequency of acute coronary accidents (12). A third VACURG study still in progress has been designed to determine especially the efficacy and the possible side effects of the natural conjugated estrogens (6).

11. Finally, the VACURG studies allowed the determination of several variables of prognostic significance for stage III and IV patients. The data collected from the clinical trials were used to develop an exponential survival model, based on several assumptions and conventions, but very useful to predict the survival of patients according to the combinations of signs and symptoms they presented and to select the best treatment for patients having characteristics associated with a high mortality rate (2,9). Although no stratification of the patients was performed in the VACURG studies, the variables of prognostic significance identified during these trials may be very helpful for the design of future studies (26).

## Therapeutic Inferences from the VACURG Clinical Trials

Stage I and II patients having undergone a radical prostatectomy need no further therapy with estrogens; actually, such a treatment may induce, in stage I patients, lethal side effects. As shown by the previous data, much more time is needed to assess the value of the radical prostatectomy itself in these patients.

Although stage III patients receiving a placebo have a faster transition rate to clinical stage IV than patients treated with 5 mg of DES daily, their survival time is longer than that of the estrogen-treated patients. This stresses the lack of necessity to start an endocrine therapy in asymptomatic patients.

Estrogen alone is a better treatment than orchiectomy and is even superior to the combination of orchiectomy and estrogen.

The 1-mg DES daily dose is as effective as the 5-mg DES daily dose while having much fewer cardiovascular side effects. However, more recent information indicates that DES at the 1-mg daily dose may be harmful in patients in a poor state of health or older than 75 years (8). Although it has been reported that a 3-mg daily dose of DES resulted in a marked decrease of the plasma testosterone level in all prostatic cancer patients (21) and that a 1-mg daily dose lowered the level only in stage III patients (19), the use of the 3-mg daily dose cannot be recommended. Its cardiovascular toxicity is unknown, but the data concerning the lethal side effects of the 1-mg dose in some patients suggest that this higher dosage may be associated with a rather important cardiovascular toxicity.

Last but not least, the VACURG studies have clearly demonstrated that the 1-mg dose is as effective as the 5-mg dose, both doses inducing in stage IV patients an equal reduction of the mortality due to cancer.

The VACURG itself suggests that stage III and IV patients in poor physical condition, with a previous history of cardiovascular disease, or older than 75 years should not be treated with estrogens unless such a treatment is required because of the presence of symptoms. On the other hand, patients with a progressive disease, large primary tumors, high-grade tumors, pain due to metastases, or a low hemoglobin level may be ameliorated from treatment at the time of diagnosis (8).

## CHEMOTHERAPY CLINICAL TRIALS

Very scanty information about chemotherapy of prostatic cancer is available (27). Only a few phase II clinical trials have been performed. At the present time, the results of two randomized studies have been published.

### National Prostatic Cancer Project Randomized Study

Five different hospitals in the United States participated to this clinical trial, the purpose of which was to investigate the activity of two cytotoxic drugs in advanced prostatic cancer (22).

Patients with histologically confirmed carcinoma of the prostate with metastases resistant or no longer responsive to an endocrine therapy were admitted to the study, provided they had evidence of a sufficient bone marrow reserve, had an expected survival of at least 90 days, and had received no previous chemotherapy nor radiation therapy on the pelvic area at a dose higher than 2,000 rads.

Patients with a second primary malignancy (except the nonmelanoma skin tumors) were not eligible.

Before starting the chemotherapy, a detailed workup including an intravenous urogram and a skeletal survey was performed. Each week, the patients were seen at the hospital and had a blood workup. The chest X-ray, intravenous urogram, and skeletal survey were repeated every 6 weeks.

The evaluation of the response to the treatment was mainly based on objective criteria: reduction of the size of the primary or metastatic tumor, decrease of the serum acid phosphatase activity, recalcification of osteolytic lesions, absence of progression of osteoblastic lesions. The responses were classified as: complete objective regression, partial objective regression, objective stabilization, objective progression.

The eligible patients were randomized to one of the following arms: (a) 5-fluorouracil, 600 mg/m², per week, intravenously; (b) cyclophosphamide, 1 g/m², every 3 weeks, intravenously; (c) standard treatment, that is, any nonchemotherapeutic treatment.

In those patients randomized to 5-fluorouracil or to cyclophosphamide, the hormonal treatment was discontinued 14 days before starting the chemotherapy. The protocol provided precise rules for reducing the dosages of the drugs, according to the type and degree of toxicity induced by the treatment.

After a 12-week interval, the response to the therapy was evaluated. Patients on 5-fluorouracil or on cyclophosphamide showing tumor progression were crossed over to the other cytotoxic drug, whereas all the other patients were continued on the same therapy until objective progression of the disease was quite evident. Patients randomized to the standard therapy were never changed to another treatment, whatever the type of response they exhibited. All patients were followed until death.

In this study, 110 patients having received a treatment for at least 3 weeks were evaluated (20,23,24). No complete objective regression was observed. Of 33 patients treated with 5-fluorouracil, 4 had a partial regression whereas 21 had a progression of their disease. Cyclophosphamide was given to 41 patients; 3 had a partial regression and 24 were progressing. No partial regression was observed among the 36 patients randomized to the standard treatment. Patients having received one of the two cytotoxic drugs showed a 50% reduction of the primary tumor size in a much higher percentage and had a longer survival than the patients on standard treatment. The difference was statistically significant ($p < 0.05$).

Crossover from 5-fluorouracil to cyclophosphamide (19 patients) resulted in 1 partial regression, whereas no regression was observed after the reversed crossover (20 patients).

Survival of the patients who showed regression or stabilization of their metastatic lesions while receiving chemotherapy was longer than the survival of the patients who had stabilization of their lesions on a standard therapy. Chemotherapy responders were found only among the patients having undergone a prior orchiectomy. Taking into account the treatment interruptions and the dose reductions due to the toxicity, cyclophosphamide appeared to have less important side effects than 5-fluorouracil. The utilization of various treatments at the several participating hospitals for what was considered as standard therapy—the third arm of the randomization process—introduced a bias in this study. In fact, some therapeutic regimens, probably ineffective in disseminated prostatic cancer, such as palliative radiotherapy or cryosurgery, were used by some investigators as standard therapy. Moreover, the additive endocrine treatments considered as standard therapy included compounds of low efficacy such as cortisone derivatives used alone or in combination with testosterone propionate, as well as more potent drugs such DES and other estrogenic compounds. These therapeutic regimens were totally ineffective, as shown by the absence of even one single partial regression in this group of 36 patients. This did not mean that all these patients were resistant to all the types of endocrine therapy. In fact, there were too many different endocrine treatments used for such a small number of patients. It would have been more useful to allocate these patients to a single endocrine treatment, such as an antiandrogen, in order to make a valid comparison with the results of the cytotoxic drugs.

As the patients entered to this clinical trial were evaluated as resistant or no longer responsive to their endocrine treatment, stabilization of the lesions, noted during the follow-up period, was considered by the investigators as an objective favorable response to the therapy.

Unfortunately, no criteria of resistance or of unresponsiveness to the previous endocrine treatment were defined in this protocol. Therefore, some patients with a tumor growing at a slow rate could have been included in the chemotherapy study. Persistence of such a process during several weeks after the start of the chemotherapy would result in a false evaluation of an objective stabilization response. This seemed to be borne out by the observation of stabilized lesions in 16 patients treated by cyclophosphamide and 8 patients treated with 5-fluorouracil, but also in 7 patients on standard therapy, although no partial objective regression response was noted in this latter group. These points stressed the necessity of considering, in these types of clinical studies, as favorable responses only cases with a partial or a complete objective regression response, the evaluation being based on well-defined rules taking into account the modifications of several clinical and laboratory parameters (13). Improvement of one single parameter might even occur in the absence of any real effect on the disease, as shown by a 6% occurrence rate of a 50% reduction in the size of the prostatic tumor in patients on the standard therapy, whereas none of these patients could be classified as responding with a partial objective regression. A much higher rate (30%) of a 50% reduction in the size of the prostatic tumor was noted in patients receiving chemotherapy. The longer survival of the patients considered as having a stabilization of their lesions was no proof of the efficacy of the treatment, as it is known that patients suffering from a slow-growing tumor have a longer survival than patients with a fast-growing tumor.

The reasons why the chemotherapy responders were found only in patients having undergone a previous orchiectomy are not obvious.

The last point to be mentioned was the more effective capacity of pain relief of the chemotherapy, the difference with the standard therapy being statistically significant.

## MAYO CLINIC STUDY

The Mayo Clinic trial was designed with a double aim: to test the value of so-called ancillary factors for estimating the response of prostatic cancer to the therapy and to evaluate the efficacy of a single chemotherapy versus a combination of two drugs in the same tumor (17).

Precise criteria of eligibility were worked out in order to avoid admission to the study of patients with marked renal insufficiency, reduced bone marrow reserve, active heart disease, or low performance status.

Only patients with a biopsy-proven, stage IV adenocarcinoma of the prostate, no longer responding to routine ablative or additive endocrine therapy, having received no previous treatment with adriamycin, 5-fluorouracil, or an alkylating agent, were eligible to the study. Patients having undergone major surgery or radiation therapy or chemotherapy with other drugs within the previous months were not eligible. Before randomization, a detailed workup, including a chest X-ray, an intravenous urogram, a bone scan, a bone marrow survey, a bone marrow biopsy, serum acid phosphatase and alkaline phosphatase determinations, and a bone marrow acid phosphatase determination, was performed. These tests were regularly repeated at stated times during the follow-up period.

Evaluation of the response to the therapy was made according to two different methods, whenever it was possible: measurement of the tumor masses excluding the primary prostatic tumor and assessment of the so-called ancillary factors. This evaluation took place after a 10-week period of treatment, unless clear-cut progression of the lesions was evident before.

In cases of measurable tumors, the response to the treatment was considered as an objective remission when a reduction in the size of the tumor of at least 50% was observed, no other lesion progressing. A reduction inferior to 50% or an increase inferior to 25% in the size of a tumor was considered as a stabilization of the disease. Appearance of a new metastase or increase in the size of the tumor greater than 25% was considered as an objective progression. Appearance of a new blastic lesion on the skeletal X-ray or of a new "hot spot" on the bone scan was also considered as progression.

The ancillary factors are specified in Table 3. In the absence of measurable tumors, only these factors were taken into account for the evaluation of the response. Based on the several factors, an overall score was established, which value determined the type of response to the chemotherapy: response, stabilization, progression. Whatever the score, the development of any new metastatic lesion was considered as indicating progression of the disease.

Eligible patients were stratified according to the following criteria:

Age: Less than 65 years
      65 years or older
Predominant lesions: Bone
                     Other sites with or without bone metastases
Previous radiation therapy: Limited: 40% or less bone marrow exposed
                                 Extensive: more than 40% bone marrow exposed

After stratification, the patients were randomly allocated to one of the two following chemotherapies:

Adriamycin, 60 mg/m$^2$, in a single i.v. dose, every 3 weeks × 2, every 4 weeks thereafter.

TABLE 3. *Mayo Clinic chemotherapy study: ancillary factors for the evaluation of response to therapy[a]* (17)

| Ancillary factors | Better | Same | Worse |
|---|---|---|---|
| Pain | 1 | 2 | 3 |
| Weight change (≥5%) | 1 | 2 | 3 |
| Hemoglobin change (≥10%) | 1 | 2 | 3 |
| Performance score change (1 level) | 1 | 2 | 3 |
| Alkaline phosphatase change (≥25%) | 1 | 2 | 3 |
| Acid phosphatase change (≥25%) | 1 | 2 | 3 |

[a] Overall score of 7 or less considered a response; overall score of 8–13 considered stable; overall score of or more than 13 considered progression.

5-Fluorouracil, 300 mg/m², + cyclophosphamide, 150 mg/m², intravenously, daily, for 5 consecutive days, repeated every 5 weeks from the first day of treatment.

Patients with an "extensive" prior radiation therapy received initially doses approximately equal to two-thirds of the above dosages. During the treatment period, the dosages were adjusted in order to keep the white blood cell nadir above 2,000 cells/mm³ and the platelet nadir above 75,000 cells/mm³.

When progression occurred during the chemotherapy, the patient was crossed over to the other regimen, provided he was still meeting the eligibility criteria to the clinical trial.

Twenty-six patients were admitted to the study. The response rate to adriamycin was 3 out of 14, whereas it was 2 out of 12 for the combined chemotherapy.

None of the 6 patients crossed over to the combination therapy showed a response; on the other hand, 2 out of 5 patients given adriamycin as second treatment had a regression. Of the 26 patients studied, 7 showed a response to one or the other of the two chemotherapy regimens. Seven patients who had an objective remission, as shown by regression of tumor masses, had an ancillary score of 9 or less. All but 2 patients showing progression of the disease had scores of at least 15; 2 other patients considered as stabilized according to their score developed a new bone metastasis and a urethral obstruction due to the tumor growth.

Although the median survival of the 7 responders was longer than that of the 19 progressing patients, the difference was not statistically significant. Patients with a better performance status seemed to respond better to the treatment. Toxicity was rather moderate and no cardiac side effects were observed in the patients treated with adriamycin.

This study was not properly designed in order to answer the two main questions concerning the reliability of the ancillary factors to evaluate the therapeutic response and the possible difference between the two chemotherapy regimens. In fact, the ancillary factor score associated a subjective criterion (pain) with objective specific and nonspecific criteria (13). Although diminution of bone pain was one of the most frequent changes observed, no scale for rating its intensity was indicated in the protocol. Two other factors rather frequently ameliorated were the performance status and the patient's weight, which modification probably resulted from the diminution of pain. Moreover, a poor correlation was observed between the changes of the serum acid and alkaline phosphatase levels and the modification of the cancer. Little information about this point, unfortunately, was given in the published report (16); in 2 cases considered as progressing, a decrease in the serum alkaline phosphatase activity was noted, but such a situation could have resulted from the stabilization of an osteoblastic metastasis, while some osteolytic or nonosseous lesions were appearing or progressing. The decrease in the serum acid phosphatase activity measured in some progressive cases was not analyzed; for instance, no information was given about the role of some factors known to influence this level, that is, fever, degradation *in vitro,* possible dedifferentiation of the tumor. Furthermore, the modifications of the prostatic tumor size, however difficult their precise measurement might be, were deliberately discarded, making the appraisal of the ancillary factors score more difficult. The lack of significant difference between the survival time of the responding and the nonresponding patients was perhaps due to a bad discrimination between the patients, because of the lack of reliability of the ancillary method.

The number of patients entered to the study was too small to allow the detection of a real difference between the single and the combination chemotherapies. The only statement that can be made is that each of them has some activity in patients with prostatic cancer.

## FINAL CONCLUSIONS

As a matter of fact, very little information is available on the objective remission rates induced in patients with prostatic cancer as a result of endocrine treatment or chemotherapy (13,27). Although several phase II clinical trials of hormone-like compounds or antiandrogens have been published, no information concerning their comparative value is available. Some large trials in this field have been designed by different cooperative groups, and it is probable that a larger amount of information on the endocrine treatment of human prostatic adenocarcinoma will be collected within the next few years.

On the other hand, very few studies testing cytotoxic compounds have been performed. The number of nonrandomized phase II trials is small. Much work remains to be done to select for randomized clinical trials the more promising drugs. Because of the frequent bone involvement present in this type of neoplasm, compounds with low bone marrow toxicity may play an important role in the future chemotherapy of prostatic cancer. Although the endocrine therapy may induce in several patients dramatic favorable responses, it has to be remembered that development of unresponsiveness or resistance to the hormonal treatment will necessitate the use of a more aggressive therapy, requiring the administration of several antimitotic compounds.

# REFERENCES

1. Bailar, J. C., III, Byar, D. P., and the Veterans Administration Cooperative Urological Research Group (1970): Estrogen treatment for cancer of the prostate. Early results with 3 doses of diethylstilbestrol and placebo. *Cancer,* 26:257–261.
2. Bayard, S., Greenberg, R., Showalter, D., and Byar, D. (1974): Comparison of treatments for prostatic cancer using an exponential-type life model relating survival to concomitant information. *Cancer Chemother. Rep.,* Part 1, 58:845–859.
3. Blackard, C. E., Doe, R. P., Mellinger, G. T., and Byar, D. P. (1970): Incidence of cardiovascular disease and death in patients receiving diethylstilbestrol for carcinoma of the prostate. *Cancer,* 26:249–256.
4. Blackard, C. E., Doe, R. P., and Seal, U. S. (1973): Serum corticosteroid-binding globulin, cortisol, and nonprotein-bound cortisol levels in patients receiving estrogen for carcinoma of the prostate. *Inv. Urol.,* 11:194–197.
5. Blackard, C. E., and Mellinger, G. T. (1972): Current status of estrogen therapy for prostatic carcinoma. *Postgrad. Med.,* 51:140–145.
6. Byar, D. P. (1972): Treatment of prostatic cancer: Studies by the Veterans Administration Cooperative Urological Research Group. *Bull. N. Y. Acad. Med.,* 48:751–766.
7. Byar, D. P. (1973): The Veterans Administration Cooperative Urological Research Group's studies of cancer of the prostate. *Cancer,* 32:1126–1130.
8. Byar, D. P. (1976): *Personal Communication.*
9. Byar, D. P., Huse, R., Bailar, J. C., III, and the Veterans Administration Cooperative Urological Research Group (1974): An exponential model relating censored survival data and concomitant information for prostatic cancer patients. *J. Natl. Cancer Inst.,* 52:321–326.
10. Byar, D. P., Mostofi, F. K., and the Veterans Administration Cooperative Urological Research Group (1972): Carcinoma of the prostate: Prognostic evaluation of certain pathologic features in 208 radical prostatectomies, examined by the step-section technique. *Cancer,* 30:5–13.
11. Byar, D. P., and the Veterans Administration Cooperative Urological Research Group (1972): Survival of patients with incidentally found microscopic cancer of the prostate: Results of a clinical trial of conservative treatment. *J. Urol.,* 108:908–913.
12. Coronary Drug Project Research Group (1970): The coronary drug project. Initial findings leading to modification of its research protocol. *JAMA,* 214:1303–1313.
13. Coune, A. (1975): Carcinoma of the prostate: Prognostic factors and criteria of response to therapy. In: *Cancer Therapy: Prognostic Factors and Criteria of Response,* edited by M. J. Staquet. Raven Press, New York.
14. Dahl, D. S., Wilson, C. S., Middleton, R. G., and Bourne, H. H. (1974): Pelvic lymphadenectomy for staging localized prostatic cancer. *J. Urol.,* 112:245–246.
15. Doe, R. P., Mellinger, G. T., and Seal, U. S. (1965): Stabilization and preservation of serum prostatic acid phosphatase activity. *Clin. Chem.,* 11:943–950.
16. Eagan, R. T., Hahn, R. G., and Myers, R. P. (1976): Adriamycin (NSC-123127) versus 5-fluorouracil (NSC-19893) and cyclophosphamide (NSC-26271) in the treatment of metastatic prostate cancer. *Cancer Treatment Rep.,* 60:115–117.
17. Eagan, R. T., Utz, D. C., Myers, R. P., and Furlow, W. L. (1975): Comparison of adriamycin (NSC-123127) and the combination of 5-fluorouracil (NSC-19893) and cyclophosphamide (NSC-26271) in advanced prostatic cancer: A preliminary report. *Cancer Chemother. Rep.,* Part 1, 59:203–207.
18. Hanash, K. A., Taylor, W. F., Greene, L. F., Kottke, B. A., and Titus, J. L. (1970): Relationship of estrogen therapy for carcinoma of the prostate to atherosclerotic cardiovascular disease: A clinicopathologic study. *J. Urol.,* 103:467–470.
19. Kent, J. R., Bischoff, A. J., Arduino, L. J., Mellinger, G. T., Byar, D. P., Hill, M., and Kozbur, X. (1973): Estrogen dosage and suppression of testosterone levels in patients with prostatic carcinoma. *J. Urol.,* 109:858–860.
20. Murphy, G. P., Saroff, J., Joiner, J. R., Prout, G. R., Gibbons, R. P., Schmidt, J. D., Johnson,

D. E., and Scott, W. W. (1976): Chemotherapy of advanced prostatic cancer by the National Prostatic Cancer Group. *Semin. Oncol.*, 3:103–106.

21. Robinson, M. R. G., and Thomas, B. S. (1971): Effect of hormonal therapy on plasma testosterone levels in prostatic carcinoma. *Br. Med. J.*, 4:391–394.

22. Scott, W. W., Gibbons, R. P., Johnson, D. E., Prout, G. R., Schmidt, J. D., Chut, M., Gaeta, J. F., Joiner, J., Saroff, J., and Murphy, G. P. (1975): Comparison of 5-fluorouracil (NSC-19893) and cyclophosphamide (NSC-26271) in patients with advanced carcinoma of the prostate. *Cancer Chemother. Rep.*, Part 1, 59:195–201.

23. Scott, W. W., Gibbons, R. P., Johnson, D. E., Prout, G. R., Schmidt, J. D., Saroff, J., and Murphy, G. P. (1976): The continued evaluation of the effects of chemotherapy in patients with advanced carcinoma of the prostate. *J. Urol.*, 116:211–213.

24. Scott, W. W., Johnson, D. E., Schmidt, J. E., Gibbons, R. P., Prout, G. R., Joiner, J. R., Saroff, J., and Murphy, G. P. (1975): Chemotherapy of advanced prostatic carcinoma with cyclophosphamide or 5-fluorouracil: Results of first national randomized study. *J. Urol.*, 114:909–911.

25. Veterans Administration Cooperative Urological Research Group (1967): Carcinoma of the prostate: Treatment comparisons. *J. Urol.*, 98:516–522.

26. Veterans Administration Cooperative Urological Research Group (1968): Factors in the prognosis of carcinoma of the prostate: A cooperative study. *J. Urol.*, 100:59–65.

27. Yagoda, A. (1973): Non-hormonal cytotoxic agents in the treatment of prostatic adenocarcinoma. *Cancer,* 32:1131–1140.

*Randomized Trials in Cancer: A Critical Review by Sites,* edited by Maurice J. Staquet, Raven Press, New York © 1978.

# Bladder Carcinoma

## Maurice J. Staquet

*Service de Médecine et Laboratoire d'Investigation Clinique Henri Tagnon, Institut Jules Bordet, and Laboratoire de Statistique Médicale, Faculté de Médecine, Université Libre de Bruxelles, Belgium*

Bladder cancer is almost unknown below the age of 40. It is more frequent in men than in women (3 to 1), and about 50% of patients have a low-stage (0, A) papillary lesion at presentation. In Europe and North America 90% of the bladder neoplasms are transitional cell carcinoma. The two most important prognostic factors are depth of infiltration (P stage) and degree of anaplasia (G stage). The growth pattern, exophytic or endophytic, also has some prognostic value.

## CLASSIFICATION AND STAGING

The two most used systems are a TNM classification (Table 1) presented in 1974 (36) and a staging procedure proposed by Jewett and Strong (14) and Marshall (17) (Table 2). The TNM classification includes P (histopathology), G (grading), and L (invasion of lymphatics) categories assessed on evidence derived from surgical operation. The Jewett-Marshall staging system is essentially designed for the description of operative specimens, but is used by many clinicians for staging patients on the basis of clinical examination and biopsies. Approximate correspondence between the two systems is given in Table 3 (2).

## INTRAVESICAL TREATMENT AND ORAL PYRIDOXINE STUDIES IN T1 CANCER

Intravesical thiotepa has been used extensively for the treatment of patients with T1 bladder cancer for the last 15 years. It was suggested that thiotepa used prophylactically after transuretheral resection (TUR) would destroy the tumor cells floating free in the bladder and prevent implantation. Without adjuvant treatment to TUR, at least 50% of the T1 patients will have a recurrence, and a certain percentage will present with high grade and stage.

The only published randomized study in T1 bladder cancer is the one of

Received September 2, 1977.

TABLE 1. *T categories of the TNM classification (1974) (36)*

T categories are based on clinical examination, urography, cystoscopy, bimanual examination under full anaesthesia, and biopsy or transurethral resection of the tumor (if indicated) prior to definitive treatment.

| | |
|---|---|
| T1S | Preinvasive carcinoma (carcinoma *in situ*) |
| TX | The minimum requirements to assess fully the extent of the primary tumor cannot be met |
| T0 | No evidence of primary tumor |
| T1 | On bimanual examination a freely mobile mass may be felt; this should not be felt after complete transurethral resection of the lesion and/or |
| | Microscopically the tumor does not extend beyond the lamina propria |
| | *Note:* This category includes papillary tumors (both infiltrating and noninfiltrating) |
| T2 | On bimanual examination there is induration of the bladder wall which is mobile. There is no residual induration after complete transurethral resection of the lesion and/or |
| | There is microscopic invasion of superficial muscle |
| T3 | On bimanual examination induration or a nodular mobile mass is palpable in the bladder wall which persists after transurethral resection of the exophytic part of the lesion and/or |
| | There is microscopic invasion of deep muscle or of extension through the bladder wall |
| | T3a  Invasion of deep muscle |
| | T3b  Extension through the bladder wall |
| T4 | Tumor fixed or invading neighbouring structures and/or |
| | There is microscopic evidence of such involvement |
| | T4a  Tumor invading prostate, uterus, or vagina |
| | T4b  Tumor fixed to the pelvic wall and/or infiltrating the abdominal wall |

Burnand et al. (7), where 51 patients were allocated at random to intravesical thiotepa or no further treatment after endoscopic loop resection or fulguration for tumors judged clinically limited to the mucosa or the submucosa. Histology later confirmed that in each case the tumor had not invaded the muscles. Ninety milligrams of thiotepa in 100 ml of sterile water was instilled into the bladder immediately after surgery and left for 30 min. No further instillation was made, unless recurrence was seen at follow-up cystoscopy. The patients were followed for between 2 and 5 years. In the 19 patients treated by thiotepa, 8 patients remained free of tumor, whereas only 1 of the 32 patients in the control group remained recurrence free, a statistically significant difference. No explanation is given for the unbalanced distribution of patients between the control and

TABLE 2. *Staging of bladder tumors (14,7)*

| | |
|---|---|
| Stage 0 | Tumor limited to mucosa |
| Stage A | Tumor not beyond submucosa |
| Stage B1 | Tumor not more than halfway through muscle |
| Stage B2 | Tumor more than halfway through muscle but not metastatic |
| Stage C | Tumor beyond muscle but not metastatic |
| Stage D1 | Tumor metastatic to points within the confines of the pelvis |
| Stage D2 | Tumor metastatic to points outside the confines of the pelvis |

TABLE 3. *Correspondance between UICC classification and Jewett system (2)*

| UICC classification | | Jewett and Strong classification |
|---|---|---|
| T1S | Preinvasive carcinoma papillary or sessile; carcinoma *in situ* | 0 |
| T1 | Tumor infiltrating subepithelial connective tissue | A |
| T2 | Tumor infiltrating superficial muscle | B1 |
| T3 | Tumor infiltrating deep muscle | B2 |
| | Tumor infiltrating perivesical tissues | C |
| T4 | Tumor fixed in pelvis or invading adjacent organs | D |
| | Tumor with lymph node invasion below the bifurcation of the iliac arteries | D1 |
| | Tumor with lymph node invasion in the peri-aortic region | D2 |

the treated group (32 versus 19 subjects), and the authors do not give the disease-free intervals nor the follow-up times for each group. In order to accept these findings as an indication that intravesical thiotepa is indeed better than no treatment, one has to assume that the median follow-up time was the same for the two groups. The mean length of time for recurrence to appear (i.e., number of months of follow-up divided by the number of recurrences) does not differ statistically in the two groups, being 2.7 months for the control and 2.2 months for thiotepa.

Intravesical prophylactic thiotepa was also tested in a randomized trial by the Veterans Administration Cooperative Urological Research Group (VACURG). Results have not been published, but the following data are available for 188 subjects (8). All patients were treated by transurethral resection for recurrences and divided randomly into three groups. One group of patients received placebo orally, the second group was given a 25-mg tablet of pyridoxine (vitamin $B_6$) daily by mouth, and the third received thiotepa instilled and kept in the bladder for 2 hr, once a week, for 4 weeks and then once a month at a dose of 60 mg. The average follow-up time was the same for the three groups, being about 31 months. The monthly recurrence rate (i.e., total number of recurrences divided by the total number of months of follow-up) was lower for thiotepa and pyridoxine than for placebo, a statistically significant difference ($p < 0.02$, one-sided test). However, the percentage of patients free of disease over the period of the study was 40% for placebo, 53% for thiotepa, and also 53% for pyridoxine, a nonsignificant difference. When the disease-free interval was calculated by the actuarial method the results of the group treated by pyridoxine were quite different from the two other groups: After an initial recurrence rate similar to that of placebo, the pyridoxine-treated group did not recur as often. It is suggested that a subgroup of about 50% of patients in the pyridox-ine-treated group was possibly cured by vitamin $B_6$ of their recurrent bladder tumor.

Pyridoxine is known to correct alterations in tryptophan metabolism, which occurs in a large percentage of patients with T1 bladder cancer. These abnormali-ties of tryptophan metabolism produce substances in the urine that are known to induce bladder cancer in mice (6).

Unfortunately, in this study, no assessment of tryptophan metabolism was possible in the pyridoxine-treated group.

Another conclusion of this trial was that whereas thiotepa does not decrease the number of patients with recurrences, it does reduce slightly the frequency of recurrence in a given patient, a conclusion opposite to the one of Burnand et al. (7).

The third randomized trial evaluating intravesical thiotepa is the one started by the E.O.R.T.C. Genito-Urinary Cooperative Group (31). Patients with T1 bladder carcinoma were randomized 1 month after transurethral resection to receive one of three treatments: 30 mg of thiotepa in 30 ml every week for 4 weeks and then every month for 1 year, or VM26, 50 mg in 30 ml, at the same schedule, or no adjuvant treatment.

Preliminary results indicate no difference between the three regimens.

## CHEMOTHERAPY IN ADVANCED CANCER

The only randomized study published to date is the one of Prout et al. (25), which was carried out as a double-blind study of 5-fluorouracil (5-FU) versus placebo in 12 centers. Surgically incurable patients who had not received any chemotherapy for the past 2 months and who were not previously treated with 5-FU or a chemical analogue were selected for the study. Patients who had pelvic irradiation from any source within 2 months of entry in the study were excluded. 5-FU was given at the dose of 15 mg/kg intravenously during a 2- to 3-hr period daily for 5 days. If toxicity had not developed after 5 days, 7.5 mg/kg was given on alternate days to day 60. Objective response was defined as a 50% decrease in the product of the two largest perpendicular diameters. Data were available for only 29 patients out of 45 admitted in the study, which might be due to the fact that too high a dose of 5-FU was utilized. The analysis of the data by matched pairs as given in the paper seems to suffer from the incompleteness of the data, since only 9 pairs of patients were available for comparison. Comparison of 5-FU and placebo in these pairs was not statistically significant. When the 29 patients were evaluated, there was 1/14 objective remis-sion in the 5-FU-treated group and 2/15 remissions in the placebo group. This striking finding is most important for the planning of future studies, since it may indicate spontaneous objective remission of the tumor in patients with advanced disease. The authors also saw toxic manifestations in the placebo-treated group, which could have been ascribed to 5-FU.

## CONCOMITANT CHEMOTHERAPY AND RADIOTHERAPY

A randomized trial was performed by Edland, Wear, and Ansfield (12) in which 36 patients stage B2, C, and D1 were allocated to radiotherapy alone or to radiotherapy and concomitant 5-FU. The average dose of radiotherapy was 6,500 rads in 47 days in the group receiving radiotherapy alone and 6,350 rads in 46 days in the other group. 5-FU was administered intravenously, 10 mg/kg, days 1–3, and 5 mg/kg, day 4, and then three times weekly until the end of the radiotherapy course, unless toxicity became too important.

The two groups were comparable in terms of clinical stage, tumor grades, prior surgical therapy, age, sex, and follow-up time. There were no patients lost to follow-up. Seventy-five percent or more regression (not defined in the article) was observed in 59% of the patients in one group and in 61% in the other. Survival curves for both treatments were almost identical. Acute morbidity was more pronounced and more frequent in the group receiving combined therapy.

## PREOPERATIVE IRRADIATION VERSUS SURGERY ALONE AND VERSUS RADIOTHERAPY ALONE (Table 4)

A randomized trial has been conducted by Prout et al. (22–24,27–30) comparing preoperative irradiation to surgery alone. The patients were stage B1 to D1, judged potentially curable, and not treated by irradiation or chemotherapy within 2 months preceding their entry in the study. Surgery was not standardized

TABLE 4. *Comparison between preoperative irradiation, surgery, and radiotherapy*

| Treatment arm | Number of patients | Survival rate | | Reference |
|---|---|---|---|---|
| A. Preoperative irradiation | | 23% | | |
| | 448 | 5 years | | 24 |
| B. Surgery alone | | 26% | | |
| | | | NS | |
| A. Preoperative irradiation | | 33% | | |
| | 199 | 5 years | | 35 |
| B. Radiotherapy alone | | 21% | | |
| | | | NS | |
| A. Preoperative irradiation | | 40% | | |
| B. Surgery alone | 72 | 3 years | 40% | 3 |
| C. Radiotherapy alone | | 40% | | |
| | | | NS | |
| A. Preoperative irradiation | | 46% | | |
| | 68 | 5 years | | 19 |
| B. Radiotherapy alone | | 16% | | |
| | | | $p < .01$ | |

between the centers, but each patient was supposed to be operated upon curatively. The patients were subject to two consecutive randomizations. The first decided whether or not the patient would be irradiated before operation, the second was carried out after surgery between 5-FU or placebo.

Preoperative irradiation was given at the dose of 4,500 rads in 28 to 32 days with an average of 1,000 rads per week. Surgery was performed 1 to 2 months after the end of irradiation.

5-FU was given intravenously in 250 to 500 ml of dextrose in no less than 2 hr at the dose of 15 mg/kg per day for 5 consecutive days beginning the 5th day following TUR or the 14th day following open surgery, after which six doses of 7.5 mg/kg per day were given on alternate days.

5-FU was dropped after it was found to be of no benefit for the survival of the patients in addition to the high toxicity it carried.

The last report available was published in 1976 and concerned 475 patients with a minimum follow-up of nearly 5 years (24).

One problem with this study is that 49% of the randomized patients were not treated as specified in the protocol or were found ineligible at surgery. Moreover, several patients were given large toxic doses of 5-FU at the beginning of the study until the protocol was modified to stop chemotherapy after surgery. Survival curves of 448 eligible patients entered in the study without taking into account whether 5-FU was administered or not were not significantly different from preoperatively irradiated patients and patients with surgery alone.

If one considers a selected group of 263 patients who completed protocol through surgery and had no disseminated disease found on operation, the 5-year survival rates are 36% for the irradiated and 28% for the others, a nonsignificant difference.

There seems to be a reduction in pathological stage in the irradiated group after radiotherapy. An exact figure, however, is impossible to obtain since the preirradiation staging is based only on the clinical and biopsy findings whereas the postsurgical assessment is made on the operative specimen or postmortem examination. By comparing the patients who are tumor-free at surgery in the irradiated group (35%) and in the nonirradiated group (8%), there is a highly significant difference between the two groups. This 8% represents a group of subjects in whom transurethral resection performed for diagnostic purposes succeeded in totally excising the tumor.

As far as survival is concerned, there was no difference in tumor-free patients between preoperative irradiation or not, but the patients with no tumors found at operation survived longer than the patients with tumor tissue in their specimen. Extreme caution is needed in interpreting these data. As pointed out by the authors, the operated irradiated group is clearly a selected group, since they must be in such a physical condition as to go far enough in the protocol to be able to receive complete radiotherapy and curative surgery. This is indicated by the fact that more patients (69%) were able to undertake curative surgery than to receive the combined treatment (50%).

The trial of Wallace and Bloom (35) was a comparison between radiotherapy and preoperative radiotherapy followed by radical cystectomy in T3 tumors. Radiotherapy alone consisted of 6,000 rads to the bladder and 4,500 to 5,000 rads to the pelvic wall in 6 weeks using five fractions per week. Preoperative radiotherapy was given at a dose of 4,000 rads in 4 weeks given at five fractions per week. Four weeks later, radical cystectomy was performed, which included complete excision of the bladder, perivesical tissue, prostate, and pelvic nodes.

A total of 199 patients were entered. Ten patients were excluded for ineligibility, leaving 189 for analysis. A statistical analysis of the whole survival curve was not done, but survival curves are identical up to 1 year and then diverge in favor of surgery after irradiation.

Another randomized trial was undertaken by the Veterans Administration Cooperative Urological Research Group (VACURG) in stage II and stage III carcinoma of the bladder (B1, B2, C, or T2 and T3)(3). Patients were randomly assigned to surgery only, or radiation therapy only, or preoperative irradiation followed by surgery. In the case of radiation therapy alone, a minimum of 5,000 rads in 4 to 5 weeks or a maximum of 6,000 rads in 5 to 6 weeks was given. When preoperative irradiation was administered the protocol specified a dosage of 4,500 rads in 4 to 5 weeks, with an interval between the end of irradiation and surgery of 4 to 6 weeks.

Surgical treatment consisted of partial or total cystectomy according to the size and location of the tumor. A few patients had pelvic lymphadenectomy. A total of 72 patients were randomized between these three groups. Only 54 completed their treatment, a 25% rate of nonevaluability. Actuarial survival curves did not show any difference between the three groups. As pointed out by the authors, the high number of nonevaluable patients (10 refused surgery) and the different surgical procedures used according to institutions could have biased the results in the two surgical groups.

Miller and Johnson (18,19) have published the results of a trial that was carried out in 68 patients with B2 and C lesions comparing preoperative radiotherapy and radiotherapy alone. The dose prescribed for the first group was 5,000 rads in 5 weeks, five fractions per week, followed by simple total cystectomy with no node dissection, whereas the second group received 7,000 rads in 7 weeks (35 fractions).

When all the patients but one (excluded for protocol violation) were taken into account, the difference in the survival rates at 5 years was statistically significant in favor of the combined modality (46% survival against 16%, $p < 0.01$). Few details about the trial are given in the publication.

## HYPERBARIC OXYGEN AND RADIATION THERAPY

The demonstration that the radiosensitivity of anoxic cells is decreased and the fact that many tumors do not have a good vascular supply has led several radiotherapists to introduce hyperbaric oxygen into clinical radiotherapy. In general, a metal tank is used in which the pressure is raised to 3 atm in 10 to 15 min with oxygen. After 15 min allowed for saturation, radiotherapy is then administered. Several randomized trials have been published comparing radiation therapy in air and oxygen.

Cade and McEwen (9), giving 6,000 rads in 8 weeks using five fractions per week, treated two groups of 20 patients each with "tumor and nodes confined to pelvis" selected at random. The two groups, however, were not comparable since the oxygen-treated group contained 4 anaplastic, 3 squamous, and 13 transitional cell carcinomas, as compared to 1 anaplastic and 19 transitional cell carcinomas in the air-treated patients. No difference in survival was seen.

van den Brenk (33) gave results of 16 cases (T2, T3, and T4) randomized in two groups of eight receiving 6 times 550 rads in air and 6 times 500 rads in oxygen. The authors said that more early deaths due to recurrent tumor have appeared in the air-treated group, but too few details are published on this small series to draw conclusions.

Plenk (20) conducted a randomized trial in 40 patients (T1 to T4), 6,000 rads in 6 weeks, five and later four fractions per week being given to both groups. Although the author claims statistical significance in favor of the hyperbaric group, the statistical method used to compare survival time does not seem adequate.

Dische in 1973 published the results (11) of two trials in patients with T1 to T4 tumor. In the first trial, 5,820 rads were given in 30 fractions over 42 days, except where only the tumor and bladder were irradiated when the same dose was given in 25 fractions over 35 days. In the second trial, 4,580 rads was given in 15 treatments over 33 days. A total of 67 patients were put in the two studies, but 6 patients randomized to oxygen were shifted to air for various reasons and in the analysis these 6 patients are considered as air allocated. This not only disrupts the balance between the number of patients in the two groups (28 versus 39), but does not permit any comparison between the two groups.

The multicenter trial carried out by the Hyperbaric Oxygen Working Party of the Medical Research Council of Great Britain (13) involved 237 patients. Subjects not over the age of 75, with tumor and nodes confined to the pelvis, were randomly allocated to the two treatment modalities. Doses, time, and fractionation schemas were different according to centers. There was no statistical difference in survival curves computed up to 5 years. Also, no effect on local control rates by hyperbaric oxygen could be demonstrated by any of the individual centers (13,16).

## CONCLUSION

Although there are more than 35 active drugs available for cancer chemotherapy, only two, thiotepa and 5-FU, have been evaluated in a randomized trial. It was shown that 5-FU was not better than placebo in advanced patients and intravesical thiotepa, tested as an adjuvant to TUR, proved to be marginally effective as a prophylactic agent in T1 tumors. Thiotepa was first used in T1 bladder cancer in 1961 (15) and since then has been recommended by most urologists in spite of extremely variable success rates (32). Sixteen years later, data are accumulating suggesting that the ratio risk-benefit is too high.

Indeed, most of the authors reporting therapeutic results have mentioned toxic effects, that is, chemical cystitis, leucopenia, thrombocytopenia, and even death due to bone marrow failure (1,5,37).

The findings that 50% of the patients with bladder cancer have an increased urinary excretion of some urinary metabolites of tryptophan (21), and the fact that oral administration of pyridoxine to patients with abnormal tryptophan metabolism restores the urinary level to normal (4), has led the VACURG to test pyridoxine as a prophylactic agent in T1 recurrent bladder after TUR. The possible cure of some patients is an important finding which needs confirmation and detailed study of tryptophan metabolism in cured and noncured patients.

Conclusions about preoperative irradiation when compared to surgery alone or about radiotherapy alone when compared to preoperative irradiation are not encouraging.

One of the problems in judging the efficacy of any therapeutic procedure is the inaccuracy of the assessment of the degree of muscular invasion and dissemination based on tumor biopsies. As shown in Table 5 (26,34,38), clinical staging assessed by biopsies after TUR is imprecise, especially for the low stages, when it is compared to pathological staging made after operation. Since once deep muscle invasion has taken place the disease is no longer localized to the pelvis (29) and since understaging is common, approaches other than regional therapies should be tried. Unfortunately, here again there is a lack of randomized trials proving the effectiveness of potentially active drugs such as *cis*-platinum, mitomycin C, adriamycin, cyclophosphamide, and methotrexate. Carter and Wasserman (10) have shown that, even in phase II nonrandomized trials, very few of the available drugs have been adequately studied.

In conclusion, it can be said that the use of randomization in the testing of treatments of bladder cancer has been finally beneficial to the patient. By this method, it has been shown that the risks of intravesical thiotepa are too large and outweigh the advantage of preventing recurrence of T1 tumor in a small

TABLE 5. *Percentage of understaging when comparing clinical staging and operative specimen (without irradiation)*

|  | Prout et al. (26) | Wajsman et al. (34) | Whitmore (38) |
|---|---|---|---|
| B1 | 46% | 42% | 7% |
| B2 | 53% | — | 21% |
| C | 31% | 21% | 45% |
| D1 | — | 8% | 81% |

percentage of patients. If randomized trials had been carried out from the beginning on the use of thiotepa, several toxic deaths would have been avoided and other drugs could have been tested adequately. In the area of preoperative irradiation, although an undefined portion of the patients could benefit from the combined modality, the need for further therapeutic research has been stressed by disappointing results. Finally, hyperbaric oxygen, a technically difficult procedure, has been abandoned.

## ACKNOWLEDGMENTS

I would like to express my gratitude to Dr. H. L. Davis, Jr. for his kind assistance with this manuscript.

This work was supported in part by grant 2 R10 CA 11488–07, awarded by the National Cancer Institute, DHEW.

## REFERENCES

1. Abbassian, A., and Wallace, D. M. (1966): Intracavity chemotherapy of diffuse non-infiltrating papillary carcinoma of the bladder. *J. Urol.,* 96:461.
2. Anderson, C. K. (1975): A comparative guide to the common systems of bladder tumor classification. Int. Bladder Conference, 1971. In: *The Biology and Clinical Management of Bladder Cancer,* edited by E. H. Cooper and R. E. Williams, p. 277. Blackwell Scientific Publications, Oxford.
3. Blackard, C. E., Byar, D. P., and the Veterans Administration Cooperative Urological Research Group (1972): Results of a clinical trial of surgery and radiation in stages II and III carcinoma of the bladder. *J. Urol.,* 108:875.
4. Brown, R. R., Price, J. M., Satter, E. J., and Wear, J. B. (1960): The metabolism of tryptophan in patients with bladder cancer. *Acta Clin. Int. Cancer,* 16:299.
5. Bruce, D. W., Edgcomb, J. H. (1967): Pancytopenia and generalized sepsis following treatment of cancer of the bladder with instillation of triethylene thiophosphoramide. *J. Urol.,* 97:482.
6. Bryan, G. T., Brown, R. R., and Price, J. M. (1964): Mouse bladder carcinogenicity of certain tryptophen metabolites and other aromatic nitrogen compounds suspended in cholesterol. *Cancer Res.,* 24:596.
7. Burnand, K. G., Boyd, P. J. R., Mayo, M. E., Shuttleworth, K. E. D., and Lloyd-Davies, R. W. (1976): Single dose intravesical thiotepa as an adjuvant to cystodiathermy in the treatment of transitional cell bladder carcinoma. *Br. J. Urol.,* 48:55.
8. Byar, D. P. (1977): *Personal communication.*
9. Cade, I. S., and Mc Ewen, J. B. (1967): Megavoltage radiotherapy in hyperbaric oxygen. *Cancer,* 20:817.
10. Carter, S. K., and Wasserman, T. H. (1975): The chemotherapy of urologic cancer. *Cancer,* 36:729.
11. Dische, S. (1973): The hyperbaric oxygen chamber in the radiotherapy of carcinoma of the bladder. *Br. J. Radiol.,* 46:13.
12. Edland, R. W., Wear, J. B., and Ansfield, F. J. (1970): Advanced cancer of the urinary bladder, an analysis of the results of radiotherapy alone vs radiotherapy and concomitant 5-fluorouracil, a prospective randomized study of 36 cases. *Am. J. Roentgenol.,* 108:124.
13. Hyperbaric Oxygen Working Party of the Medical Research Council (1977): *Personal communication.*
14. Jewett, H. J., and Strong, G. H. (1946): Infiltrating carcinoma of bladder: Relation of depth of penetration of bladder wall to incidence of local extension and metastases. *J. Urol.,* 55:366.
15. Jones, H. C., and Swinney, J. (1961): Thiotepa in the treatment of tumors of the bladder. *Lancet,* ii:615.

16. Kirk, J., Wingate, S. W., and Walson, E. R. (1976): High dose effects in the treatment of carcinoma of the bladder under air and hyperbaric oxygen condition. *Clin. Radiol.,* 27:137.
17. Marshall, V. F. (1952): Relation of preoperative estimate to pathologic demonstration of extent of vesical neoplasms. *J. Urol.,* 68:714.
18. Miller, J. S., and Johnson, D. E. (1973): Megavoltage irradiation of bladder cancer: Alone, postoperative or preoperative? *Proc. 7th Natl. Cancer Conf.,* p. 771. J. B. Lippincott, Philadelphia.
19. Miller, L. S. (1977): Bladder cancer: Superiority of preoperative irradiation and cystectomy in clinical stage B2 and C. *Cancer,* 39:973.
20. Plenk, H. P. (1972): Hyperbaric radiation therapy. *Am. J. Roentgenol.,* 114:152.
21. Price, J. M., and Brown, R. R. (1962): Studies on the etiology of carcinoma of the urinary bladder. *Acta Clin. Int. Cancer,* 18:684.
22. Prout, G. R., Jr. (1967): The development of a cooperative study and its preliminary observations on adjuvants (5-FU and irradiation) in the surgical treatment of bladder carcinoma. In: *Inter-American Conference on Toxicology and Occupational Medicine. Bladder Cancer,* A symposium edited by K. F. Lampe, p. 270. Aesculapius Publishing Co., Birmingham, Ala.
23. Prout, G. R., Jr. (1968): Adjuvants in the surgical treatment of bladder carcinoma. In: *Cancer Therapy by Integrated Radiation and Operation,* edited by B. Rush, Jr., and R. H. Greenlaw. Charles C Thomas, Springfield, Ill.
24. Prout, G. R. (1976): The surgical management of bladder carcinoma. *Urol. Clin. N. Am.,* 3:149.
25. Prout, G. R., Bross, I. D. J., Slack, N. H., and Ausman, R. K. (1968): Carcinoma of the bladder, 5-fluorouracil and the cutical role of a placebo. *Cancer,* 22:926.
26. Prout, G. R., Hollow, J., and Free, E., III (1973): *The Bladder in Cancer Medicine.* Lea & Febiger, Philadelphia.
27. Prout, G. R., Jr., Slack, N. H., and Bross, I. D. J. (1970): Irradiation and 5-fluorouracil as adjuvants in the management of invasive bladder carcinoma. A cooperative group report after 4 years. *J. Urol.,* 104:116.
28. Prout, G. R., Slack, N. H., and Bross, I. D. J. (1970): Preoperative irradiation as an adjuvant in the surgical management of invasive bladder carcinoma. *Trans. Am. Assoc. Genito-Urinary Surg.,* 62:160.
29. Prout, G. R., Slack, N. H., and Bross, I. D. J. (1971): Preoperative irradiation as an adjuvant in the surgical management of invasive bladder carcinoma. *J. Urol.,* 105:223.
30. Prout, G. R., Slack, N. H., and Bross, I. D. J. (1973): Preoperative irradiation and cystectomy for bladder carcinoma, IV: Results in a selected population. *Proc. 7th Natl. Cancer Conf.,* p. 783. J. B. Lippincott, Philadelphia.
31. Schulman, C. C., Rozencweig, M., Staquet, M., Kenis, Y., and Sylvester, R. (1976): EORTC randomized trial for the adjuvant therapy of T1 bladder carcinoma. *Eur. Urol.,* 2:271.
32. Staquet, M. (1976): The randomized clinical trial: A prerequisite for rational therapy. *Eur. Urol.,* 2:265.
33. van den Brenk, H. A. S. (1968): Hyperbaric oxygen in radiation therapy. *Am. J. Roentgenol.,* 102:8.
34. Wajsman, Z., Merrin, C., Moore, R., and Murphy, S. P. (1975): Current results from treatment of bladder tumors with total cystectomy at Roswell Park Memorial Institute. *J. Urol.,* 113:806.
35. Wallace, D. M., and Bloom, H. J. G. (1976): The management of deeply infiltrating (T3) bladder carcinoma: controlled trial of radical radiotherapy versus preoperative radiotherapy and radical cystectomy (First Report). *Br. J. Urol.,* 48:587.
36. Wallace, D. M., Chisholm, G. D., and Hendry, W. F. (1975): TNM classification for urological tumours (UICC)—1974. *Br. J. Urol.,* 47:1.
37. Watkins, W. E., Kozak, J. A., and Flanagan, M. J. (1967): Severe pancytopenia associated with the use of intravesical thiotepa. *J. Urol.,* 98:470.
38. Whitmore, W. F., Jr. (1977): Assessment and management of deeply invasive and metastatic lesions. *Cancer Res.,* 37:2756–2758.

*Randomized Trials in Cancer: A Critical Review by Sites*, edited by Maurice J. Staquet, Raven Press, New York © 1978.

# Renal Adenocarcinoma

## M. Staquet

*Service de Médecine et Laboratoire d'Investigation Clinique, Institut Jules Bordet et Laboratoire de Statistique Médicale, Faculté de Médecine, Université Libre de Bruxelles, Belgium*

In spite of innumerable publications on hormonal therapy of renal cell carcinoma, there is only one randomized prospective trial, which was undertaken by the Renal Cell Carcinoma Cooperative Study Group. This trial, cited by Prout (1), is a comparison among testosterone, medroxyprogesterone, and placebo (doses not stated). The results available on 100 patients indicate no difference among the three regimens.

Another randomized trial was performed (2,3) to test the value of preoperative irradiation. A total of 141 patients with clinically operable tumor were randomized between surgery alone or surgery preceded by 3,000 rads in 3 weeks to the area including the regional lymph nodes.

The nephrectomy specimens were classified according to the P category of the TNM classification, allowing poststratification of the patients. P1 are patients with tumors infiltrating only the parenchyma, P2 are neoplasms extending beyond the kidneys but not infiltrating intrarenal or extrarenal veins and/or lymph vessels, and P3 are cancers infiltrating veins and/or lymph vessels.

There was no difference in the actuarial survival curves in any of the P categories.

## REFERENCES

1. Prout, G. R. (1973): The kidney and ureter. In: *Cancer Medicine*, edited by Holland and E. Frei, p. 1665. Lea & Febiger, Philadelphia.
2. Van Der Werf-Messing, B. (1973): Carcinoma of the kidney. *Cancer*, 32:1056.
3. Van Der Werf-Messing, B. (1974): Carcinome du rein: un essai thérapeutique. *J. Radiol. Electrol.*, 55:785.

Received June 30, 1977.

# Subject Index

## A

Abdominoperitoneal resection, 177,178
Actinomycin D, 12,133-143,220,280,351,
    363,365,366,368,370,373,374
  single vs. multiple courses of, 134-136
  single vs. multiple courses of in Wilms'
    tumor, 136-138
  vs. vincristine, 139-140
  vs. vincristine vs. actinomycin D +
    vincristine in groups II and III
    nephroblastoma, 140-143
  + vincristine vs. no chemotherapy,
    143-145
Adenocarcinoma, 178
  ductal, 162
  gastrointestinal, 175
  prostatic, 396,407
  renal, 423
  of small bowel, 218
ADIC, 364,366,372
ADR, 279,282
Adrenalectomy, 247,249,264
Adriamycin (ADM), 39,91,120,196,207,
    214,220,253,257,258,261,264,282,
    283,292,294,334,350,359,362,365,
    366,368-370,405,406,419
Alkaline phosphatase, 205,405
Alopecia, 364
7-Alpha-methyl-19-nortestosterone, 252
Amenorrhea, drug-induced, 246
Amethopterin, 40
Aminoglutethimide, 249
Aminopterin, 1
Ampulla of Vater, 163
Anal verge, 177
Anaplasia, 149,166
  Broder's degree of, 167
Androgenotherapy, 59
Anemia, 57,63
  aplastic, 55
  hemolytic, 55
  refractory, 65
Angiosarcoma, 371
Anterior resection, 177
Antiestrogens, 253
Aorta, 399
Arteries, 235,399
Ascites, 205
L-Asparaginase, 1,21,43

Aspirin, 164
Atherosclerosis, 399
Avian myxovirus (influenza A), 48
Axilla, 235,238,239,243,245,246,263
  ipsilateral, 239
  irradiation of, 240
5-Aza-acytidine, 41
Azarine, 66
Azaserine, 66
Azotemia, 69

## B

BACON, 334
BACOP, 97
Baker's Antifol, 220
BCG (Bacillus Calmette-Guerin), 12,42,45,
    46,120,264,334,341-343,352,353
  allogenic leukemia cells with, 44
  glaxo-freeze-dried, 44
  intradermal, 44,65
  intravenous glaxo-, 46
  lyophylized Pasteur, 47
  MER-, 202
  side effects of, 46
  Tice-strain, 47
BCNU-P, comparison with CTX-P, 90, 150-
    172,196,200,220,264
BCVPP, 120,123
Berkson-Gage projections, 276
BHD, 350, 352, 353
Bilirubin, serum levels, 166,205
Biopsy, 377
  bone
    microradiography of, 75
    marrow, 405
1,3-Bishchloro-ethyl nitrosourea (BCNU),
    6,10,15,47,74,75,90,114,115,119,
    120,121,166,350,351,353,354
Bleomycin, 91,120,121,212,214,220,294,
    331-334
Blood
  lymphocyte level, 58
  white count, 21, 65
Bone
  marrow aspirate, 55
  metastasis, 406
  scan, 405

Pyridoxine, 413,414,419
Pyrimidines, fluorinated, 12

## R

Radiotherapy, 58,61,82-83,95,98,111,123,
147-219,241,246,262,263,274,275,
276,277,278,284,285,286,292,303-
306,313,331-337,345,348,377-380,
402,403
and chemotherapy, 92-94
combined surgery and, 236-241
hyperbaric oxygen and, 417-418
megavoltage, 107
photon, 335
preoperative vs. postoperative in treatment of Wilms' tumor, 136-138
prophylactic, 103
or therapeutic castration by, 241,
242,243
and surgery, *see* Surgery and radiotherapy
techniques, trials comparing, 105-107
trials involving, 136,137,334-335
Rappaport scheme, 77
Relapse, hematological, 15
Remission, complete (CR), 25,26,36,39,42,
46,48,49,55,89,90,95,192,280,282,
343,348,350,352,353,367
Remission, partial (PR), 89,90,192,343,348-
353,367
Rhabdomyosarcomas, 143-145

## S

Sarcoma
of colon, rectum, anus, 204
Ewing's, 370,371,372
Kaposi's, 373,374
osteogenic, 370-372
reticulum cell (RCS), 77,79,83,89
soft tissue in adults, 359-375
undifferentiated, 371
Sepsis, bacterial, 27
SGOT, serum levels of, 205
Sodium fluoride, effect on bone recalcifica-
tion, 74
Spironolactone, 221
Spleen
enlargement of, 55,56
treatment of, 61-63
Splenectomy, 58,59,67,103
early, 62-63
Splenic pedicle, 109
Splenomegaly, 63,65
Stilbestrol, 249
Streptonigrin, 56,114,265
Streptozotocin, 167,207,218,219,221
Studies
ALB 6606, 29

ALGB, 348
ALGB 6503, 41
ALGB-ECOG, 73
Austrian Study Group, 301
Baltimore Cancer Research Center, 109,
110
BIKE, 5
British Medical Research Council, 45,
303
British National Lymphoma Investiga-
tion Group, 111,118,119
Cancer and Leukemia Cooperative
Group B (CALGB), 7,8,48,200,
313
Cancer Research Campaign, 236
Central Oncology Group, 260,352
Children's Cancer Study Group (CCSG),
132,133,140$n$
Children's Cancer Study Group A
(CCSGA), 2,10,11,12,134-136,
138,140,143-145
COG 7030, 195,196
COG-RTOG, 185
Cooperative Breast Cancer Group, 249,
250,252,253
Coronary Drug Project Research Group,
398,401
Eastern Cooperative Oncology Group
(ECOG), 69,115,118,120,153,
207,217,258,280,285,345,348,
350,351,362,370
randomized dose-response, 196
0-4, 192
1274B, 159
1276, 185
1574, 316
1575, 313
2276, 185
3272, 218
3275, 157
4275, 200
European Organization Research on the
Treatment of Cancer (EORTC),
32,33,42,107,109,212,216,252
Brain Tumor Group, 381,385
Genito-Urinary Cooperative Group,
414
Head and Neck Cooperative Group,
332
Leukaemia and Hematosarcoma
Cooperative Group, 32,57
Gastrointestinal Tumor Study Group
(GITSG), 167
6175, 185
8174, 157
8274, 159
Gynecologic Oncology Group (GOG),
276,291,292